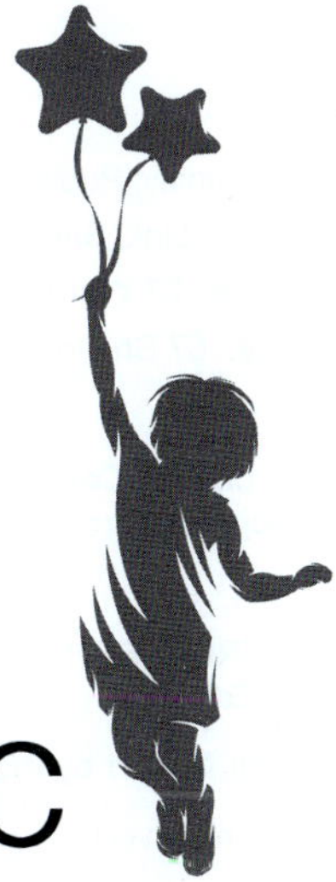

Pediatric Nephrology

On-The-Go

FOURTH EDITION

Editors

Hui-Kim Yap

Sharon Teo

Kar-Hui Ng

National University Hospital, Singapore

World Scientific

NEW JERSEY • LONDON • SINGAPORE • BEIJING • SHANGHAI • HONG KONG • TAIPEI • CHENNAI • TOKYO

Published by

World Scientific Publishing Co. Pte. Ltd.
5 Toh Tuck Link, Singapore 596224
USA office: 27 Warren Street, Suite 401-402, Hackensack, NJ 07601
UK office: 57 Shelton Street, Covent Garden, London WC2H 9HE

British Library Cataloguing-in-Publication Data
A catalogue record for this book is available from the British Library.

PEDIATRIC NEPHROLOGY ON-THE-GO
Fourth Edition

First Edition 2012
Second Edition 2015
Third Edition 2018
Fourth Edition 2021

This information aims to guide physicians in the management of children's kidney diseases and reflects current practice at the Khoo Teck Puat–National University Children's Medical Institute, National University Hospital, Singapore. Considerable care has been taken to ensure that the contents are accurate and current at the time of publication, but the reader is advised to check the drug doses, indications and precautions carefully. The authors are not responsible for any errors which may result from this publication. Application of the information in a particular situation remains the professional responsibility of the practitioner.

Cover Art by Chuan Ming Loo and Aidan Lui Ming Xian

ISBN 978-981-124-644-9 (hardcover)
ISBN 978-981-124-851-1 (paperback)
ISBN 978-981-124-825-2 (ebook for institutions)
ISBN 978-981-124-826-9 (ebook for individuals)

For any available supplementary material, please visit
https://www.worldscientific.com/worldscibooks/10.1142/12531#t=suppl

Printed in Singapore

PREFACE TO THE FOURTH EDITION

As is tradition, *Pediatric Nephrology On-The-Go* is launched at the triennial Primer in Pediatric Nephrology for Asia. Since the 3rd Primer in 2018, the global pandemic has ruthlessly invaded many facets of our lives — although we are physically more distant because of travel restrictions, we are, in fact, more connected now through cloud-powered platforms. Attendance at conferences is now possible from the comfort of our homes. 2021 marks the inaugural fully virtual 4th Primer in Pediatric Nephrology for Asia, and we welcome our esteemed colleagues and friends from geographical locations far beyond Asia. To keep up with the times, we are, for the first time, also introducing an e-Book version of *Pediatric Nephrology On-The-Go*.

It has always been our intention for *Pediatric Nephrology On-The-Go* to be a hands-on and practical reference for pediatricians, pediatric nephrologists, dialysis nurses, and physicians in training. Much emphasis has been placed on the portability of this pocket-sized book, now made even more compact with the e-Book version. In addition to extensive updates to existing chapters, this edition contains 7 new chapters, encompassing key topics such as glomerulonephritis associated with anti-neutrophil cytoplasmic antibody (ANCA) positive vasculitis, membranous nephropathy, neurogenic bladder, immunosuppressive medications, anti-CD20 monoclonal antibody therapy, recurrent focal segmental glomerulosclerosis post kidney transplantation, and prolonged intermittent kidney replacement therapy (PIKRT).

With heartfelt appreciation, we would like to honor and thank each and every one of our colleagues and international fellows, past and present, who have been part of the Shaw NKF-NUH Children's Kidney Center family at the National University Hospital, Singapore, for your contributions. You have all left footprints throughout the pages, making *Pediatric Nephrology On-The-Go* the unique and trusted reference it is today.

We dedicate this book to you, our readers. Stay Safe.

Hui-Kim Yap
Sharon Teo
Kar-Hui Ng

CONTRIBUTORS

From the Staff of the Department of Pediatrics, Yong Loo Lin School of Medicine, National University of Singapore, and the Khoo Teck Puat–National University Children's Medical Institute, National University Hospital, Singapore

Division of Pediatric Nephrology, Dialysis and Renal Transplantation Shaw-NKF-NUH Children's Kidney Centre:

- **Cahyani Gita Ambarsari**
  Clinical Fellow (2013–2014)
- **Eric Emmanuel T. Aragon**
  Clinical Fellow (2006–2009)
- **Alona R. Arias-Briones**
  Clinical Fellow (2019–2020)
- **Swasti Chaturvedi**
  Consultant (2014–2016)
- **Qiao Zhi Chee**
  Senior Resident
- **Manu Chhabra**
  Resident
- **Rachelle C. Dela Cruz**
  Clinical Fellow (2011–2012)
- **Sudha Ekambaram**
  Clinical Fellow (2013–2014)

- **Noor Haziah Hussain**
  Nurse Manager
- **Prithi R. Inamdar**
  Clinical Fellow (2017)
- **Simple Kakar**
  Clinical Fellow (2014–2015)
- **Chee Teck Koh**
  Resident
- **Lee Jin Koh**
  Clinical Fellow (2014–2016), Resident Physician (2018–2020)
- **Khine Wut Yee Kyaw**
  Clinical Fellow (2019–present)
- **Mahantesh V. Patil**
  Clinical Fellow (2010–2012)
- **Perry Yew-Weng Lau**
  Assistant Professor, Senior Consultant
- **Esther Hui Min Leow**
  Associate Consultant (2018–2019)
- **Isaac Desheng Liu**
  Consultant (2006–2020)
- **Shraddha Lohia**
  Clinical Fellow (2021–present)
- **David Liangjian Lu**
  Senior Resident
- **Kar-Hui Ng**
  Associate Professor, Senior Consultant
- **Khin Myat Lwin Nyein**
  Clinical Fellow (2008–2009)
- **Archana Pinapala**
  Clinical Fellow (2018–2019)

- **Risky Vitria Prasetyo**
  Clinical Fellow (2010–2011)
- **Md Abdul Qader**
  Clinical Fellow (2016–2018)
- **Lourdes Paula R. Resontoc**
  Clinical Fellow (2009–2012)
- **Subhankar Sarkar**
  Clinical Fellow (2017–2018)
- **Kiran P. Sathe**
  Clinical Fellow (2013)
- **Khin Le Le Shein**
  Clinical Fellow (2013–2014)
- **Annushkha Sharanya Sinnathamby**
  Senior Resident
- **Azmeri Sultana**
  Clinical Fellow (2015)
- **Sharon Sher Leen Teo**
  Consultant
- **Vivek Kumar Todi**
  Clinical Fellow (2014–2015)
- **Kyaw Thu Ya**
  Clinical Fellow (2012–2015)
- **Hui-Kim Yap**
  Professor, Head and Senior Consultant
- **Wee-Song Yeo**
  Consultant (2005–2017)

Division of Pediatric Critical Care:

- **Poi-Lin Koh**
  Senior Consultant

- **Jacqueline Soo-May Ong**
  Head and Senior Consultant
- **Ryan Richard Taylor**
  Consultant

Division of Pediatric Endocrinology:

- **Kah-Yin Loke**
  Associate Professor, Head and Senior Consultant
- **Andrew Anjian Sng**
  Consultant

Division of Pediatric Infectious Diseases:

- **Mas Suhaila Isa**
  Consultant (2004–2017)

Department of Diagnostic Imaging:

- **Yi-Ming Teo**
  Consultant

Department of Pediatric Surgery:

- **Krishnan Prabhakaran**
  Professor, Emeritus Consultant
- **Yoke Lin Nyo**
  Consultant

Department of Pharmacy:

- **Sok Hoon Lim**
  Senior Pharmacist

Ministry of Health Holdings, Singapore:

- **Brandon Yi Da Hoong**
  House Officer (2021)

CONTENTS

F. Tubular Disease

G. Glomerular Disease

H. Chronic Kidney Disease

K. Transplantation

L. Procedures

M. Appendices

1 Management of Acute Kidney Injury

Resontoc LP, Prasetyo RV, Ng KH, Teo S and Yap HK

A. Definitions

1. Acute kidney injury (AKI):
   a. Rapid decline in glomerular filtration rate, resulting in impairment of excretion of nitrogenous waste product, and loss of water and electrolyte regulation as well as acid-base regulation.
   b. Kidney Disease Improving Global Outcomes (KDIGO):
      - Increase in serum creatinine by ≥26.5 μmol/L within 48 hours
        OR
      - Increase in serum creatinine ≥1.5 times baseline, within the prior 7 days
        OR
      - Urine volume <0.5 ml/kg/hour for 6 hours.
2. Oliguric versus non-oliguric AKI:
   - Oliguric: Urine volume <400 ml/m^2/day.
   - Non-oliguric: Urine volume is normal.

B. Staging of AKI

1. KDIGO criteria of mild (Stage 1), moderate (Stage 2), and severe (Stage 3) AKI:

Stage	Serum Creatinine	Urine Volume
1	Increase to 1.5–1.9x baseline* OR Increase of ≥26.5 μmol/L	<0.5 ml/kg/hour for 6–12 hours
2	Increase to 2.0–2.9x baseline	<0.5 ml/kg/hour for ≥12 hours
3	Increase to 3x times baseline OR Increase in creatinine to ≥353.6 μmol/L OR Initiation of kidney replacement therapy OR Decrease in eGFR to <35 ml/min/1.73m^2 in patients <18 years	<0.3 ml/kg/hour for >24 hours OR anuria for ≥12 hours

*If baseline serum creatinine is unknown, it is generally recommended to use a presumed baseline of 120 ml/min/1.73m^2 or the published minimum and maximum normative serum creatinine values for age and gender.

2. RIFLE criteria in adults define the severity of AKI (Acute Dialysis Quality Initiative):
   a. Risk, Injury and Failure based on changes in serum creatinine or urine output.
   b. Clinical outcome classes based on persistence of kidney failure, namely, Loss and End stage kidney disease.
3. pRIFLE criteria for pediatric patients and nRIFLE criteria for neonates are based on the estimated glomerular filtration rate (eGFR) and urine output.
4. Acute Kidney Injury Network (AKIN) staging system in adults:
   a. Mild AKI (stage 1), moderate AKI (stage 2) and severe AKI (stage 3) are comparable to the risk, injury and failure categories in RIFLE.
   b. Kidney replacement therapy is classified as stage 3.

Class	Creatinine			Urine Output Criteria (ml/kg/hour)		
RIFLE [AKIN]	AKIN	RIFLE	pRIFLE and nRIFLE	RIFLE/ AKIN	pRIFLE	nRIFLE
Risk [1]	Increased creatinine ≥1.5–2x OR increase by ≥26.5 μmol/L	Increased creatinine 1.5x OR GFR decrease >25%	Increased creatinine 1.5x OR eGFR decrease by 25%	<0.5 for 6 hours	<0.5 for 8 hours	<1.5 for 24 hours

(*Continued*)

Class	Creatinine			Urine Output Criteria (ml/kg/hour)		
RIFLE [AKIN]	AKIN	RIFLE	pRIFLE and nRIFLE	RIFLE/ AKIN	pRIFLE	nRIFLE
Injury [2]	Increased creatinine >2–3x	Increased creatinine 2x or GFR decrease >50%	Increased creatinine 2x or eGFR decrease by 50%	<0.5 for 12 hours	<0.5 for 16 hours	<1.0 for 24 hours
Failure [3]	Increased creatinine >3x OR creatinine ≥354 μmol/L (acute rise ≥44 μmol/L) OR on RRT	Increased creatinine 3x OR GFR decrease >75% OR creatinine >354 μmol/L (acute rise >44 μmol/L)	Increased creatinine 3x OR eGFR decrease by 75% OR eGFR <35 ml/min/ 1.73m^2	<0.3 for 24 hours OR Anuria for 12 hours	<0.3 for 24 hours OR anuria for 12 hours	<0.7 for 24 hours OR anuria for 12 hours
Loss	Persistent failure > 4 weeks					
End stage	Persistent failure > 3 months					

5. All these classification systems are based on identifying a minimal change in kidney functional parameters that are related to an outcome and a gradation of severity that associates with incremental risk of worse outcomes.
    - For AKIN, the increase in creatinine must occur in <48 hours.
    - For RIFLE, the AKI should be both abrupt (within 1–7 days) and sustained (>24 hours).

C. Etiology

Pre-renal	Renal	Post-renal
True volume depletion • Gastrointestinal losses, hemorrhage, burns, renal salt-wasting conditions Effective renal hypoperfusion • Decreased arterial pressure (cardiac failure) • Systemic vasodilatation (septic shock, neurogenic shock, cirrhosis) • Intestinal obstruction Intrarenal vasoconstriction • Hepatorenal syndrome • Cardiorenal syndrome • Medications: non-steroidal anti-inflammatory agents (NSAIDs), angiotensin-converting enzyme inhibitors, angiotensin receptor blockers, calcineurin inhibitors	Glomerulonephritis (GN) • Post-infectious GN • Systemic lupus erythematosus • IgA vasculitis • Membranoproliferative GN • Anti-neutrophil cytoplasmic antibody-associated GN • Anti-glomerular basement membrane disease • Idiopathic rapidly progressive GN • Hypertension • Diabetes mellitus Vascular • Hemolytic-uremic syndrome • Renal artery thrombosis • Renal vein thrombosis • Thrombotic microangiopathies Acute tubulointerstitial nephritis • Infections such as Epstein–Barr virus, cytomegalovirus, human immunodeficiency virus and leptospirosis • Drugs including herbal preparations	Structural • Posterior urethral valve • Ureteric obstruction • Neurogenic bladder • Retroperitoneal fibrosis Crystalluria • Tumorlysis syndrome • Melamine Calculi Blood clot Medications that cause urinary retention such as first-generation anti-histamines, anti-cholinergics, epidural anesthesia

(*Continued*)

Pre-renal	Renal	Post-renal
	Acute pyelonephritis Tumor infiltration Tubular nephrotoxins • Aminoglycosides, furosemide, vancomycin, acyclovir • Wasp sting • Plant toxins • Snake-bite • Pigments such as hemoglobin (hemolysis in G6PD deficiency, falciparum malaria), myoglobin (rhabdomyolysis) • Radiocontrast agents	

D. Clinical Manifestations

1. Children presenting with conditions associated with severe hypovolemia:
   a. Children with vomiting, diarrhea and decreased oral intake are at risk of developing severe hypovolemia and AKI.
   b. In some conditions associated with polyuria, such as diabetic ketoacidosis, renal tubular acidosis, and chronic tubulopathies, if fluid intake is insufficient to keep up with urine loss, severe hypovolemia and pre-renal AKI can develop.
   c. Physical signs of hypovolemia: Tachycardia, poor capillary refill, decreased skin turgor, dry mucous membranes, sunken eyes, and orthostatic blood pressure changes.
2. Children presenting acutely with symptoms suggestive of kidney disease:
   a. Acute onset of oliguria, edema and gross hematuria, with a preceding history of pharyngitis or impetigo is consistent with post-infectious glomerulonephritis.
   b. Bloody diarrhea with oliguria or anuria suggests diarrhea-associated hemolytic-uremic syndrome, whereas, in children with

pneumonia, development of oliguria accompanied by anemia and thrombocytopenia is indicative of pneumonia-associated hemolytic-uremic syndrome.

c. Systemic signs and symptoms of vasculitis such as purpuric or malar rash, joint pain or swelling and hemoptysis, suggest the possibility of rapidly progressive GN associated with systemic vasculitis.

3. Detection of abnormal laboratory parameters (raised urea, creatinine, hyperkalemia, abnormal urinalysis) in patients at risk of AKI:
   a. Critically ill children with sepsis and hypotension, frequently have multiorgan failure resulting in AKI with oligoanuria, especially with the use of inotropes such as noradrenaline or adrenaline.
   b. Infants and children post-cardiopulmonary bypass.
   c. Immunosuppressed or neutropenic children such as oncology patients undergoing chemotherapy or bone marrow transplantation in the presence of:
      - Sepsis.
      - History of nephrotoxic medications including antibiotics such as aminoglycosides, vancomycin, acyclovir or amphotericin-B, furosemide, chemotherapeutic agents such as cisplastin, and calcineurin inhibitors.
4. Newborn infants with oliguria or anuria:
   a. Oliguria in the newborn beyond 72 hours is worrying and should be investigated.
   b. In the absence of ischemic injury, anuria or oliguria suggests a major congenital malformation such as posterior urethral valves, or genetic disease such as autosomal recessive polycystic kidney disease.
   c. In the sick neonate with hematuria, bilateral renal vein thrombosis should be suspected.

E. Diagnostic Approach

I. Recognize the presence of AKI

1. AKI should be defined and staged using the KDIGO criteria.
2. Intensive urine output monitoring is associated with increased detection of moderate to severe AKI and reduced incidence of fluid overload.

3. Using serum creatinine alone may delay the recognition of AKI especially in the presence of fluid overload.

$$\text{Corrected creatinine} = \text{Measured creatinine} \times \left(1 + \frac{\text{Net fluid balance}}{\text{Total body water}}\right)$$

where total body water = 0.6 × Weight (kg)

Note: Utilization of 0.6 as the constant to estimate total body water may be confounded by age, gender and fluid overload states.

II. Establish etiology of AKI

1. Early diagnosis of pre-renal and obstructive causes is important as prompt corrective measures may prevent the onset of established kidney injury.
2. Urinary sediment:
   a. Microscopic examination for cells, crystals, cellular debris, and casts.
      - Presence of hematuria associated with dysmorphic red cells and red cell casts suggests a diagnosis of glomerulonephritis.
      - Renal tubular epithelial cells, tubular cell casts or coarsely granular pigmented casts suggest acute tubular necrosis.
      - Pyuria suggests pyelonephritis or tubulointerstitial disorders (sterile pyuria).
      - Presence of eosinophils is highly suggestive of acute allergic interstitial nephritis.

   b. Crystals in the urine may be useful indicators of the underlying etiology in the appropriate clinical setting with AKI:
      - Uric acid crystals in tumor lysis syndrome.
      - Calcium oxalate crystals in ethylene glycol poisoning.

   c. Scant findings may be consistent with pre-renal or obstructive causes of AKI.
3. Blood and urinary indices to differentiate between pre-renal and established kidney failure:
   a. Based on the premise that the proximal renal tubular transport mechanisms are still able to respond to the hypovolemic stimulus in pre-renal failure as compared to the failure of these transport mechanisms in acute tubular necrosis.

b. Indices used with caution in premature neonates <32 weeks gestation, since a high urinary sodium excretion is commonly observed.

c. Fractional sodium excretion:
FE_{Na} = (urine/plasma sodium)*(plasma/urine creatinine)*100%

d. Fractional urea excretion:
FE_{urea} = (urine/plasma urea)*(plasma/urine creatinine)*100%

Indices	Pre-renal*	Intrinsic Renal*
Urine sodium (mmol/L)	<20 (<20)	>40 (>50)
Urine osmolality (mOsm/kg)	>500 (>400)	<350 (<400)
Urine/plasma urea	>8	<3
Urine/plasma osmolality	>1.15 (>1.2)	<1.1 (<1.2)
Urine/plasma creatinine	>40	<20
Fractional sodium excretion (FE_{Na}) (%)	<1 (<2.5)	>1 (>2.5)
Fractional urea excretion (FE_{urea}) (%)	<35	>50

*Values in parenthesis are the criteria for neonates.

4. Other laboratory tests:
   a. Full blood count to look for anemia, thrombocytopenia and reticulocytosis, suggestive of hemolytic-uremic syndrome or vasculitis-associated GN.
   b. Peripheral blood smear to look for schistocytes in hemolytic-uremic syndrome, or spherocytes in lupus nephritis.
   c. Urine hemoglobin or serum myoglobin to exclude pigment nephropathy, if the history is suggestive of intravascular hemolysis or rhabdomyolysis.
   d. Serum complement levels (C3 and C4), anti-nuclear antibodies, anti-neutrophil cytoplasmic antibodies, and anti-glomerular basement membrane antibodies to distinguish the various glomerular diseases.
      - Serum complement C3 is low at presentation in post-infectious GN, lupus nephritis, membranoproliferative GN and some forms of familial hemolytic-uremic syndrome.

e. Specific patterns of biochemical abnormalities may be seen in certain causes of AKI.
   - Elevated lactate dehydrogenase levels in hemolytic-uremic syndrome or other causes of hemolysis.
   - Hypocalcemia, hyperphosphatemia and hyperuricemia occur in tumor lysis syndrome.
   - Elevation of the serum creatine kinase levels in rhabdomyolysis.
   - An increase in the anion and osmolar gaps in the presence of AKI is suggestive of ethylene glycol poisoning.

f. Factors H, I, B, CD46, anti-factor H antibodies, and ADAMTS13 activity for atypical hemolytic-uremic syndrome.

5. Imaging:

a. Ultrasonography:
   - Initial imaging modality to detect bilateral upper tract obstruction, bladder outlet obstruction or obstruction of a solitary functioning kidney.
   - Dilatation of the pelvicalyceal system can be detected within 24 to 36 hours of the onset of acute urinary obstruction.
   - Dilatation of the upper tract may not be seen in the acute stage of ureteral obstruction if this is accompanied by a decrease in urine output.
   - In lower tract obstruction, ureteral dilatation, bladder size and wall hypertrophy, as well as the presence of associated lesions such as ureterocele can be identified by ultrasonography.
   - An increase in echogenicity is seen in both acute and chronic kidney disease.
   - In neonates with renal vein thrombosis, Doppler flow scanning will be able to demonstrate decreased blood flow.

b. Radionuclide imaging:
   - ^{99m}Technetium mercaptoacetyltriglycine (MAG3) is used to assess blood flow and the severity of functional obstruction.

c. Computed tomography (CT) scan of abdomen:
   - Non-contrast CT scans can demonstrate the renal pelvis and proximal ureter, and may be helpful in identifying sites of ureteral obstruction, stones, tumors or congenital abnormalities.
   - Contrast-enhanced scans should be avoided in AKI due to the risk of contrast-induced AKI.

d. Magnetic resonance urogram (MRU):
   - Static MRU is useful to identify collecting system morphology in obstructive uropathies, regardless of excretory function.
   - Risk of nephrogenic systemic fibrosis following gadolinium-based contrast agents in patients with kidney failure limits the use of the dynamic scan in AKI.

6. Indications for kidney biopsy:
   a. Clinical suspicion of a rapidly progressive form of GN or acute allergic interstitial nephritis.
   b. Etiology is unclear.
   c. Prolonged AKI for assessing extent of damage, differentiating between acute tubular necrosis and acute cortical necrosis.

F. Medical Management

1. Guiding principles:
   a. Management of AKI should be focused on modifiable factors:
      - Preventing additional kidney injury.
      - Optimizing nutrition.
      - Minimizing the sequelae of electrolyte abnormalities and fluid overload.
   b. Because of the availability and efficacy of dialysis, patients with AKI often succumb not to AKI, but to other comorbidities.
2. Maintain adequate renal perfusion:
   a. In severely ill patients who are at risk of ischemic AKI, correction of pre-renal factors such as dehydration, poor cardiac output, hypovolemia, and acid-base and electrolyte abnormalities is important to prevent the development of AKI.
   b. Unless contraindicated due to fluid overload or cardiac failure, a child with clinical evidence of hypovolemia and oliguria should be administered an intravenous fluid challenge over 20 to 30 minutes, with either crystalloid solutions such as normal saline (10 to 20 ml/kg) or 5% albumin if hypotensive.
   c. This can be repeated if the child is still hypovolemic.
   d. Restoration of adequate urine flow and improvement in kidney function with fluid resuscitation is consistent with pre-renal disease.

   e. If urine output does not increase and kidney function fails to improve with restoration of intravascular volume, invasive monitoring may be required to adequately assess the child's fluid status and help guide further therapy.
   f. If oliguria persists despite adequate correction of pre-renal factors, give a trial of loop diuretics to promote diuresis in order to facilitate fluid management:
      - Intravenous furosemide bolus 2–5 mg/kg/dose (maximum 240 mg) or infusion 0.1–1 mg/kg/hr.
      - Intravenous bumetanide 0.02–0.1 mg/kg/dose (maximum 3 mg).
3. Prevent fluid overload and hypertension:
   a. Volume status should be assessed by history, physical examination, hematocrit, and imaging such as focused transthoracic ultrasound evaluation of the heart and inferior vena cava (IVC).
   b. Vasopressors should be considered as soon as possible if volume repletion has not achieved the hemodynamic goal to avoid excessive fluid therapy.
   c. In critically ill children, the degree of fluid overload is an independent risk factor for mortality.
   d. Peak percentage fluid overload exceeding 10% during Pediatric Intensive Care Unit (PICU) admission is associated with:
      - Higher mortality.
      - Chronic lung disease in premature neonates.
      - Prolonged mechanical ventilation.
   e. Equations for percent fluid overload:
      i. 2017 updated American College of Critical Care Medicine Clinical Practice Parameters for Hemodynamic Support of Pediatric and Neonatal Septic Shock:

$$\%\ \text{Fluid overload} = \frac{\text{Total fluid in (L)} - \text{Total fluid out (L)}}{\text{Admission weight (kg)}} \times 100$$

      ii. Weight-based determination for fluid overload:

$$\%\ \text{Fluid overload} = \frac{\text{Daily weight (kg)} - \text{Admission weight (kg)}}{\text{Admission weight (kg)}} \times 100$$

   f. Fluid volume should be restricted to insensible water loss calculated at 400 ml/m^2 per day or 30 ml/100 kcal, in addition to replacing urine, gastrointestinal and other losses.

g. Restrict sodium intake to 2–3 mmol/kg/day.
h. Therapy should be aimed at decreasing the body weight by 0.5 to 1% daily.
i. Fluid overload may aggravate hypertension in patients with glomerulonephritis, resulting in hypertensive emergencies.
   - Treat with intravenous antihypertensive agents that can produce a controlled reduction of blood pressure in order to avoid worsening of the cerebral edema due to disruption of cerebral autoregulation.

4. Maintain normal electrolytes and acid-base status:
   a. In oligoanuric AKI, do not give potassium and phosphate unless there is significant hypokalemia or hypophosphatemia.
   b. Hyperkalemia:
      i. Hyperkalemic emergencies where serum potassium levels ≥7 mmol/L are accompanied by electrocardiographic changes such as peaked T waves, flattened P waves, increased PR interval, and widening of the QRS complex:
         - Intravenous calcium given slowly over 15–30 minutes:
           - 10% calcium gluconate 0.5 ml/kg up to a maximum of 20 ml.
           - 10% calcium chloride 0.2 ml/kg up to a maximum of 10 ml.
         - Nebulized salbutamol:
           - Body weight <25 kg: 2.5 mg.
           - Body weight ≥25 kg: 5 mg.
         - Intravenous salbutamol 4 mg/kg.
         - Intravenous insulin 1 IU/5 g dextrose:
           - 0.1 IU/kg insulin and dextrose 0.5 g/kg.
           - Monitor blood glucose at 15 minutes and every 30 minutes subsequently until blood glucose is stable.
      ii. Less urgent elevations of serum potassium 6 to <7 mmol/L:
         - Oral or rectal sodium polystyrene sulfonate (Resonium) 1g/kg to a maximum of 30 g.
         - Correction of concomitant acidosis.
   c. Hyponatremia:
      i. Fluid restriction and loop diuretics if due to fluid overload.
      ii. Sodium supplementation if there is renal salt wasting.

d. Hypocalcemia and hyperphosphatemia:
   - Calcium-based phosphate binders.

e. Severe metabolic acidosis where serum bicarbonate <15 mmol/L or pH <7.2:
   i. Intravenous sodium bicarbonate (1–3 mmol/kg) or
   ii. Oral sodium citrate.

   Note: Use with caution in patients with fluid overload and hypertension.

5. Ensure adequate nutrition:

a. Caloric requirement:
   i. Increase caloric intake to 150% of maintenance needs.

Body wt (kg)	Daily Maintenance Caloric Requirements (kcal)
3–10	100 × (body wt)
10–20	50 × (body wt) + 1000
>20	20 × (body wt) + 1500

   ii. Because of the necessity for fluid restriction, increasing the concentration of the enteral feeds or parenteral hyperalimentation will improve caloric delivery.
      - Often limited by an increase in osmolarity of the feeds with consequent hypernatremia.
      - For patients on milk feeds, the potassium load of milk can be reduced by mixing milk with Resonium and decanting.
      - 1g of Resonium should be added for every mmol of potassium in the milk.
   iii. Early institution of dialysis will allow better optimization of nutrition in these patients.

b. Protein intake:
   i. Ensure adequate caloric intake with carbohydrates and/or fats.
   ii. Aim for a protein intake of 3 g/kg/day.
   iii. Additional amino acid supplementation (approximately 20%) should be given to children on hemodialysis or continuous kidney replacement therapy to compensate for the loss of amino acids.

6. Dosage adjustment of medications primarily excreted through the kidneys.
   - Drug levels should be routinely monitored where therapeutic levels are available.

7. Avoid further nephrotoxic insults:
   a. NSAIDs.
   b. Nephrotoxic antibiotics, antivirals and antifungals.
      - A combination of Piperacillin-Tazobactam and Vancomycin is more nephrotoxic than either drug alone.
   c. Angiotensin-converting enzyme inhibitors or angiotensin receptor blockers.
   d. Calcineurin inhibitors.
   e. High osmolality contrast agents
8. Algorithm:

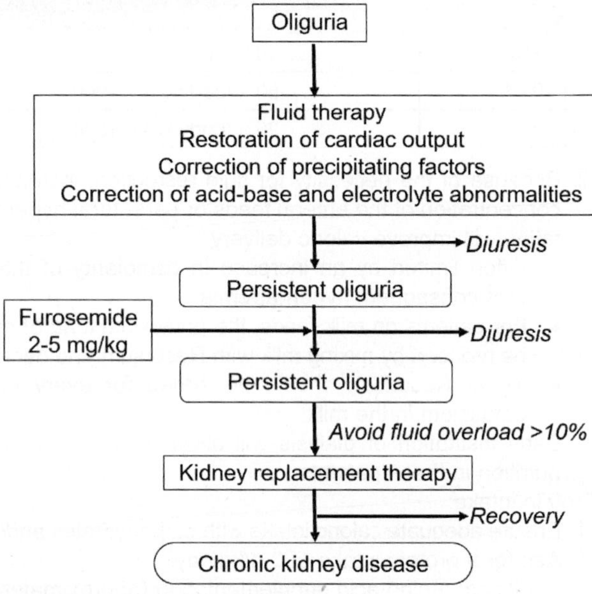

G. Acute Kidney Replacement Therapy

1. Indications:
   a. Traditional indications:
      i. Severe hyperkalemia unresponsive to conservative therapy.

ii. Uncontrolled acidosis that cannot be safely corrected because of the risk of sodium or volume overload.
iii. Severe volume overload with uncontrolled hypertension, pulmonary edema or cardiac failure.
iv. Progressive uremia with deterioration in the general condition.
v. Hypercatabolic states with an increase in blood urea by >10 mmol/L per day.

b. Early institution of dialysis in the critically ill child with AKI:
i. Percent fluid overload ≥10% especially in children post-cardiac surgery or on extracorporeal membrane oxygenation (ECMO).
ii. Create enough volume space so that the nutritional and therapeutic needs may be met, as severe fluid restriction results in:
- Inadequate nutrition.
- Propensity to hypoglycemia.
- Insufficient volume space for blood products.
- Difficulty in drug delivery, such as inotropic support and antibiotic infusions.

2. Strategies for acute kidney replacement therapy:

	Peritoneal Dialysis	Hemodialysis	Prolonged Intermittent Kidney Replacement Therapy	Continuous Kidney Replacement Therapy
Vascular access required	No	Yes	Yes	Yes
Anticoagulation required	Not required	Required	Required	Required
Continuous therapy	Yes	No	No	Yes
Easy to perform	Yes	No	No	Relative

(*Continued*)

(*Continued*)

	Peritoneal Dialysis	Hemodialysis	Prolonged Intermittent Kidney Replacement Therapy	Continuous Kidney Replacement Therapy
Hemodynamic stability	Good	Poor	Fair	Good
Fluid balance achieved	Yes (variable)	Yes (as tolerated)	Yes	Yes
Metabolic stability	Good	Poor	Fair	Good
Risk of cerebral edema	Low	High	Intermediate	Low
Nutrient removal	Fair	Less significant	Fair	Very significant
Drug removal (unbound)	Less significant	Significant	Significant	Significant
Speed of toxin removal	Slow	Fast	Intermediate	Intermediate
Patient mobilization	Convenient	Convenient	Fairly convenient	Difficult
Cost of procedure	Low	Intermediate	Intermediate	High

- **In patients with acute brain injury or increased intracranial pressure, we recommend the use of continuous kidney replacement therapy or peritoneal dialysis.**

Recommended Reading

1. Ellis EN, Arnold WC. (1982) Use of urinary indexes in renal failure in the newborn. *Am J Dis Child* **136**:615–617.
2. Patel HP. (2006) The abnormal urinalysis. *Pediatr Clin North Am* **35**:958–962.
3. Ackan-Arikan A, Zappitelli M, Loftis LL, Washburn KK, Jefferson LS, Goldstein SL. (2007) Modified RIFLE criteria in critically ill children with acute kidney injury. *Kidney Int* **10**:963–964.

4. Bellomo R, Kellum JA, Ronco C. (2007) Defining and classifying acute renal failure: From advocacy to consensus and validation of the RIFLE criteria. *Intensive Care Med* **33**:409–413.
5. Agarwal R, Brunelli SM, Williams K, Mitchell MD, Feldman HI, Umscheid CA. (2009) Gadolinium-based contrast agents and nephrogenic systemic fibrosis: A systematic review and meta-analysis. *Nephrol Dial Transplant* **24**:856–863.
6. Askenazi DJ, Ambalavanam N, Goldstein SL. (2009) Acute kidney injury in critically ill newborns: What do we know? What do we need to learn? *Pediatr Nephrol* **24**:265–274.
7. Pickering JW, Endre ZH. (2009) GFR shot by RIFLE: Errors in staging acute kidney injury. *Lancet* **373**:1318–1319.
8. Yap HK. (2011) Acute kidney insufficiency. In: *Textbook of Clinical Pediatrics*. Edited by: Elzouski AY, Stapleton FB, Whitley RJ, Oh W, Harfi HA, Nazer H. Springer. pp 2907–2920.
9. Kidney Disease: Improving Global Outcomes (KDIGO) Acute Kidney Injury Work Group. (2012) KDIGO clinical practice guideline for acute kidney injury. *Kidney Int* **2**:S1–S138.
10. Mehta R, Bagga A, Patibandla R, Chakravarthi R. (2017) Detection and management of AKI in the developing world: The 18th Acute Disease Quality Initiative (ADQI) International Consensus Conference. *Kidney Int Rep* **2**:515–518.
11. Davis AL, Carcillo JA, Aneja RK, Deymann AJ, Lin JC, Nguyen TC, Okhuysen-Cawley RS, Relvas MS, Rozenfeld RA, Skippen PW, Stojadinovic BJ, Williams EA, Yeh TS, Balamuth F, Brierley J, de Caen AR, Cheifetz IM, Choong K, Conway E Jr, Cornell T, Doctor A, Dugas MA, Feldman JD, Fitzgerald JC, Flori HR, Fortenberry JD, Graciano AL, Greenwald BM, Hall MW, Han YY, Hernan LJ, Irazuzta JE, Iselin E, van der Jagt EW, Jeffries HE, Kache S, Katyal C, Kissoon NT, Kon AA, Kutko MC, MacLaren G, Maul T, Mehta R, Odetola F, Parbuoni K, Paul R, Peters MJ, Ranjit S, Reuter-Rice KE, Schnitzler EJ, Scott HF, Torres A Jr, Weingarten-Abrams J, Weiss SL, Zimmerman JJ, Zuckerberg AL; American College of Critical Care. (2017) Medicine clinical practice parameters for hemodynamic support of pediatric and neonatal septic shock. *Crit Care Med* **45**:1061–1093.
12. Selewski DT, Goldstein SL. (2018) The role of fluid overload in the prediction of outcome in acute kidney injury. *Pediatr Nephrol* **33**:13–24.
13. Devarajan P. (2020, updated) Prevention and management of acute kidney injury (acute renal failure) in children. *UpToDate ONLINE*. http://www.uptodateonline.com.
14. Devarajan P. (2020, updated) Acute kidney injury in children: Clinical features, etiology, evaluation, and diagnosis. *UpToDate ONLINE*. http://www.uptodateonline.com.
15. Liu KD, Goldstein SL, Vijayan A, Parikh CR, Kashani K, Okusa MD, Agarwal A, Cerdá J; *AKI!Now* Initiative of the American Society of Nephrology. (2020) *AKI!Now* Initiative: Recommendations for awareness, recognition, and management of AKI. *Clin J Am Soc Nephrol* **15**:1838–1847.

2 Preventing Contrast-Induced Acute Kidney Injury

Teo S, Ng KH and Yap HK

A. Definition

1. Contrast-induced acute kidney injury (CI-AKI):
   - Condition in which impairment in kidney function, that is, a decrease in estimated glomerular filtration rate (eGFR) by ≥25% from the baseline, within 24–48 hours following the intravascular administration of a contrast medium in the absence of an alternative etiology.
   - Typically, the serum creatinine peaks 3–5 days after contrast medium administration and returns to baseline or near baseline within 1–3 weeks.
2. Contrast-associated acute kidney injury (CA-AKI):
   - Any AKI occurring within 48 hours after administration of contrast media.
   - Applies to situations in which clinical evaluation for other potential causes of AKI has not been performed or cannot be excluded.

B. Risk Factors

1. Patient-related:
   a. Chronic kidney disease (CKD):
      - Highest risk if eGFR <30 ml/min/1.73m^2.

   b. Diabetes mellitus with CKD.
   c. Volume depletion, including use of diuretics.
   d. Hypotension and/or sepsis.
   e. Anemia.

f. Low cardiac output:
   - New York Heart Association (NYHA) class 3–4.

g. Concomitant use of nephrotoxic drugs.

2. Procedure-related:
   a. Dose of contrast media.
      - Multiple contrast injections within 72 hours.
      - Volume of contrast media.
   b. Route of contrast media:
      - Intra-arterial.
   c. Choice of contrast media:
      - Osmolality.
      - Viscosity.

C. Commonly Used Contrast Media

1. First-generation agents such as ioxagate are hyperosmolal, ionic monomers (1400–1800 mOsm/kg).
2. Second-generation agents such as iohexol are low osmolal, non-ionic monomers (500–850 mOsm/kg).
3. Third-generation agents such as iodixanol are iso-osmolal, non-ionic dimers (approximately 290 mOsm/kg).

Compound	Name	Type	Iodine Content (mgl/ml)	Osmolality (mOsm/kg)	Level
Ionic	Diatrizoate (Hypaque 50)	Monomer	300	1550	High osmolal
Ionic	Metrizoate (Isopaque 370)	Monomer	370	2100	High osmolal
Ionic	Ioxaglate (Hexabrix)	Dimer	320	580	High osmolal
Non-ionic	Iopamidol (Isovue 370)	Monomer	370	796	Low osmolal
Non-ionic	Iohexol (Omnipaque 300, 350)	Monomer	300 350	647.1 755	Low osmolal

(*Continued*)

(Continued)

Compound	Name	Type	Iodine Content (mgI/ml)	Osmolality (mOsm/kg)	Level
Non-ionic	Ioxilan (Oxilan 350)	Monomer	350	695	Low osmolal
Non-ionic	Iopromide (Ultravist 370)	Monomer	370	774	Low osmolal
Non-ionic	Iodixanol (Visipaque 270, 320)	Monomer	270 320	290 (lower viscosity) 290	Iso-osmolal

D. Indications for Prophylactic Strategy

1. Patients with abnormal kidney function who received a non-steroidal anti-inflammatory drug (NSAID) or other nephrotoxic agents within 24 hours of the procedure.
2. Volume-depleted patients at risk of AKI.
3. Patients with ongoing AKI.
4. Patients with a previous history of CA-AKI.
5. Intra-arterial contrast:
   a. Patients with eGFR <60 ml/min/1.73m^2 AND proteinuria.
   b. Patients with eGFR <60 ml/min/1.73m^2 AND other comorbidities including diabetes, heart failure and liver failure.
   c. Patients with eGFR <45 ml/min/1.73m^2 even in the absence of proteinuria or any other comorbidities.
6. Intravenous iodinated contrast:
   a. Stable eGFR <30 ml/min/1.73m^2 and not on dialysis.
   b. Patients with stable eGFR 30–44 ml/min/1.73m^2 who have multiple other potential risk factors.
   c. Patients on maintenance dialysis with significant residual kidney function.

E. Preventive Measures

1. Investigation-related:
   a. Use alternative tests without iodine-based contrast media, particularly in high-risk patients.
   b. Use lower doses of contrast media:
      - Dose in grams of iodine = eGFR in ml/min.
      - Ratio of contrast media volume (ml):eGFR should be <3.7.
   c. Use of iso-osmolal non-ionic contrast media with low viscosity such as Visipaque 270 or 320.
   d. Avoid repetitive studies that are closely spaced within 48 to 72 hours.
      - Ideally the interval between procedures should be 2 weeks (expected recovery time of AKI).
2. Patient-related:
   a. Avoid volume depletion.
   b. Discontinue nephrotoxic agents, including NSAIDs, loop diuretics and aminoglycosides, at least 24–48 hours before and after contrast media administration.
   c. Hold metformin 48 hours before and after the procedure.
   d. Volume expansion with isotonic saline.
   e. Consider administering antioxidant N-acetylcysteine (optional, no strong evidence in randomized controlled trials) in selected high-risk patients.

F. Volume Expansion with Isotonic Saline

1. For outpatient adolescents with eGFR ≥45 ml/min/1.73m^2:
   - Infuse 5 ml/kg/hour isotonic 0.9% saline for at least 1 hour before the procedure and 3 ml/kg/hour for 6 hours after the procedure.
2. For high-risk patients with eGFR <45 ml/min/1.73m^2, infuse isotonic 0.9% saline at a rate of 2–3 ml/kg/hour starting at least 12 hours before the procedure, and continuing for 12 hours after the procedure.
   - For acidotic patients, correct the acidosis with sodium bicarbonate 8.4% or 4.2% (infancy) prior to the procedure followed by maintenance bicarbonate infusion.

G. N-Acetylcysteine Protocol

1. There is no clear benefit from recent randomized control trials and meta-analysis for the use of N-acetylcysteine in preventing CI-AKI.
2. Oral N-acetylcysteine can be used together with volume expansion in patients at increased risk of CI-AKI:
   - 1200 mg/1.73m^2 twice daily on the day before and the day of the procedure for a total of 4 doses.

H. Monitoring of Kidney Function

1. Check kidney function (urea, creatinine, sodium, potassium, bicarbonate, chloride):
   - Baseline prior to procedure.
   - 2, 24 and 48–72 hours after procedure.
   - If there is no increase in serum creatinine, the patient can be discharged.
2. Monitor urine output:
   - Intake/output chart.
3. Metformin and other nephrotoxic agents such as loop diuretics may be restarted at least 48–72 hours after the procedure if there is no CI-AKI.

I. Need for Dialysis after Contrast Administration

1. Patients with CKD stage 4 or 5 who are not on maintenance dialysis do not require acute dialysis after contrast administration.
2. Dialysis immediately post-contrast administration in patients on maintenance dialysis has no benefit in:
   - Preservation of residual kidney function.
   - Limiting the risk of allergic-like reactions.
   - Preventing volume overload.
   - Preventing osmotic-induced electrolyte shifts.
3. Dialysis can be done within 72 hours post-contrast administration but should be done earlier if there are concerns of volume overload.

Recommended Reading

1. Solomon R. (2005) The role of osmolality in the incidence of contrast-induced nephropathy: A systematic review of angiographic contrast media in high risk patients. *Kidney Int* **68**:2556–2563.
2. Kidney Disease: Improving Global Outcomes (KDIGO) Acute Kidney Injury Work Group. (2012) KDIGO clinical practice guideline for acute kidney injury. *Kidney Int Suppl* **2**:69–88.
3. Cruz DN, Goh CY, Marenzi G, Corradi V, Ronco C, Perazella MA. (2012) Renal replacement therapies for prevention of radiocontrast-induced nephropathy: A systematic review. *Am J Med* **125**(1):66–78
4. Weisbord SD, Gallagher M, Jneid H, Garcia S, Cass A, Thwin SS, Conner TA, Chertow GM, Bhatt DL, Shunk K, Parikh CR, McFalls EO, Brophy M, Ferguson R, Wu H, Androsenko M, Myles J, Kaufman J, Palevsky PM; PRESERVE Trial Group. (2018) Outcomes after angiography with sodium bicarbonate and acetylcysteine. *N Eng J Med* **378**:603–614.
5. Davenport MS, Perazella MA, Yee J, Dillman JR, Fine D, McDonald RJ, Rodby RA, Wang CL, Weinreb JC. (2020) Use of intravenous iodinated contrast media in patients with kidney disease: Consensus statements from the American College of Radiology and the National Kidney Foundation. *Radiology* **294**:660–668.
6. ACR Committee on Drugs and Contrast Media. (2021) ACR manual of contrast media. Version 10.3. ACR Committee on Drugs and Contrast Media, pp. 33–44.

1 Fluid and Electrolyte Therapy for Infants and Children

Lau PYW, Resontoc LP, Koh PL and Yap HK

A. Introduction

1. The goals of intravenous (IV) fluid therapy are to prevent:
   a. Dehydration.
   b. Deficiencies of sodium and potassium.
   c. Ketoacidosis.
   d. Protein degradation.
2. There is no "one-size-fits-all" approach to IV fluid therapy, as the prescription needs to be individualized to take into account the following:
   a. Medical condition of the child
   b. Initial fluid, electrolyte and acid-base status.
   c. Therapeutic goal.
   d. Changes in the fluid, electrolyte and acid-base status with ongoing IV fluid therapy and losses.

B. Fluid Requirements for Children with Normal Hydration

I. Daily maintenance fluid requirements via IV route:

1. Association between metabolic rate and fluid requirement:
   a. Fluid maintenance volume is the volume of daily fluid intake, which replaces the insensible losses (from skin, lungs and

stools) and the fluid required to excrete excess solute load (urea, creatinine, electrolytes) in a child with normal kidneys.

b. In a child with average normal kidney response: **1 ml of water is required for each kilocalorie consumed**:

	Daily Fluid Volume (ml per 100 kcal)
Insensible loss (IL)	50
Obligatory urine volume required to excrete a solute load (renal solute load) (RSL)	66.7
Water of oxidation (WO)	16.7
Total fluid requirement = IL + RSL – WO	**100**

2. Caloric requirements:

Body Weight (kg)	Daily Caloric Requirements (kcal/day)
3–10	100 kcal/kg
10–20	1000 + 50 kcal/kg for each kg >10kg
>20	1500 + 20 kcal/kg for each kg >20kg

Note: **IL – WO = 30 ml/100 kcal or 400 ml/m^2**.

3. Maintenance fluid requirements for a clinically well child with normal hydration but no oral intake (e.g., prior to elective surgery):

a. Calculated using **Holliday–Segar method**, which estimates caloric expenditure from weight:

Body Weight (kg)	Daily Maintenance Fluid
3–10	100 ml/kg
10–20	1000 ml + 50 ml/kg for each kg >10kg
>20	1500 ml + 20 ml/kg for each kg >20kg
Normal maximum amount	2500 ml per day

b. This method is **NOT** used for:
   i. Babies who are <28 days old.
   ii. Calculating oral maintenance fluid requirements.
   iii. Patients who are overweight.

4. Fluid requirement of an overweight patient is based on age and **ideal body weight (IBW) (kg)**:

a. Weight for 50% percentile for the patient's age
OR
b. Formula to get the IBW (in adolescent and adults)
Male: 50 + 2.3*(height in cm/2.5 – 60)
Female: 45.5 + 2.3*(height in cm/2.5 – 60)

5. Maintenance fluid requirements for term neonates (<28 days old):

Age	Daily Fluid Requirements (ml/kg)
Day 1	50–60
Day 2	70–80
Day 3	80–100
Day 4	100–120
Day 5–28	120–150

6. Adjustment of maintenance fluid requirements may be needed in the following:
   a. Factors affecting insensible water loss:

Increased Losses	% Change	Decreased Losses	% Change
Prematurity	100–300	Enclosed incubator	25–50
Radiant warmer	50–100	Humidified air	15–30
Phototherapy	25–50	Sedation	5–25
Hyperventilation	20–30	Decreased activity	5–25
Increased activity	5–25	Hypothermia	5–15
Hyperthermia	12% per °C		

   Example: A sick child on mechanical ventilation with humidified gases may need 50% less fluid than a clinically well child due to inactivity and the humidified air.

   b. Maintenance fluid requirements may be reduced to 50–80% in inappropriate anti-diuretic hormone (ADH) secretion:
      i. Post-surgery.
      ii. Stress, pain, nausea or vomiting.
      iii. Central nervous system disease.

iv. Liver disease.
v. Nephrotic syndrome.
vi. Pulmonary disease.
vii. Hypothyroidism.
viii. Hypoadrenalism.
ix. Medications, e.g., carbamazepine, cyclophosphamide, vincristine, selective serotonin reuptake inhibitors.

c. Underlying medical conditions with specific fluid requirements, e.g., kidney failure and cardiac failure.

II. Daily electrolyte requirements:

Sodium (Na)	3–4 mmol/kg
Potassium (K)	2–3 mmol/kg
Chloride (Cl)	2–4 mmol/kg
Calcium (Ca)	0.5–1.0 mmol/kg (maximum 2 g/day in infants, and 3–4 g/day in older children)
Magnesium (Mg)	0.25 mmol/kg
Phosphate (PO_4)	2 mmol/kg

III. Types of solutions for IV maintenance fluids:

1. Considerations:
   a. Increasing reports of iatrogenic hyponatremia with catastrophic neurological outcomes seen in hospitalized children receiving hypotonic maintenance fluid therapy.
   b. Cause of hyponatremia is due to a combination of a positive balance of electrolyte-free water (from the administration of hypotonic fluid) and the impaired ability in sick patients to excrete hypotonic urine secondary to ADH secretion.
   c. Data supporting isotonic 0.9% saline solution as maintenance fluid therapy include several meta-analyses based on small clinical trials.

i. American Academy of Pediatrics (AAP) recommends that patients from 28 days to 18 years of age requiring maintenance IV fluids should receive isotonic solutions, which significantly decrease the risk of developing hyponatremia.
ii. NICE 2015 guidelines recommend the initial use of isotonic crystalloids that contain sodium in the range of 131–154 mmol/L as maintenance fluid.

d. Physiologically, IV fluids, according to their tonicity, redistribute mainly to the interstitial fluid (isotonic fluids) or the interstitial and intracellular fluid compartments (hypotonic fluids).
   i. Isotonic fluids are typically employed in fluid resuscitation to correct an acute intravascular fluid deficit.
   ii. Administration of hypotonic fluids generates the necessary osmotic driving force needed to allow the movement of water from the extracellular to intracellular compartment, hydrating both compartments, which is the goal of maintenance fluid therapy in hemodynamically stable fasting children.
e. There is increasing evidence that the administration of Cl-rich IV fluids (e.g., 0.9% saline that contains Cl exceeding that of plasma by approximately 60%) is associated with:
   i. Increased risk of mortality.
   ii. Direct effect on intrarenal perfusion, vasoconstriction, and glomerular filtration.
   iii. Impaired coagulation (Cl-rich resuscitation fluid)
   iv. Risk of fluid overload as compared to a balanced crystalloid solution (e.g., PlasmaLyte with a Cl concentration closer to plasma Cl concentration).
   v. Hypertension.

   Note: Children with impaired kidney functions are particularly at risk of the above sequelae due to the reduced ability to excrete excess Cl.
f. 0.9% saline solution delivers Na and Cl loads 2x more than a 0.45% saline solution ml for ml, which can potentially result in Na and Cl overload in children.

2. Choice of maintenance fluids:
   a. Children <40 kg: Use 0.45% saline solution (hypotonic solution) as an initial maintenance fluid therapy for clinically well children

and adjusted in response to monitoring during intravenous fluid therapy.

b. Children ≥40 kg: Use 0.9% saline solution as 0.45% saline delivers a Na load of <4 mmol/kg/day, except in children who cannot tolerate Na or Cl overload.

c. Recommended fluid to be infused as maintenance therapy for clinically well children with normal hydration is:

Children <40 kg: 0.45% saline with 5% dextrose. **Children ≥40 kg: 0.9% saline with 5% dextrose.** **Add 1–2 mmol/kg/day of KCl (if there is no hyperkalemia or kidney impairment).**

d. Do **NOT** use 0.45% saline with 5% dextrose solution in the following situations:
   i. Serum Na is low (<130 mmol/L).
   ii. Initial treatment of acute neurological conditions, e.g., meningitis and head injury.
   iii. Conditions associated with syndrome of inappropriate antidiuretic hormone secretion (SIADH).
   iv. Volume resuscitation.

e. Neonates:
   i. For term neonates who are ≤7 days old, 0.45% saline with 5% dextrose solution can provide excessive Na and inadequate glucose.
      - Consider a combination drip consisting of dextrose and an added 20% sodium chloride (NaCl) to provide 4 mmol/kg/day of Na and a glucose delivery rate of 4–6 mg/kg/min.
   ii. For term neonates ≥8 days old, 0.45% saline with 5 to 10% dextrose solution can be used safely.

IV. Daily maintenance fluid requirements via ORAL route:

1. Due to the low caloric density of milk (67 kcal/ml) and significant water loss in feces from oral feeding, the recommended oral maintenance fluid volume is higher than the intravenous requirement.

Age		Recommended Daily Oral Fluid
1st day		60 ml/kg/day
2nd day		90 ml/kg/day
3rd day		120 ml/kg/day
4th day to 6 months		150 ml/kg/day
7 months to 1 year		100–120 ml/kg/day
1 to 3 years		900 ml/day
4 to 8 years		1200 ml/day
9 to 13 years	Boys Girls	1800 ml/day 1600 ml/day
14 to 18 years	Boys Girls	2600 ml/day 1800 ml/day

2. Types of oral fluids:
   a. Age ≤6 months old: Mainly milk.
   b. Age >6 months old: Water, milk and other fluids (once solid feeds are established).

C. Fluid Requirements for Children with Dehydration

The fluid requirements for a dehydrated child should include
- Maintenance requirements +
- Deficit +
- Ongoing losses

I. Estimation of severity of dehydration:

Clinical Signs	Magnitude of Dehydration (Body Weight Loss)		
	Mild (3–5%)	Moderate (6–9%)	Severe (≥10%)
Behavior	Normal	Irritable or lethargic	Hyperirritable, drowsy or comatose
Breathing	Normal	Increased	Increased, deep

(*Continued*)

(*Continued*)

Clinical Signs	Magnitude of Dehydration (Body Weight Loss)		
	Mild (3–5%)	Moderate (6–9%)	Severe (≥10%)
Thirst	Slight	Moderate	Intense
Mucous membrane	Dry	Very dry	Parched
Tears	Present	+/–	Absent
Skin turgor	Normal	Tenting	Severe tenting
Skin colour and temperature	Normal	Cool	Cool and mottled
Capillary refill	<2 sec	2–3 sec	>3 sec
Anterior fontanelle	Normal	+/–	Sunken
Eyes	Normal	Slightly sunken	Sunken
Urine output	Decreased	Oliguric	Azotemic
Blood pressure (BP)	Normal	Normal or postural drop	Decreased
Heart rate	±Increased	Increased	Marked increase

II. Initial resuscitation (in established or impending shock):

1. Initial resuscitation should be: **Fluid bolus** of **20 ml/kg of 0.9% saline, Ringer's lactate, or PlasmaLyte solution**.
   - Hypotensive: Give over 10 minutes.
   - Compensated shock: Give over 20–30 minutes.

   Note: Patients should **not** have signs of fluid overload.
2. Limit crystalloid fluid boluses in specific pre-existing conditions (e.g., cardiac or kidney disease), diabetic ketoacidosis, or trauma.
   - In trauma, give blood products early (bolus 10 ml/kg), preferentially over crystalloids.
3. The child should be reassessed (heart rate, perfusion, blood pressure, urine output) immediately after the fluid bolus, and additional fluid bolus may be needed.
   - Seek expert advice early (e.g., from intensivists) if >40–60 ml/kg of IV bolus fluids are needed and/or inotropes are required.

III. Maintenance volume requirement:

1. Most children will tolerate standard fluid requirements as recommended by the Holliday–Segar method mentioned above.
2. Some acutely ill children with increased ADH secretion may benefit from their maintenance fluid requirement being restricted to 50–80% of the normal recommended volume.

IV. Deficit volume replacement:

1. Fluid deficit in ml can be calculated following an estimation of the degree of dehydration expressed as a percentage of body weight.

Volume of fluid deficit (ml) = % dehydration/100 × weight (kg) × 1000

2. Recommended fluid to replace volume deficit:

For patients <40 kg and without hyponatremia: 0.45% saline with 5% dextrose **For patients ≥40 kg: 0.9% saline with 5% dextrose**

3. Rate of replacement of fluid deficit depends on the child's illness:
   a. Replacement may be rapid in most cases of gastroenteritis.
      - Give the first half of the total volume (fluid deficit + maintenance – initial resuscitation volume) over the first 8 hours, followed by half of the total volume over the next 16 hours.

   b. Replacement has to be slower in diabetic ketoacidosis and meningitis.
      - Replace the total volume over 48 hours.

V. Ongoing losses

1. Ongoing losses (e.g., from diarrhea, nasogastric suction, and drains) should be measured and replaced regularly if the above combined fluid deficit/maintenance approach fails to correct the dehydration.
2. Replacement may be based on each previous hour or 4-hour period, depending on the situation.

3. Type of fluid used to replace ongoing losses depends on the electrolyte composition of the fluid being lost.
   - For example, nasogastric suction losses should be replaced with IV 0.45% saline with KCl 10 mmol added to each 500 ml of 0.45% saline.

Body Fluid	Na mmol/L	K mmol/L	Cl mmol/L	HCO_3 mmol/L
Gastric juice	20–80	5–30	100–140	0
Pancreas	120–140	5–15	90–120	110
Bile	130–160	5–15	80–120	40
Small intestine	100–140	5–25	90–135	30
Ileostomy	45–135	3–15	20–115	30–110
Diarrhea	10–90	10–80	10–110	15–50
Sweat normal	10–30	3–10	10–35	0
Sweat cystic fibrosis	50–130	5–25	50–110	0
Burn exudate	140	5	110	20

VI. Example of fluid therapy for severe isonatremic dehydration:

A 10-month-old boy with a body weight of 10 kg was admitted for gastroenteritis with initial hypotension due to 15% dehydration. Laboratory results revealed Na 138 mmol/L, K 3 mmol/L, and Cl 95 mmol/L.

a. Initial management of hypovolemic shock:
   0.9% saline 20 ml/kg (200 ml) was given over 10 minutes. BP returned to normal after this.

b. Subsequent fluid regime:
   Maintenance fluid (ml) = 100 ml/kg × 10
   = 1000 ml
   Fluid deficit (ml) = % dehydration/100 × weight (kg) × 1000
   = 1500 ml
   Remaining fluid deficit volume after fluid bolus = 1500 – 200 = 1300 ml
   Total volume to give = Remaining fluid deficit + maintenance volume
   = 1300 + 1000 = 2300 ml
   Give the first half of 2300 ml over the first 8 hours and the rest over the next 16 hours.

(*Continued*)

Fluid orders: *IV 5% dextrose + 0.45% saline 1150 ml over the first 8 hours, Followed by IV 5% dextrose + 0.45% saline 1150 ml over the next 16 hours. Add IV 7.45% KCl 2 mmol/kg/day to the 5% dextrose + 0.45% saline solution if there are no contraindications.*

D. Rehydration of Children with Severe Acute Malnutrition

1. Severe acute malnutrition (SAM) is defined as a mid-upper arm circumference <11.5 cm or weight-for-height Z-score <–3.
2. Rehydration of dehydrated children with SAM should be done orally rather than intravenously, when possible, to reduce the risk of overhydration and heart failure.
3. Rehydrate initially using standard WHO low-osmolality oral rehydration salt (ORS) solution (glucose 125 mmol/L, Na 45 mmol/L, K 40 mmol/L, Cl 70 mmol/L, osmolality 300 mmol/L).
   a. Give 5 ml/kg every 30 minutes for the first 2 hours.
   b. If the child is still dehydrated, give F-75 (starter formula with 75 kcal and 0.9 g protein per 100 ml) 5–10 ml/kg/hour every alternate hour for a maximum of 10 hours.
   c. Assess frequently: Every 30 minutes for the first 2 hours and hourly thereafter.
4. If in shock, give IV resuscitation fluid at 15 ml/kg/hour using any of the following:
   a. Ringer's lactate solution with 5% dextrose.
   b. 5% dextrose + 0.45% saline solution with KCl 20 mmol/L.
   c. Monitor every 5–10 minutes for signs of overhydration and congestive heart failure.
      - If signs develop, stop IV fluid therapy immediately.
5. Monitor serum electrolytes at baseline and 6-hourly until the child is fully hydrated.

E. Correction of Electrolyte and Acid-Base Abnormalities

I. Hyponatremia:

1. Management of hyponatremia must take into consideration the patient's fluid status:
   a. Fluid restriction in SIADH.
   b. Diuretics in congestive heart failure, nephrotic syndrome, liver cirrhosis.
   c. Na and water deficit replacement in hypovolemic hyponatremia.
2. In acute hyponatremia (<48 hours), Na correction can be done quickly.
3. **Recommended target rate of Na correction in chronic hyponatremia (>48 hours): <8–10 mmol/L per day.**
   - Most reported cases of osmotic demyelination occurred after rates of correction that exceeded 12 mmol/L per day, although isolated cases occurred only after 9–10 mmol/L per day.
4. Na equivalent in fluid preparations:
   Normal saline = 154 mmol/L Na
   D/S(R) or 0.45% saline = 77 mmol/L Na
   D/S(M) or 0.23% saline = 38.5 mmol/L Na
   3% saline = 513 mmol/L Na
   Note: Saline concentration should not exceed 3% in an IV infusion.
5. Na equivalent in oral preparations:
   NaCl tablet = 8.5 mmol Na + 8.5 mmol Cl
   20% NaCl solution = 3.42 mmol Na/ml
   Sodium bicarbonate ($NaHCO_3$) tablet 500 mg = 137 mg Na = 6 mmol Na + 6 mmol HCO_3
   Shohl's solution (Na citrate) = 1 mmol Na + 1 mmol citrate (= 3 mmol HCO_3) per ml

II. Hyponatremic dehydration:

Na Deficit (mmol) = 0.6 × body wt (kg) × (135 – serum [Na])

1. Example of fluid therapy of asymptomatic hyponatremic dehydration with serum [Na] >120 mmol/L:

A 10-month-old boy with a body weight of 10 kg was admitted for vomiting and diarrhea with 10% dehydration. Laboratory results revealed Na 125 mmol/L, K 3.0 mmol/L, and Cl 94 mmol/L.

a. Calculate the total fluid volume required.
   Fluid deficit (ml) = % dehydration/100 × weight (kg) × 1000 = 1000 ml
   Maintenance fluid (ml) = 100 ml/kg × 10 = 1000 ml
   Total fluid volume = fluid deficit + maintenance = 2000 ml
b. Calculate the estimated Na load required to correct the hyponatremia.
   - Maintenance Na = 4 mmol/kg/day = 4 × 10 = 40 mmol
   - Na deficit associated with isonatremic volume loss (mmol) = 140 mmol/L × fluid deficit volume (L) = 140 mmol
   - Na deficit on top of isonatremic volume loss (mmol) = 0.6 × weight (kg) × (135 – serum Na) = 0.6 × 10 × (135 – 125) = 60 mmol
   - Total Na required = 40 + 140 + 60 = 240 mmol
c. Giving 2 L of 0.45% saline would give a Na load of 154 mmol, which is insufficient to correct the hyponatremia.
   - Hence, in this case, to ensure adequate Na load to correct hyponatraemia, 2 L of **0.9% saline will be used**, and this would give a Na load of 308 mmol.
d. Using the **sequential deficit/maintenance approach**:
   - Give the fluid deficit volume over the first 8 hours, followed by a maintenance volume in the next 16 hours.

Fluid orders:
IV 5% dextrose + 0.9% saline 1000 ml over the first 8 hours.
Followed by IV 5% dextrose + 0.9% saline 1000 ml over the next 16 hours.
Add IV 7.45% KCl 2 mmol/kg/day to the 5% dextrose + 0.9% saline if there is urine output.

2. Adrogué–Madias equation:
   a. Can be used to predict the change in serum Na concentration [Na] (mmol/L) following a therapeutic maneuver to avoid overly rapid correction of hyponatremia:

$$\Delta\,[\mathbf{Na}] = \frac{\textbf{Infusate }[\mathbf{Na}] - \textbf{serum }[\mathbf{Na}]}{[\mathbf{0.6} \times \textbf{body wt (kg)}] + \mathbf{V}} \times \mathbf{V}$$

where Δ [Na] = change in serum [Na}, and V = infusate volume (L)

b. Example of use of the Adrogué–Madias equation:

A 10-month-old boy with a body weight of 10 kg was admitted for vomiting and diarrhea with 10% dehydration. Laboratory results revealed Na 125 mmol/L, K 3.0 mmol/L, and Cl 94 mmol/L.

Fluid orders:

IV 5% dextrose + 0.9% saline 1000 ml over the first 8 hours.

Followed by IV 5% dextrose + 0.9% saline 1000 ml over the next 16 hours.

Add IV 7.45% KCl 2 mmol/kg/day to the 5% dextrose + 0.9% saline solution if there is urine output

Using the Adrogué–Madias equation:

a. In the first 8 hours, the change in serum [Na] will be from 125 mmol/L to 129 mmol/L (increase [Na] at 0.5 mmol/L per hour).

b. In the next 16 hours, the change in serum [Na] will be from 129 mmol/L to 133 mmol/L (increase [Na] at 0.25 mmol/L per hour).

c. An improved Adrogué–Madias equation has recently been derived to determine the volume of any infusate (V) to correct hyponatremia to target [Na]:

$$\mathbf{V\ (L)} = \frac{\mathbf{\Delta\ [Na] \times [0.6 \times body\ wt\ (kg)]}}{\mathbf{Infusate\ [Na] - target\ [Na]}}$$

3. Management of symptomatic acute hyponatremic dehydration with serum [Na] <120 mmol/L:
   a. Hyponatremia is seldom symptomatic unless the serum [Na] is <120 mmol/L and if hyponatremia occurs quickly.
   b. In a child with hyponatremic seizures, give 3–5 ml/kg of 3% saline over 10–15 minutes.
      - Monitor serum [Na], and if seizures are ongoing, the infusion should be repeated.
   c. To prevent further hyponatremic seizures, aim for a serum [Na] target of 120–125 mmol/L.
      - Calculate the Na deficit and give the balance of the 3% saline infusion **over the next 60 minutes**.
   d. When a serum [Na] of 120 mmol/L is achieved, embark on further correction of fluid deficit and Na deficit gradually **over the next 48 hours**.
      - Include maintenance Na requirement AND

- Correction of Na deficit associated with isonatremic volume loss (mmol)
  $= 140$ mmol/L $\times$ fluid deficit volume (L) AND
- Correction of Na deficit on top of isonatremic volume loss (mmol)
  $= 0.6 \times$ weight (kg) $\times$ (target [Na] – serum [Na]).

e. Monitor the serum Na and fluid status every 4–6 hours and adjust the rehydration drip as needed to achieve correction of fluid deficit and gradual correction of hyponatremia.

f. Example of fluid therapy for symptomatic acute hyponatremia:

A 10-month-old boy with a body weight of 10 kg was admitted for vomiting and diarrhea with 10% dehydration. He is having a generalized tonic-clonic seizure. Laboratory results revealed Na 110 mmol/L, K 3.5 mmol/L, and Cl 95 mmol/L.

a. Emergency management of hyponatremic seizure:
   Give 3–5 ml/kg of 3% saline over 10–15 minutes.
   *In this case, **50 ml of 3% saline was given over 15 minutes** with resolution of seizure.*

b. Aim for a target serum [Na] of 120–125 mmol/L to prevent further seizures:
   Na deficit (mmol) $= 0.6 \times$ weight (kg) $\times$ (120 – serum [Na]) $= 60$ mmol
   This is equal to 117 ml of 3% saline.
   50 ml of 3% saline had been given earlier to stop the fits.
   *Hence another 67 ml of 3% saline can be given **over the next 60 minutes**.*

c. Further correction of the serum [Na] over the next 48 hours after 120 mmol/L has been achieved:
   I. Determine the Na load in IV therapy to correct serum Na from 120 to 125 mmol/L over next 24 hours.
      - Maintenance Na requirement $= 4$ mmol/kg/day $= 4 \times 10 = 40$ mmol
   ii. Correct Na deficit associated with isonatraemic volume loss (mmol)
      $= 140$ mmol/L $\times$ fluid deficit volume (L) $= 140$ mmol
   iii. Correct Na deficit on top of isonatraemic volume loss (mmol)
      $= 0.6 \times$ weight (kg) $\times$ (125 – serum Na)
      $= 0.6 \times 10 \times (125 - 120) = 30$ mmol
   iv. Total Na required in hyponatremic dehydration $= 40 + 140 + 30 = 210$ mmol
      - Amount of IV 5% dextrose + 0.9% saline to deliver 210 mmol Na in next 24 hours = 1370 ml
   v. With 117 ml of 3% NaCl given earlier to correct severe hyponatraemia, the total fluid received in 24 hours will be 1487 ml.
      - This volume can correct 50% of the fluid deficit volume and covers the daily maintenance fluid volume in the next 24 hours.

Fluid orders using a combined deficit/maintenance approach:
IV 5% dextrose + 0.9% saline 1370 ml over the next 24 hours.

4. In hyponatremic patients with **severe symptoms (obtundation, coma)**, the **initial correction rate can be 1–2 mmol/L per hour for several hours**.
   - This limit can be cautiously exceeded if severe symptoms are not responding to correction according to the specified target.
5. Recommended indications for stopping the rapid correction of symptomatic hyponatremia are:
   a. Cessation of life-threatening manifestations.
   b. Moderation of other symptoms.
   c. Achievement of serum [Na] of 125–130 mmol/L, or even lower, i.e., 120 mmol/L, if the baseline serum [Na] was <100 mmol/L.

III. Asymptomatic hyponatremia (<135 mmol/L) developing on IV fluid therapy:

1. If a child is receiving a hypotonic solution, change to an isotonic fluid.
2. Restrict maintenance IV fluids in children who are hypervolemic or at risk of hypervolemia by either:
   a. Restricting maintenance fluids to 50–80% of their routine maintenance needs OR
   b. Reducing maintenance fluids, calculated on the basis of insensible losses within the range of 300–400 ml/m²/day plus urinary output.

IV. Hypernatremic dehydration:

Free Water Deficit (L) = 0.6 × body wt (kg) × {1 – (serum [Na]/140)}

1. Fluid resuscitation if hypovolemic:
   a. If the patient is in shock, give 10–20 ml/kg of 0.9% saline over 20–30 minutes.
   b. If oliguric, give 10–20 ml/kg of 0.45% saline hourly till urine flow is established.

2. Correction of free water deficit should be done over at least 48 hours, lowering the serum [Na] by not more than 10 mmol/L per day.
   a. Maintenance fluid requirements should be added to the calculation.
   b. Do not correct too rapidly as this will result in cerebral edema due to the presence of intracellular idiogenic osmoles.
   c. Choose solutions that are not too relatively hypotonic to the current serum [Na].
      - Never use pure dextrose solution as IV correction.
   d. Monitor serum [Na] every 4–6 hours.
      - If hypernatremia worsens or is unchanged in 4–6 hours, review the fluid and consider changing it to fluids with more free water content.
3. Correct for hypocalcemia (seen in 10%).
4. Serum [Na] >180 mmol/L is an indication for peritoneal dialysis, using a dialysate fluid containing 150 mmol/L [Na].
5. Example of fluid therapy in hypernatremic dehydration:

> A 6-month-old boy was admitted for fever, vomiting and poor feeding. He was irritable with sunken eyes. Capillary refill was 2 seconds. His weight was 5 kg (<3rd percentile). Laboratory results revealed Na 170 mmol/L, K 4 mmol/L, and Cl 125 mmol/L.
>
> a. Calculate the free water deficit:
> Free water deficit (L) = 0.6 x weight (kg) x [1 – (serum [Na]/140)]
> = 0.6 x 5 x [1 – (170/140)] = 0.64 L
> *To bring down his serum [Na] from 170 mmol/L to 140 mmol/L by 10 mmol/L/day, we aim to give this* ***free water deficit volume over 3 days****.*
>
> b. Maintenance volume = 100 ml/kg x 5 = 500 ml per day
>
> c. Volume of fluid per day = maintenance + 1/3 of free water deficit
> = 500 + 213 = 713 ml
>
> d. Decide on the type of fluid for correction:
> Can start with 5% dextrose + 0.45% saline.
>
> ***Fluid orders:***
> *IV 5% dextrose + 0.45% saline 713 ml over 24 hours.*
> *After 4 hours, the repeat serum [Na] was 172 mmol/L, and there was polyuria past 4 hours.*
> *Use fluid of increased free water content instead. Change to IV 5% dextrose + 0.23% saline.*
> *Consider adding replacement urine losses ml for ml.*

V. Potassium (K) deficit:

K Deficit (mmol) ≈ 0.6 × body wt (kg) × (4 – serum K)

1. For severe hypokalemia (serum [K] ≤2.5 mmol/L) with symptoms (cardiac arrhythmia, paralysis, severe muscle weakness), give K infusion at 0.2 mmol/kg/hour for 2–3 hours with cardiac monitoring and recheck serum [K] at the end.
   a. **Maximum infusion rate in the general ward is 0.2 mmol/kg/hour while the maximum infusion rate in thc intensive care unit is 0.4 mmol/kg/hour**.
   b. Infusion of >40 mmol/L K solutions via the peripheral vein may result in phlebitis; hence, infusion via central line is preferred with ECG monitoring.
2. For serum [K] between 2.5 and 3.5 mmol/L, give enteral or slow IV K supplementation.
   a. Use an enteral route for K supplementation whenever possible due to the risk of cardiac arrhythmia with rapid IV administration.
   b. Oral KCl 0.5–1 mmol/kg/dose (maximum 20 mmol) and repeated at 4–6 hours:
      - Age ≤5 years: Maximum 1 mmol/kg
      - Age >5 years: Maximum 0.5 mmol/kg

   OR
   c. Oral KCl 0.5–1 mmol/kg/dose (maximum 10 mmol) hourly until serum [K] normalizes:
      - Check serum [K] after every 3 doses.
3. K replacement should only be given when urine output is established.
4. Contraindications to adding K additive into IV fluids include:
   a. Presence of hyperkalemia (serum K >5 mmol/L)
   b. At risk of hyperkalemia:
      - Use of potassium-sparing diuretics or renin-angiotensin system blockers.
      - Adrenal insufficiency.

- Severe tissue damage, e.g., burns or crush injury.
- Tumor lysis syndrome.

c. Abnormal kidney function as suggested by elevated serum creatinine.
d. At the risk of kidney impairment suggested by anuria for at least 12 hours or oliguria for at least 16 hours:
   - Acute glomerulonephritis.
   - Acute kidney injury.

5. K equivalent in oral preparations:
   Span K tablet = 600 mg, K = 8 mmol K.
   Mixture KCl = 500 mg K per 5 ml = 1.34 mmol K + 1.34 mmol Cl per ml.
   Mixture K citrate 30% = 2.8 mmol K + 0.9 mmol citrate per ml.
   K citrate tablet = 1080 mg = 10 mmol K + 3.3 mmol citrate.

VI. Metabolic acidosis:

Bicarbonate (HCO_3) deficit (mmol)
= 0.3 × (Base Deficit) × body wt (kg)
OR
= 0.3 × (Desired [HCO_3] – Actual [HCO_3]) × body wt (kg)

1. This formula accounts for half correction of the HCO_3 deficit.
2. Treatment of acute metabolic acidosis:
   a. Consider giving IV $NaHCO_3$, especially if serum [HCO_3] <12 mmol/L.
   - In acidosis secondary to volume depletion, target a desired [HCO_3] of 15 mmol/L, as volume replacement is sufficient to correct the remaining acidosis.
   - In renal tubular acidosis, correct the acidosis to a desired [HCO_3] of 24 mmol/L.
   - In diabetic ketoacidosis, correct the acidosis with $NaHCO_3$ if pH is ≤7.0, and target a pH of at least 7.1.

b. Rate of correction depends on the target [HCO_3] and clinical situation.
   - Give half of the HCO_3 deficit as a bolus dose if pH is ≤7.0 followed by the other half as an infusion over 2–4 hours.

c. Use 4.2% $NaHCO_3$ in neonates and infants.

3. Formulations:
   - 1 ml 8.4% $NaHCO_3$ = 1 mmol Na + 1 mmol HCO_3.
   - $NaHCO_3$ tablet 500 mg
     = 137 mg Na = 6 mmol Na + 6 mmol HCO_3.
   - Shohl's solution = 1 mmol Na + 1 mmol citrate (3 mmol HCO_3) per ml.
4. Correct simultaneously K and Ca deficits during the correction of metabolic acidosis.

F. Monitoring

1. Monitoring regime is essential for all children on IV hydration.
2. An accurate daily intake and output record should be kept.

Time	Parameters To Be Monitored
Prior to IV fluid administration	• Weight • Serum Na, K, Cl, HCO_3, urea, creatinine.
Patient receiving replacement IV fluids for ongoing losses 24 hours later and subsequent days of IV therapy	• Daily weight. • Daily serum Na, K. (Note: More frequent monitoring 4–6 hourly if serum electrolytes are abnormal).
Patient still receiving IV maintenance fluids at >50% of calculated maintenance levels 24 hours later and subsequent days of IV therapy	• Daily weight. • Periodic serum Na, K. (Note: More frequent monitoring if serum electrolytes are abnormal).

G. Osmolality and Tonicity of Available Intravenous Solutions

IV Solution	Glucose mmol/L	Na* mmol/L	Cl mmol/L	Lactate mmol/L	K mmol/L	Osmolality mOsm/L	Tonicity
0.9% saline	—	154	154	—	—	308	Isotonic
0.45% saline	—	77	77	—	—	154	Hypotonic
3% saline	—	513	513	—	—	1026	Hypertonic
5% dextrose	278	—	—	—	—	278	Very hypotonic
10% dextrose	555	—	—	—	—	555	Very hypotonic
0.9% saline + 5% dextrose	278	154	154	—	—	586	Isotonic
0.45% saline + 5% dextrose	278	77	77	—	—	432	Hypotonic
0.23% saline + 5% dextrose	278	38	38	—	—	355	Very hypotonic
Ringer's lactate	—	130	110	28	4	280	Almost isotonic
5% albumin	—	140	125	—	—	260	Isotonic
PlasmaLyte	23	140	98	Acetate: 27 mmol/L Gluconate: 23 mmol/L	5	295	Isotonic
Plasma (reference)		135–145	95–108		3.5–5.3	275–295	

*Solutions that contain [Na] in the range of 131–154 mmol/L are considered isotonic.

Recommended Reading

1. Chesney RW, Batisky DL. (1995) Fluid and electrolyte therapy in infants and children. In: *Fluid, Electrolyte and Acid-Base Disorders*, 2nd edition. Edited by: Arieff AI, Defronzo RA. pp. 896.
2. Moritz ML, Ayuz JC. (2010) New aspects in the pathogenesis, prevention, and treatment of hyponatremic encephalopathy in children. *Pediatr Nephrol* **25**:1225–1238.
3. Cavari Y, Pitfield AF, Kissoon N. (2013) Intravenous maintenance fluids revisited. *Pediatr Emer Care* **29**:1225–1231.
4. WHO. (2013) Fluid management. In: *WHO Pocket Book of Hospital Care for Children*, 2nd edition. pp. 304–305.
5. Green J, Lillie J. (2017) Intravenous fluid therapy in children and young people in hospital N29. *Arch Dis Child Educ Pract Ed* **102**:327–331.
6. Feld LG, Neuspiel DR, Foster BA, Leu MG, Garber MD, Austin K, Basu RK, Conway EE Jr, Fehr JJ, Hawkins C, Kaplan RL, Rowe EV, Waseem M, Moritz ML; Subcommittee on fluid and electrolyte therapy. (2018) Clinical practice guideline: Maintenance intravenous fluids in children. *Pediatrics* 142:e20183083. doi:10.1542/peds.2018-3083.
7. Anigilaje EA. (2018) Management of diarrhoeal dehydration in childhood: A review for clinicians in developing countries. *Front Pediatr* **6**:1–19.
8. Hayes W. (2019) Abnormal saline in abnormal kidney function: Risks and alternatives. *Pediatr Nephrol* **34**:1191–1199.
9. NICE. (2020) 2020 Surveillance of intravenous fluid therapy in children and young people in hospital (NICE guideline NG29). https://www.nice.org.uk/guidance/ng29/resources/2020-surveillance-of-intravenous-fluid-therapy-in-children-and-young-people-in-hospital-nice-guideline-ng29-pdf-11284810779589
10. Chen S, Shieh M, Chiaramonte R, Shey J. (2021) Improving on the Adrogué–Madias formula. *Kidney* **2**:360–365.

2 Evaluation of Acid-Base Disorders

Lau PYW and Yap HK

A. Definitions

Acidemia	Arterial pH below the normal range of 7.35–7.45
Alkalemia	Arterial pH above the normal range of 7.35–7.45
Acidosis	Process that tends to lower the extracellular fluid pH (increase in hydrogen ion concentration $[H^+]$) by: • Fall in serum bicarbonate $[HCO_3^-]$ and/or • Increase in partial pressure of carbon dioxide $[pCO_2]$
Alkalosis	Process that tends to raise the extracellular fluid pH (decrease in $[H^+]$) either by: • Increase in serum $[HCO_3^-]$ and/or • Decrease in pCO_2
Simple acid-base disorder	Presence of an acid-base disorder with the appropriate respiratory or renal compensation for that disorder
Mixed acid-base disorder	Simultaneous presence of more than one acid-base disorder

B. Approach to Acid-Base Disorders

1. Check the internal consistency of the blood gas results using Kassirer–Bleich equation.

$$[H^+] = 24 \times \frac{pCO_2}{[HCO_3^-]}$$

a. Methods for estimating [H⁺]:

pH	True [H⁺] (nmol/L)	Estimated [H⁺] (nmol/L)	
		0.8/1.25	"Limited Linear"
7.00	100	98	
7.10	79	78	
7.20	63	63 (50 × 1.25)	60
7.30	50	50 (10 × 1.25)	50
7.40	40	40	40
7.50	32	32 (40 × 0.8)	30
7.60	25	26 (32 × 0.8)	
7.70	20	20	

"Limited Linear" method:
Last 2 digits of pH – 40 = factor to be added or subtracted from 40

b. Internal consistency is present when the values on both sides of the Kassirer–Bleich equation are not different from each other by more than 10%.

2. Diagnose the type of primary acid-base disorder:

a. Normal ranges for blood gas interpretation:

	Acceptable Normal Range
pH	7.35–7.45
pCO_2	35–45 mmHg
$[HCO_3^-]$	22–26 mmol/L
Standard base excess (SBE)	–2 to +2 mmol/L

b. Acid-base disorders:

Type of Disorder	pCO_2	$[HCO_3^-]$	pH
Metabolic acidosis	↓	↓↓	↓
Respiratory alkalosis	↓↓	↓	↑
Metabolic alkalosis	↑	↑↑	↑
Respiratory acidosis	↑↑	↑	↓

3. Determine whether it is a simple acid-base disorder or a mixed acid-base disorder:
   a. Evaluate the adequacy of compensation of the primary disorder (a physiological approach based on kidney and lung acid-base interaction).

Primary Disorder	Initial Chemical Change	Compensatory Response		Expected Compensation
Metabolic acidosis	$[HCO_3^-]\downarrow$	$pCO_2\downarrow$		$\Delta pCO_2 = 1.2 \times \Delta[HCO_3^-]$ OR Winter's formula: Expected pCO_2(mmHg) = $(1.5 \times [HCO_3^-]) + 8 \pm 2$
Metabolic alkalosis	$[HCO_3^-]\uparrow$	$pCO_2\uparrow$		$\Delta pCO_2 = 0.7 \times \Delta[HCO_3^-]$ OR Expected pCO_2(mmHg) = $(0.7 \times \{[HCO_3^-] - 24\}) + 40 \pm 2$
Respiratory Acidosis	$pCO_2\uparrow$	$[HCO_3^-]\uparrow$	Acute	$[HCO_3^-]$ increase by 1 mmol/L for every 10 mmHg increase in pCO_2
			Chronic	$[HCO_3^-]$ increase by 3.5 mmol/L for every 10 mmHg increase in pCO_2
Respiratory alkalosis	$pCO_2\downarrow$	$[HCO_3^-]\downarrow$	Acute	$[HCO_3^-]$ decrease by 2 mmol/L for every 10 mmHg fall in pCO_2
			Chronic	$[HCO_3^-]$ decrease by 4 mmol/L for every 10 mmHg fall in pCO_2

b. Base excess approach: In an acute care setting where the measured plasma [HCO_3^-] level is not available, SBE obtained from most blood gas printouts can be used in acid-base evaluation.

Primary Disorder	Initial Chemical Change	Compensatory Response		Expected Compensation
Metabolic acidosis	SBE ↓	pCO_2 ↓		$\Delta pCO_2 = SBE$
Metabolic alkalosis	SBE ↑	pCO_2 ↑		$\Delta pCO_2 = 0.6 \times SBE$
Respiratory acidosis	pCO_2 ↑	SBE ↑	Acute	$SBE = 0 \pm 2$
			Chronic	$SBE = 0.4 \times (pCO_2 - 40)$
Respiratory alkalosis	pCO_2 ↓	SBE ↓	Acute	$SBE = 0 \pm 2$
			Chronic	$SBE = 0.4 \times (pCO_2 - 40)$

4. For metabolic acidosis, calculate the serum anion gap.

$$\text{Serum anion gap (AG)} = [Na^+] - \{[Cl^-] + [HCO_3^-]\}$$

where [Na^+] = sodium concentration, [Cl^-] = chloride concentration.

a. Normal AG: 12 ± 2 mmol/L.

b. High AG is the "footprint" of retained organic acid.
   - A pragmatic approach is to actively seek out causes of high AG metabolic acidosis in patients with serum AG >14 mmol/L.

c. Correct for hypoalbuminemia, which can reduce the AG.
   - Each 10 g/L reduction in serum albumin decreases the AG by 2.5 mmol/L.
   - Figge equation:

$$\text{Corrected AG} = \text{AG} + 0.25 \times \{40 - \text{measured albumin (g/L)}\}$$

d. AG is a relatively insensitive indicator of the presence of lactic acidosis and has limited usefulness for monitoring its course.
   - A direct measurement of lactate is essential for detecting and monitoring for lactic acidosis.

5. In cases of high AG metabolic acidosis, exclude the presence of concomitant normal AG metabolic acidosis or metabolic alkalosis by analyzing the ratio of the increase in AG from 12 mmol/L (ΔAG) to the decrease in the $[HCO_3^-]$ from 24 mmol/L ($\Delta[HCO_3^-]$).

Mixed Acid-Base Disorders	$\Delta AG - \Delta[HCO_3^-]$	$\Delta AG/\Delta[HCO_3^-]$ Ratio
High AG metabolic acidosis only	–6 to +6	1–1.6
High AG metabolic acidosis + Normal AG metabolic acidosis	>–6 $\Delta AG < \Delta[HCO_3^-]$	<1
High AG metabolic acidosis + Metabolic alkalosis	>+6 $\Delta AG > \Delta[HCO_3^-]$	>1.6

6. In cases of high AG metabolic acidosis, it is useful to calculate the serum osmolar gap (SOG).

> Calculated serum osmolality (mOsm/L) =
> $2[Na^+]$ + [glucose (mmol/L)] + [urea (mmol/L)]
> OR
> $2[Na^+]$ + {[glucose (mg/dL)]/18} + {[urea (mg/dL)]/2.8}
> SOG = Measured serum osmolality – Calculated serum osmolality

a. Actual measured serum osmolality should be close to the calculated serum osmolality in normal circumstances.
b. SOG is helpful to determine whether additional unmeasured osmotically active molecules are present.
c. Normal SOG <10 mOsm/L.
d. Causes of elevated SOG: refer to the mnemonic "MAE DIE".

M	methanol
A	acetone
E	ethanol
D	diuretics (mannitol)
I	isopropyl alcohol
E	ethylene glycol

7. In cases of normal AG metabolic acidosis, it is useful to calculate the urine anion gap (UAG) and look at the urine pH.
   a. Urine pH reflects the concentration of free H^+ in the urine.
      - Normal individuals subject to acute acid loading have a urine pH <5.5, whereas individuals with impaired acidification have a urine pH >5.5.
   b. Urine anion gap (UAG) is also known as the urine net charge.

      $$\text{Urine anion gap (UAG)} = \{[U_{Na+}] + [U_{K+}]\} - [U_{Cl-}]\}$$

      i. UAG measures the difference between unmeasured anions and unmeasured cations in the urine.
      ii. UAG is an indirect method of measuring the rate of ammonium (NH_4^+) excretion.
         - A positive UG between 20 and 90 mmol/L is indicative of low or normal NH_4^+ excretion.
      iii. As the rate of NH_4^+ excretion increases, UAG becomes progressively negative.
      iv. UAG is useful to clarify whether the kidney response to acidosis is appropriate.
         - A negative UAG between –20 and –50 mmol/L is indicative of increased NH_4^+ excretion during metabolic acidosis, e.g., in severe diarrhea.

- Patients with type 1 renal tubular acidosis (dRTA) and type 4 RTA typically show impaired renal NH_4^+ excretion and a positive urine anion gap >40 mmol/L (see chapter "Renal Tubular Acidosis").

v. NH_4^+ excretion decreases as the glomerular filtration rate declines; hence, the absence of acute kidney injury or chronic kidney disease is a requirement for a meaningful interpretation of UAG.

8. Urine osmolal gap (UOG) is an indirect surrogate of the urinary NH_4^+ concentration irrespective of the accompanying anion.

$$\text{Calculated urine osmolality} = 2[U_{Na+}] + 2[U_{K+}] + [U_{urea}] + [U_{glucose}]$$
$$\text{UOG} = \text{Measured urine osmolality} - \text{Calculated urine osmolality}$$

a. UOG >400 mosmol/kg: This is expected with NAG metabolic acidosis due to chronic diarrhea, inhalation of toluene, and other disorders in which the kidney response to acidemia remains intact.

b. UOG <150 mosmol/kg in a patient with chronic metabolic acidosis: Suggests NH_4^+ excretion is impaired, e.g., distal RTA and type 4 RTA.

C. Metabolic Acidosis

I. Clinical manifestations:

1. Acute acidemia:
   - Tachypnea.
2. Chronic acidemia:
   - Nausea.
   - Anorexia.

- Poor weight gain.
- Muscle weakness.

II. Evaluation of metabolic acidosis:

1. Causes of high anion gap (HAG) metabolic acidosis:
   a. Kidney failure.
   b. Ketoacidosis:
      i. Diabetic ketoacidosis.
      ii. Starvation.
      iii. Ketotic hypoglycemia.
      iv. Defect in carbohydrate metabolism.
      v. Alcohol.
   c. Lactic acidosis:
      i. Type A:
         - Hypoxia.
         - Shock.
         - Carbon monoxide poisoning.
      ii. Type B:
         - Inborn error of metabolism.
         - Drugs, e.g., salicylates.
         - Methanol.
         - Ethylene glycol.
         - Isopropyl alcohol.
         - Paraldehyde.
   d. Organic acidurias.
   e. Aminoacidopathies.
2. Causes of normal anion gap (NAG) metabolic acidosis:
   a. Normal or low serum chloride:
      - Severe gastroenteritis.
      - Carbonic anhydrase inhibitors.
      - Post-hypocapnic acidosis.
      - Early kidney failure.
   b. High serum chloride:
      - Renal tubular acidosis (RTA).
      - Ureteral diversions, e.g., ureterosigmoidostomy.
      - Chloride administration.

3. Algorithm for approach to NAG metabolic acidosis:

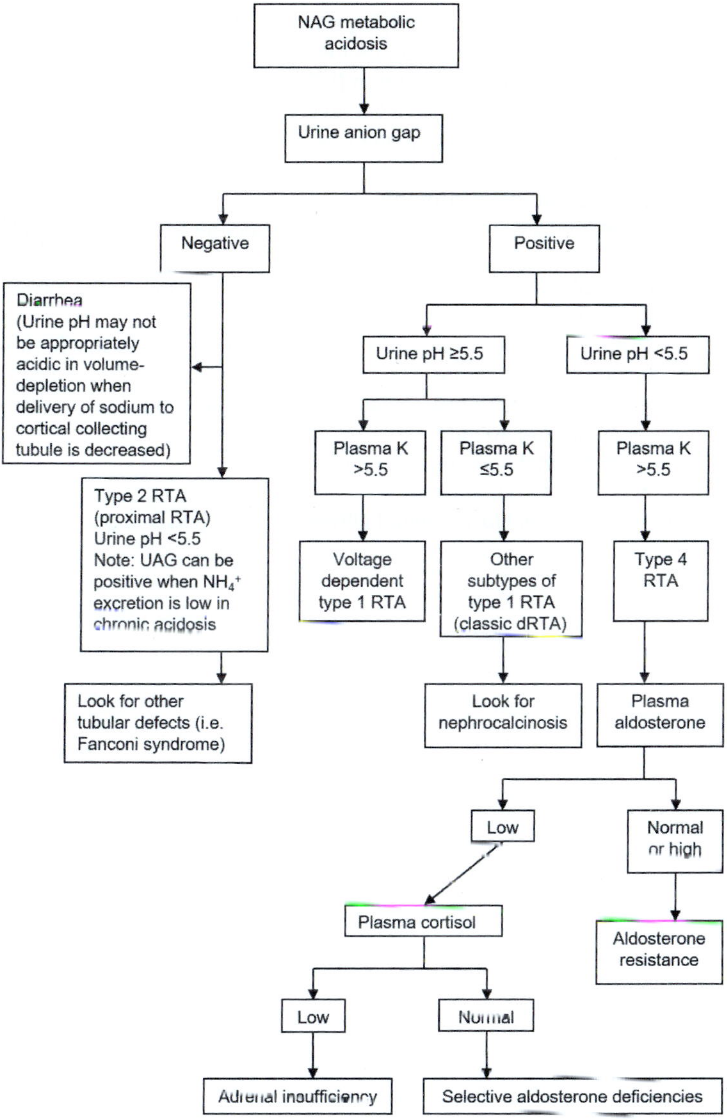

III. Management:

1. Look for and treat the underlying cause of acidosis.
2. Acute metabolic acidosis can be treated with IV sodium bicarbonate replacement, especially if serum $[HCO_3^-]$ <12.
   Note: This does not apply to diabetic ketoacidosis.
3. In infants, use only 4.2% sodium bicarbonate.
4. Replace the calculated deficit:
   a. Bicarbonate deficit (mmol)
      = {desired plasma $[HCO_3^-]$ – present plasma $[HCO_3^-]$} × weight × 0.3.
   b. Rate of correction depends on a target $[HCO_3^-]$ and clinical scenario.
   c. Oral replacement (either tablet or liquid) can be in the form of bicarbonate or citrate.
      - Sodium bicarbonate ($NaHCO_3$) tablet 500 mg
        = 137 mg sodium
        = 6 mmol sodium + 6 mmol $[HCO_3^-]$.
      - Shohl's solution
        = 1 mmol Na + 1 mmol citrate (3 mmol $[HCO_3^-]$) per ml.

D. Metabolic Alkalosis

I. Approach to metabolic alkalosis:

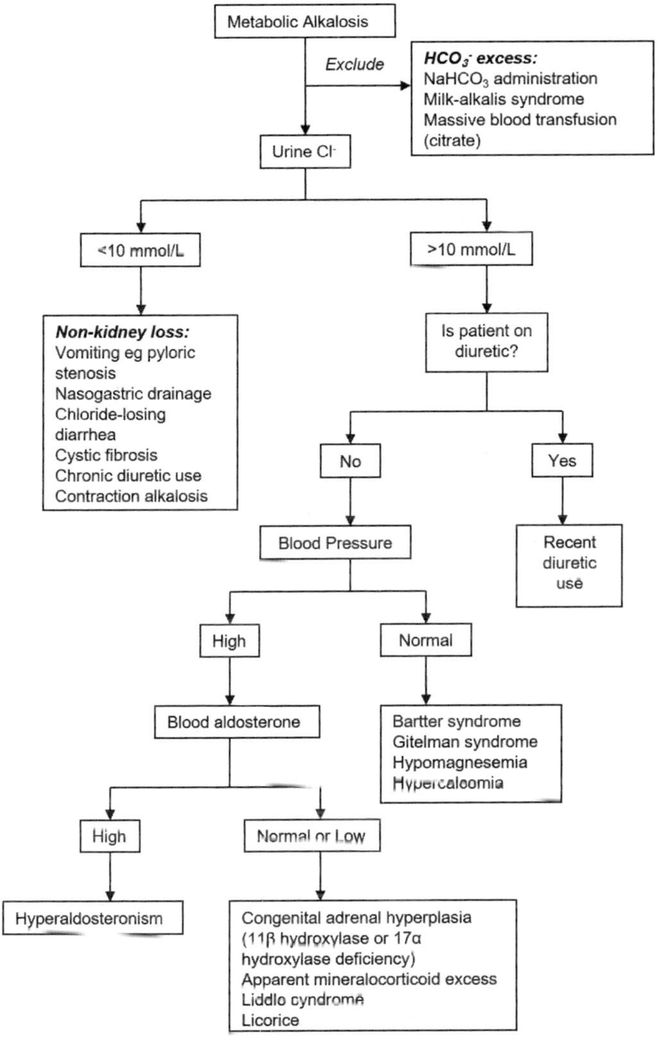

II. Management:

1. If untreated, compensatory hypoventilation may occur, resulting in increased pCO_2 but is limited by a strong competing interest (oxygenation).
2. Complications:
   a. Mental confusion.
   b. Obtundation.
   c. Seizures.
   d. Paresthesia.
   e. Hypokalemia.
   f. Cardiac arrhythmias.
3. Saline-responsive alkalosis:
   a. Causes:
      i. Vomiting of gastric secretion, e.g., congenital hypertrophic pyloric stenosis.
      ii. Nasogastric drainage.
      iii. Diuretics.
   b. Replete extracellular fluid volume with sodium chloride infusion and potassium chloride replacement.
4. Saline-resistant alkalosis:
   a. Causes:
      i. Bartter syndrome.
      ii. Gitelman syndrome.
      iii. Conn syndrome.
   b. Identify and treat the underlying cause.

E. Respiratory Acidosis

I. Causes:

1. Breathing problem (mechanics):
   a. Central control of breathing:
      i. Drugs:
         - Anesthetics.
         - Sedatives.
         - Opioids.

   ii. Brain injury.
   iii. Congenital central hypoventilation syndrome.

b. Respiratory muscle weakness:
   i. Spinal cord injury.
   ii. Spinal cord tumors.
   iii. Spinal muscular atrophy.
   iv. Botulism.
   v. Tetanus.
   vi. Guillain-Barré syndrome.
   vii. Myasthenia gravis.
   viii. Muscular dystrophy.
   ix. Organophosphate poisoning.

c. Chest wall restriction:
   i. Kyphoscoliosis.
   ii. Contracted chest from burn scars.

d. Lung failure:
   i. Lung restriction:
      - Pneumothorax.
      - Massive pleural effusion.
      - Hemothorax.
      - Pulmonary fibrosis.
      - Sarcoidosis.
   ii. Parenchyma:
      - Pneumonia.
      - Pulmonary edema.
   iii. Airway:
      - Severe acute asthma.
      - Chronic obstructive pulmonary disease.

II. Clinical manifestations:

1. Central nervous system manifestations:
   a. Drowsiness.
   b. Somnolence.
   c. Irritability.
   d. Restlessness.
   e. Confusion.
   f. Headache.

2. Respiratory symptoms:
   a. Compensatory tachypnea.
   b. Irregular breathing.
   c. Cyanosis.
3. Tachycardia.

III. Management:

1. Support ventilation.
2. Identify and treat the underlying cause.

F. Respiratory Alkalosis

I. Causes:

1. Anxiety.
2. Central nervous system disorders:
   a. Encephalopathy.
   b. Tumors.
   c. Infection.
   d. Cerebrovascular accident.
3. Inborn errors of metabolism: Urea cycle disorders with associated hyperammonemia.
4. Hormones/Drugs:
   a. Salicylates.
   b. Catecholamines.
   c. Progesterone.
   d. Analeptic overdosage (e.g., doxapram).
5. Fever.
6. Endotoxaemia.
7. Hyperthyroidism.
8. Hypoxia.
9. Liver insufficiency.
10. Lung disease:
    a. Early restrictive disorders.
    b. Pulmonary emboli.

   c. Pneumonia.
   d. Mild pulmonary edema.
   e. Acute asthma exacerbation.

11. Overventilation with a mechanical ventilator.

II. Clinical manifestations:

1. Increase in ventilation.
2. Risk of respiratory muscle fatigue with prolonged increase work of breathing.

III. Management of respiratory alkalosis:

1. Identify and treat the underlying cause.

Recommended Reading

1. Wrenn K. (1990) The delta (delta) gap: An approach to mixed acid-base disorders. *Ann Emerg Med* **19**(11):1310–1313.
2. Adrogue HJ, Madias NE. (2010) Secondary responses to altered acid-base status: The rules of engagement. *J Am Soc Nephrol* **21**:920–923.
3. Kraut JA, Nagami GT. (2013) The serum anion gap in the evaluation of acid-base disorders: What are its limitations and can its effectiveness be improved? *Clin J AM Soc Nephrol* **8**:2018–2024.
4. Berend K, deVries APJ, Gans ROB. (2014) Physiological approach to assessment of acid-base disturbances. *N Engl J Med* **371**:1434–1445.
5. Berend K. (2018) Diagnostic use of base excess in acid-base disorders. *N Engl J Med* **378**:1419–1428.
6. Batlle D, Aqeel SHB, Marquez A. (2018) The urine anion gap in context. *Clin J Am Soc Nephrol* **13**(2):195–197.
7. Emmett M, Palmer BF. (2020, updated) The delta anion gap/delta HCO3 ratio in patients with a high anion gap metabolic acidosis. Edited by: Sterns RH, Forman JP. *UpToDate ONLINE*. http://www.uptodateonline.com.
8. Emmett M, Palmer BF. (2020, updated) Simple and mixed acid-base disorders. Edited by: Sterns RH, Forman JP. *UpToDate ONLINE*. http://www.uptodateonline.com.

3 Evaluation and Treatment of Magnesium Deficiency

Lohia S, Lu L, Teo S, Lau PYW and Yap HK

A. Introduction

1. Only a very small proportion of total body magnesium (Mg) exists extracellularly in the ionized form, where it acts as a membrane stabilizer and also has a role in nerve conduction.
   a. 1% of Mg is extracellular, of which 60% is ionized, 30% is protein-bound, and the rest is part of salt complexes.
   b. The remaining 99% of Mg is intracellular: 60% in bones, 20% in muscles, and the rest in the remaining tissues.
2. Mg handling:
   a. In the kidneys, 95% of the filtered Mg is reabsorbed in the proximal convoluted tubule (10–25%), thick ascending limb (50–70%), and distal convoluted tubule (5–10%).
   b. Mg is also present in gastrointestinal secretions, predominantly in the lower gastrointestinal tract (7.5 mmol/L) with smaller amounts in the upper gastrointestinal tract (0.5 mmol/L).
3. Hypomagnesemia is defined as serum magnesium (Mg) <0.70 mmol/L (1.7 mg/dL).

B. Suspect Hypomagnesemia

1. Hypomagnesemia may be an incidental finding.
2. Neuromuscular:
   a. Seizures, including generalized seizures and multifocal seizures.
   b. Tetany, including positive Trousseau and Chvostek sign, spasms and cramps.
   c. Muscle weakness, including respiratory muscles in severe cases.

   d. Vertical nystagmus (rare, in severe cases).
   e. Involuntary movements, including tremors, athetosis and chorea.
   f. Altered mental state, including apathy, delirium and coma.
3. Cardiovascular:
   a. Unexplained tachycardia.
   b. Premature atrial complexes and/or premature ventricular complexes.
   c. Atrial fibrillation (severe deficiency).
   d. Ventricular arrhythmias, including Torsades de pointes (severe deficiency).
   e. ECG changes including:
      - QRS complex widening and peaked T-waves (moderate deficiency).
      - PR prolongation, progressive QRS prolongation, and reduced T-waves amplitude (severe deficiency).
4. Refractory biochemical abnormalities:
   a. Refractory hypocalcemia:
      - Mechanisms include hypoparathyroidism, parathyroid hormone (PTH) resistance, and reduced 1-hydroxylation of 25-hydroxyvitamin D.
      - Has been associated with normomagnesemic magnesium depletion, i.e., intracellular magnesium depletion not severe enough to result in hypomagnesemia.
   b. Refractory hypokalemia:
      - Proposed mechanism includes reducing in the Mg-mediated tonic inhibition of luminal ROMK channels in the distal convoluted tubules.

C. Causes of Mg Deficiency

1. Gastrointestinal causes:
   a. Diarrhea of any cause.
   b. Severe vomiting, including large volume nasogastric aspiration.
   c. Acute pancreatitis, due to saponification of Mg in fat.
   d. Long-term proton pump inhibitor use, especially with concomitant diuretic use.
   e. Marked dietary deprivation (rare).

2. Kidney causes:
   a. Drug-induced tubular dysfunction or injury:
      - Loop and thiazide diuretics.
      - Nephrotoxic drugs: Aminoglycosides, amphotericin B, cisplatin.
      - Calcineurin inhibitors: Tacrolimus, cyclosporine.
      - Monoclonal antibodies antagonists of epidermal growth factor receptor, e.g., cetuximab.
      - Pentamidine.
      - Digoxin
      - Alcohol.
   b. Other causes of tubular injury:
      - Acute tubular necrosis.
      - Post-obstructive diuresis.
      - Interstitial nephritis.
   c. Increased tubular Mg delivery:
      - Volume-expanded states, including primary hyperaldosteronism and syndrome of inappropriate antidiuretic hormone secretion.
      - Uncontrolled diabetes mellitus.
      - Chronic metabolic acidosis, by increasing ionized (and hence filtered) Mg.
   d. Hypercalcemia (by competing with Mg for tubular reabsorption).
   e. Inherited renal magnesium wasting:

Disorder	Gene (Inheritance)	Other Features
I. Hypercalciuric hypomagnesemias		
FHHNC types 1 and 2 (Familial hypomagnesemia with hypocalcemia and nephrocalcinosis)	*CLDN16* (AR), *CLDN19* (AR)	• Hypercalciuria, hypocitraturia, hyperuricemia, nephrocalcinosis, nephrolithiasis, polyuria, elevated PTH, kidney failure. • Ocular abnormalities in type 2.
Bartter syndrome type 5	*CASR* (AD)	• Hypocalcemia with normal or low PTH. • Severe cases with Na and K wasting.

(*Continued*)

Disorder	Gene (Inheritance)	Other Features
Bartter syndrome type 3	*CLCNKB* (AR)	• Bartter-like phenotype in infancy, with Ca, Na, K wasting. • Subsequently hypocalciuric (Gitelman-like phenotype).
II. Hypocalciuric (Gitelman-like) hypomagnesemias		
Gitelman syndrome	*SLC12A3* (AR)	• Hypocalciuria, hypokalemia, metabolic alkalosis. • Chondrocalcinosis at an older age.
Bartter syndrome, type 4	*BSND* (AR)	• Antenatal presentation. • Progression to kidney failure. • Sensorineural deafness.
EAST syndrome (Epilepsy, ataxia, sensorineural deafness and tubulopathy)	*KCNJ10* (AR)	• Sensorineural deafness, seizures (generalized tonic-clonic), motor delay, ataxia. • Gitelman-like dyselectrolytemia.
Isolated dominant hypomagnesemia	*FXYD2* (AD)	• Hypocalciuria without Gitelman-like dyselectrolytemia.
HNF1β nephropathy	*HNF1B* (AD)	• Hypocalciuria without Gitelman-like dyselectrolytemia. • Varyingly associated with CAKUT, hyperuricemic nephropathy, maturity-onset diabetes of the young (MODY).
Hyperphenylalaninemia, tetrahydrobiopterin deficient (HPABH4D)	*PCBD1* (AD)	• Transient neonatal hyperphenylalaninemia. • Can be associated with MODY, but not CAKUT. • May have hypocalciuria.

(*Continued*)

(*Continued*)

Disorder	Gene (Inheritance)	Other Features
III. Mitochondrial hypomagnesemias		
Hypertension, hypercholesterolemia and hypomagnesemia (HHH)	*MTTI* (Mt)	• Hypertension and hypercholesterolemia. • Associated with hypocalciuria.
Hyperuricemia, pulmonary hypertension, kidney failure and alkalotic syndrome (HUPRAS)	*SARS2* (AR)	• Hyperuricemia, pulmonary hypertension, kidney failure, and alkalosis.
Kearns-Sayre syndrome (KSS)	Mitochondrial DNA deletion (Mt)	• External ophthalmoplegia, retinopathy, cardiac conduction defects. • Can have weakness, ataxia, endocrinopathies.
IV. Other hypomagnesemias		
Hypomagnesemia with secondary hypocalcemia (HSH)	*TRPM6* (AR)	• Severe hypomagnesemia, often presenting with neonatal seizures. • Hypocalcemic with low PTH. • Due in part to a reduced colonic Mg uptake.
Isolated recessive hypomagnesemia (IRH)	*EGF* (AR)	• Intellectual disability (possibly secondary to hypomagnesemic seizures).
Neonatal inflammatory skin and bowel disease, type 2 (NISBD2)	*EGFR* (AR)	• Severe inflammation of skin, bowel, lungs.
Hypomagnesemia with seizures and mental retardation (HSMR)	*CNNM2* (AD/AR)	• May be associated with intellectual disability, seizures, impaired brain development.

(*Continued*)

Disorder	Gene (Inheritance)	Other Features
Autosomal dominant hypomagnesemia (ADH)	*KCNA1* (AD)	• May be associated with myokymia. • Mutations in *KCNA1* have also been associated with ataxia and seizures.
Kenny-Caffey syndrome type 2 (KCS2)	*FAM111A* (AD)	• Severe short stature with bone abnormalities, ocular abnormalities, hypoparathyroidism with hypocalcemia.

AD: Autosomal dominant, AR: Autosomal recessive, Mt: Mitochondrial inheritance, CAKUT: Congenital anomaly of kidney and urinary tract.

3. Other causes:
    a. Refeeding syndrome.
    b. Ketogenic diet.
    c. Intravenous chelation by:
        - Foscarnet.
        - Citrate-containing blood products when there is citrate accumulation due to inadequate hepatic function for citrate metabolism.
    d. Hungry bone syndrome following:
        - Parathyroidectomy.
        - Thyroidectomy for hyperthyroidism.
        - Correction of severe metabolic acidosis.
    e. Cutaneous losses in severe burns.

D. Evaluation of Hypomagnesemia

1. Determining kidney vs. non-kidney magnesium loss:
    a. Urine Mg:creatinine ratio (see chapter "Reference Ranges for Urinary Solute Excretion").
        i. May be used as a screening tool.
        ii. Significant intra-individual variability and may be falsely low in the presence of severe hypomagnesemia.

b. Fractional excretion of Mg (FE_{Mg}):
   i. $FE_{Mg} = (U_{Mg} \times P_{Creatinine})/(0.7 \times P_{Mg} \times U_{Creatinine}) \times 100\%$, where U and P refer to urine and plasma, respectively.
   ii. Coefficient of 0.7 for P_{Mg} is because only 70% of the magnesium can be filtered at the glomerulus.
   iii. In the presence of hypomagnesemia and normal kidney function:
      - $FE_{Mg} \geq 4\%$: Consistent with kidney magnesium wasting.
      - $FE_{Mg} \leq 2\%$: Consistent with non-kidney losses.

c. 24-hour urine Mg excretion (adults):
   - >1 mmol/day: Consistent with kidney Mg wasting.
   - ≤0.41 mmol/day: Consistent with non-kidney losses.

2. Genetic analysis:
   - If an inherited renal Mg wasting disorder is clinically suspected, genetic analysis should be offered to establish a molecular diagnosis.

3. Algorithm for evaluation of hypomagnesemia:

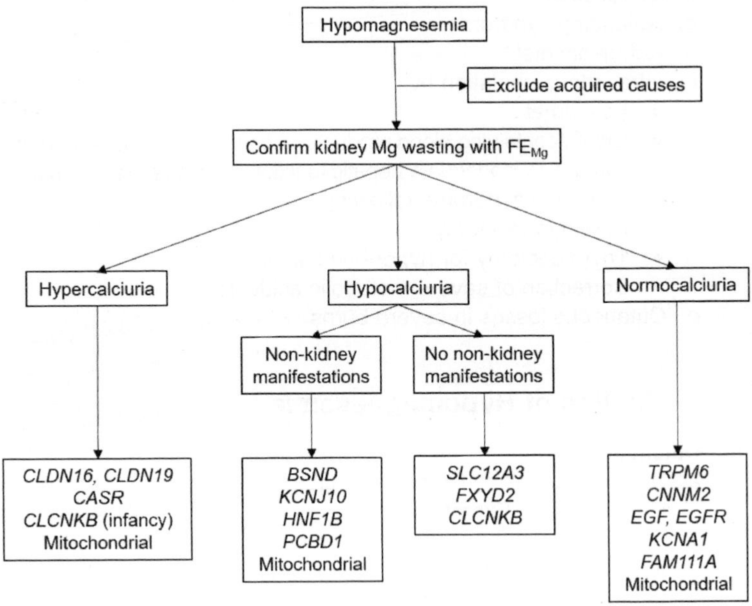

E. Treatment of Hypomagnesemia

1. Magnitude of Mg deficit is difficult to gauge clinically or deduced from the serum Mg concentration.
2. Oral administration of Mg supplements is the preferred way to correct Mg deficiency.
   - Intravenous (IV) Mg causes a temporary elevation in plasma Mg, which partially inhibits stimulus to Mg reabsorption in the loop of Henle, resulting in up to 50% of the infused Mg being excreted.
   - If IV infusions are required, slow infusions are better than bolus doses to replete Mg stores.
3. IV Mg is reserved for:
   a. Acute, severe complications of hypomagnesemia.
   b. Intolerable gastrointestinal side effects to oral supplements.
4. Dosing:

Indication	Dose
Hemodynamic compromise	• IV Mg sulfate 25–50 mg/kg (maximum 2 g) in 0.9% saline (diluted to 200 mg/ml) over 2–15 minutes, repeated as necessary. • Subsequently, IV 100–200 mg/kg (maximum 8 g) over 12–24 hours, repeated daily until plasma Mg >0.4 mmol/L and for least 3–5 days if there is concomitant hypocalcemia.
Severe symptoms	• IV Mg sulfate 25–50 mg/kg (maximum 2 g) in 0.9% saline (diluted to 200 mg/ml) over 5–60 minutes. • Subsequent infusion as for hemodynamic compromise.
No or minimal symptoms, oral route unavailable	• Mg <0.4 mmol/L: IV Mg sulfate 100–200 mg/kg (maximum 8 g) over 12–24 hours. • Mg 0.4–0.6 mmol/L: IV Mg sulfate 50–100 mg (maximum 4 g) over 4–12 hours. • Mg 0.7–0.8 mmol/L: IV Mg sulfate 25–50 mg/kg (maximum 2 g) over 1–2 hours. • Continue for 1–2 days after normalization of plasma Mg.
No or minimal symptoms	• 10–20 mg/kg/dose of elemental Mg up to 4×/day (800–1600 mg/day) with a preference for sustained release formulations. • Continue for 1–2 days after normalization of plasma Mg.
Special considerations	• eGFR <30 ml/min/1.73m^2: Reduce the dose by 50% and carefully monitor plasma Mg.

5. Monitoring for IV infusion of Mg:
   a. Watch for signs of hypermagnesemia:
      - Facial flushing.
      - Loss of deep tendon reflexes.
      - Hypotension.
      - Atrioventricular block.
   b. Measure plasma Mg only 6–12 hours after the end of infusion to allow for equilibration with intracellular compartment.
6. Formulations:
   a. 50% Mg sulfate (IV formulation):
      - 2 mmol/ml = 4 mEq/ml = ~50 mg/ml elemental Mg.
      - 0.2 ml/kg/dose = 0.4 mmol/kg/dose = 0.8 mEq/kg/dose = ~10 mg/kg/dose elemental Mg.
   b. Oral formulations:
      - Dosing is limited by gastrointestinal discomfort and diarrhea.
      - Oral bioavailability of magnesium is approximately one-third in patients with normal intestinal function.
      - Bioavailability may be enhanced and gastrointestinal side effects reduced with sustained-release (SR) preparations.

Salt	Elemental Magnesium Content		
	(mg)	(mmol)	(mEq)
GNC® Magnesium 250 mg tablet	250	10.4	20.8
Magnesium oxide 140 mg tablet	84.5	3.5	7
Magnesium lactate 833 mg tablet (SR)	84	3.5	7
Magnesium sulfate 35% solution	354	1.46	2.92

7. Other therapies:
   a. Potassium-sparing diuretics, e.g., amiloride, may be considered in kidney magnesium wasting or in cases in which high doses of oral magnesium result in diarrhea.
      - By reducing electrogenic sodium reabsorption in the collecting tubule, potassium-sparing diuretics attenuate luminal electronegativity, thus enabling paracellular Mg reabsorption.

   b. Use with caution in conditions associated with salt wasting, e.g., Gitelman syndrome.
8. Increase dietary intake of high Mg-containing foods.
   a. Nuts (almond, cashew, peanut).
   b. Green vegetables (spinach).
   c. Tofu and Soya beans.
   d. Beans.
   e. Dark chocolate.
   f. Whole grain (brown rice, whole wheat).

Recommended Reading

1. Konrad M, Schlingmann KP. (2016) Disorders of calcium and magnesium metabolism In: *Pediatric Kidney Disease*. Edited by: Geary DF, Schaefer F. Springer-Verlag Berlin Heidelberg. pp. 921–952.
2. Viering DHHM, de Baaij JHF, Walsh SB, Kleta R, Bockenhauer D. (2017) Genetic causes of hypomagnesemia, a clinical overview. *Pediatr Nephrol* **32**:1123–1135.
3. Yu ASL, Yarlagadda SG. (2019, updated) Hypomagnesemia: Clinical manifestations of magnesium depletion. Edited by: Goldfarb S, Lam AQ. *UpToDate ONLINE*. http://www.uptodateonline.com.
4. Yu ASL. (2020, updated) Hypomagnesemia: Causes of hypomagnesemia. Edited by: Goldfarb S, Lam AQ. *UpToDate ONLINE*. http://www.uptodateonline.com.
5. Yu ASL. (2021, updated) Hypomagnesemia: Evaluation and treatment. Edited by: Goldfarb S, Lam AQ. *UpToDate ONLINE*. http://www.uptodateonline.com.

1 Approach to Diagnosis of Hypertension

Prasetyo RV, Sarkar S, Sng A, Ng KH, Loke KY and Yap HK

A. Clinic Blood Pressure (BP)

1. Timing of clinic BP measurements:

a. Children ≥3 years should have their BP measured:
   i. At least annually in otherwise healthy children.
   ii. At every health encounter specifically for those with:
      - Obesity.
      - Kidney disease.
      - Diabetes.
      - Aortic arch obstruction or coarctation.
      - Intake of medications known to increase BP.

b. Children <3 years should have their BP measured in the following circumstances:
   - History of prematurity, i.e., <32 weeks of gestation, being small for gestational age, very low birth weight (VLBW), other problems requiring neonatal intensive care, or umbilical artery line.
   - Congenital heart disease (repaired or unrepaired).
   - Recurrent urinary tract infection, hematuria or proteinuria.
   - Known kidney disease or urologic malformations.
   - Family history of congenital renal disease.
   - Solid organ transplant.
   - Malignancy or bone marrow transplant.
   - Treatment with drugs known to raise BP.
   - Systemic diseases associated with hypertension (neurofibromatosis, tuberous sclerosis, sickle cell disease).
   - Evidence of elevated intracranial pressure.

2. Method of clinic BP measurement:

a. Child should have avoided stimulant drugs or foods, has been sitting quietly for 5 minutes, is seated with his/her back supported, feet on the floor and right arm supported, and cubital fossa at heart level.

b. The right arm is preferred for consistency and comparison with standard tables and because of the possibility of coarctation of the aorta, which might lead to falsely low readings in the left arm.

c. Appropriate cuff size:
   i. Cuff with an inflatable bladder width that is at least 40% of the arm circumference with a point midway between the olecranon and the acromion.
   ii. Bladder length should cover 80–100% of the arm circumference.

d. Dinamap (oscillometric device) may be used for the screening of BP in children:
   i. Cuff should cover at least 80% of the arm circumference, as measurements tend to be higher than the auscultatory method by about 10 mmHg for systolic BP (SBP) and 5 mmHg for diastolic BP (DBP).
   ii. Oscillometric devices measure the mean arterial pressure (MAP) and the SBP and DBP are derived using various algorithms based on the measured MAP.
   iii. If BP is >90th percentile, perform auscultation with an aneroid sphygmomanometer.
   iv. Repeat BP that visit, and at least 2 other occasions before diagnosing hypertension.

e. Sphygmomanometer (aneroid):
   i. Gold standard for diagnosis of hypertension in young patients.
   ii. Measurement technique:
      - Bell of stethoscope should be placed over the brachial artery 2–3 cm above the antecubital fossa.
      - Cuff should be inflated 20–30 mmHg above the point at which the radial pulse disappears.
      - Cuff should be deflated at the rate of 2–3 mmHg per second.
   iii. The SBP is determined by the onset of the tapping Korotkoff sounds (K1).
   iv. The DBP is determined by the disappearance of the Korotkoff sounds (K5).

- In some children, Korotkoff sounds can be heard to 0 mmHg, then BP measurement should be repeated with less pressure on the head of the stethoscope.
- Only if very low K5 persists should K4 (muffling of the sounds) be recorded as the DBP.

f. Infants:
   i. BP measurement using the auscultation method may be difficult. Hence, practically, BP obtained by Dinamap may be used instead.
   ii. Infants should be supine during BP measurement.
   iii. Normative data for this age group is based on K4 rather than K5.

g. Measurement of BP in the legs by the auscultatory method:
   i. Patient should be in prone position.
   ii. An appropriately sized cuff should be placed mid-thigh and the stethoscope placed over the popliteal artery.
   iii. The SBP in the legs is usually 10–20% higher than the brachial artery pressure.

3. Criteria for diagnosis and staging of hypertension using clinic BP:

a. For the diagnosis of hypertension, use the *mean of 2 consecutive* BP measurements taken by auscultation, repeated at 3 different visits.

Criteria / Diagnosis or Stage	Age 1 to <13 years	Age ≥13 years
	SBP or DBP (percentile)	SBP/DBP (mmHg)
Normal	<90th	<120/<80
Elevated BP	≥90th to <95th OR 120/80 mmHg to <95th (whichever is lower)	120–129/<80
Stage 1 hypertension	≥95th to <(95th + 12) mmHg OR 130/80 to 139/89 mmHg (whichever is lower)	130–139/80–89
Stage 2 hypertension	≥(95th + 12) mmHg OR ≥140/90 mmHg (whichever is lower)	≥140/90

b. Severe acute hypertension is defined as a rise in BP >30 mmHg above the 95th percentile:

Hypertensive urgency	• No end-organ damage. • No or minimal symptoms.
Hypertensive emergency	• Symptomatic with complaints such as nausea, dyspnea, headaches and blurred vision. • End-organ damage such as cerebral infarction, cerebral hemorrhage, encephalopathy (altered mental status, seizures), pulmonary edema and kidney failure.

c. Estimated BP in well infants > 2 weeks old with a post-conceptional age of 26–44 weeks:

Post-conceptual Age		50th Percentile	95th Percentile	99th Percentile
44 weeks	SBP	88	105	110
	DBP	50	68	73
	MAP	63	80	85
42 weeks	SBP	85	98	102
	DBP	50	65	70
	MAP	62	76	81
40 weeks	SBP	80	95	100
	DBP	50	65	70
	MAP	60	75	80
38 weeks	SBP	77	92	100
	DBP	50	65	70
	MAP	60	75	80
36 weeks	SBP	72	87	92
	DBP	50	65	70
	MAP	59	72	71
34 weeks	SBP	70	85	90
	DBP	40	55	60
	MAP	50	65	70
32 weeks	SBP	68	83	88
	DBP	40	55	60
	MAP	48	62	69
30 weeks	SBP	65	80	85
	DBP	40	55	60
	MAP	48	65	68

(*Continued*)

Post-conceptual Age		50th Percentile	95th Percentile	99th Percentile
28 weeks	SBP DBP MAP	60 38 45	75 50 58	80 54 63
26 weeks	SBP DBP MAP	55 30 38	72 50 57	77 56 63

d. Age-specific 90th centile of clinic BP (K4 used for DBP):

i. Boys 0–12 months old:

Height (cm)	51	59	63	66	68	70	72	73	74	76	77	78	80
Weight (kg)	4	4	5	5	6	7	8	9	9	10	10	11	11
SBP (mmHg)	87	101	106	106	106	105	105	105	105	105	105	105	105
DBP (mmHg)	68	65	63	63	63	65	66	67	68	68	69	69	69

ii. Girls 0–12 months old:

Height (cm)	54	55	56	58	61	63	66	68	70	72	74	75	77
Weight (kg)	4	4	4	5	5	6	7	8	9	9	10	10	11
SBP (mmHg)	76	98	101	104	105	106	106	106	106	106	106	105	105
DBP (mmHg)	68	65	64	64	65	65	66	66	66	67	67	67	67

- These diastolic pressures were obtained based on K4. Normative data for K5 diastolic pressures are not available for this age group.
- Those data are for children who are <u>awake</u>. If BP is taken when the infant is sleeping, 7 mmHg should be added to the SBP and 5 mmHg to the DBP before comparison with this data.

e. Clinic BP normative data by age and height centiles (Flynn *et al.*, 2017):

i. Boys 1–17 years old:

Age (year)	BP Percentile (+mmHg)	SBP (mmHg) Percentile of Height							DBP (mmHg) Percentile of Height						
		5th	10th	25th	50th	75th	90th	95th	5th	10th	25th	50th	75th	90th	95th
1	50th	85	85	86	86	87	88	88	40	40	40	41	41	42	42
	90th	98	99	99	100	100	101	101	52	52	53	53	54	54	54
	95th	102	102	103	103	104	105	105	54	54	55	55	56	57	57
	95th + 12	114	114	115	115	116	117	117	66	66	67	67	68	69	69
2	50th	87	87	88	89	89	90	91	43	43	44	44	45	46	46
	90th	100	100	101	102	103	103	104	55	55	56	56	57	58	58
	95th	104	105	105	106	107	107	108	57	58	58	59	60	61	61
	95th+ + 12	116	117	117	118	119	119	120	69	70	70	71	72	73	73
3	50th	88	89	89	90	91	92	92	45	46	46	47	48	49	49
	90th	101	102	102	103	104	105	105	58	58	59	59	60	61	61
	95th	106	106	107	107	108	109	109	60	61	61	62	63	64	64
	95th + 12	118	118	119	119	120	121	121	72	73	73	74	75	76	76
4	50th	90	90	91	92	93	94	94	48	49	49	50	51	52	52
	90th	102	103	104	105	105	106	107	60	61	62	62	63	64	64
	95th	107	107	108	108	109	110	110	63	64	65	66	67	67	68
	95th + 12	119	119	120	120	121	122	122	75	76	77	78	79	79	80
5	50th	91	92	93	94	95	96	96	51	51	52	53	54	55	55
	90th	103	104	105	106	107	108	108	63	64	65	65	66	67	67
	95th	107	108	109	109	110	111	112	66	67	68	69	70	70	71
	95th + 12	119	120	121	121	122	123	124	78	79	80	81	82	82	83

6	50th	93	93	94	95	96	97	98	54	54	55	56	57	57	58
	90th	105	105	106	107	109	110	110	66	66	67	68	68	69	69
	95th	108	109	110	111	112	113	114	69	70	70	71	72	72	73
	95th + 12	120	121	122	123	124	125	126	81	82	82	83	84	84	85
7	50th	94	94	95	97	98	98	99	56	56	57	58	58	59	59
	90th	106	107	108	109	110	111	111	68	68	69	70	70	71	71
	95th	110	110	111	112	114	115	116	71	71	72	73	73	74	74
	95th + 12	122	122	123	124	126	127	128	83	83	84	85	85	86	86
8	50th	95	96	97	98	99	99	100	57	57	58	59	59	60	60
	90th	107	108	109	110	111	112	112	69	70	70	71	72	72	73
	95th	111	112	112	114	115	116	117	72	73	73	74	75	75	75
	95th + 12	123	124	124	125	127	128	129	84	85	85	86	87	87	87
9	50th	96	97	98	99	100	101	101	57	58	59	60	61	62	62
	90th	107	108	109	110	112	113	114	70	71	72	73	74	74	74
	95th	112	112	113	115	116	118	119	74	74	75	76	76	77	77
	95th + 12	124	124	125	127	128	130	131	86	86	87	88	88	89	89
10	50th	97	98	99	100	101	102	103	59	60	61	62	63	63	64
	90th	108	109	111	112	113	115	116	72	73	74	74	75	75	76
	95th	112	113	114	116	118	120	121	76	76	77	77	78	78	78
	95th + 12	124	125	126	128	130	132	133	88	88	89	89	90	90	90
11	50th	99	99	101	102	103	104	106	61	61	62	63	63	63	63
	90th	110	111	112	114	116	117	118	74	74	75	75	75	76	76
	95th	114	114	116	118	120	123	124	77	78	78	78	78	78	78
	95th + 12	126	126	128	130	132	135	136	89	90	90	90	90	90	90

(*Continued*)

(*Continued*)

Age (year)	BP Percentile (+mmHg)	SBP (mmHg) Percentile of Height							DEP (mmHg) Percentile of Height						
		5th	10th	25th	50th	75th	90th	95th	5th	10th	25th	50th	75th	90th	95th
12	50th	101	101	102	104	106	108	109	61	62	62	62	62	63	63
	90th	113	114	115	117	119	121	122	75	75	75	75	75	76	76
	95th	116	117	118	121	124	126	128	78	78	78	78	78	79	79
	95th + 12	128	129	130	133	136	138	140	90	90	90	90	90	91	91
13	50th	103	104	105	108	110	111	112	61	60	61	62	63	64	65
	90th	115	116	118	121	124	126	126	74	74	74	75	76	77	77
	95th	119	120	122	125	128	130	131	78	78	78	78	80	81	81
	95th + 12	131	132	134	137	140	142	143	90	90	90	90	92	93	93
14	50th	105	106	109	111	112	113	113	60	60	62	64	65	66	67
	90th	119	120	123	126	127	128	129	74	74	75	77	78	79	80
	95th	123	125	127	130	132	133	134	77	78	79	81	82	83	84
	95th + 12	135	137	139	142	144	145	146	89	90	91	93	94	95	96
15	50th	108	110	112	113	114	114	114	61	62	64	65	66	67	68
	90th	123	124	126	128	129	130	130	75	76	78	79	80	81	81
	95th	127	129	131	132	134	135	135	78	79	81	83	84	85	85
	95th + 12	139	141	143	144	146	147	147	90	91	93	95	96	97	97
16	50th	111	112	114	115	115	116	116	63	64	66	67	68	69	69
	90th	126	127	128	129	131	131	132	77	78	79	80	81	82	82
	95th	130	131	133	134	135	136	137	80	81	83	84	85	86	86
	95th + 12	142	143	145	146	147	148	149	92	93	95	96	97	98	98
17	50th	114	115	116	117	117	118	118	65	66	67	68	69	70	70
	90th	128	129	130	131	132	133	134	78	79	80	81	82	82	83
	95th	132	133	134	135	137	138	138	81	82	84	85	86	86	87
	95th + 12	144	145	146	147	149	150	150	93	94	96	97	98	98	99

ii. Girls 1–17 years old:

Age (year)	BP Percentile (+mmHg)	SBP (mmHg) Percentile of Height							DBP (mmHg) Percentile of Height						
		5th	10th	25th	50th	75th	90th	95th	5th	10th	25th	50th	75th	90th	95th
1	50th	84	85	86	83	87	88	88	41	42	42	43	44	45	46
	90th	98	99	99	100	101	102	102	54	55	56	56	57	58	58
	95th	101	102	102	103	104	105	105	59	59	60	60	61	62	62
	95th + 12	113	114	114	115	116	117	117	71	71	72	72	73	74	74
2	50th	87	87	88	89	90	91	91	45	46	47	48	49	50	51
	90th	101	101	102	103	104	105	106	58	58	59	60	61	62	62
	95th	104	105	106	106	107	108	109	62	63	63	64	65	66	66
	95th + 12	116	117	118	118	119	120	121	74	75	75	76	77	78	78
3	50th	88	89	89	90	91	92	93	48	48	49	50	51	53	53
	90th	102	103	104	104	105	106	107	60	61	61	62	63	64	65
	95th	106	106	107	103	109	110	110	64	65	65	66	67	68	69
	95th + 12	118	118	119	120	121	122	122	76	77	77	78	79	80	81
4	50th	89	90	91	92	93	94	94	50	51	51	53	54	55	55
	90th	103	104	105	106	107	108	108	62	63	64	65	66	67	67
	95th	107	108	109	109	110	111	112	66	67	68	69	70	70	71
	95th + 12	119	120	121	121	122	123	124	78	79	80	81	82	82	83
5	50th	90	91	92	93	94	95	96	52	52	53	55	56	57	57
	90th	104	105	106	107	108	109	110	64	65	66	67	68	69	70
	95th	108	109	109	110	111	112	113	68	69	70	71	72	73	73
	95th + 12	120	121	121	122	123	124	125	80	81	82	83	84	85	85

(Continued)

(Continued)

Age (year)	BP Percentile (+mmHg)	SBP (mmHg) Percentile of Height 5th	10th	25th	50th	75th	90th	95th	DBP (mmHg) Percentile of Height 5th	10th	25th	50th	75th	90th	95th
6	50th	92	92	93	94	96	97	97	54	54	55	56	57	58	59
	90th	105	106	107	108	109	110	111	67	67	68	69	70	71	71
	95th	109	109	110	111	112	113	114	70	71	72	72	73	74	74
	95th + 12	121	121	122	123	124	125	126	82	83	84	84	85	86	86
7	50th	92	93	94	95	97	98	99	55	55	56	57	58	59	60
	90th	106	106	107	109	110	111	112	68	68	69	70	71	72	72
	95th	109	110	111	112	113	114	115	72	72	73	73	74	74	75
	95th + 12	121	122	123	124	125	126	127	84	84	85	85	86	86	87
8	50th	93	94	95	97	98	99	100	56	56	57	59	60	61	61
	90th	107	107	108	110	111	112	113	69	70	71	72	72	73	73
	95th	110	111	112	113	115	116	117	72	73	74	74	75	75	75
	95th + 12	122	123	124	125	127	128	129	84	85	86	86	87	87	87
9	50th	95	95	97	98	99	100	101	57	58	59	60	60	61	61
	90th	108	108	109	111	112	113	114	71	71	72	73	73	73	73
	95th	112	112	113	114	116	117	118	74	74	75	75	75	75	75
	95th + 12	124	124	125	126	128	129	130	86	86	87	87	87	87	87
10	50th	96	97	98	99	101	102	103	58	59	59	60	61	61	62
	90th	109	110	111	112	113	115	116	72	73	73	73	73	73	73
	95th	113	114	114	116	117	119	120	75	75	76	76	76	76	76
	95th + 12	125	126	126	128	129	131	132	87	87	88	88	88	88	88
11	50th	98	99	101	102	104	105	106	60	60	60	61	62	63	64
	90th	111	112	113	114	116	118	120	74	74	74	74	74	75	75
	95th	115	116	117	118	120	123	124	76	77	77	77	77	77	77
	95th + 12	127	128	129	130	132	135	136	88	89	89	89	89	89	89

12	50th	102	102	104	105	107	108	108	61	61	61	62	64	65	65
	90th	114	115	116	118	120	122	122	75	75	75	75	76	76	76
	95th	118	119	120	122	124	125	126	78	78	78	78	79	79	79
	95th + 12	130	131	132	134	136	137	138	90	90	90	90	91	91	91
13	50th	104	105	106	107	108	108	109	62	62	63	64	65	65	66
	90th	116	117	119	121	122	123	123	75	75	75	76	76	76	76
	95th	121	122	123	124	126	126	127	79	79	79	79	80	80	81
	95th + 12	133	134	135	136	138	138	139	91	91	91	91	92	92	93
14	50th	105	106	107	108	109	109	109	63	63	64	65	66	66	66
	90th	118	118	120	122	123	123	123	76	76	76	76	77	77	77
	95th	123	123	124	125	126	127	127	80	80	80	80	81	81	82
	95th + 12	135	135	136	137	138	139	139	92	92	92	92	93	93	94
15	50th	105	106	107	108	109	109	109	64	64	64	65	66	67	67
	90th	118	119	121	122	123	123	124	76	76	76	77	77	78	78
	95th	124	124	125	126	127	127	128	80	80	80	81	82	82	82
	95th + 12	136	136	137	138	139	139	140	92	92	92	93	94	94	94
16	50th	106	107	108	109	109	110	110	64	64	65	66	66	67	67
	90th	119	120	122	123	124	124	124	76	76	76	77	78	78	78
	95th	124	125	125	127	127	128	128	80	80	80	81	82	82	82
	95th + 12	136	137	137	139	139	140	140	92	92	92	93	94	94	94
17	50th	107	108	109	110	110	110	111	64	64	65	66	66	66	67
	90th	120	121	123	124	124	125	125	76	76	77	77	78	78	78
	95th	125	125	126	127	128	128	128	80	80	80	81	82	82	82
	95th + 12	137	137	138	139	140	140	140	92	92	92	93	94	94	94

B. Ambulatory Blood Pressure (ABP)

1. Usefulness of ABP monitoring in children

a. More accurate for diagnosis of hypertension than clinic BP.
b. More reproducible than casual or home BP measurements.
c. More predictive of future BP.
d. Correlates more strongly than clinic BP with target organ injury, in particular, left ventricular hypertrophy.

2. Indications

a. ABP should be performed for the confirmation of hypertension in children and adolescents with:
   - Elevated BP for ≥1 year.
   - Stage 1 hypertension over 3 clinic visits.

b. Recommended in children with high-risk conditions:
   - Assess the severity of hypertension.
   - Abnormal circadian BP patterns may indicate an increased risk of target organ damage.

c. Monitoring for response to antihypertensive medications.

3. Procedure

a. ABP machine is worn for 24 hours.
b. Activities for that day are recorded, including sleep and wake times.
c. Select the appropriate cuff size for the non-dominant arm.
d. This is an oscillometric BP machine set to measure BP once every ½ hour during waking hours, and once every hour during sleep.
e. Data is divided into a 24-hour period (overall summary), and wake and sleep periods.
f. Minimum requirements for a successful report:
   - At least 40–50 readings for a full 24-hour report.
   - Minimum of 1 reading every hour.
   - 65–75% of all possible BP readings for a partial day report.

4. Parameters in an ABP report

Example of ABP report of a girl

Overall Summary

	AVG	STD		MIN		MAX		Dipping
Systolic:	128	12.65	mmHg	104	(09:29 Thu)	149	(07:25 Fri)	-0.7%
Diastolic:	75	13.02	mmHg	50	(08:55 Fri)	97	(16:25 Thu)	-2.6%
MAP:	93	12.11	mmHg	70		114		-3.2%
Pulse Pressure:	52	4.57	mmHg	42		60		
Heart Rate:	88	12.38	bpm	72		119		

	Reading(s)	Time
Percent of Systolic above limits:	82.1%	87.7 %
Percent of Diastolic above limits:	35.9%	43.9 %

Wake Period(s) 08:00 - 22:00

	AVG	STD		MIN		MAX	
Systolic:	127	12.39	mmHg	104	(09:29 Thu)	144	(16:25 Thu)
Diastolic:	75	12.97	mmHg	50	(08:55 Fri)	97	(16:25 Thu)
MAP:	92	12.04	mmHg	70		114	
Pulse Pressure:	53	4.35	mmHg	45		60	
Heart Rate:	93	12.75	bpm	75		119	

	Reading(s)	Time
Percent of Systolic readings > 120mmHg:	75.9%	81.1 %
Percent of Diastolic readings > 84mmHg:	24.1%	22.4 %

Number of Wake Period(s) readings: 29

Sleep Period(s) 22:00 - 08:00

	AVG	STD		MIN		MAX	
Systolic:	128	14.06	mmHg	108	(01:25 Fri)	149	(07:25 Fri)
Diastolic:	77	13.80	mmHg	56	(22:25 Thu)	96	(07:25 Fri)
MAP:	95	12.82	mmHg	78		113	
Pulse Pressure:	52	5.36	mmHg	42		59	
Heart Rate:	81	4.97	bpm	72		89	

	Reading(s)	Time
Percent of Systolic readings > 107mmHg:	100.0%	100.0%
Percent of Diastolic readings > 66mmHg:	70.0%	72.2%

Number of Sleep Period(s) readings: 10

a. **BP index = Average ABP/95th percentile of the normative data**
To obtain this, divide the values in rectangles by the corresponding 95th percentile of normative values.
Hypertension defined as BP index >1.0
In the above example:

SBP index (24h)	= 128/113	= 1.13
DBP index (24h)	= 75/73	= 1.03
SBP index (day)	= 127/120	= 1.06
DBP index (day)	= 75/84	= 0.89
SBP index (night)	= 128/107	= 1.20
DBP index (night)	= 77/66	= 1.17

This girl has hypertension, as most of the indices are more than 1.0.

b. **BP load = Percentage of BP recordings > normative value**
   - These are the values in the ovals and relate to target organ damage.
   - There is no consensus on the acceptable limit of BP load, although a BP load of >25–30% should be considered abnormal.
   - The BP load is useful for staging of hypertension (see below).

c. **Dipping = [(mean wake BP – mean sleep BP)/mean wake BP] × 100%**
   - These are the numbers in the triangle.
   - Normal dipping is at least 10%.
   - Hypertensive patients have dipping <10% and may even have negative values (sleep BP higher than wake BP).
   - It is less certain how to interpret and weigh the importance of nocturnal dipping in children. In adults, "non-dippers" have a greater risk for left ventricular hypertrophy and cardiovascular morbidity.

5. Normative data:

a. Infants and Adults:

Height (cm)	Percentile for a 24-hour Period		Daytime Percentile		Nighttime Percentile	
	90th	95th	90th	95th	90th	95th
Infants and Toddlers (2 to 30 months)#						
55–95	114.7/75.2	**118.9/79.1**	116.7/79.7	**120.9/83.9**	111.2/71.7	**115.1/75.2**
Adults (≥21 years old)*						
		130/80		**135/85**		**120/70**

#Based on data from 97 subjects (Varda *et al.*, 2005)
*Based on European Society of Hypertension, 2013

b. Normal values for ABP (mmHg) for healthy boys (5–20 years old) by height:*

24 hour ABP — SBP/DBP (MAP)			
Height (cm)	50th	90th	95th
120	104.5/65.6 (77.5)	113.8/73.9 (86.3)	116.8/76.7 (89.3)
125	105.3/65.9 (78.1)	114.8/74.1 (86.7)	117.8/76.8 (89.6)
130	106.2/66.1 (78.7)	115.9/74.2 (87.2)	118.9/76.9 (89.9)
135	107.2/66.4 (79.3)	116.9/74.4 (87.6)	120.0/76.9 (90.2)
140	108.3/66.6 (79.9)	118.2/74.5 (88.0)	121.2/77.0 (90.5)
145	109.5/66.9 (80.5)	119.5/74.7 (88.5)	122.5/77.1 (90.9)
150	110.9/67.1 (81.1)	121.0/74.8 (89.1)	124.0/77.1 (91.4)
155	112.5/67.2 (81.7)	122.6/74.8 (89.7)	125.7/77.2 (91.9)
160	114.2/67.3 (82.3)	124.4/74.9 (90.3)	127.4/77.3 (92.6)
165	116.1/67.5 (83.1)	126.3/75.1 (91.1)	129.3/77.5 (93.3)
170	118.0/67.6 (83.9)	128.1/75.3 (91.9)	131.1/77.7 (94.0)
175	119.7/67.8 (84.7)	129.8/75.4 (92.7)	132.6/77.8 (94.8)
180	121.5/68.0 (85.5)	131.3/75.5 (93.5)	134.1/77.9 (95.6)
Daytime ABP — SBP/DBP (MAP)			
120	110.8/72.3 (83.8)	121.7/80.2 (92.9)	125.2/82.4 (95.6)
125	111.1/72.3 (84.1)	121.9/80.1 (93.0)	125.3/82.2 (95.6)
130	111.5/72.2 (84.3)	122.2/79.9 (93.1)	125.5/82.0 (95.6)
135	112.0/72.1 (84.5)	122.5/79.7 (93.1)	125.7/81.8 (95.5)
140	112.7/72.1 (84.7)	123.0/79.5 (93.1)	126.0/81.5 (95.5)
145	113.7/72.1 (85.0)	123.9/79.4 (93.2)	126.9/81.4 (95.5)
150	115.1/72.1 (85.4)	125.3/79.3 (93.4)	128.3/81.2 (95.7)
155	116.8/72.1 (85.8)	127.1/79.3 (93.8)	130.2/81.2 (96.0)
160	118.6/72.2 (86.4)	129.4/79.4 (94.5)	132.7/81.3 (96.7)
165	120.6/72.3 (87.1)	131.9/79.7 (95.4)	135.3/81.7 (97.7)
170	122.6/72.6 (88.0)	134.1/80.0 (96.5)	137.6/82.1 (98.8)
175	124.4/72.8 (89.0)	136.1/80.5 (97.7)	130.6/82.6 (100.1)
180	126.2/73.1 (90.0)	138.0/80.9 (99.0)	141.6/83.1 (101.4)

(*Continued*)

(*Continued*)

24 hour ABP — SBP/DBP (MAP)			
Height (cm)	50th	90th	95th
Nightime ABP — SBP/DBP (MAP)			
120	93.6/54.3 (66.8)	103.3/60.7 (75.9)	106.3/62.6 (79.5)
125	94.6/54.8 (67.6)	104.8/61.4 (76.6)	107.9/63.4 (80.0)
130	95.6/55.1 (68.3)	106.3/62.1 (77.3)	109.7/64.2 (80.5)
135	96.7/55.5 (69.0)	107.8/62.7 (77.9)	111.4/64.8 (80.9)
140	97.9/55.8 (69.6)	109.3/63.2 (78.3)	113.0/65.4 (81.2)
145	99.0/56.0 (70.1)	110.6/63.5 (78.6)	114.4/65.8 (81.3)
150	100.1/56.2 (70.6)	111.8/63.7 (78.9)	115.7/66.0 (81.4)
155	101.3/56.2 (71.2)	113.0/63.8 (79.2)	116.8/66.0 (81.5)
160	102.6/56.3 (71.9)	114.3/63.8 (79.7)	118.1/66.0 (81.9)
165	104.1/56.5 (72.7)	115.7/63.9 (80.3)	119.4/66.0 (82.3)
170	105.6/56.7 (73.6)	117.2/63.9 (80.9)	120.9/66.1 (82.8)
175	107.2/56.9 (74.5)	118.8/64.0 (81.5)	122.4/66.1 (83.3)
180	108.7/57.1 (75.4)	120.3/64.1 (82.1)	123.9/66.1 (83.8)

c. Normal values for ABP (mmHg) for healthy girls (5–20 years old) by height:*

24-hour ABP — SBP/DBP (MAP)			
Height (cm)	50th	90th	95th
120	104.0/65.9 (77.2)	112.0/70.9 (83.6)	114.3/72.2 (85.3)
125	105.0/65.9 (77.8)	113.2/71.4 (84.2)	115.6/72.8 (86.0)
130	106.0/66.0 (78.3)	114.3/71.9 (84.9)	116.7/73.4 (86.7)
135	106.8/66.1 (78.7)	115.3/72.4 (85.5)	117.7/74.1 (87.4)
140	107.8/66.2 (79.2)	116.2/72.9 (86.1)	118.7/74.7 (88.0)
145	108.7/66.3 (79.7)	117.4/73.4 (86.7)	119.9/75.3 (88.6)
150	109.0/66.5 (80.2)	118.7/73.8 (87.3)	121.2/75.7 (89.2)
155	111.2/66.7 (80.8)	120.0/74.0 (87.9)	122.5/76.0 (89.7)
160	112.4/67.0 (81.5)	121.0/74.1 (88.4)	123.3/76.1 (90.2)
165	113.7/67.4 (82.3)	121.8/74.2 (88.9)	124.1/76.2 (90.6)

(*Continued*)

	24-hour ABP — SBP/DBP (MAP)		
Height (cm)	**50th**	**90th**	**95th**
170	115.0/68.0 (83.1)	122.8/74.4 (89.5)	124.9/76.2 (91.1)
175	116.4/68.6 (84.0)	123.8/74.5 (90.1)	125.8/76.2 (94.5)
	Daytime ABP — SBP/DBP (MAP)		
120	110.0/73.2 (73.2)	118.2/80.1 (80.1)	120.4/81.9 (81.9)
125	110.5/72.8 (72.8)	119.0/79.9 (79.9)	121.3/81.8 (81.8)
130	111.0/72.4 (72.4)	119.7/79.8 (79.8)	122.1/81.8 (81.8)
135	111.6/72.1 (72.1)	120.4/79.8 (79.8)	122.9/81.8 (81.8)
140	112.2/71.8 (71.8)	121.3/79.7 (79.7)	123.8/81.9 (81.9)
145	113.1/71.7 (71.7)	122.5/79.8 (79.8)	125.1/82.0 (82.0)
150	114.3/71.8 (71.8)	123.9/79.9 (79.9)	126.5/82.0 (82.0)
155	115.6/72.0 (72.0)	125.2/79.9 (79.9)	127.9/82.0 (82.0)
160	117.0/72.4 (72.4)	126.4/79.9 (79.9)	129.1/82.0 (82.0)
165	118.3/73.1 (73.1)	127.3/80.0 (80.0)	129.8/81.9 (81.9)
170	119.8/73.9 (73.9)	128.1/80.2 (80.2)	130.5/82.0 (82.0)
175	121.2/74.8 (74.8)	128.9/80.5 (80.5)	131.0/82.0 (82.0)
	Nighttime ABP — SBP/DBP (MAP)		
120	95.0/55.4 (68.0)	103.3/63.1 (76.8)	105.6/65.2 (79.5)
125	95.7/55.3 (68.2)	104.4/63.3 (76.9)	106.9/65.5 (79.4)
130	96.4/55.1 (68.4)	105.5/63.4 (77.0)	108.1/65.7 (79.6)
135	96.9/54.8 (68.5)	106.5/63.4 (77.2)	109.3/65.8 (79.7)
140	97.5/54.6 (68.7)	107.5/63.3 (77.4)	110.4/65.7 (79.9)
145	98.1/54.5 (69.0)	108.5/63.1 (77.7)	111.6/65.6 (80.2)
150	98.9/54.3 (69.3)	109.5/63.0 (78.0)	112.7/65.5 (80.4)
155	100.0/54.4 (69.8)	110.5/62.9 (78.3)	113.6/65.5 (80.6)
160	101.1/54.6 (70.4)	111.2/62.9 (78.6)	114.1/65.5 (80.8)
165	102.2/54.9 (71.2)	111.8/62.9 (79.1)	114.4/65.5 (81.2)
170	103.4/55.1 (72.0)	112.4/66.9 (79.6)	114.8/70.8 (81.6)
175	104.6/55.4 (72.8)	113.1/63.1 (80.3)	115.3/65.6 (82.2)

*Based on data of 949 subjects (Wuhl *et al.*, 2002)

6. Staging of hypertension according to ABP level:

a. Children (aged 5–16 years, height: boys [120–180 cm], girls [120–175] cm):

Classification	Clinic BP Hypertension	Ambulatory Hypertension (Both criteria must be satisfied, in either the awake or sleep period, or both)	
	Clinic BP	Mean Ambulatory SBP or DBP	24-hour SBP or DBP load (%)
Normal BP	<90th percentile	<95th percentile	<25
Elevated BP	≥90th but <95th percentile OR >120/80 mmHg to <95th percentile (whichever is lower)	<95th percentile	≥25
Ambulatory hypertension	>95th percentile	>95th percentile OR >130/80 (mean) >135/85 (awake) >125/75 (sleep) (whichever is lower)	25–50
Severe ambulatory hypertension	>95th percentile	>95th percentile	>50

b. ABP in adults (≥21 years old):

Classification	Clinic BP Hypertension	Ambulatory Hypertension
	Clinic BP	Mean Ambulatory SBP/DBP
Normal BP	<120/80 mmHg	24-hour <115/<75 mmHg Awake <120/<80 mmHg Sleep <100/<65 mmHg
Elevated BP	120–129/<80 mmHg	24-hour 115–<125/<75 mmHg Awake 120–<130/<80 mmHg Sleep 100–<110/<65 mmHg
Ambulatory hypertension	Not applicable	24-hour ≥125/≥75 mmHg Awake ≥130/≥80 mmHg Sleep ≥110/≥65 mmHg

(Continued)

Classification	Clinic BP Hypertension	Ambulatory Hypertension
	Clinic BP	Mean Ambulatory SBP/DBP
Stage 1 hypertension	130–139/80–89 mmHg	24-hour 125–<130/75–<80 mmHg Awake 130–<135/80–<85 mmHg Sleep 110–<120/65–<70 mmHg
Stage 2 hypertension	≥140/≥90 mmHg	24-hour ≥130/≥80 mmHg Awake ≥135/≥85 mmHg Sleep ≥120/≥70 mmHg

7. Definitions based on comparison of clinic BP and ABP:

a. White coat hypertension:
   - Clinic BP that is consistently elevated (≥95th percentile for children) but ABP remains normal.

b. Masked hypertension:
   - Normal clinic BP but elevated ABP.
   - Carries a significant risk of hypertensive end-organ damage.

8. Value of ABP monitoring in high-risk patients:

a. Target organ damage despite normal clinic BPs such as proteinuria and left ventricular hypertrophy.
b. Apparent drug-resistant hypertension.
c. Unusual BP variability or episodic hypertension.
d. Chronic kidney disease.
e. Diabetes mellitus.
f. Determining the efficacy of drug treatment over 24 hours.
g. Hypotensive symptoms with antihypertensive drugs.
h. Obstructive sleep apnea where there may be non-dipping and accentuated morning BP surge.
i. Obesity.
j. Solid organ transplantation.
k. Genetic syndromes such as neurofibromatosis, Turner syndrome, Williams syndrome.
l. Coarctation of the aorta repair.
m. History of prematurity to evaluate for non-dipping.

C. Home Blood Pressure (HBP)

1. Usefulness of HBP monitoring in children:

a. Good screening tool in children and adjunct to office BP:
   - Initial evaluation of untreated children with suspected hypertension.
   - Children with treated hypertension before each follow-up visit.

b. Confirmatory out-of-office BP monitoring method after ABP monitoring or when ABP is unavailable or not tolerated.

c. Comparison of HBP and office BP:
   - In normotensive children and adolescents, HBP readings are similar to office BP measurements.
   - In hypertensive children, systolic (not diastolic) HBP appears to be lower than office BP.

d. Treatment decisions can be made using HBP measurements if these are in agreement with office measurements.

e. Can identify children with white coat and masked hypertension but needs confirmation with ABP.

2. Normative data for home SBP/DBP in children and adolescents by gender and height:

Height (cm)	Boys		Girls	
	50th centile	95th centile	50th centile	95th centile
120–129	105/64	119/76	101/64	119/74
130–139	108/64	121/77	103/64	120/76
140–149	110/65	125/77	106/65	122/77
150–159	112/65	126/78	108/66	123/77
160–169	115/65	128/78	110/66	124/78
170–179	117/66	132/78	112/66	125/79
180–189	121/67	134/79	114/67	128/80

3. Use validated home BP monitors:

- Check online registries for home BP monitors, which are validated.

Registries	Website
General (international registries) STRIDE BP (European) Medaval	 https://stridebp.org/ https://medaval.ie/blood-pressuremonitors/
Regional registries American Medical Association British and Irish Hypertension Society Hypertension Canada Japanese Society of Hypertension	 https://www.validatebp.org/ https://bihsoc.org/bp-monitors/ https://hypertension.ca/bpdevices http://www.jpnsh.jp/com_ac_wg1.html

4. Procedure:

a. Minimum of 12 readings required with a minimum duration of 3 to 7 days to improve association of HBP and ABP:
   - Averaging up to 12 readings in 3 days OR
   - A 7-day HBP with at least 3 days of duplicate morning and evening measurements after 5 minutes of sitting/rest and 1 minute between measurements, a total of at least 12 readings.

b. Use electronic devices that have been clinically validated to avoid the observer-induced errors of the manual auscultatory method.

c. Ensure the availability of different cuff sizes to accommodate the wide range of arm circumference of children and adolescents.

d. Nocturnal HBP monitoring:
   - Night-time BP during sleep predicts cardiovascular risk.
   - May be more preferable in children and is comparable to nocturnal ABP, providing a similar association with indices of preclinical target organ damage.
   - Particularly important for children with diabetes, nephropathy and sleep apnea.

D. Algorithm for Diagnosis of Hypertension

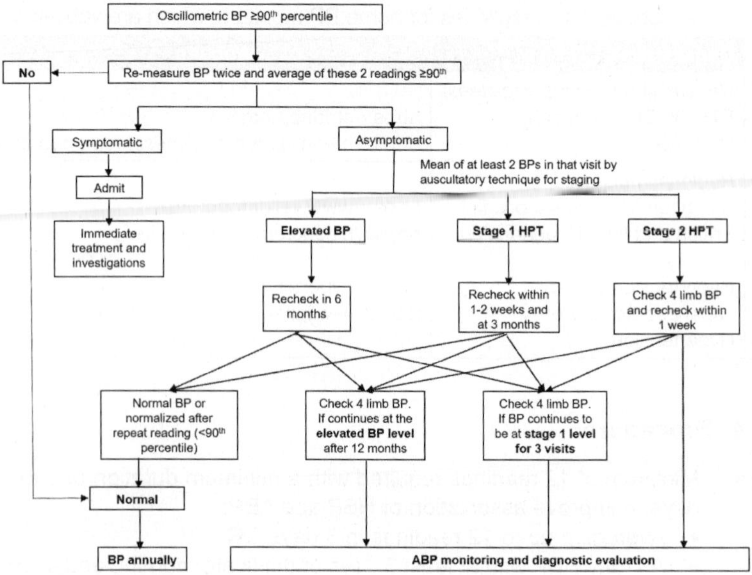

1. The urgency of laboratory evaluation is based on the child's age, history, physical examination findings, and level of BP elevation.
2. Stage 1 hypertension allows time for evaluation before initiating treatment unless the patient is symptomatic.
3. Stage 2 hypertension requires more prompt evaluation and pharmacologic therapy.
4. Stage 1 and Stage 2 hypertension require investigations for target organ injury.

E. Evaluation

I. Evaluation of primary hypertension:

1. Primary hypertension is the most common cause of hypertension in children and adolescents.

2. Elevation in SBP is more predictive of primary hypertension while elevation in DBP is more predictive of secondary hypertension.
3. Children with suspected primary hypertension do not require extensive evaluation for secondary causes of hypertension.
4. History taking should include:
   - Nutritional history.
   - Physical activity.
   - Psychosocial factors including stress.
   - Family history.
5. Characteristics of primary hypertension in children include:
   a. Age ≥6 years.
   b. Positive family history of hypertension in parents and/or grandparents.
   c. Overweight or obesity.
   d. No history or physical signs suggestive of a secondary cause of hypertension.
6. Assessment for comorbidities:
   a. Cardiovascular risk factors:
      - Smoking.
      - Alcohol.
   b. Sleep history (risk of obstructive sleep apnea).
   c. Physical signs suggesting insulin resistance:
      - Truncal obesity.
      - Acanthosis nigricans.
   d. Initial investigations:
      - Fasting glucose.
      - Fasting lipids.
      - Serum uric acid.
      - Aspartate transaminase and alanine transaminase.
      - Sleep study (if loud frequent snoring).

II. Evaluation of secondary hypertension:

1. All children and adolescents who do not fulfill the characteristics of primary hypertension should be evaluated for the causes of secondary hypertension.

2. Clinical approach:

	Etiology	Associated Findings
History	Bronchopulmonary dysplasia. Umbilical artery catheterization.	Perinatal history.
	Anabolic steroids. Substance abuse (cocaine, amphetamines). Nasal ephedrine.	Drug history including herbal medicine, nutritional supplements and recreational drugs.
	Heavy metals, e.g., lead, cadmium, mercury. Phthalates.	Environmental exposure to toxins.
	Pheochromocytoma. Thyrotoxicosis.	Triad of a headache, sweating and tachycardia.
Physical examination	Thyrotoxicosis.	Tachycardia, proptosis, goiter.
	Chronic kidney failure.	Growth retardation, pallor.
	Cushing syndrome or disease.	Obesity, moon facies, acne, striae.
	Coarctation of aorta.	Radiofemoral delay.
	Obstructive sleep apnea.	Adenotonsillar hypertrophy.
	Neurocutaneous syndromes.	Café-au-lait spots, adenoma sebceum.
	Renal artery stenosis.	Renal bruit.
	Congenital adrenal hyperplasia.	Ambiguous or virilized genitalia.
	Wilms tumor. Neuroblastoma.	Abdominal mass.
	Hydronephrosis. Polycystic kidney disease. Hepatorenal fibrocystic disease.	Palpable kidney.
	Renal parenchymal disease.	Hematuria, edema, fatigue.

3. Initial general investigations:
   a. To rule out chronic kidney disease and chronic pyelonephritis:
      - Blood urea, creatinine, sodium, potassium, chloride, bicarbonate, calcium, phosphate, and uric acid.
      - Urine dipstick, microscopy and culture.
      - Full blood count.
   b. To rule out congenital anomaly of the kidneys or disparate kidney size:
      - Kidney ultrasonography.

- Doppler kidney ultrasonography may be used as a non-invasive screening study for the evaluation of possible renal artery stenosis in normal children and adolescents ≥8 years of age who are suspected of having renovascular hypertension and who will cooperate with the procedure.

III. Evaluation for target organ injury:

	Target Organ Injury
Target Patients	Patients with BP ≥95th percentile. Patient with elevated BP with diabetes mellitus or kidney disease. Patients at risk of hypertension, e.g., chronic kidney disease, long-term steroids.
History	Headache. Blurring of vision. Exertional dyspnea.
Physical Examination	Cardiomegaly with heaving apex beat. Hypertensive retinopathy.
Initial General Investigations	Evaluation for left ventricular hypertrophy (LVH): a. No need to do ECG for the evaluation of LVH in children with hypertension. b. 2D-echocardiography: i. Timing of procedure: • At initiation of treatment. • Repeat at 6–12 month intervals in persistent hypertension despite treatment, concentric hypertrophy or reduced LV ejection fraction. • If results are initially normal, repeat at yearly intervals in secondary hypertension, Stage 2 or chronic Stage 1 hypertension that is incompletely treated. ii. Definitions. • In children >8 years of age, LVH is defined as LV mass index (LVMI) >51 $g/m^{2.7}$ (boys and girls) or by LV mass >115 g/m^2 for boys and >95 g/m^2 for girls. • LV wall thickness >1.4 cm is abnormal. • Concentric hypertrophy is defined as LV relative wall thickness >0.42 cm. • LV ejection fraction <53% is considered decreased. Urine microalbuminuria in those with secondary causes of hypertension.

IV. Workup for hypertensive patients with hypokalemia:

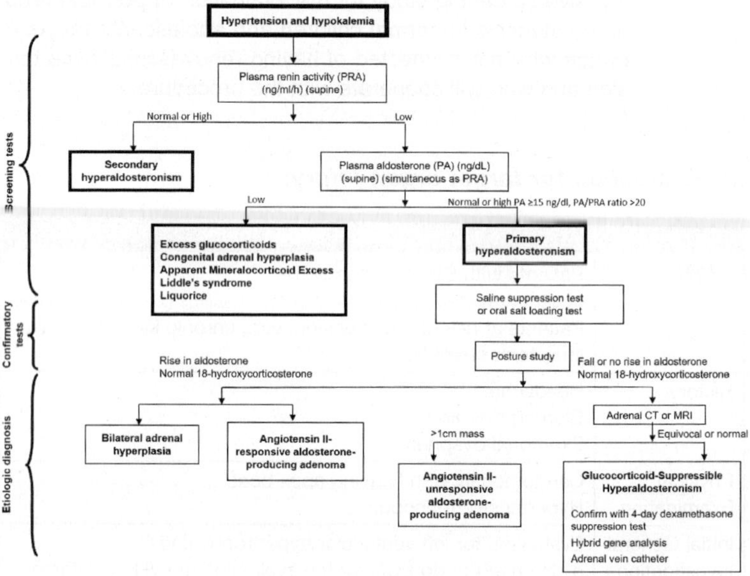

Note: For calculation of plasma aldosterone (PA)/renin (PRA) ratio, conversion of PA is as follows: 1 pmol/L = 0.04 ng/dL.

V. Principles of investigations in suspected aldosterone excess states:

1. Primary hyperaldosteronism:
   a. Hypokalemia.
   b. Metabolic alkalosis.
   c. Increased 24-hour urinary potassium excretion.
   d. Decreased 24-hour urinary sodium excretion.
   e. Hypertension that is usually moderate-to-severe and refractory to treatment.
2. Optimization of the patient for evaluation for hyperaldosteronism:
   a. Drugs that alter aldosterone or renin secretion should be avoided if possible.

- Beta-blockers and spironolactone should be withdrawn for 2–4 weeks before testing.
- Beta-blockers lower PRA secretion and often produce a false positive PA/PRA ratio in patients with essential hypertension.
- Spironolactone inhibits the actions of aldosterone on the mineralocorticoid receptor, thereby increasing serum concentrations of PRA.
- If the screening test is performed while on ACE inhibitors, angiotensin receptor blockers, calcium channel antagonists, or alpha-blockers, and aldosterone levels remain frankly elevated in the setting of suppressed renin activity, the likelihood of primary aldosteronism remains high.

b. Hypokalemia should be corrected as it directly inhibits aldosterone release.
c. Patient should not be dehydrated as this stimulates the renin-aldosterone system (RAS).

3. Saline suppression test:
   a. Acute intravascular volume expansion with isotonic saline normally suppresses the RAS.
   b. Isotonic saline is infused over 4–6 hours. This test should not be performed in patients with compromised cardiac function due to the risk of pulmonary edema.
   c. In normal subjects, PA levels normally decrease below 166 pmol/L (6 ng/dL) at the end of the saline infusion:
      - Levels >277 pmol/L (10 ng/dL) are diagnostic of autonomous aldosterone production.
      - Values between 166–277 pmol/L (6–10 ng/dL) are considered indeterminate but are highly suspicious for this disorder.
4. Oral salt loading test:
   a. Oral salt loading for 3 days results in extra and intravascular volume expansion and RAS suppression in normal individuals.
   b. Patients are instructed to eat a high (200 mmol) sodium diet for 3 days, or take four 500 mg sodium chloride tablets (1 tablet = 8.2 mmol sodium) with each meal (3 meals) for 3 days.
   c. On the 3rd day of the high sodium diet, a 24-hour urine collection for aldosterone excretion, creatinine, and sodium is collected.
   d. Aldosterone excretion greater than 39 nmol/d (14 µg/d), in the presence of a urinary sodium excretion greater than 200 mmol

per 24 hours, is 96% sensitive and 93% specific for the diagnosis of primary hyperaldosteronism.

e. Oral salt loading can be performed on an outpatient basis. However, BP and potassium levels should be monitored during the testing to avoid the acceleration of hypertension or the precipitation of severe hypokalemia.

5. Posture study:
   a. The principle here is that adrenal adenomas producing aldosterone are sensitive to the adrenocorticotrophic hormone (ACTH), whereas bilateral idiopathic adrenal hyperplasia is sensitive to angiotensin II.
   b. Patients have blood tests at 8 am for aldosterone, cortisol, renin, and 18-hydroxycorticosterone.
   c. After 4 hours of being upright and walking around (which stimulates angiotensin II production due to blood pressure changes, not affecting ACTH), the blood tests are repeated.
   d. Patients should be well hydrated for this test, with urine sodium >20 mmol/L.
   e. Adrenal adenomas will show very little change in aldosterone levels whereas the benign adrenal hyperplasia cases will show increased aldosterone (due to stimulation by the increased angiotensin II).
6. Hybrid gene study:
   a. Diagnosis of autosomal dominant familial hyperaldosteronism type 1 or gloucocorticoid-remediable aldosteronism.
   b. Characterized by hybrid or chimeric gene on chromosome 8q: *CYP11B1* (regulatory region of the 11β-hydroxylase gene), coupled with *CYP11B2* (structural region of the aldosterone synthase gene).

VI. Principles of investigations in suspected excess glucocorticoid states:

1. Hypercortisolism:
   a. Features of Cushing syndrome are usually apparent.
   b. Screening tests:
      i. 24-hour urine free cortisol.
      ii. Overnight standard (low-dose) dexamethasone suppression test:
         - 1 mg of dexamethasone to be taken at 11 pm.

   iii. Serum cortisol at 8 am and 8 pm for assessment of diurnal variation.
      - Ensure plug is set beforehand, otherwise stress at blood-taking may spuriously increase serum cortisol.
   c. Etiologic diagnostic test:
      i. Overnight high-dose dexamethasone suppression test.
         - Differentiates Cushing's disease (pituitary ACTH hypersecretion) from other causes of Cushing's syndrome (ectopic ACTH or adrenal tumors).

2. Congenital adrenal hyperplasia:
   a. Perform the following hormone analysis:
      - Aldosterone.
      - Cortisol.
      - Deoxycorticosterone (DOC).
      - 11-deoxycortisol.
      - 17-hydroxyprogesterone.
      - Dehydroepiandosterone (DHEAS).
      - Testosterone.
      - ACTH.
   b. 11-β-hydroxylase deficiency (*CYP11B1* mutation):
      - Mildly virilized.
      - Hypoglycaemic due to decreased/absent cortisol.
   c. 17-α-hydroxylase deficiency (CYP17 mutation):
      - Inadequate virilization.

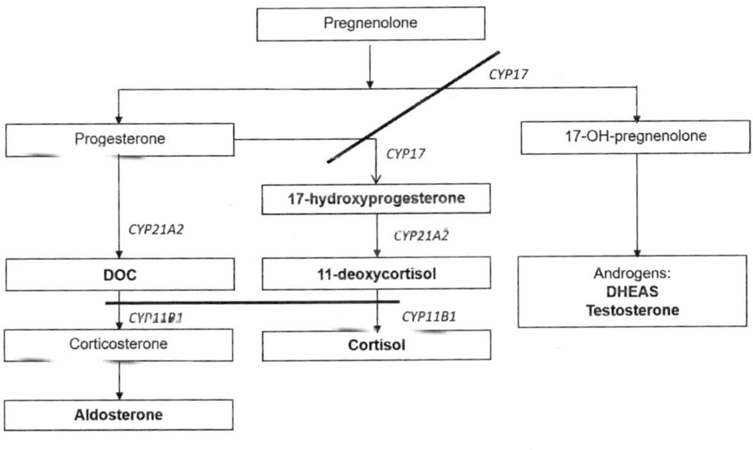

VII. Principles of investigations for catecholamine excess states:

1. Catecholamine secreting tumors:
   a. Pheochromocytoma (80%): Arises from chromaffin cells of the adrenal medulla.
   b. Paraganglioma (20%): Extra-adrenal origin.
2. Consider associated familial syndromes:
   a. Von Hippel–Landau syndrome.
   b. Neurofibromatosis type 1.
   c. Multiple Endocrine Neoplasia type 2A or 2B (MEN2).
   d. Familial Paraganglioma Syndrome:
      - Associated with mutations in the succinate dehydrogenase subunit genes (*SDHx*: *SDHA, SDHAF2, SDHB, SDHC, SDHD*).
3. Biochemical screening:
   a. 24-hour urine fractionated metanephrines (metanephrine and normetanephrine) and catecholamines (adrenaline, noradrenaline, dopamine) for 3 days (3 samples).
   b. 24-hour urine vanillylmandelic acid for 3 days (3 samples).
   c. Plasma-fractionated metanephrines (drawn from indwelling cannula following 30 minutes of supine rest): if high index of suspicion.
   d. Protocol for a 24-hour urine collection:
      i. Withhold interfering drugs for at least 2 weeks:
         - Drugs that increase catecholamine secretion (cocaine, amphetamines, caffeine).
         - Sympathomimetics (phenylephrine, pseudoephedrine, dobutamine, isoprenaline, terbutaline, salbutamol).
         - Alpha-2 blockers (phenoxybenzamine, phentolamine).
         - L-dopa (precursor of catecholamines).
         - Drugs that inhibit catecholamine reuptake or metabolism (tricyclic antidepressants, bupropion, reboxetine, viloxazine, antipsychotics, monoamine oxidase inhibitors, prochlorperazine, reserpine).
         - Drugs that influence the spectrometry measurements (labetalol, sotalol, isoproterenolol, acetaminophen).

ii. Dietary restrictions for 2 days prior to urine collection (no coffee, tea, bananas, cocoa products, vanilla products).
iii. Avoid stress and strenuous exercise, during the urine collection.
iv. Urine should be collected in a bottle containing added acid (to ensure stability of urinary catecholamines).

4. Indications for localization of tumor:
   a. Increase in urine catecholamines at least 2 times above the upper limit.
   b. Increase in urine fractionated metanephrines above the upper limit of normal.
   c. Significant increase in fractionated plasma metanephrine levels.
5. Imaging techniques:
   a. Adrenal/abdominal CT scan or MRI for screening for tumors.
   b. Scinitiscan [$^{123 \text{ or } 131}$I] meta-iodo-benzylguanidine (MIBG) or ^{111}In pentetreotide:
      i. Specific for adrenaline-producing tumors.
      ii. Patients should receive oral non-radioactive iodine before the administration of radiolabeled MIBG to compete with free radioactive iodine, minimizing radioactive exposure to the thyroid gland.
      iii. Avoid drugs that inhibit the uptake of MIBG prior to the scan:
         - Propranolol
         - Labetolol
         - Calcium channel blockers
         - Phenylephrine
         - Pseudoephedrine
         - Phenothiazines
         - Tricyclic antidepressants
         - Monoamine oxidase Inhibitors.
      iv. False negative rate of 10%.
   c. Positron emission tomography (PET)-CT scan:
      i. Identifies metabolically active lesions.
      ii. Types of PET-CT scan include:
         - Gallium (^{68}Ga) 1,4,7,10-tetraazacyclododecane-1,4,7,10-tetraacetic acid (DOTA)-octreotate (DOTATATE).
         - Fluoro (^{18}F)-3,4-dihydroxyphenylalanine (DOPA).

- Fluoro (^{18}F)-2-deoxy-glucose (FDG).

iii. ^{18}F-FDG PET-CT has the greatest sensitivity for identifying paragangliomas and recurrent tumors.

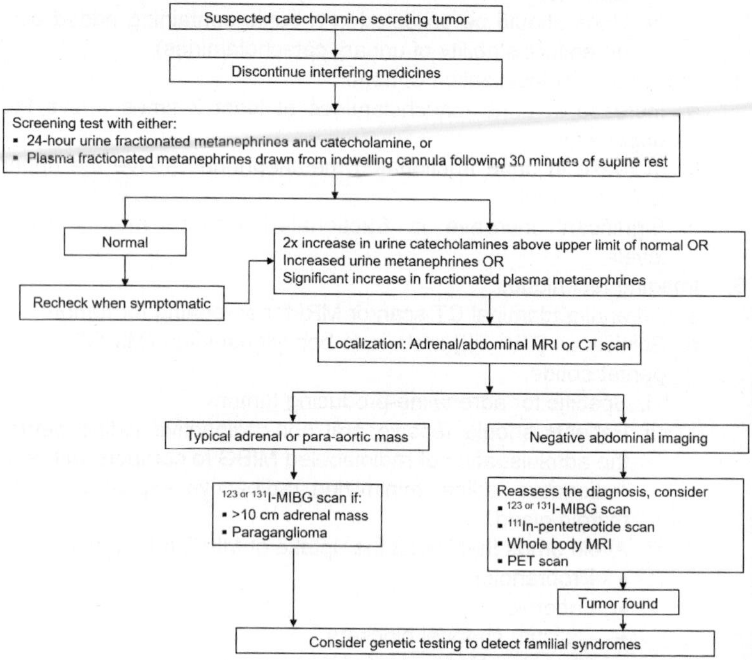

VIII. Workup for patients with suspected renal artery stenosis:

1. Causes of renovascular hypertension:
   a. Fibrous and fibromuscular dysplasia.
   b. Vasculitis:
      - Takayasu disease.
      - Kawasaki disease.
      - Moyamoya disease.
   c. Vascular malformations:

- Thromboembolism, e.g., prior umbilical catheterization.
- Arteriovenous malformation.
- Renal artery aneurysm.

d. Inherited conditions:
- Neurofibromatosis.
- Williams syndrome.
- Klippel–Trenaunay–Weber syndrome.

e. Others:
- Congenital rubella.
- Compression by extrinsic masses.
- Congenital fibrous bands.
- Post-traumatic.
- Retroperitoneal fibrosis.

2. Indications for renovascular imaging:
   a. Young children with hypertension.
   b. Children or adolescents with Stage 2 hypertension.
   c. Children or adolescents with significant diastolic hypertension (especially on ABP monitoring).
   d. Children or adolescents with renal bruit detected on physical examination.
   e. Children and adolescents with notable size discrepancy between the kidneys on standard ultrasound imaging.
   f. Any child or adolescent with hypertension and hypokalemia on screening laboratory investigations.
   g. Any child at risk of renovascular hypertension.
   Note: Even if the peripheral renin activity (PRA) is normal, renovascular imaging should be performed if clinical suspicion is high, as about 15% of children with arteriographically evident renal artery stenosis have normal PRA values.
3. Types of renovascular imaging
   a. Doppler renal ultrasound
      i. Good screening test for renal artery stenosis in normal weight children and adolescents ≥8 years of age.
      ii Can be used to assess the severity of renal artery stenosis by measuring:
         - Peak systolic velocity at stenotic site.
         - Resistive index in the post-stenotic arteries.
   b. Captopril renal scan (MAG3 or DMSA):

i. Less useful in children with RAS as they often have more complicated vascular abnormalities, and should generally be avoided.
ii. Allows comparison between two kidneys.
iii. Captopril is expected to cause a decline in the glomerular filtration rate of the stenotic kidney, often accompanied by an increase in GFR in the contralateral kidney due to the removal of angiotensin II-mediated vasoconstriction. The net effect is that the difference between the two kidneys is enhanced.
iv. MAG3 may be more reliable in patients with renal insufficiency.
v. DMSA has the advantage of being able to demonstrate segmental involvement.
vi. Procedure:
   - Do a baseline DMSA/MAG3 scan before the captopril test.
   - Do a baseline serum creatinine before the captopril test.
   - Patient should stop taking angiotensin-converting enzyme (ACE) inhibitors at least 1 week before the test.
   - Existing non-ACE inhibitor antihypertensive should be omitted on the morning of the test.
   - Ensure normal hydration by non-restrictive fluid intake. Also, give the patient 10 ml/kg of water 30 minutes before the scan.
   - Patient is to lie supine 1 hour before the test.
   - Give oral captopril 1 hour before the test, as per following dose:

Size	Dose
<10 kg	6.25 mg
10–20 kg	12.5 mg
21–40 kg	25 mg
>40 kg	50 mg

   - Do post-captopril DMSA/MAG3 scan.
   - Closely monitor the BP during the scan.
   - Do post-captopril serum creatinine.

c. MR or CT angiography:
   i. Accurate alternative to renal arteriogram but may miss stenosis of accessory renal arteries and more distal portions of renal arteries.
   ii. Limited CT scan prior to angiography also provides information of structure of kidneys, adrenals and surrounding structures.
   iii. MR has the advantage of avoiding ionizing radiation but is contraindicated in children with chronic renal failure due to the use of gadolinium.
d. Selective renal arteriography:
   i. Gold standard for the diagnosis of renal artery stenosis.
   ii. An added advantage is that therapeutic transluminal balloon angioplasty or the placement of bridging stents can be performed.
   iii. Disadvantage of exposing the child to the risk of contrast-induced nephropathy.
   iv. Incidence of severe complications is rare:
      - Intimal tear or injury.
      - Renal artery thrombosis or branch embolus.
e. Selective sampling of renal vein renin:
   i. Performed at the time of renal angiogram to provide evidence of unilateral or bilateral disease.
   ii. Inferior vena cava (IVC) above and below the renal veins should be sampled at the same time as the renal veins.
   iii. Interpretation:
      - Selective renal vein renin concentration ≥1.5 times the concentration in the contralateral kidney indicates renin-mediated hypertension from that kidney.
      - Ratio between renal vein renin from contralateral kidney and caudal IVC <1.3 indicates the suppression of renin production in the contralateral kidney, which occurs if the contralateral kidney is normal.

Recommended Reading

1. Task Force on Blood Pressure Control in Children. (1987) Report of the Second Task Force on blood pressure control in children. *Pediatrics* 79: 1–25.

2. Garovic VD, Hilliard AA, Turner ST. (2006) Monogenic forms of low-renin hypertension. *Nat Clin Pract Nephrol* **2**:624–630.
3. Dionne JM, Abitbol CL, Flynn JT. (2012) Hypertension in infancy: Diagnosis, management and outcome. *Pediatr Nephrol* **27**:17–32.
4. Flynn JT, Daniels SR, Hayman LL, Maahs DM, McCrindle BW, Mitsnefes M, Zachariah JP, Urbina EM. (2014) On behalf of the American Heart Association Atherosclerosis, Hypertension and Obesity in Youth Committee of the Council on Cardiovascular Disease in the Young. Update: Ambulatory blood pressure monitoring in children and adolescents: A scientific statement from the American Heart Association. *Hypertension* **63**:1116–1135.
5. Lurbe E, Agabiti-Rosei E, Cruickshank JK, Dominiczak A, Erdine S, Hirth A, Invitti C, Litwin M, Mancia G, Pall D, Rascher W, Redon J, Schaefer F, Seeman T, Sinha M, Stabouli S, Webb NJ, Wuhl E, Zanchetti A. (2016) European Society of Hypertension guidelines for the management of high blood pressure in children and adolescents. *J Hypertens* **34**:1887–1920.
6. Flynn JT, Kaelber DC, Baker-Smith CM, Blowey D, Carroll AE, Daniels SR, de Ferranti SD, Dionne JM, Falkner B, Flinn SK, Gidding SS, Goodwin C, Leu MG, Powers ME, Rea C, Samuels J, Simasek M, Thaker VV, Urbina EM. (2017) Subcommittee on screening and management of high blood pressure in children. Clinical practice guideline for screening and management of high blood pressure in children and adolescents. *Pediatrics* **140**:e20171904.
7. Whelton PK, Carey RM, Aronow WS, Casey DE Jr, Collins KJ, Dennison Himmelfarb C, DePalma SM, Gidding S, Jamerson KA, Jones DW, MacLaughlin EJ, Muntner P, Ovbiagele B, Smith SC Jr, Spencer CC, Stafford RS, Taler SJ, Thomas RJ, Williams KA Sr, Williamson JD, Wright JT Jr. (2018) ACC/AHA/AAPA/ABC/ACPM/AGS/APhA/ASH/ASPC/NMA/PCNA Guideline for the prevention, detection, evaluation, and management of high blood pressure in adults: A report of the American College of Cardiology/American Heart Association Task Force on clinical practice guidelines. *Hypertension* **71**:1269–1324.
8. Stergiou G, Stambolliu E, Bountzona I, Ntineri A, Kollias A, Vazeou A, Soldatou A. (2019) Home blood pressure monitoring in children and adolescents: Systematic review of evidence on clinical utility. *Curr Hypertens Rep* **21**:64. doi: 10.1007/s11906-019-0967-2.
9. Young WF. (2020, updated) Pheochromocytoma and paraganglioma in children. Edited by: Pappo AS, Geffner ME AG. *UpToDate ONLINE*. http://www.uptodateonline.com.
10. Picone DS, Padwal R, Campbell NRC, Boutouyrie P, Brady TM, Olsen MH, Delles C, Lombardi C, Mahmud A, Meng Y, Mokwatsi GG, Ordunez P, Phan HT, Pucci G, Schutte AE, Sung KC, Zhang XH, Sharman JE. (2020) Accuracy in Measurement of Blood Pressure (AIM-BP) collaborative. How to check whether a blood pressure monitor has been properly validated for accuracy. *J Clin Hypertens (Greenwich)* **22**:2167–2174.
11. Kidney Disease: Improving Global Outcomes (KDIGO) Blood Pressure Work Group. (2021) Clinical practice guideline for the management of blood pressure in chronic kidney disease. *Kidney Int* **99(3S):**S1–S87.

2 Treatment of Hypertension

Prasetyo RV, Sarkar S, Qader MA, Teo S, Lim SH and Yap HK

A. Management of Confirmed Hypertension

1. Stage 1 hypertension allows time for evaluation before initiating treatment unless the patient is symptomatic.
2. Patients with stage 2 hypertension may need more prompt evaluation and pharmacologic therapy.
3. Symptomatic patients with stage 2 hypertension require immediate evaluation and treatment.
4. All children with chronic kidney disease (CKD) and mean arterial pressure (MAP) consistently above the 50th percentile.

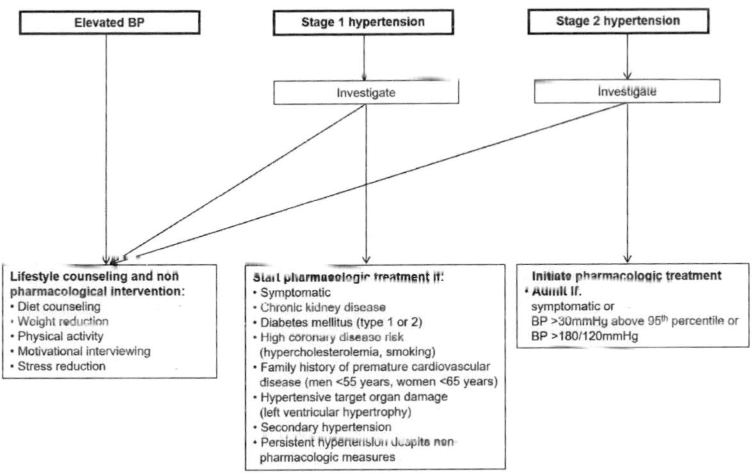

B. Lifestyle and Non-pharmacological Intervention

1. Dietary counseling including Dietary Approaches to Stop Hypertension (DASH) approach:
   - Diet that is high in fruits, vegetables, low-fat milk products, whole grains, fish, poultry, nuts, and lean red meats.
   - Limited intake of sugar and sweets.
   - Lower sodium intake (<2300 mg/day for adults).
2. Physical activity:
   - Moderate to vigorous physical activity at least 3 to 5 days per week (30–60 minutes per session).
   - This helps to reduce systolic blood pressure (BP) by an average of 6.6 mmHg and prevents vascular dysfunction.
3. Motivational interviewing combined with other behavioral techniques to address being overweight and to improve adherence to antihypertensive medications.
4. Stress reduction.
5. Good sleep habits.
6. Avoid smoking and alcohol.

C. Antihypertensive Drug Therapy

I. Principles:

1. Acceptable drug classes in children include angiotensin-converting enzyme (ACE) inhibitors, angiotensin receptor blockers (ARBs), beta-blockers, calcium channel blockers, and diuretics.
2. Recommendations for the initiation of pharmacologic treatment in children and adolescents with hypertension include:
   a. ACE inhibitors.
   b. ARBs.
   c. Long-acting calcium channel blockers.
   d. Thiazide diuretics.
3. Specific classes of antihypertensive drugs should be used in specific clinical circumstances:
   a. ACE inhibitors or ARBs in those with diabetes and microalbuminuria, or proteinuric kidney diseases to prevent left ventricular hypertrophy and proteinuria progression.

   b. Beta-blockers or calcium channel blockers in those with migraines.
4. Initiation of pharmacologic treatment:
   a. Start at the lowest recommended dose, and then increase every 2–4 weeks till the desired BP is reached.
   b. Once the highest recommended dose is reached or if the child experiences side effects, then a second drug from a different class should be added.
   c. Thiazide diuretic is the preferred second agent if there is salt and water retention associated with the hypertensive medication.
5. Certain combinations of drugs have complementary mechanisms of actions, e.g., ACE inhibitors with diuretics, vasodilators with diuretic or beta-blockers.
   a. Routine use of combination therapy is not recommended.
   b. Can be considered once BP control has been achieved to reduce the cost and improve compliance.
6. Monitor electrolytes and serum creatinine periodically in those treated with ACE inhibitors or diuretics.
7. Pure beta-blockers should not be used alone without prior adequate alpha-adrenergic blockade in children with hyperadrenergic states such as pheochromocytoma and metamphetamine overdose.
8. In patients with CKD, the control of proteinuria is important, as this is strongly associated with poor BP control and worsening BP over time.

II. Blood pressure goal:

1. To achieve a BP level that not only reduces the risk for target organ damage in childhood but also reduces the risk for hypertension and related cardiovascular disease in adulthood.
2. To achieve ≤50th percentile 24-hour MAP for age, sex and height in CKD patients, especially in those with proteinuria.

	Uncomplicated Primary Hypertension With No Target Organ Damage	Chronic Kidney Disease
<13 years old	<90th percentile	24-hour mean arterial pressure (MAP) <50th percentile by ambulatory BP monitoring
≥13 years old	<130/80 mmHg	

III. Resistant hypertension

1. Defined in adults as persistently elevated BP despite treatment with 3 or more antihypertensive agents of different classes and all at maximally effective doses, at least one should be a diuretic.
2. Etiology:
   a. Office hypertension.
   b. Poor adherence to medical treatment.
   c. Ingestion of substances that elevate BP:
      - Excess salt
      - Alcohol
      - Sympathomimetic drugs
      - Amphetamines
      - Cocaine
      - Steroids
      - Hormonal contraceptives
      - Calcineurin inhibitors
      - Some antidepressants
      - Non-steroidal anti-inflammatory drugs (NSAIDs).
   d. Lack of administration of more effective drugs (ineffective doses in poor kidney function).
3. Management of resistant hypertension:
   a. Dietary sodium restriction.
   b. Limitation of substances known to elevate BP.
   c. Identification of previously undiagnosed secondary causes of hypertension.
   d. Optimization of current therapy.
   e. Addition of an agent such as an aldosterone receptor antagonist helps address volume excess as well as untreated hyperaldosteronism.

IV. Monitoring of therapy:

1. Monitor BP every 3 to 6 months with standardized auscultatory office BP in children with CKD.
2. ABP monitoring should be done once a year.

V. *Step-down of drug therapy:*

1. Gradual reduction of the drug dosages after an extended course of good BP control.
2. Eventual aim is to completely discontinue the drug.
3. Best candidates are children with uncomplicated hypertension, especially those who were overweight but have successfully lost weight.
4. Continue BP monitoring after cessation of the drug.

VI. *Oral anti-hypertensive drug doses in children and adolescents:*

Drug	Dose	Maximum Dose	Maximum Adult Dose	Comments
ACE inhibitors and Angiotensin II receptor blockers				
Captopril Infants:	0.05 mg/kg/dose 6–24 hourly	6 mg/kg/day		Teratogenic. Check potassium and creatinine within 1 week regularly. FDA approval for child ≥6 years and creatinine clearance ≥30 ml/min/1.73m^2.
Children:	0.5 mg/kg/dose 8 hourly	6 mg/kg/day	50 mg 8 hourly to 450 mg/day	
Enalapril ≥1 month:	0.08 mg/kg/day 12–24 hourly	0.6–1 mg/kg/day 12–24 hourly	40 mg/day 12–24 hourly	
Lisinopril ≥6 years	0.07 mg/kg/day 24 hourly (up to 5 mg)	0.6 mg/kg/day 24 hourly	40 mg/day 24 hourly	
Ramipril	1.6 $mg/m^2/day$ 24 hourly	6 $mg/m^2/day$ 24 hourly	10 mg/day 24 hourly	
Losartan potassium	0.5–0.7 mg/kg/dose 24 hourly	1.4 mg/kg/dose 24 hourly	100 mg/day 24 hourly	

(*Continued*)

(Continued)

Drug	Dose	Maximum Dose	Maximum Adult Dose	Comments
Candesartan 1–5 years	0.02 mg/kg/day 12–24 hourly (up to 4 mg)	0.4 mg/kg/day 12–24 hourly	16 mg/day 12–24 hourly	
≥6 years <50 kg	4 mg/day 12–24 hourly	16 mg/day 12–24 hourly	32 mg/day 12–24 hourly	
≥50 kg	8 mg/day 12–24 hourly	32 mg/day 12–24 hourly	32 mg/day 12–24 hourly	
Irbesartan 6–12 years	75 mg/day 24 hourly	150 mg/day 24 hourly	300 mg/day 24 hourly	
≥13 years	150 mg/day 24 hourly	300 mg/day 24 hourly		
Telmisartan	1 mg/kg/day 24 hourly	2 mg/kg/day 24 hourly	80 mg/day 24 hourly	
Valsartan ≥6 years	1.3 mg/kg/day 24 hourly	2.7 mg/kg/day 24 hourly	160 mg/day 24 hourly	
Beta-blockers				
Atenolol	0.5–1 mg/kg/day 12–24 hourly	2 mg/kg/day 12–24 hourly	100 mg/day	Contraindicated in asthma, heart failure, and diabetes mellitus. Discontinue treatment in event of severe (heart rate <80/minute) or symptomatic bradycardia.
Propranolol	0.2–0.5 mg/kg/dose 6–12 hourly	1.5 mg/kg/dose 6–12 hourly	640 mg/day 6–12 hourly	
Labetolol	1–2 mg/kg/dose 12 hourly	10 mg/kg/dose 6 hourly	600 mg/dose 6 hourly	

(*Continued*)

Drug	Dose	Maximum Dose	Maximum Adult Dose	Comments
Carvedilol	0.1 mg/kg/ dose 12 hourly Increase by 0.1 mg/kg/ dose every 1–2 weeks	0.8 mg/kg/ dose 12 hourly	25 mg 12 hourly	
Calcium channel antagonists				
Amlodipine 1–5 years ≥6 years	 0.1 mg/kg/ day 2.5 mg/day	 0.6 mg/kg/day (up to 5 mg) 10 mg/day	 10 mg/day	
Nifedipine	0.04–0.25 mg/kg/dose 4–6 hourly	1–2 mg/kg/ day 4–6 hourly	10 mg 4–6 hourly	Contraindicated in patients with heart failure and reduced ejection fraction.
Nifedipine Extended Release	0.25–0.5 mg/ kg/day 12–24 hourly	3 mg/kg/day 12–24 hourly	120 mg/day	
Peripheral alpha-antagonists				
Prazosin	Test dose: 5 μg/kg (maximum 0.25 mg); 0.025 mg/kg/ dose 6–12 hourly	0.5 mg/kg/ day 6–12 hourly	40 mg/day 6–12 hourly	Hypotension or syncope may occur especially after first dose.
Terazosin	Test dose: 0.02 mg/kg/ dose; 0.04 mg/kg/ day 12–24 hourly	0.4 mg/kg/ day	20 mg/day	If hypotension occurs at 2–4 hours following dose, change to 12-hourly dosing.

(*Continued*)

(*Continued*)

Drug	Dose	Maximum Dose	Maximum Adult Dose	Comments
Clonidine	2–5 μg/kg/dose 6–12 hourly	10 μg/kg/dose 6–12 hourly	2.4 mg/day	Drowsiness.
>6 years	0.1 mg/24 hourly patch applied every 7 days (= total oral daily dose after titration)	0.3 mg/24 hourly patch applied every 7 days	0.3 mg/24 hourly patch applied every 7 days	Beta-blockers may potentiate bradycardia and may increase rebound hypertension during withdrawal.
Diuretics				
Hydrochlorothiazide	1 mg/kg/day 12–24 hourly	2 mg/kg/day 12–24 hourly	50 mg/day 12–24 hourly	Check electrolytes and creatinine within 1 week and regularly. Potassium supplementation may be required.
Furosemide	0.5–1 mg/kg/dose 6–24 hourly	12 mg/kg/day	240 mg 4–6 hourly (maximum 600 mg/day)	
Bumetanide	0.015 mg/kg/dose 6–24 hourly	0.1 mg/kg/dose 6–24 hourly	10 mg/day	
Vasodilators				
Minoxidil	0.1–0.2 mg/kg/dose 8–24 hourly	10 mg/dose 8–24 hourly		
Hydralazine	0.25 mg/kg/dose 6–12 hourly	25 mg/dose 6–12 hourly		

D. Management of Hypertensive Urgencies and Emergencies

I. Cerebral autoregulation:

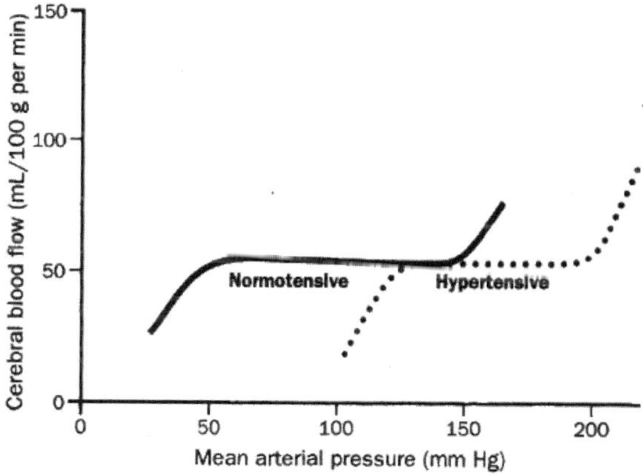

1. As systemic arterial pressure rises progressively, the ability of cerebral vessels to constrict and thereby maintain constant cerebral blood flow, is eventually overcome and these vessels suddenly dilate, inducing hyperperfusion and cerebral edema (PRES — posterior reversible encephalopathy syndrome).
2. A shift to the right in the autoregulation curve occurs with chronic hypertension.
3. In previously normotensive subjects, the upper limit of autoregulation can be as low as a MAP of 120mmHg, equivalent to a BP of 160/100 mmHg.
4. In hypertensive patients, a rapid lowering of BP may result in decreased cerebral perfusion at a higher mean arterial BP than in normotensive subjects.

II. Definitions:

1. Severe acute hypertension is defined as:
   a. Pediatrics: Rise in BP >30 mmHg above the 95th percentile.
   b. Adult: Systolic BP ≥180 mmHg and/or diastolic BP ≥120 mmHg.
2. Hypertensive urgencies (severe asymptomatic hypertension):
   a. Significant elevation of BP without acute end-organ injury.
   b. Minimal or no symptoms, usually a mild headache.
   c. More common in the pediatric population.
3. Hypertensive emergencies:
   a. Defined as an elevation of both the systolic and diastolic BPs with acute end-organ injury including cerebral infarction, cerebral hemorrhage, encephalopathy (altered mental state, seizures), left heart failure and pulmonary edema, and Grade III–IV retinopathy (exudates, hemorrhage and papilledema).
   b. Patients are symptomatic with complaints of headaches, epistaxis, blurred vision, nausea and vomiting.

III. Initial management:

1. Admit the patient to the pediatric intensive care unit.
2. Monitor the patient's vital signs, including:
   a. Glasgow coma scale.
   b. Continuous arterial BP monitoring.
   c. ECG monitoring.
3. Investigations:
   a. Full blood count.
   b. Urea, creatinine, sodium, chloride, bicarbonate, calcium, phosphate, and uric acid.
   c. Arterial blood gas.
   d. Urine microscopy.
   e. ECG.
   f. Chest X-Ray.
   g. CT head if neurological signs present.

4. Identify possible predisposing factors for acute hypertension:
   a. Medication nonadherence.
   b. Ingestion of a salt load.
5. Identify the specific causes of hypertension that may require other management approaches:
   a. Coarctation of the aorta.
   b. Intracranial trauma.
   c. Intracranial mass lesion.
   d. Sympathomimetic drug overdose.
   e. Severe pain.
6. Consider sedation or pain relief with IV midazolam or IV fentanyl.
7. Start the patient on nifedipine (adalat) 5–10 mg stat (oral or sublingual) while preparing for parenteral medications.
8. Choice of parenteral medications depends on the etiology of hypertension and potential complications.

IV. Initial goal of therapy:

1. Hypertensive emergencies:
   a. Treat with intravenous antihypertensive that can produce a controlled reduction of BP, aiming to decrease the systolic BP by ≤25% over the first 8 hours after presentation, and then gradually normalizing the BP over 24 to 48 hours.
   b. Initial rapid decrease in BP may be harmful because there may be disrupted cerebral autoregulation in raised intracranial pressure (ICP), such as in hypertensive encephalopathy or cerebrovascular disease.
   c. The goal is not normalization of BP, but a reduction to a safe level to limit further end-organ damage.
2. Hypertensive urgencies.
   a. The goal of therapy is a reduction in BP within a 24-hour period.
   b. Oral therapy can be considered although parenteral therapy is often preferred.

V. *Anti-hypertensive medications in hypertensive urgencies or emergencies:*

Drug	Dosage	Onset	Duration	Advantages	Caveats
Nifedipine	Oral or sublingual 0.25–0.50 mg/kg q30 mins. Increase dose if ineffective (maximum dose 20 mg).	15–20 mins	2–5 hours		**Only if patient is conscious.** Contraindicated in heart failure with reduced ejection fraction.
Glyceryl trinitrite	Continuous IV infusion 1–10 μg/kg/min (maximum dose 400 μg/min)	At once	3–5 mins	Rapid onset and cessation. Relieves coronary spasm. Reduces preload and to a lesser extent afterload.	Bradycardia. Tachycardia. Headache. Methemoglobinemia. Vomiting.
Sodium nitroprusside	Continuous IV infusion 0.25–8.0 μg/kg/min. Increase the dose by 25% every 5–10 mins until the desired BP control is obtained. Maximum final concentration: 200 μg/ml. If maximum dose is used for >10 mins without good BP control, stop the drug because of toxicity risk.	2 mins	1–10 mins		Contraindicated: • Coarctation of aorta. • Closed head injury. • High ICP. • Intracranial hemorrhage. Chronic use may cause cyanide and thiocyanate accumulation. Do thiocyanate levels if used >48 hours. Toxicity risk increases with decreased kidney or liver function.

Labetalol	IV 0.2 mg/kg over 2 mins. If no response in 5–10 mins, increase to 0.4–1.0 mg/kg (maximum bolus dose 20 mg) OR continuous IV infusion 0.4–1.0 mg/kg/hour (maximum dose 3mg/kg/hour).	5 mins	0.3–23 hours	Favorable cardiac effect. Favorable CNS effect: Use in patients with raised intracranial pressure.	Contraindicated in acute heart failure. Adverse effects: • Reactive airway disease • Heart failure • Heart block • Paradoxical hypertension • Postural hypotension • Hepatitis • Muscle weakness • Urinary retention • Scalp tingling • Burning in throat.
Furosemide	IV 1–5 mg/kg/dose 6 hourly (maximum dose 240 mg) OR continuous IV infusion 0.1–1.0 mg/kg/hour	2–5 mins	2 hours	Drug of choice in acute glomerulo-nephritis with fluid overload.	Hyponatremia. Hypokalemia.
Hydralazine	0.1–0.3 mg/kg (maximum 10 mg) slow IV over 3–5 mins. Repeat every 4–6 hours OR continuous infusion 4–6 µg/kg/min (maximum 300 µg/min)	10–20 mins	3–8 hours	Effective and doses can be repeated if necessary.	Increases ICP. May cause non-homogeneous cerebral perfusion. Tachycardia. Severe headache. Fluid retention.

(Continued)

(Continued)

Drug	Dosage	Onset	Duration	Advantages	Caveats
Nicardipine	Continuous IV infusion 1–3 µg/kg/min (maximum 250 µg/min)	1–2 hours	2–4 hours	Similar to nifedipine without the deleterious risk of depressing myocardial function. Promotes natriuresis.	Elevation of ICP **(avoid in those at risk of raised ICP).** Tachycardia. Flushing. headache. Hypotension. Peripheral edema. Gastrointestinal disturbance.
Esmolol	IV 0.5 mg/kg over 1 min, repeat every 5–10 mins if required. IV infusion of 1.5–18 mg/kg/hour (undiluted 10 mg/ml)	1–2 mins	10–20 mins	Useful during anesthesia to prevent post-intubation hypertension and tachycardia. Useful in acute aortic dissection.	Hypotension. Nausea. Rarely given for >48 hours. ***Avoid in patients where the cause of hypertension is unknown.**
Phentolamine	0.5–0.1 mg/kg stat (maximum dose 5 mg), THEN 5–50 µg/kg/min.	1–2 mins	3–10 hours	Drug of choice in catecholamine excess.	Postural hypotension. Tachycardia. Cerebral vascular spasm. Nausea.

***Avoid pure beta-blockers prior to adequate alpha-blockade in patients with hyperadrenergic states (pheochromocytoma, metamphetamine overdosage).**

VI. Algorithm for treatment of hypertensive urgencies and emergencies:

Hypertensive urgencies or emergencies

If conscious:
Consider **oral/sublingual nifedipine** 0.25-0.50 mg/kg q30 min
Increase dose if ineffective (maximum dose 10 mg)

If no contraindications (allergy):
IV GTN continuous infusion (neat)
1-10 μg/kg/min (maximum 400 μg/min)

If no contraindications (asthma, heart disease, allergy):
IV labetolol push 0.2 mg/kg over 2 min
If no response in 5-10 mins, increase to 0.4-1.0 mg/kg (maximum bolus dose 20 mg)
Continue with continuous IV infusion
0.4-1.0 mg/kg/hr (max 3 mg/kg/hr)
Avoid pure beta-blockers prior to adequate alpha-blockade in patients with hyperadrenergic states (phaeochromocytoma and metamphetamine overdose)

If inadequate response, consider other drugs such as **IV sodium nitroprusside and IV hydralazine**

If acute glomerulonephritis or fluid overload, consider:
IV furosemide 1-5 mg/kg/dose 6H (maximum 240 mg)
OR
Continuous IV infusion 0.1-1.0 mg/kg/hr
Higher dose needed in renal impairment

OR

IV bumetanide 0.02-0.1 mg/kg/dose 6H (maximum 3mg 8H or 10 mg/day)

Recommended Reading

1. Shann F., ed. (2017) *Drug Doses.* 17th Edition. Collective Pty Limited.
2. Lurbe E, Agabiti-Rosei E, Cruickshank JK, Dominiczak A, Erdine S, Hirth A, Invitti C, Litwin M, Mancia G, Pall D, Rascher W, Redon J, Schaefer F, Seeman T, Sinha M, Stabouli S, Webb NJ, Wuhl E, Zanchetti A. (2016) 2016 European Society of Hypertension guidelines for the management of high blood pressure in children and adolescents. *J Hypertens* **34**:1887–1920.
3. Flynn JT, Kaelber DC, Baker-Smith CM, Blowey D, Carroll AE, Daniels SR, de Ferranti SD, Dionne JM, Falkner B, Flinn SK, Gidding SS, Goodwin C, Leu MG, Powers ME, Rea C, Samuels J, Simasek M, Thaker VV, Urbina EM. (2017) Subcommittee on screening and management of high blood pressure in children. Clinical practice guideline for screening and management of high blood pressure in children and adolescents. *Pediatrics* **140**:e20171904.
4. Lexicomp, Inc. (n.d.) Pediatric drug information. *UpToDate ONLINE*. http://www.uptodateonline.com.
5. Kidney Disease: Improving Global Outcomes (KDIGO). (2021) 2021 clinical practice guideline for the management of blood pressure in chronic kidney disease. *Kidney Int* 99(3):S1–S87

1 Management of Childhood Urinary Tract Infection

KWY Kyaw, Teo S, Resontoc LP, Ng KH, Lau PYW and Yap HK

A. Definition of Terms

Urinary tract infection (UTI)	Presence of proliferating bacteria in the urinary tract causing tissue invasion and inflammation.
Upper UTI or pyelonephritis	Infection involving the kidney parenchyma causing systemic and local symptoms.
Lower UTI or cystitis	Infection limited to the lower urinary tract (with acute voiding symptoms as the major feature).
Asymptomatic or covert bacteriuria	Colonization of the urinary tract by uropathogens without causing any symptoms.
Uncomplicated UTI	UTI occurring in a structurally and functionally normal upper and lower urinary tract, with normal kidney function, and a competent immune system.
Complicated UTI	UTI associated with anatomical or functional abnormalities of the urinary tract: a) Evidence of obstructive uropathy: i. Poor urine flow. ii. Abdominal or bladder mass. b) Being seriously ill (toxic). c) Septicemia. d) Raised creatinine. e) Failure to respond to antibiotic treatment within 48 hours.
Recurrent UTI	a) ≥2 episodes of acute pyelonephritis OR b) 1 episode of acute pyelonephritis/upper UTI + ≥1 episode of cystitis/lower UTI OR c) ≥3 episodes of cystitis/lower UTI.

B. Diagnosis of UTI

I. Guidelines for suspecting UTI:

1. All infants and children with unexplained fever ≥38.5°C.
2. Infants and children with alternative site of infection who remain unwell.
3. Infants and children with signs and symptoms suggestive of UTI.

II. Signs and symptoms:

1. Signs and symptoms of UTI differ according to age:

Infants present with non-specific signs and symptoms and therefore the diagnosis of a UTI requires a HIGH INDEX of suspicion.

Age Group		Signs and Symptoms*		
		Most Common ◄——► Least Common		
Infants <3 months		Fever. Vomiting. Lethargy. Irritability.	Poor feeding. Failure to thrive.	Abdominal pain. Jaundice. Hematuria. Offensive urine.
Infants and children ≥3 months	Preverbal	Fever.	Abdominal pain. Loin tenderness. Vomiting. Poor feeding.	Lethargy. Irritability. Hematuria. Offensive urine. Failure to thrive.
	Verbal	Frequency. Dysuria.	Dysfunctional voiding. Changes to continence. Abdominal pain. Loin tenderness.	Fever. Malaise. Vomiting. Hematuria. Offensive urine. Cloudy urine.

*NICE guidelines 2007, updated 2018.

2. Differentiating between upper and lower tract UTI:

Clinical	Upper Tract	Lower Tract
Age	<2 years	≥2 years
Temperature ≥38°C	+	–
Voiding dysfunction	–	+
Suprapubic pain	–	+
Loin pain	+	–
C-reactive protein	Raised	Normal
Kidney involvement: • Raised creatinine • Area of edema on a power Doppler ultrasound • Photopenic area on DMSA scan	+	–

III. Work-up:

1. Urine dipstick:

	Leucocyte (+)	Leucocyte (–)
Nitrite (+)	Send for urine culture. Treat as UTI. Start antibiotics.	Send for urine culture. Start antibiotics (if freshly voided sample was obtained).
Nitrite (–)	Send for microscopy and culture. Start antibiotics only if with good evidence of UTI.	Not UTI. Explore other causes of fever. Send for microscopy if known structural abnormalities of the kidney.

*Dipstick (positive leucocyte esterase and nitrite) is useful to ***rule in*** UTI in children ≥2 years.

2. Urine microscopy:
   a. Standard microscopy (centrifuged sample):

	WBC >5/hpf	WBC 0–5/hpf
Bacteriuria (+)	Send for culture. Treat as UTI.	Send for culture. Treat as UTI.
Bacteriuria (–)	Send for culture. Start antibiotics only if clinically (+) UTI.	Not UTI.

*Microscopy is useful to ***rule out*** disease in all age groups.

b. Enhanced microscopy (uncentrifuged sample using hemocytometer or flow imaging analysis technology):
   - Pyuria defined as ≥10 WBC/mm³.

3. Urine culture is the gold standard in diagnosing UTI.

Method of Collection	Colony Count/ml (Pure Culture)	Probability of Infection (%)*
Suprapubic aspiration	Gram-negative bacilli: Any number Gram-positive cocci: $>10^3$.	>99%.
Transurethral catheterization	$>10^5$. $\geq 5 \times 10^4$. 10^3 to $<5 \times 10^4$. $<10^3$.	95%. Infection likely. Suspicious, repeat. Infection unlikely.
Clean void Boy Girl	$>10^4$. 3 specimens $\geq 10^5$. 2 specimens $\geq 10^5$. 1 specimen $\geq 10^5$. 5×10^4 to 10^5. 10^4 to 5×10^4. $<10^4$.	Infection likely. 95%. 90%. 80%. Suspicious, repeat. Symptomatic: Suspicious, repeat. Asymptomatic: Infection unlikely. Infection unlikely.

*Criteria from the American Academy of Pediatrics, 2011.

a. The following should be considered indeterminate and be repeated:
   i. Significant growth of 2 pathogens.
   ii. A predominant pathogen with a contaminant.
   iii. Intermediate growth of a single pathogen.
b. Contamination rate of urine obtained by the following are:
   i. Bag specimen: 50–60%.
   ii. Clean catch urine (CCU) sample: 26%.
   iii. Transurethral catheterization: 10%.
   iv. Suprapubic aspiration (SPA): 1%.
c. For urine collection, the anterior urethra should be cleaned with an antiseptic solution (0.1% chlorhexidine or povidone-iodine solution).

d. Transurethral catheterization or SPA sample for culture is recommended when a bag or single CCU culture sample is positive on screening.
e. Urine samples for culture should be sent immediately to the laboratory as bacteria continue to proliferate in warm temperatures.
    - If there is a delay in transport, the urine sample should be transported in iced water and stored at 4°C.

4. Diagnosis of UTI:
    a. Definitive diagnosis should be based on both urinalysis results that suggest infection (pyuria and/or bacteriuria) and a positive urine culture.
    b. UTI may be present in the absence of pyuria if the urine is collected early in the disease before the inflammatory response has developed.

C. Imaging

- The prevalence of structural abnormalities in the urinary tract in infants and children with UTI ranges from 10 to 75%.
- About 5–35% have significant obstruction that requires surgery.

I. Goals of imaging:

1. To identify those with underlying structural kidney abnormalities, especially **obstructive uropathies** requiring surgery.
2. To identify those with factors predisposing them to an increased risk of recurrent UTI.
3. To identify those with kidney parenchymal damage (primarily in those with severe or bilateral disease), predisposing them to an increased risk of:
    - Hypertension (38%).
    - Pre-eclampsia in pregnancy

II. Kidney and bladder ultrasound:

1. Non-invasive procedure.
2. Gives information on:
   a. Kidney size and shape.
   b. Bladder size and configuration and bladder wall thickness.
   c. Presence or absence of pelvicalyceal and ureteral dilatation.

Recommendation:
Kidney and bladder ultrasound scan should be done as an initial investigation to detect dilatation secondary to obstruction and other abnormalities in:

- All infants and children aged <24 months following a first febrile UTI.
- All children with presumptive upper tract UTI.
- Children with recurrent UTIs.
- All children with a UTI who have poor growth, hypertension, symptoms suggestive of urinary tract obstruction, or a family history of urinary tract abnormalities.
- Children who do not respond as expected to the appropriate antimicrobial therapy.

III. Micturating cystourethrogram (MCUG):

1. Gives information on:
   a. Bladder lesions.
   b. Urethral lesions, especially posterior urethral valves in boys.
   c. Competence of the vesicoureteric junction, and the grade of vesicoureteric reflux (VUR) if present.
2. Radiation minimization protocols should be used in infants and young children.
3. Can be performed after the acute phase of infection, once the urine has become sterile.

Recommendation:
MCUG is considered in:
- All children aged <2 years with a first febrile UTI, and especially infants whose infections were serious at presentation.
- Boys of all ages with presumptive upper or lower tract UTI and ultrasound abnormalities (to exclude posterior valves).
- Girls aged ≥2 to <6 years with complicated UTI or recurrent UTI.
- Girls aged ≥6 years with complicated UTI or recurrent UTI plus a scar on a DMSA scan.

IV. Contrast-enhanced voiding urosonography (CeVU):

1. Uses an ultrasonographic contrast agent to image the lower urinary tract and detect VUR whilst avoiding radiation.
2. May be more sensitive in detecting some low-grade reflux and can image the urethra in males.

V. ^{99m}Technetium Dimercaptosuccinic acid (DMSA) scan:

1. Gives information on:
   a. Focal areas of decreased uptake indicating:
      i. Acute pyelonephritis in the acute stage.
      ii. Established scars when DMSA scan is done ≥3 months later.
         - 50% of children with scarring had normal MCUGs.
   b. Differential function of the 2 kidneys.
2. Established scars can only be diagnosed 3 months after an acute pyelonephritic episode.
   - If DMSA scan is done within 3 months of the acute infection in young children and demonstrates focal photopenic areas, consider repeating after the child is 5 years old, when IV sedation is not required for the procedure, to confirm the presence of scars.

> *Recommendation*:
> DMSA scan is considered in:
> - All children aged <2 years with febrile UTI.
> - Children aged ≥2 years with clinical evidence of acute pyelonephritis or complicated UTI or recurrent UTI.
>
> Note: Procedure can be delayed until the child is >5 years old when sedation is not required.

VI. Diuretic renography with ^{99m}Technetium Mercaptoacetyltriglycine (MAG3)

1. Gives information on:
   a. Kidney perfusion.
   b. Uptake, excretion and drainage of the radiotracer.
      - T½ >20 minutes suggests true mechanical obstruction rather than nonobstructive pelvicalyceal dilatation.
   c. Differential function of both kidneys.
2. If there is delayed excretion, frusemide at 1 mg/kg is given after 15 minutes.

> *Recommendation*:
> MAG3 renogram is indicated when:
> - Pelvicalyceal dilatation is ≥1.5 cm on ultrasound examination.
> - Vesicoureteric stenosis is suspected in the presence of ureteric dilatation on ultrasound examination, and the absence of VUR on MCUG (requires an empty bladder with a free-draining urine catheter to visualize the vesicoureteric junction).

VII. Algorithm for investigation of UTI:

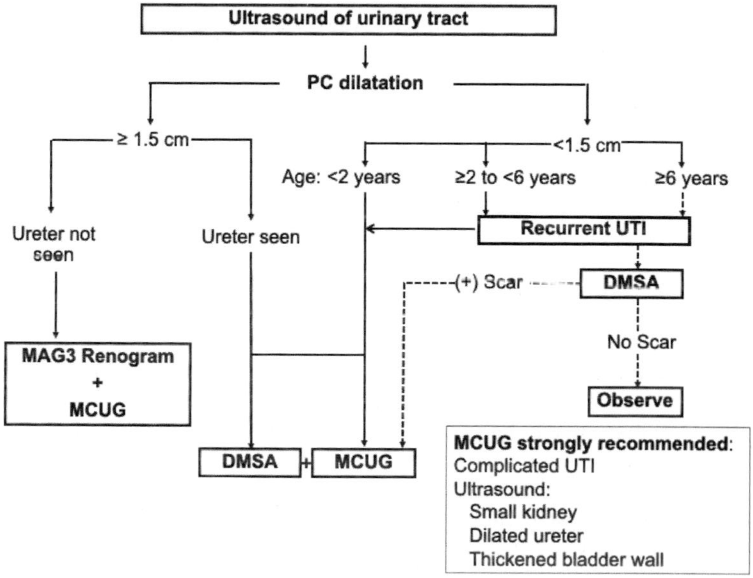

D. Treatment

I. Guiding principles:

1. The drug of choice should be based on the local resistance patterns of the uropathogens as well as recent antibacterial treatment received by the patient.
   - Empiric therapy should also provide adequate coverage for *Escherichia coli*, the most common uropathogen in children.
2. The drug should have minimal adverse effects on the major organ systems.
3. A high concentration of the drug should be present in the urine after administration.
4. Second and third-generation cephalosporins should be avoided as empiric therapy in uncomplicated UTI to avoid increase in antibiotic resistance.

5. Urinary antiseptics such as nitrofurantoin and nalidixic acid should not be the initial drug of choice in upper tract UTI.
6. Duration of therapy should be 10 days for upper tract UTI and febrile complicated cystitis and 5 days for uncomplicated afebrile cystitis in children ≥2 years old.
7. Repeat urine culture is required if:
   - Fever persists after 72 hours of appropriate antibiotic therapy based on antibiotic susceptibility of uropathogen.
   - Uropathogen demonstrates only intermediate sensitivity or resistance to the initial empiric antibiotic.

II. Oral therapy:

1. Oral antibiotics are efficacious in both lower and upper tract UTI, provided the child is adept in taking medicine orally.
2. Oral therapy can be considered in infants >1 month with uncomplicated UTI.
3. Oral amoxicillin-clavulanic acid should be used as first-line empiric therapy in stable children presenting with uncomplicated UTI.
4. Oral cefaclor or cephalexin can be used as first-line empiric therapy in stable children with kidney abnormalities.
5. Ciprofloxacin should be limited to UTI caused by *Pseudomonas aeruginosa* or other multidrug-resistant gram-negative bacteria to minimize bacterial resistance to the fluoroquinolones.
6. In children with penicillin and cephalosporin allergies, treatment with co-trimoxazole or ciprofloxacin is recommended.
7. Commonly used oral antibiotics:

Antibiotic	Frequency	Therapeutic Dose (mg/kg/dose)	Prophylactic Dose (mg/kg ON)
Amoxicillin	Q8 hourly	• 10–25 (maximum 1 g)	• 10
Amoxicillin-Clavulanic acid (Augmentin 7:1)	Q12 hourly	• 10–25 (amoxicillin) (maximum 1 g)	
Ampicillin-sulbactam (Unasyn)	Q12 hourly	• 15–25 (ampicillin) (maximum 2 g)	

(*Continued*)

Antibiotic	Frequency	Therapeutic Dose (mg/kg/dose)	Prophylactic Dose (mg/kg ON)
Cephalexin	Q6 hourly	• 12.5–25 (maximum 500 mg)	• 12.5 (maximum 250 mg)
	Q12 hourly	• 25–50 (maximum 1 g)	
Cefaclor	Q8 hourly	• 10–15 (maximum 500 mg)	• 10
Cefuroxime	Q12–24 hourly	• 10–15 (maximum 500 mg)	
Ciprofloxacin	Q12 hourly	• 5–10 (maximum 500 mg)	
Co-trimoxazole* Trimethoprim (TMP 1 mg) Sulphamethoxazole (SMX 5 mg)	Q12 hourly	• 3–4 (TMP)	• 2
Trimethoprim	Q12 hourly	• 3–4	• 2
Fosfomycin@	Q48–72 hourly^	• ≤1 year: 1 g • >1 to <15 years: 2 g • ≥15 years: 3 g	• Age-adjusted dose given Q7–10 days
Nalidixic acid*#	Q6 hourly	• 7.5–15 (maximum 100 mg) • Reduce to 7.5 after 2 weeks (maximum 50 mg)	• 15 Q12 hourly
Nitrofurantoin*#	Q6 hourly Q8 hourly	• 1.5 (maximum 100 mg) • 2 (maximum 100 mg)	• 1–2 (maximum 100 mg)

*Contraindicated in patients with glucose-6-phosphate dehydrogenase (G6PD) deficiency.
#Avoid in infants <3 months.
@Should not be used for upper tract UTI due to poor systemic absorption.
^Single dose therapy is recommended for uncomplicated cystitis.

III. Intravenous antibiotics:

1. Intravenous antibiotics are indicated in:
   a. Infants ≤1 month of age.
   b. Poor oral intake.
   c. Organisms resistant to effective oral antibiotics.
   d. Complicated UTI.
   e. Immunocompromised patients.
2. Intravenous single high dose gentamicin is the empiric treatment of choice in all age groups with no known kidney abnormalities, changing to oral antibiotics depending on culture results.
3. Intravenous gentamicin and ampicillin should be used in neonates until culture results are available.
   - Ampicillin is included in the regimen to cover the small percentage of infants with enterococcal UTI.
4. Intravenous ceftriaxone is the drug of choice in complicated UTI.
   - Ceftriaxone should be avoided in neonates as it may affect bilirubin transport in the liver.
5. Aminoglycosides should be avoided in patients with abnormal urinary tracts or raised serum creatinine.
6. In complicated UTI, if an aminoglycoside is required based on antibiotic sensitivity results, amikacin is the aminoglycoside of choice as its nephrotoxic potential may be lower than gentamicin.
7. Commonly used parenteral antibiotics — intravenous (IV) and intramuscular (IM):

Antibiotic	Route	Frequency	Dose (mg/kg/dose)	Comment
Amikacin	IV, IM	Single daily dose	• Term neonate: 15 • 1 week to 10 years: 25 (D1), then 18 • >10 years: 20 (D1), then 15 (maximum 1.5 g/day)	• Monitor levels • Trough level <5 mg/L • Renal adjustment
Ampicillin	IV, IM	Q12 hourly (Week 1) Q6 hourly (Weeks 2–4) Q4–6 hourly (Week 4+)	• 10–25 • Severe: 50 (maximum 2 g)	• Renal adjustment

(*Continued*)

Antibiotic	Route	Frequency	Dose (mg/kg/dose)	Comment
Amoxicillin-Clavulanic acid	IV, IM	Q8 hourly	• 30 (maximum 1.2 g/dose)	• Renal adjustment
Cefazolin	IV, IM	Q8 hourly	• 10–15 (adult 500 mg)	• Renal adjustment
		Q6 hourly	• Severe: 50 (maximum 2 g)	
Cefuroxime	IV	Q8 hourly	• 25 (adult 1 g)	
		Q12 hourly (Week 1) Q8 hourly (Week 2) Q6 hourly (>Week 2)	• 25 (adult 1 g)	
Cefotaxime	IV	Q8 hourly (≥Week 4) Q12 hourly (<Week 4)	• 25 (adult 1 g)	
		Q8 hourly (Week 1) Q6 hourly (Weeks 2–4) Q4–6 hourly (>Week 4)	• Severe: 50 (adult 2–3 g)	
Ceftriaxone	IV, IM	Q24 hourly	• 50 (adult 1 g)	• Use with caution in neonates
		Q12 hourly	• Severe: 50 (maximum 2 g)	
Ceftazidime	IV, IM	Q8 hourly Q12 hourly (Week 1)	• 25 (adult 0.5–1 g)	• Renal adjustment
		Q8 hourly	• Severe: 50 (maximum 2 g)	
Ertapenem	IV, IM	Q12 hourly (<12 years)	• 15 (maximum 500 mg) • (Adolescents: 1 g/day)	• Renal adjustment

(*Continued*)

(*Continued*)

Antibiotic	Route	Frequency	Dose (mg/kg/dose)	Comment
Gentamicin	IV, IM	Q24 hourly	• Term neonate to Week 1: 5 • Week 1–10 years: 6 • >10 years: 5 (maximum 240–360 g/day) • Synergistic use: 3	• Monitor levels • Trough level <1 mg/L • Renal adjustment
Meropenem	IV	Q8 hourly	• 10–20 (adult 0.5–1 g)	• Renal adjustment
		Q12 hourly (Week 1) Q8 hourly (>Week 1)	• Severe: 20–40 (maximum 2 g)	
Piperacillin-Tazobactam	IV	Q8 hourly (<6 months) Q6–8 hourly (≥6 months)	• 100	• Renal adjustment

IV. Treatment algorithm for first UTI or uncomplicated UTI:

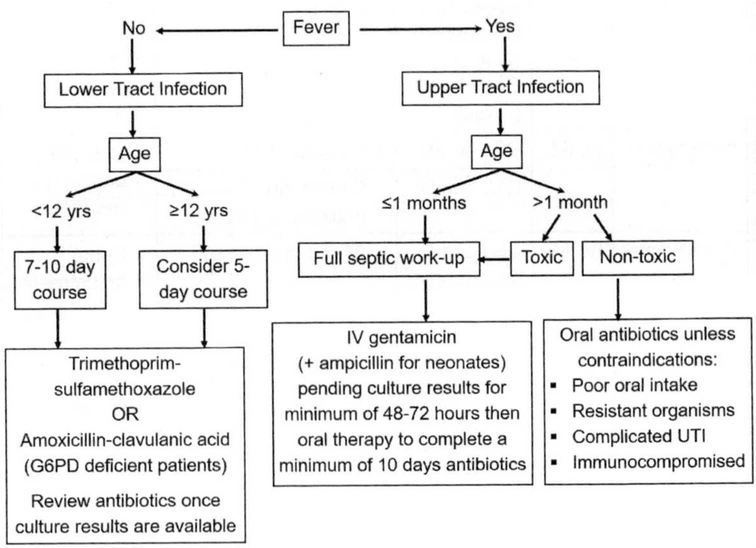

E. Antibiotic Prophylaxis

1. Not routinely recommended in infants and children following first-time UTI.
2. Recommended in:
   a. Infants and children prior to MCUG or other investigations requiring bladder catheterization, starting on the day of procedure for 3 days.
   b. Children aged ≤2 years with dilating VUR (Grades III to V), until at least 2 years after a febrile UTI.
   c. Children aged >2 years with dilating VUR (Grades III to V) and febrile UTI, until at least 2 years after a febrile UTI.
   d. Children with recurrent UTI and non-dilating VUR (Grades I and II), until 2 years after a febrile UTI.
   e. Children with troublesome recurrent UTI, until 6–12 months infection-free.

F. General Measures

1. Infrequent voiding, constipation, phimosis, and poor perineal hygiene increase the likelihood of bacteriuria and predispose to recurrent UTI.
2. Treatment involves the following:
   a. High fluid intake and timed voiding.
   b. Prevention and management of constipation.
   c. Perineal hygiene involving:
      i. Proper wiping of perineum from front to back in girls.
      ii. Keeping the perineal region dry.
      iii. Wearing cotton underwear.
      iv. Avoiding bubble baths if it causes vulval irritation and itch.
3. Cranberry juice has not been shown to be useful for the prevention of recurrent UTI in adult women.
4. Release of preputial adhesions:
   a. 1% hydrocortisone cream applied once daily after bath with gentle pressure, for 3 to 4 weeks for tight foreskin.
      - The prepuce should be retractable after 4–6 weeks.
      - Do not forcefully retract as this will irritate the foreskin.
      - Do not use steroids for more than 3 months, as this may predispose to lichen chronicus et atrophicus.

b. Circumcision can be considered in boys with recurrent UTI.
   - Systemic review has shown that 111 circumcisions would be required to prevent 1 episode of UTI.

Recommended Reading

1. Njoku J, van Schooneveld T. (n.d.) Fosfomycin: Review and use criteria. The Nebraska Medical Center. https://www.nebraskamed.com/sites/default/files/documents/for-providers/asp/Fosfomycin-Drug-REVIEW.pdf.
2. Chu CC, Chen KC, Diau GY. (1999) Topical steroid treatment of phimosis in boys. *J Urol* **162**:861–863.
3. Michael M, Hodson EM, Craig JC, Martin S, Moyer VA. (2003) Short versus standard duration oral antibiotic therapy for acute urinary tract infection in children. *Cochrane Database Syst Rev* (1):CD003966. doi:10.1002/14651858. CD003966.
4. Singh-Grewal D, Macdessi J. Craig JC. (2005) Circumcision for the prevention of urinary tract infection in boys: A systematic review of randomized trials and observational studies. *Arch Dis Child* **90**:853–858.
5. National Institute of Health and Care Excellence (NICE). (2007) Clinical guideline and management of urinary tract infection under 16s — Diagnosis and management. Updated in: 2018.
6. Subcommittee on Urinary Tract Infection; Steering Committee on Quality Improvement and Management. (2011) Urinary tract infection: Clinical practice guideline for the diagnosis and management of the initial UTI in febrile infants and children 2 to 24 months. *Pediatrics* **128**:595–610.
7. Williams G, Craig JC. (2011) Long-term antibiotics for preventing recurrent urinary tract infection in children. *Cochrane Database Syst Rev* (3):CD001534. doi:10.1002/14651858. CD001534.pub3. Updated in: *Cochrane Database Syst Rev* **4**(2019):CD001534.
8. Nagler EVT, Williams G, Hodson EM, Craig JC. (2011) Interventions for primary vesicoureteric reflux. *Cochrane Database Syst* Rev **6**:CD001532.
9. Jepson RG, Williams G, Craig JC. (2012) Cranberries for preventing urinary tract infections. *Cochrane Database Syst Rev* **10**:CD001321. doi: 10.1002/14651858.CD001321.pub5.
10. The RIVUR Trial Investigators, Hoberman A, Greenfield SP, Mattoo TK, Keren R, Mathews R, Pohl HG, Kropp BP, Skoog SJ, Nelson CP, Moxey-Mims M, Chesney RW, Carpenter MA. (2014) Antimicrobial prophylaxis for children with vesicoureteral reflux. *N Engl J Med* **370**:2367–2376.
11. Strohmeier Y, Hodson EM, Willis NS, Webster AC, Craig JC. (2014) Antibiotics for acute pyelonephritis in children. *Cochrane Database Syst Rev* (7):CD003772. doi: 10.1002/14651858.CD003772.pub4.
12. Shaikh N, Hoberman A. (2021) Urinary tract infections in infants older than one month and young children: Acute management, imaging, and prognosis. Edited by: Mattoo TK, Edwards MS, Torchia MM. *UpToDate ONLINE*. http://www.uptodateonline.com.
13. Hoen LA, Bogaert G, Radmayr C, Dogan HS, Nijman RJM, Quaedackers J, Rawashdeh YF, Silay MS, Tekgul S, Bhatt NR, Stein R. (2021) Update of the EAU/ESPU guidelines on urinary tract infections in children. *J Pediatr Urol* **17**:200–207.

2 Management of Primary Vesicoureteral Reflux

Prasetyo RV, Teo S, Resontoc LP and Yap HK

A. Definition of Vesicoureteric Reflux (VUR)

1. Retrograde passage of urine from the bladder into the upper urinary tract.
2. Types of VUR:
   a. Primary VUR: Maturational abnormality of the ureterovesical junction that results in retrograde passage of urine up the ureter during voiding.
   b. Secondary VUR: Due to abnormally high voiding pressures as a result of obstruction or dysfunction of the lower urinary tract, resulting in failure of closure of the ureterovesical junction during bladder contractions.
      - Posterior urethral valve.
      - Neurogenic bladder.
      - Bladder bowel dysfunction (BBD).

B. Prevalence of Primary VUR

1. About 1–3% of healthy children have primary VUR.
2. Age and gender ratios:
   - Infants up to 6 months: M>F (3:1).
   - Infants from 21 to 24 months: F=M (1:1).

	Prevalence of VUR (%)	Sex
After febrile UTI	8–50	F>M (2:1)
Antenatal hydronephrosis	10–17	M>F (2:1)
Sibling/parent with VUR	25/35	

C. Grading of VUR on Micturating Cystourethrogram (MCUG)

1. International Reflux Study Group (IRSG) Classification System

I	II	III	IV	V

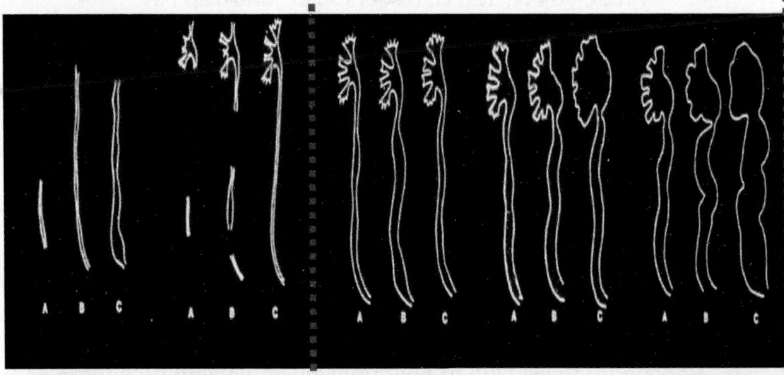

Ureter only	Ureter, pelvis, calyces, no dilatation	Mild dilatation of pelvis	Loss of sharp angle of fornices	Loss of papillary impression with gross dilatation
		Dilating VUR		

2. Ureteral diameter ratio (UDR):
   - Pelvic ureteral width measured at its greatest diameter divided by the distance from the bottom of the L1 vertebral body to the top of the L3 vertebral body.

D. Natural History of VUR

1. VUR occurs in 30–50% of children aged <2 years with urinary tract infections (UTIs).
2. Risk of recurrent UTI:
   a. Meta-analysis showed that antibiotic prophylaxis lowered the risk of UTI in children with VUR, regardless of whether the VUR grade was dilating or non-dilating.

b. Combined surgical and antibiotic treatment versus antibiotics alone did not reduce the risk of febrile UTI for up to 2 years but caused a 57% reduction in febrile UTI by 5 years, but did not result in reduced risk of new or progressive kidney damage at any time point.

3. Rates of spontaneous resolution of VUR after medical management:

VUR Grade	5-year Resolution Rate (%)
I	72.0–87.5
II	61.0–77.6
III	49.0–52.8
IV	12.2–32.0
V	11.0–32.0

- High likelihood of spontaneous resolution of VUR with correction of BBD, which decreases recurrent UTI.

4. Association with kidney scarring:
   a. Development of new scars in children with VUR:

Age of Patient (years)	Frequency of New Scars (%)
<2	19.8
2–4	9.8
≥5	4.6

   b. Kidney scarring is associated with hypertension.
   c. Females, especially those with severe and bilateral scarring, are at risk of pre-eclampsia and hypertension during pregnancy.

E. Diagnosis of VUR

1. VUR can be diagnosed in 5 possible settings:
   a. Following a febrile UTI.
   b. Newborns antenatally detected to have moderate to severe hydronephrosis.

c. Asymptomatic siblings of a patient diagnosed with VUR are at a higher risk of VUR:
   i. Postnatal kidney ultrasound scan may be useful to look for pelvicalyceal and ureteral dilatation.
   ii. Those with dilatation should be monitored closely for 2 years for UTI.
   iii. Those with UTI should be investigated further (see chapter "Management of Childhood Urinary Tract Infections" for age-appropriate investigations).
d. Investigation of congenital abnormality of the kidney and urinary tract (CAKUT), e.g., cystic-dysplastic kidneys.
e. History suggestive of BBD:
   i. Secondary VUR should be excluded.
   ii. May require further urologic investigations including urodynamic studies.
   iii. BBD is associated with:
      - Higher UTI incidence while on antibiotic prophylaxis.
      - Lower rates of resolution of VUR (reflux persistence).
      - Reduced success of endoscopic treatment of VUR.
      - New scarring.

2. MCUG or contrast-enhanced voiding urosonography (CeVUS) is recommended for diagnosis in the following children with presumptive upper tract infection, once bacteriuria has resolved:
   a. Children aged <2 years with first febrile UTI, especially in early infancy.
   b. Girls aged ≥2 to <6 years with complicated UTI or recurrent UTI.
   c. Girls aged ≥6 years with complicated UTI or recurrent UTI, with a scar on DMSA scan.
   d. All boys with febrile UTI.

F. Management of VUR

I. Goal of treatment:

1. Prevention of recurrent UTI.
2. Prevention of kidney damage (kidney scarring).
   - Importance of prompt antibiotic therapy for all febrile UTI.

- Adequate antibiotic treatment in the first 2–3 days of fever significantly reduces the risk of kidney scarring (see chapter "Management of Childhood Urinary Tract Infection" for choices of appropriate antibiotics).

II. Indications for continuous antibiotic prophylaxis:

1. Age ≤2 years with dilating VUR (Grades III–V), until at least 2 years after a febrile UTI.
2. Age >2 years with dilating VUR (Grades III–V) and febrile UTI, until at least 2 years after a febrile UTI.
3. Recurrent UTI and non-dilating VUR (Grades I–II), until 2 years after a febrile UTI.

III. Choice of prophylactic antibiotics:

1. Properties of antibiotics used for urinary prophylaxis:
   a. Should be effective against the majority of the uropathogens.
   b. Do not alter the intestinal flora significantly.
   c. Cause minimal side effects.
   d. Do not lead to the development of bacterial resistance.
2. Antibiotic options:
   a. Trimethoprim 2 mg/kg ON.
   b. Co-trimoxazole 2 mg/kg (Trimethoprim) ON.
   c. Nitrofurantoin 1–2 mg/kg ON.
   d. First- and second-generation cephalosporins:
      - Cephalexin 12.5 mg/kg ON.
      - Cefaclo 10 mg/kg ON.
   e. Fosfomycin: Given once in 7–10 days
      - ≤1 year: 1 g.
      - >1 to <15 years: 2 g.
      - ≥15 years: 3 g.

IV. Surgical interventions:

1. Surgical correction of VUR, namely ureteric reimplantation, has not been shown to be superior to long-term antibiotic prophylaxis in preventing kidney scarring, cortical thinning, or poor kidney growth.

2. Surgery may be best reserved for children with VUR who have recurrent breakthrough UTIs despite adequate antibiotic prophylaxis.
3. Endoscopic correction of VUR such as, subureteric transurethral endoscopic injection (STING) of dextranomer/hyaluronic acid copolymer (Deflux), and its modification technique, hydrodistension implantation technique (HIT), offers an alternative method of correcting VUR.
   a. Success rates for correction of VUR Grades I–V after one treatment:

VUR Grade	Success Rate (%)
I	78.5
II	72.0
III	63.0
IV	51.0
V	51.0

   b. Overall success rate after the second treatment is 68%.
4. Post-surgical radiological investigations should include:
   a. Kidney ultrasound scan at 3 months.
   b. MCUG or CeVUS at 3 months.

G. Follow-up

1. All children with dilating VUR must be closely followed up:
   a. 3 to 4-monthly while still on antibiotic prophylaxis.
   b. 3 to 4-monthly for one year after stopping antibiotic prophylaxis, then 6-monthly for 2 years, then annually thereafter.
2. Parameters to be monitored:
   a. Height, weight and blood pressure at each visit.
   b. Routine urinalysis and cultures in asymptomatic children while on antibiotics and up to one year after stopping antibiotics.
   c. Urine dipstick for protein annually.
   d. Urine protein:creatinine ratio annually when:
      - Urine dipstick is positive for protein.

   - Patients with bilateral kidney scars or a single kidney with scars.
   - From puberty onwards.

   e. Annual kidney ultrasound scans to monitor for kidney growth until the age of 16 years.

   f. Annual kidney function assessment in patients at high risk of progressive kidney disease:
   - Bilateral kidney scars.
   - Single kidney with scars.
   - Low glomerular filtration rate at presentation.

3. Advice to parents/caregivers:
   a. Perform urinalysis, microscopy and cultures whenever symptoms suggestive of UTI occur.
   b. Avoid potentially nephrotoxic drugs such as non-steroidal anti-inflammatory drugs (NSAIDs) if the child has kidney scarring.
   c. Long-term follow-up is necessary for children with cortical scarring or congenital dysplasia, mainly to prevent the development of VUR-related sequelae such as hypertension, pregnancy complications, UTI, or chronic kidney disease.
4. Consider repeat DMSA scan if:
   a. Recurrent acute pyelonephritis.
   b. Photopenic areas are present on the initial early DMSA scan performed within 3 months of UTI.
   - DMSA scans can be performed after the age of 5 years to avoid intravenous sedation.

Recommended Reading

1. Craig JC, Simpson JM, Williams GJ, Lowe A, Reynolds GJ, McTaggart SJ, Hodson E, Carapetis JM, Cranswick NE, Smith G, Irwig LM, Caldwell PHY, Hamilton S, Roy LP; Prevention of Recurrent Urinary Tract Infection in Children with Vesicoureteric Reflux and Normal Renal Tracts (PRIVENT) Investigators. (2009) Antibiotic prophylaxis and recurrent urinary tract infection in children. *N Engl J Med* **361**:1748–1759.
2. Estrada CR Jr, Passerotti CC, Graham DA, Peters CA, Bauer SB, Diamond DA, Cilento BG Jr, Borer JG, Cendron M, Nelson CP, Lee RS, Zhou J, Retik AB, Nguyen HT (2009) Nomograms for predicting annual resolution rate of primary vesicoureteral reflux: Results from 2,462 children. *J Urol* **182**:1535–1541.
3. Skoog SJ, Peters CA, Arant BS Jr, Copp HL, Elder JS, Hudson RG, Khoury AE, Lorenzo AJ, Pohl HG, Shapiro E, Snodgrass WT Diaz M. (2010) Pediatric Vesicoureteral

Reflux Guidelines Panel summary report: Clinical practice guidelines for screening siblings of children with vesicoureteral reflux and neonates/infants with prenatal hydronephrosis. *J Urol* **184**:1145–1151.

4. The RIVUR Trial Investigators, Hoberman A, Greenfield SP, Mattoo TK, Keren R, Mathews R, Pohl HG, Kropp BP, Skoog SJ, Nelson CP, Moxey-Mims M, Chesney RW, Carpenter MA. (2014) Antimicrobial prophylaxis for children with vesicoureteral reflux. *N Engl J Med* **370**:2367–2376.
5. de Bessa J Jr, de Carvalho Mrad FC, Mendes EF, Bessa MC, Paschoalin VP, Tiraboschi RB, Sammour ZM, Gomes CM, Braga LH, Netto JMB. (2015) Antibiotic prophylaxis for prevention of febrile urinary tract infections in children with vesicoureteral reflux: A meta-analysis of randomized, controlled trials comparing dilated to nondilated vesicoureteral reflux. *J Urol* **193**:1772–1777.
6. Wang HHS. (2015) Efficacy of antibiotic prophylaxis in children with vesicoureteral reflux: Systematic review and meta-analysis. *J Urol* **193**:963–969.
7. Williams G, Hodson EM, Craig JC. (2019) Interventions for primary vesicoureteric reflux. *Cochrane Database Syst Rev* **2**(2):CD001532. doi:10.1002/14651858.CD001532.pub5.
8. Edwards A, Peters CA. (2019) Managing vesicoureteral reflux in children: Making sense of all the data. *F1000 Research* **8**:29.
9. Smiljana BK, Selim G. (2020) Vesicoureteral reflux, etiology, diagnostics, treatment and complications-review article. *JMS* **3**(3):93–99.
10. Mattoo TK, Greenfield Sp. (2021, updated) Clinical presentation, diagnosis and course of primary vesicoureteral reflux. Edited by: Baskin LS, Stapleton FB, Kim S. *UpToDate ONLINE*. http://www.uptodateonline.com.
11. Mattoo TK, Greenfield Sp. (n.d.) Management of vesicoureteric reflux. Edited by: Baskin LS, Stapleton FB, Kim S. *UpToDate ONLINE*. http://www.uptodateonline.com.

3 Management of Neurogenic Bladder

Nyo YL, Hoong BYD, Teo S, Lau PYW and Yap HK

A. Definition

1. Neurogenic bladder refers to the impairment of bladder filling or voiding arising from dysfunction or discoordination of the detrusor muscle and external urethral sphincter, which results from a neurological insult affecting detrusor and sphincter innervation.

B. Etiology

1. Spinal dysraphisms:
   - Myelomeningocele (accounts for 80% of neurogenic bladder cases).
   - Lipomeningocele.
   - Sacral agenesis.
   - Diastematomyelia.
   - Tethered cord.
2. Spinal cord lesions:
   - Trauma.
   - Neoplasia.
   - Transverse myelitis.
   - Ischemia.
3. Brain lesions:
   - Cerebral palsy.
   - Trauma.
   - Meningoencephalitis.

4. Pelvic surgery or irradiation:
   - Hirschsprung's disease.
   - Ureteric reimplantation.
   - Bladder rhabdomyosarcoma.
5. Non-neurogenic neurogenic bladder (Hinman's Syndrome).

C. Pathophysiology

1. Neurological control of micturition:
   a. Voluntary control of micturition involves the interplay of the sympathetic, parasympathetic and somatic nervous systems.
   b. Filling phase:
      i. Sympathetic supply from T12–L2 spinal segments travels via the hypogastric nerve to:
         - Inhibit bladder contraction via β-adrenergic inhibitory receptors.
         - Stimulate urethral and bladder neck smooth muscle contraction via α-adrenergic receptors, which increases bladder outlet resistance to facilitate bladder filling.
      ii. Somatic control via the pudendal nerve, arising from Onuf's nucleus in the sacral cord, contributes to contraction of the external sphincter striated muscles to ensure continence.
   c. Voiding phase:
      i. Mechanoreceptors lining the bladder wall send afferent signals to the pontine micturition center.
      ii. After integrating input from higher cerebral centers of micturition control, efferent signals descend the spinal cord to:
         - Inhibit the sympathetic and somatic neurons, resulting in relaxation of the bladder neck and external urethral sphincter.
         - Stimulate parasympathetic activity via the pelvic splanchnic nerves (S2–4), which contracts the detrusor muscles, allowing micturition.
   d. Higher centers of micturition control develop later in childhood, enabling the child to voluntarily void at a socially acceptable time and place.

2. Typical patterns of neurogenic bladder:

	Detrusor Overactivity (DO)	Detrusor Underactivity (DU)
Sphincter Overactivity (SO)	Detrusor/sphincter dyscoordination • Deleterious to kidney function	Incomplete bladder emptying • May be deleterious to kidney function
Sphincter Underactivity (SU)	Urinary incontinence • Not deleterious to kidney function	Urinary incontinence with incomplete bladder emptying • Risk of kidney impairment induced by urinary tract infection (UTI)

*Poor correlation between the etiology and spinal level of neurological insult with the type and severity of bladder dysfunction.

3. Mechanism of bladder and kidney deterioration:
   a. Sustained high intravesical pressure (>40 cmH_2O) due to:
      - Hypertonia or hyperreflexia, with or without the presence of vesicoureteric reflux (VUR).
      - Increase in bladder outlet resistance, e.g., from detrusor-sphincter dyssynergia (DSD), bladder outlet injury and fibrosis, and bladder outlet procedures.
   b. High post-void residual urine predisposing to chronic cystitis and recurrent UTI.

D. Clinical Evaluation

I. Points in history:

1. Assessment of lower urinary tract (LUT) symptoms:
   a. Storage symptoms:
      - Incontinence, nocturia, enuresis, daytime frequency, and urgency

      Note: Differentiate between abnormal storage symptoms and polyuria: Polyuria is defined as urine output >2 $L/m^2/day$ in children.

b. Voiding symptoms:
    - Hesitancy.
    - Straining.
    - Intermittency.
    - Post-void dribbling.
    - Poor urinary stream.
    - Urinary retention.
2. Assessment of bowel habits:
    a. Frequency of stools.
    b. Consistency of stools.
    c. Fecal continence.
3. Determination of etiology.
    a. Antenatal history.
    b. History of neurological impairment.
    c. Psychosocial history and history of urinary retention and constipation to suggest a non-neurogenic neurogenic bladder.
4. Look for complications:
    - Symptoms suggestive of UTI: Urinary frequency, dysuria, abdominal/back pain, nausea, vomiting, fever, foul-smelling urine, and hematuria.

II. Physical examination:

1. Assess growth:
    - Height, weight and head circumference.
2. Assess for complications of urinary tract obstruction:
    a. Measure blood pressure.
    b. Examine the abdomen for ballotable kidneys and palpable bladder.
    c. Look for signs of chronic kidney disease (CKD).
3. Assess for level of neurological lesion:
    a. Skin/back: Midline dimples, tufts of hair, hemangiomata, sinus tracts, scoliosis, kyphosis, vertebral defects.
    b. Neurological examination and gait: Limb atrophy, foot deformities, motor or sensory deficits.
        - In sacral myelomeningocele, bladder dynamics may be affected even if the lower extremity function is preserved.
    c. Anal sphincter tone.

   d. Associated hydrocephalus: Head shape, cranial sutures, fontanelles.
4. Look for features of associated genetic syndromes.
5. Assess for associated bowel dysfunction: Fecal loading.

E. Investigations

1. Assessment of kidney function:
   a. Urea, creatinine, sodium, potassium, chloride, bicarbonate, calcium, phosphate, and uric acid:
      - Renal tubular acidosis type 4 may be associated with obstructive uropathy.
   b. Urine protein:creatinine ratio (UPCR) or a 24-hour urine protein excretion:
      - Consider urine albumin:creatinine ratio (UACR) or 24-hour urine albumin excretion to exclude glomerular proteinuria.
2. Exclude urinary tract infection:
   a. Urine dipstick for leukocytes and nitrites.
   b. Urine microscopy for pyuria, hematuria and bacteriuria.
   c. Urine culture:
      - Interpretation of culture results should be done in conjunction with the presence of symptoms, degree of pyuria on urinalysis as well as the presence of intervention, e.g., clean intermittent catheterization (CIC) and prophylactic antibiotics.
3. Assessment of bladder function/structure:
   a. Bladder diary/frequency volume chart:
      i. Functional capacity vs. expected bladder capacity (EBC)
         - EBC (ml) = 30 x (Age + 1)
         - Maximum capacity: 500 ml.
         - Determination of functional capacity whilst on CIC can contribute towards decisions regarding frequency of CIC and the necessity of augmentation.
      ii. Voiding frequency:
         - Frequent small volume voiding suggests overflow incontinence: Check for high post-void residual urine (PVRU).
      iii. Volume of urine production (day vs. night vs. total):
         - Determination of polyuria or nocturnal polyuria as cause of "incontinence".

b. Stool chart to assess for constipation:
   - Can occur if there is concurrent neurogenic bowel.
   - Can contribute to poor bladder emptying.

c. Uroflowmetry:
   - Non-invasive screening tool for bladder function that can be performed in toilet-trained children.
   - Measures urine volume voided over time.

Parameters	Findings and Interpretation	Flow Rates and Flow Curves
Maximum flow rate (Qmax)	• Normal values for adult size patients: ▪ Males: >25 ml/s. ▪ Females: 30–40 ml/s. • Low Qmax is reflective of outflow obstruction or poor detrusor contractility. • Can be influenced by the voluntary use of abdominal pressure.	• Normogram for children (5–15 years)*: ▪ Girls: 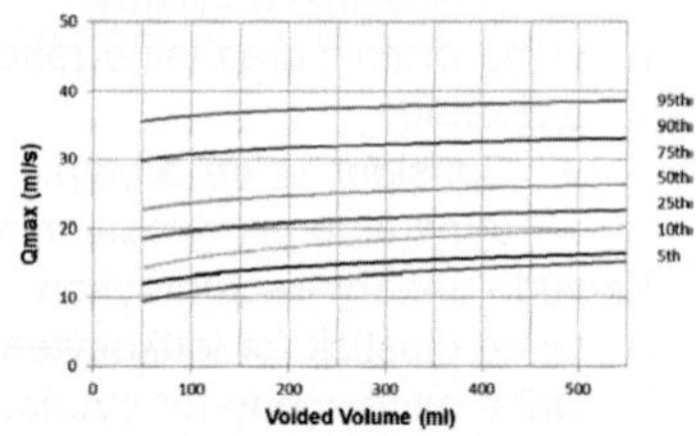 ▪ Boys: 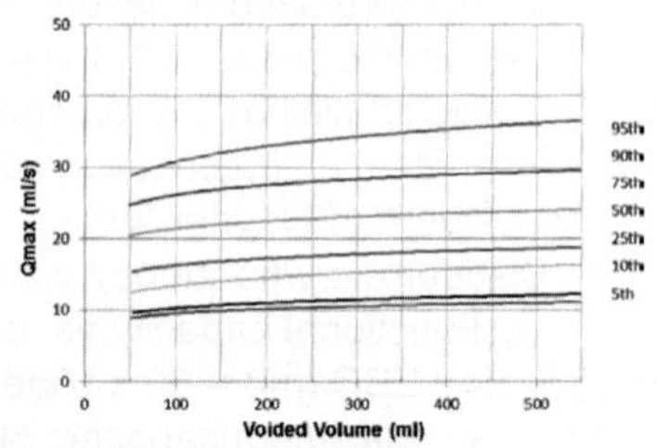
Voided volume	Generally has to be at least 50 ml for the uroflow test to be valid for interpretation.	
PVRU	Considered significant when >10% of EBC or 25 ml.	

(*Continued*)

Parameters	Findings and Interpretation	Flow Rates and Flow Curves
Flow curves	Bell-shaped curve: • Normal.	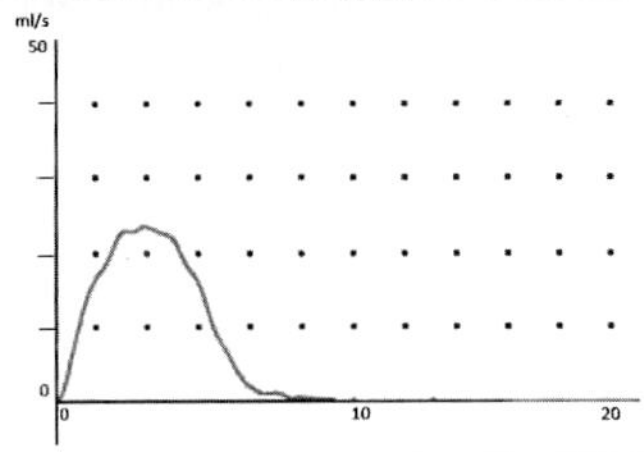
	Plateau-shaped curve: • Suggest outflow resistance or poor detrusor contractility.	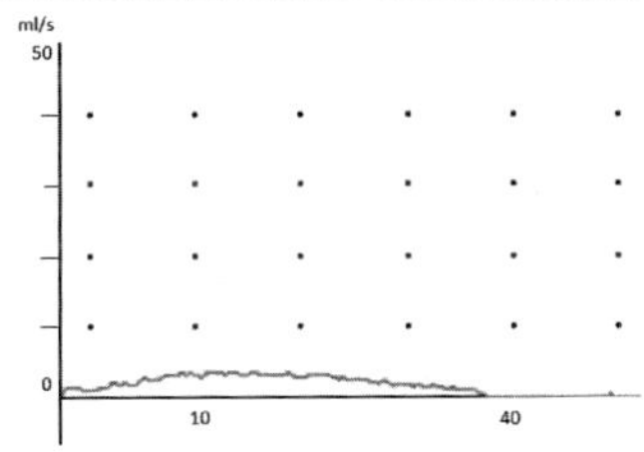
	Intermittent/ interrupted flow pattern: • Suggest dysfunctional voiding.	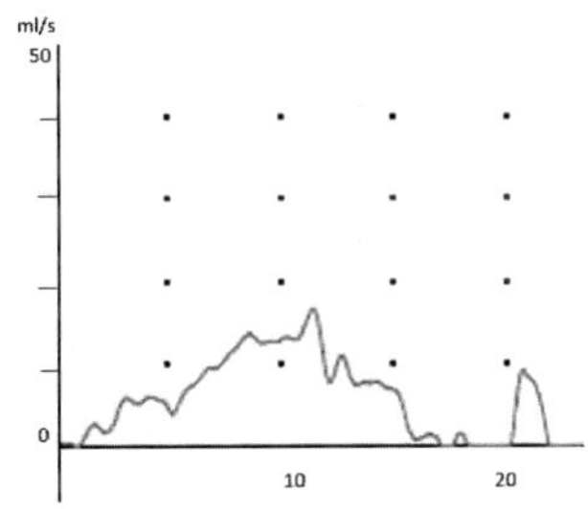

*See (Gupta *et al.*, 2013).

4. Look for structural abnormalities of the urinary tract:
   a. Ultrasound of the kidneys, ureters and bladder (KUB).
      i. Pelviectasis/hydronephrosis and/or hydroureter:
         - Good surrogate indicator of high pressure; If it is new or progressive, it suggests a sustained high-pressure system (>40 cmH_2O).

- If high pressure is suspected, recommend urodynamics study (UDS).

ii. Bladder wall thickness:
- ≥4 mm is significant.
- Poor indication of severity.

iii. Bladder volume:
- Estimated volume (ml) = (3.142 × length × breadth × height)/6

b. Micturating cystourethrogram (MCUG):
i. Bladder size and shape.
ii. Bladder contours: smooth vs. trabeculated.
iii. Presence and grade of VUR.
iv. PVRU.
v. Can be done together with UDS (video UDS).

c. ^{99m}Tc-MAG3 renogram with bladder catheterization:
i. Split kidney function >5% indicates a significant difference.
ii. $T_{1/2}$ >20 minutes with hydroureter may suggest ureterovesical junction obstruction.

d. ^{99m}Tc-DMSA scan:
i. Assess differential kidney function.
ii. Photopenic areas to suggest scarring.

5. UDS +/– electromyography (EMG) +/– contrast (video UDS):
a. UDS: Bladder volume, bladder pressure, detrusor leak point pressure.
b. EMG: Sphincter activity.

Abnormal Findings	UDS/EMG
• Small volume • High pressure • High detrusor leak point pressure (dLPP) • Low compliance	• Normal filling pressure does not exceed 15–20 cmH_2O at capacity. • Sustained pressure above 40 cmH_2O is contributory to upper tract deterioration. • dLPP >40 cmH_2O is a poor prognostic factor for kidney deterioration. • Compliance = Pressure/Volume (steep gradient of the UDS curve)

(*Continued*)

Abnormal Findings	UDS/EMG
	Normal compliance curve: 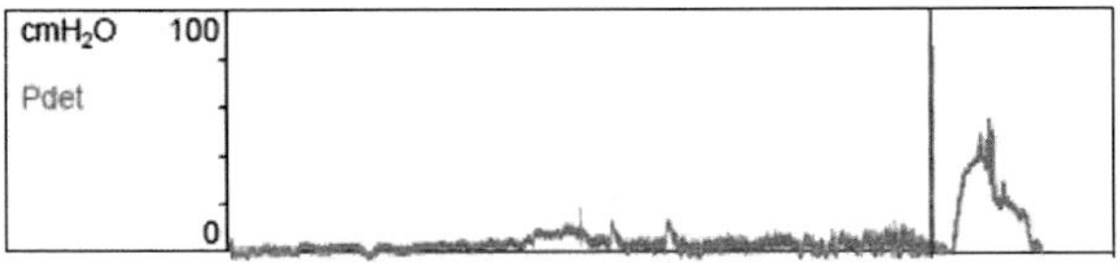 Low compliance curve: 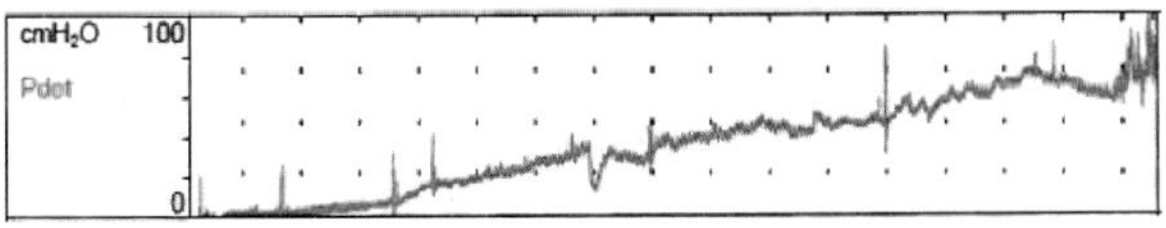
Detrusor/ bladder overactivity (OAB)	• OAB characteristic of neurogenicity. • Can take different forms: Phasic, intermittent, low or high amplitude, etc. • Can be provoked in a normal bladder, e.g., by fast infusion.

F. Management

I. Aims of treatment:

1. Maintaining a stable bladder to preserve kidney function.
   a. Good capacity bladder with compliant detrusor muscle.
   b. Periodic and complete emptying of bladder at low pressure (safe emptying with no post-void residue).
2. Management of bladder and bowel symptoms and maintaining dryness (culturally/socially appropriate).
3. Maximizing independent function and quality of life.

II. General principles of management:

1. Low threshold for adopting CIC with early institution of CIC.
2. Early institution of aggressive anti-cholinergic usage to optimize functional capacity and minimize the need for bladder augmentation.

3. Encourage bladder cycling to optimize functional capacity and minimize the need for bladder augmentation.
4. Regular surveillance with ultrasound KUB to monitor and institute timely intervention to minimize kidney damage.
5. VUR and urinary incontinence secondary to a small volume and a poorly compliant bladder usually improve with bladder augmentation alone.
   - Anti-reflux procedures and bladder neck procedures are usually not separately indicated.

III. CIC:

1. Aims:
   - Eliminate residual urine to reduce UTI risk.
   - Prevent overdistension of the bladder, which can cause hydronephrosis, VUR and CKD.
2. Recommended for all patients with a neurogenic bladder.
3. Early institution of CIC is recommended:
   a. Most children will require CIC for continence by the age of 3.
   b. Initiation of CIC during the neonatal period or infancy improves acceptance, compliance and success, marked by reduced kidney deterioration.
   c. Proper education and training of the caregiver (and patient), clean and atraumatic technique, and good compliance are important for the success of CIC.
   d. Frequency of CIC: This is a function of the degree of compliance and the risks to mitigate.
      - Depends on the objectives of clearance of residual/static urine vs. alleviation of pressure risks vs. achievement of dryness.
      - Usually 4–5x a day with or without an overnight drain to mitigate the risk of sustained high-pressure bladder.
   e. By the ages of 7 to 8 years, children possess sufficient motor skills to perform self-catheterization.
4. Hydronephrosis and VUR develop in $<10\%$ of patients, and social continence is achieved in $>50\%$ of patients on CIC.
5. UTI risk is low as long as complete bladder emptying is achieved.
   - Asymptomatic bacteriuria is to be expected.

IV. *Medical therapy:*

1. Anticholinergics:
   a. Mechanism of action:
      i. Blocks the M3 muscarinic receptor, which mediates detrusor contraction.
      ii. Reduces the frequency of uninhibited detrusor contractions and increases bladder capacity.
   b. Appropriate for patients with high bladder pressures, detrusor hyperreflexia, or VUR.
   c. Early treatment with anticholinergics minimizes the rate of kidney deterioration and the need for bladder augmentation.
   d. Side effects: Dry mouth, dry eyes, constipation, facial flushing, blurred vision, heat intolerance, urinary retention.
   e. Common agents:
      i. Oxybutynin (Ditropan):
         - Infants: 0.1 mg/kg 3×/day.
         - Children 1–5 years: 0.2 mg/kg 2–3×/day (maximum 5 mg/dose).
         - Children >5 years: 5 mg 2–3×/day (maximum 5 mg 4×/day).
      ii. Tolterodine (Detrusitol):
         - Longer-acting anticholinergic suitable for school-going children.
         - Dose: 0.05 mg/kg (adult 2 mg) 12 hourly (maximum 8 mg/day).
         - For kidney and liver impairment: 1 mg 12 hourly (or 2 mg daily).
         - Fewer side effects compared to oxybutynin.
      iii. Solifenacin
         - Dose:
           - 9–15 kg: 2 mg daily (maximum 4 mg/day)
           - 15.1–30 kg: 3 mg daily (maximum 5 mg/day)
           - 30.1–45 kg: 3 mg daily (maximum 6 mg/day)
           - 45.1–60 kg: 4 mg daily (maximum 8 mg/day)
           - >60 kg: 5 mg daily (maximum 10 mg/day)

- For patients with kidney and liver impairment: Keep at the starting dose and do not increase to the recommended maximum dose.
- Side effects: Constipation is more common.

iv. Trospium
- 0.4 mg/kg 12 hourly (maximum 20 mg).

2. Beta-3 Adrenergic agonist (β3-agonist):
   a. Mechanism of action:
      - β3-selective receptor agonist relaxes the detrusor muscle to manage detrusor overactivity.
   b. Side effects: Hypertension, dry mouth, constipation.
   c. Mirabegron:
      i. Use mainly in adolescents and young adults.
      ii. Dose: 25 mg daily
         - Increase to 50 mg after 4–8 weeks (maximum 100 mg daily).
3. Alpha antagonist:
   a. Indication:
      - Use in sphincter overactivity (SO).
   b. Mechanism of action:
      - Smooth muscle relaxants at the bladder neck and proximal urethra.
   c. Common agents:
      i. Prazosin:
         - Dose: 0.005 mg/kg test dose, then 0.025–0.1 mg/kg (adult 1–5 mg) 6–12 hourly.
         - Side effects: Hypotension, palpitations, dizziness, nausea, drowsiness.
      ii. Terazosin:
         - Dose: 0.02 mg/kg test dose, then 0.04–0.4 mg/kg (adult 2–20 mg) daily.
         - Side effects: Hypotension, dizziness, drowsiness, nausea, peripheral edema.
      iii. Tamsulosin:
         - Oral dosage: 0.2 mg once daily (maximum 0.8 mg/day).
         - Side effects: Orthostatic hypotension, dizziness, rhinitis, diarrhea, nausea.

V. Endoscopic botulinum toxin A injections:

1. Indications:
   - Failure of treatment with anticholinergics/antimuscarinics to achieve low pressure, adequate volume.
2. Effects:
   a. Reduction of maximum detrusor pressure by 32–54%.
   b. Increase of bladder volume by 27–162%.
3. Side effects/Disadvantages:
   a. Unable to void to completion with high residual urine necessitating CIC.
   b. Transient effect requiring repeat injections.
   c. Require cystoscopy and general anesthesia.
4. Onabotulinum toxin A:
   a. Maximum dose: 300 IU.
   b. Injected into 20–30 different sites in bladder wall, avoiding the trigone

VI. Management of complications and co-morbidities:

1. UTI
   a. Up to 70% of patients performing CIC have asymptomatic bacteriuria.
   b. Only symptomatic patients should be investigated (urinalysis and cultures) and treated:
      i. Pain with CIC.
      ii. Gross hematuria.
      iii. Back or abdominal pain.
      iv. Fever, lethargy, nausea, vomiting.
   c. Evaluate for the cause of UTI:
      i. Treatment non-compliance, in particular, the frequency of CIC.
      ii. Ineffective treatment.
      iii. Constipation.
      iv. Change in bladder dynamics.
   d. Prophylactic antibiotics are reserved for patients with recurrent symptomatic UTI.

2. VUR:
   a. VUR is secondary to underlying bladder dysfunction.
   b. Adequate treatment of bladder dysfunction is necessary to control VUR.
      - Primary treatment with CIC +/– augmentation should be sufficient and anti-reflux procedures are not usually required.
3. Bowel management:
   a. Neurogenic bowel commonly co-occurs with neurogenic bladder, manifesting as chronic constipation with stool incontinence.
   b. Stool impaction can impair bladder filling and cause urine retention, while stool incontinence increases the risk of bladder contamination and UTI.
   c. Aims of treatment:
      i. Regular bowel emptying.
      ii. Prevention of constipation.
   d. Treatment:
      i. Oral laxatives.
      ii. Enemas.
      iii. Digital evacuation.
      iv. Advanced modalities:
         - Transanal irrigation.
         - Antegrade continence enema (Malone).
4. Psychosexual dysfunction:
   a. Assess the psychological impact of the condition on the child.
   b. Addressing sexuality and fertility should begin before/during puberty.
   c. Thorough counseling should be done before conception.
   d. Females attempting conception should receive folic acid supplementation and maintain adequate vitamin B12 levels.

VII. Role of surgery:

1. Bladder augmentation:
   a. Indication:
      i. Failure of non-operative or conservative management with anticholinergic medications and botox injections.
      ii. High-pressure system with evidence of upper tract deterioration as seen on ultrasound KUB and UDS parameters.

- Not responding to anticholinergics or botox injections OR
- Progressive decline in compliance despite maximal anticholinergics and botox.
- Fast progression/late discovery.

iii. Small incontinent bladder in a patient with maturity and desire for social continence.

b. Types:

i. Enteric bladder augmentation:

- Small bowel.
- Sigmoid or ascending colon.

ii. Ureter:

- Dilated ureter with a non-functioning ipsilateral kidney.

c. Recommend continent diversion procedure (Mitrofanoff procedure) at the same time, as the augmented bladder will require lifelong CIC for emptying.

d. Complications of enterocystoplasty:

i. Accumulation of mucous in an augmented bladder:

- More mucous in the colonic segment compared to the ileal segment.
- Mucus accumulation reduces with time in ileal segment augmentations.
- Consider regular (daily to weekly) bladder washout during the time of CIC with sterile normal saline (in aliquots of 20 ml) to manage excessive mucus accumulation.

ii. Hyperchloremic metabolic acidosis with colonic segment:

- Associated with ammonia reabsorption in patients with severe kidney impairment.

iii. Vitamin B12 deficiency:

- Associated with the use of the terminal part of the ileum for the augmentation
- Avoidable when the last 15 cm of the terminal ileum is not used for the augmentation.

iv. Bladder calculi:

- Associated with mucous production and recurrent urinary tract infections.

v. Secondary malignancies in the augmented bladder.

- Associated with small bowel and large bowel augmentation.

- Annual endoscopic surveillance is recommended to commence 10 years after augmentation.

vi. Perforation:

- Possible contributing factors include overdistension and false passage.

2. Bladder neck/outlet surgery:
   a. Indicated when the bladder outlet is weak, to increase resistance and allow urinary continence.
   b. Should not be done without first achieving a low-pressure reservoir as this can predispose to upper tract deterioration.
   c. Options:
      i. Endoscopic bulking agents.
      ii. Artificial urinary sphincters.
      iii. Bladder neck slings.
      iv. Bladder neck reconstruction at the time of augmentation.
3. Cutaneous urinary diversion:
   a. Types of diversion depend on whether the patient is continent or incontinent.
   b. Continent (Mitrofanoff vs. Monti):
      i. Indications:
         - Patients who are unable or unwilling to perform urethral catheterization.
         - Difficulty for self-catheterization such as female patients who are wheelchair-bound.
         - To improve CIC adherence.
      ii. Can be done at the time of augmentation or on its own if augmentation is not indicated.
      iii. Complications:
         - Stenosis.
         - Leakage.
         - False passage.
         - Malignancy: Squamous cell carcinoma (rare).
   c. Incontinent diversion:
      i. Type:
         - Vesicostomy.
         - Ureterostomy.
      ii. Temporary or permanent.
      iii. No bladder cycling and will promote continued bladder deterioration in exchange for upper tract protection.

iv. Indications:
- When the patient and/or carer are not able to perform CIC at all.
- Major premorbid, intellectually disabled, bed-bound, activities of daily living (ADL) dependent.

v. Complications of vesicostomy:
- Mucosal prolapse.
- Bleeding.
- Skin irritation.
- Malignancy: Squamous cell carcinoma (rare).

VIII. Long-term follow-up:

1. Lifelong multidisciplinary follow-up is required.
2. At every visit, a complete medical history and physical examination should be performed, with a focus on LUT symptoms, bowel habits, treatment compliance/side effects, and psychosexual issues.
3. Regular evaluation of the upper and lower tract is required.
   a. Serum creatinine and UPCR/UACR:
      - 6-monthly for the first year, then
      - Annually if stable.

   b. Ultrasound KUB:
      - 3-monthly in the first year, then
      - 6-monthly in the second year, then
      - Annually thereafter if stable ultrasound findings and bladder management is unchanged.
      - Frequency of surveillance should be increased if there are changes in urinary continence or recurrent UTI.

   c. UDS:
      i. For infants with spina-bifida:
         - UDS should be done at age 3–6 months and 1 year, and then 2-yearly thereafter.

      ii. For new-onset neurogenic bladder or newly discovered neurogenic bladder:
         - UDS should be done at diagnosis as a baseline, then 1–2-yearly depending on the presence of poor prognostic parameters such as high dLPP.

d. MCUG should be done at diagnosis and repeated when:
   i. Planning for surgery.
   ii. Progressive hydronephrosis from ultrasound KUB surveillance with recurrent febrile UTI.

e. DMSA may help monitor patients with recurrent febrile UTI.

4. In patients with worsening LUT symptoms or kidney function, a complete neurological evaluation should be performed, including magnetic resonance imaging (MRI) of the whole spine to exclude a secondary tethered cord or hydrocephalus, or syringomyelia.
5. New neurological changes also mandate a complete investigation of the urinary tract.

Recommended Reading

1. Verpoorten C, Buyse GM. (2008) The neurogenic bladder: Medical treatment. *Pediatr Nephrol* **23**:717–725.
2. Bauer SB. (2008) Neurogenic bladder: Etiology and assessment. *Pediatr Nephrol* **23**:541–551.
3. Fowler CJ, Griffiths D, de Groat WC. (2008) The neural control of micturition. *Nat Rev Neurosci* **9**:453–466.
4. Gupta DK, Sankhwar SN, Goel A. (2013) Uroflowmetry nomograms for healthy children 5 to 15 years old. *J Urol* **190**(3):1008–1013.
5. Stein R, Bogaert G, Dogan HS, Hoen L, Kocvara R, Nijman RJM, Quadackers JSLT, Rawashdeh YF, Silay MS, Tekgul S, Radmayr C. (2020) EAU/ESPU guidelines on the management of neurogenic bladder in children and adolescent part I diagnostics and conservative treatment. *Neurourol Urodyn* **39**:45–57.
6. Stein R, Bogaert G, Dogan HS, Hoen L, Kocvara R, Nijman RJM, Quaedackers J, Rawashdeh YF, Silay MS, Tekgul S, Radmayr C. (2020) EAU/ESPU guidelines on the management of neurogenic bladder in children and adolescent part II operative management. *Neurourol Urodyn* **39**:498–506.
7. Baskin LS. (2021, updated) Myelomeningocele (spina bifida): Urinary tract complications. Edited by: Patterson MC, Wilcox D. *UpToDate ONLINE*. http://www.uptodate.com.
8. Nepple KG. (2021, updated) Management of bladder dysfunction in children. Edited by: Baskin LS, Mattoo TK, Kim MS. *UpToDate ONLINE*. http://www.uptodate.com.

1 Management of Antenatally Diagnosed Hydronephrosis

Pinapala A, Yap HK, Teo S, K Prabhakaran, Nyo YL, Ng KH and Resontoc LP

A. Prevalence

1. Urinary tract dilation (hydronephrosis, hydroureteronephrosis, pyelectasis, and pyelocaliectasis) is detected on prenatal ultrasound in 1–5% of all pregnancies.
2. 90% of antenatal hydronephrosis are detected by 18 weeks gestation and 95% by 22 weeks.
3. 60% of antenatal hydronephrosis are physiological and will resolve before the end of pregnancy or within the first year of life.
4. Fetal urine flow is 4–6 times greater than neonatal urine production, due to differences in renovascular resistances, glomerular filtration rate, and concentrating ability before and after birth. These differences may contribute to ureteric dilatation in-utero in the absence of functionally significant obstruction.
5. 20% of infants with antenatal hydronephrosis have significant uropathy. If diagnosis and treatment are delayed, persistent hydronephrosis can lead to permanent kidney destruction.
6. Mild hydronephrosis detected in the second trimester is more common in fetuses with Down's syndrome compared with normal fetuses.

B. Definitions

1. Renal pelvic diameter (RPD):
   a. Measurement of the maximum anteroposterior diameter (APD) of the renal pelvis.

b. Antenatal hydronephrosis is defined as RPD ≥5 mm at any gestation age and requires postnatal evaluation.

c. The severity of antenatal hydronephrosis is classified based on the RPD measurement of each kidney:

Severity of Hydronephrosis	RPD (mm)		Risk of Kidney Abnormality (%)
	2nd Trimester	3rd Trimester	
Mild	<7	<9	11.9
Moderate	7–10	9–15	45.1
Severe	>10	>15	88.3

2. Society for Fetal Urology (SFU) hydronephrosis grading system:
   - Based on the degree of pelvic dilation, presence of calyceal dilation, and the presence and severity of parenchymal thinning or atrophy.

Grade	Features	IVU	Ultrasound Variants
0	No splitting 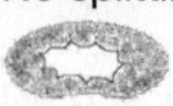		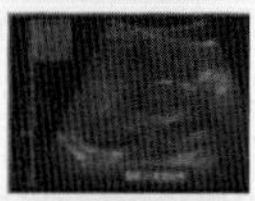
1	Urine in pelvis barely split sinus 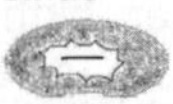		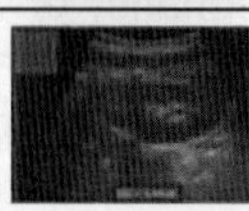
2	Urine fills intrarenal pelvis 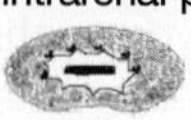	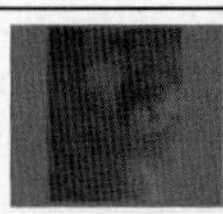	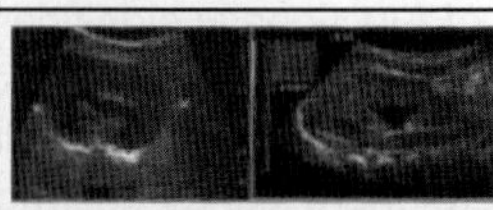
	Urine fills extrarenal pelvis, major calyces dilated 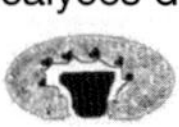	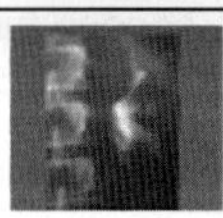	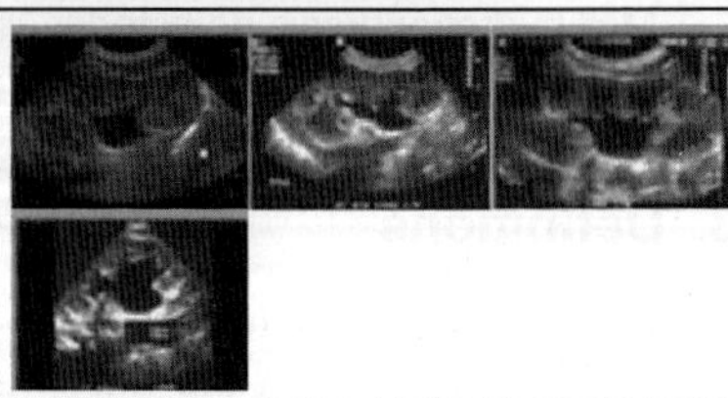

(*Continued*)

Grade	Features	IVU	Ultrasound Variants
3	SFU grade 2 and minor calyces uniformly dilated and parenchyma preserved 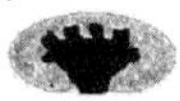	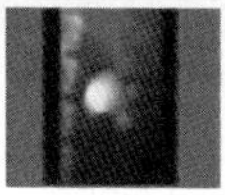	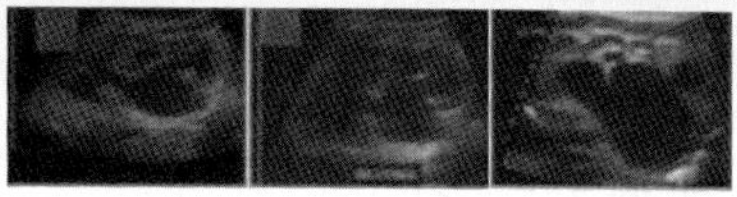
4	SFU grade 3 and thin parenchyma 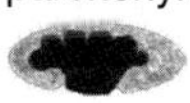	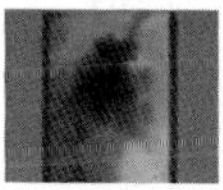	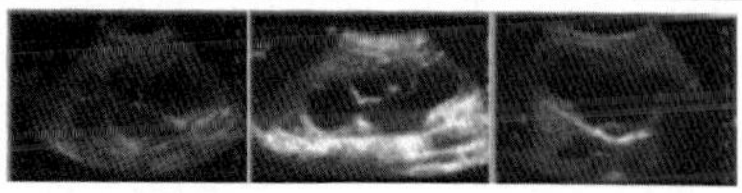

Urinary tract dilation (UTD) classification system:

a. Applies to urinary tract dilation that presents either antenatally or postnatally.
b. Based on 6 ultrasound findings:
   i. Anterior-posterior RPD.
   ii. Calyceal dilatation:
      - Distinguish between central and peripheral after the third trimester.
   iii. Renal parenchymal thickness.
   iv. Parenchymal appearance with respect to echogenicity, presence or absence of cortical cysts and corticomedullary differentiation.
   v. Urologic abnormalities:
      - Ureteral dilatation (transient visualization of ureter postnatally is considered normal).
      - Presence of ureterocele.
      - Dilated posterior urethra.
   vi. Bladder abnormalities including increased wall thickness.

   Note: In antenatal studies, unexplained oligohydramnios is an additional criterion.
c. Stratification is based on the most concerning ultrasound finding.

Grade	APD (mm)		Other Anomalies
	Gestation 16–27 weeks	Gestation ≥28 weeks	
Antenatal Presentation:			
Normal	<4	<7	None
A1 (Low risk)	4 to <7	7 to <10	With or without central calyceal dilation
A2–3 (Increased risk)	≥7	≥10	OR Peripheral calyceal dilation OR Ureteral dilation OR Bladder or renal parenchymal abnormalities OR Unexplained oligohydramnios

Grade	APD (mm)	Other Anomalies
Postnatal Presentation (After 48 Hours of Life):		
Normal	<10	None
P1 (Low risk)	10 to <15	OR Central calyceal dilation
P2 (Intermediate risk)	≥15	OR Peripheral calyceal dilation OR Ureteral dilatation
P3 (High risk)	Any size	AND Abnormal renal parenchymal echogenicity or cysts OR Decreased corticomedullary differentiation OR Bladder abnormalities

C. Evaluation

1. Look for high risk features on the antenatal ultrasound:
   - Any parenchymal abnormality.
   - Calyceal dilatation.
   - Ureterocele.
   - Bladder wall thickening.
   - Bilateral findings.
   - Ureteral dilatation.
   - Oligohydramnios.
   - Lack of urine in bladder.
2. Differential diagnosis of antenatal hydronephrosis:

Etiology	Incidence (%)
Transient hydronephrosis	41–88
Pelviureteric junction (PUJ) obstruction	10–30
Vesicoureteral reflux (VUR)	10–20
Vesicoureteric junction (VUJ) obstruction/megaureter	5–10
Multicystic dysplastic kidney	4–6
Posterior urethral valve/urethral atresia	1–2
Ureterocele/ectopic ureter/duplex system	5–7
Others: Prune belly syndrome, congenital ureteric strictures, megalourethra	Uncommon

3. Important clinical features suggesting specific underlying causes:
   - Abdominal mass due to enlarged kidney: PUJ obstruction or multicystic dysplastic kidneys.
   - Palpable bladder and/or poor stream and dribbling: Posterior urethral valves in a male infant.
   - Abnormalities in the spine and lower limb with patulous anus: Neurogenic bladder.
   - Single umbilical artery: Congenital abnormalities of the kidney and urinary tract (CAKUT), particularly vesicoureteric reflux.
   - Examination for other associated congenital anomalies should also be carried out to exclude syndromic associations such as VACTERL association, prune belly syndrome, branchial-renal-oto syndrome, and retinal-renal syndrome.

- Deformities secondary to oligohydramnios may be present in newborns with severe bilateral urinary tract obstruction: Hip dislocation, talipes equinovarus, and the Potter facies, comprising a receding chin, low set ears, hypertelorism with epicanthic folds, and a compressed broad flat nose.

4. Kidney function should be assessed in general after 48 hours, as serum creatinine values obtained in the first 48 hours may reflect maternal levels.

D. Management

I. Principles

1. In general, antenatal interventions are not required except for watchful monitoring.
2. Pregnancy should be allowed to proceed to term and normal delivery can be allowed in the absence of other complications like severe oligohydramnios or other fetal anomalies.
3. Severe intrauterine urinary obstruction affecting both kidneys in the first trimester can lead to fetal lung hypoplasia presenting clinically at birth as severe respiratory distress that is incompatible with life.
4. Such severe bilateral urinary tract obstruction may also compromise kidney development, resulting in bilateral renal dysplasia and abnormal kidney function, typically described in infants with posterior urethral valves.

II. Unilateral hydronephrosis

1. Most cases of hydronephrosis are not detected by physical examination and, therefore, require kidney ultrasound evaluation postnatally.
2. In prenatally diagnosed severe unilateral hydronephrosis and males with distended bladder and mild to moderate hydronephrosis, ultrasound evaluation should be done after 48 hours of age and within the first week of life.
3. In prenatally diagnosed mild to moderate hydronephrosis, an ultrasound should be done after 7 days to allow increased urine

production to fill the dilated systems and increase the accuracy of the imaging.

4. If postnatal kidney ultrasound demonstrates severe hydronephrosis defined as renal pelvis diameter (RPD) ≥15 mm, a diuretic (furosemide) renogram (MAG3) and micturating cystourethrogram (MCUG) should be performed.
5. If RPD <15 mm, then a repeat ultrasound evaluation should be done at 6 weeks, 3 months and 6 months, then 6-monthly till age 2 years, then yearly.
6. If postnatal kidney ultrasound demonstrates moderate hydronephrosis, defined as RPD >10 mm, associated with dilated calyces and/or parenchymal thinning (SFU Grade 3 or 4), a MAG3 and MCUG should be performed.
7. If postnatal kidney ultrasound demonstrates a dilated ureter, the MCUG should be performed first to exclude primary VUR. If there is VUR, a DMSA scan should then be performed. If there is no VUR, proceed on to a MAG3 renogram with a bladder catheter *in-situ* to exclude VUJ obstruction. Magnetic resonance urography (MRU) can also be considered if VUJ obstruction is suspected.
8. Antibiotic prophylaxis with amoxicillin 10 mg/kg nightly should be given to neonates with RPD ≥15 mm, or those with RPD >10 mm and SFU Grade 3 or 4, or those with a dilated ureter during the evaluation. The amoxicillin dose should be increased to 10 mg/kg 8 hourly on the day of the MCUG or for a MAG3 renogram if there is a bladder catheter *in-situ*. The antibiotics should be continued for 3 days at therapeutic doses.

III. Bilateral hydronephrosis

1. In prenatally diagnosed moderate to severe bilateral hydronephrosis and males with distended bladder with mild to moderate bilateral hydronephrosis, the following procedures should be performed on the first postnatal day:
   a. Ultrasound evaluation, including a detailed evaluation of the bladder for the presence of bladder wall thickening, dilated posterior urethra, and ureterocele.
   b. Renal function test including serum creatinine, electrolytes and acid-base evaluation.

   c. Monitoring of urine output.
   d. Urine microscopy and urine culture, before starting on antibiotic prophylaxis with amoxicillin 10 mg/kg nightly.
2. If postnatal kidney ultrasound demonstrates moderate hydronephrosis, defined as RPD >10 mm or the presence of dilated ureter(s), the MCUG should be performed followed by a MAG3 renogram or DMSA scan to assess the relative kidney function. A MAG3 renogram with bladder catheter *in-situ* or MRU should be considered if VUJ obstruction is suspected, especially in the presence of a dilated ureter.
3. If RPD ≤10 mm with no dilated ureter(s), then antibiotics can be discontinued and a repeat ultrasound evaluation should be done at 1 week, 6 weeks, 3 months and 6 months, then 6-monthly till age 2 years, then yearly. If the subsequent kidney ultrasound demonstrates persistent hydronephrosis defined as RPD >10 mm or the presence of dilated ureter(s), the MCUG should be performed. Monitoring for urinary tract infection should also be done for the first year of life.
4. In prenatally diagnosed mild bilateral hydronephrosis, an ultrasound should be done after 7 days to allow the increased urine production to fill the dilated systems and increase the accuracy of the imaging.

IV. Referral for surgical intervention

1. The decision for surgical intervention should be made by the age of 6 months in infants with PUJ obstruction, as kidney function has been shown to increase significantly in those undergoing surgery at <1 year of age, but normalized in only 1 of 6 patients >1 year of age.
2. Indications for referral for surgical intervention in patients with hydronephrosis include:
   a. Reduced differential function <40%.
   b. Deterioration of differential function >5% from baseline.
   c. Sustained (SFU Grades 3 or 4) or increasing hydronephrosis with half time of drainage of tracer following furosemide injection (T½) >20 minutes.
   d. Suspected VUJ obstruction.
   e. Febrile breakthrough infection or symptoms such as loin pain.

V. Algorithm for management of prenatally diagnosed hydronephrosis

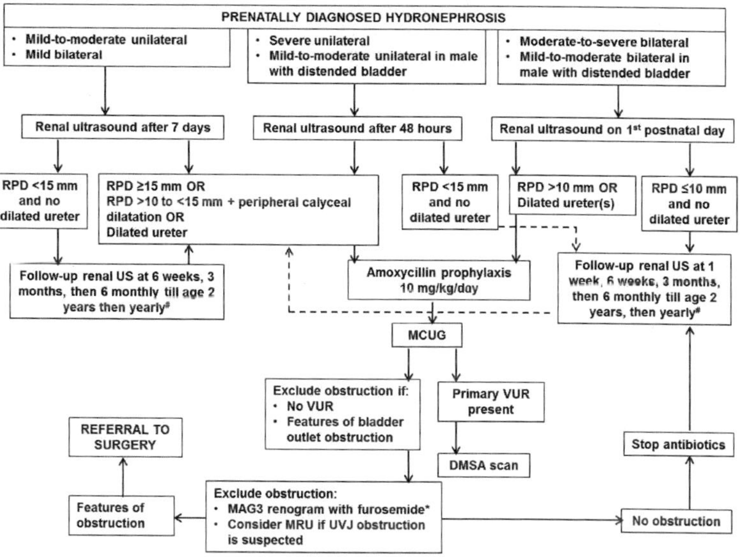

Note: *A MAG3 renogram should be performed with a bladder *catheter in-situ* if VUJ obstruction is suspected.
#Monitoring for urinary tract infection should be performed at least thrice monthly or whenever febrile in the first year of life.

Recommended Reading

1. Nguyen HT, Herndon CDA, Cooper C, Gatti J, Kirsch A, Kokorowski P, Lee R, Perez-Brayfield M, Metcalfe P, Yerkes E, Cendron M, Campbell JB. (2010) The Society for Fetal Urology Consensus statement on the evaluation and management of antenatal hydronephrosis. *J Pediatr Urol* **6**:212–231.
2. Nguyen HT, Benson CB, Bromley B, Campbell JB, Chow J, Coleman B, Cooper C, Crino J, Darge K, Herndon CD, Odibo AO, Somers MJ, Stein DR. (2014) Multidisciplinary consensus on the classification of prenatal and postnatal urinary tract dilation (UTD classification system). *J Pediatr Urol* **10**:982–990.

3. Yalçınkaya F, Özçakar ZB. (2020) Management of antenatal hydronephrosis. *Pediatr Nephrol* **35**:2231–2239.
4. Baskin LS. (2020, updated) Postnatal management of fetal hydronephrosis. Edited by: Wilcox D, Kim MS. *UpToDate ONLINE.* http://www.uptodateonline.com.
5. Baskin LS. (2020, updated) Congenital ureteropelvic junction obstruction. Edited by: Wilcox D, Kim MS. *UpToDate ONLINE*. http://www.uptodateonline.com.

2 Approach to Cystic Kidney Diseases in Children

Liu ID, Chee QZ, Chee QZ, Qader MA, Ng KH, Sultana A, Teo YM, Teo S and Yap HK

A. Introduction

1. Cystic kidney diseases are a group of heterogeneous conditions and can be broadly classified into genetic and non-genetic causes.
2. Renal cysts may arise from different parts of the nephron, or be of non-nephron origin such as tumors.
3. Many cystic kidney diseases occur as part of ciliopathies, which are defects involving the structure or function of cilia.
   - Ciliopathies can affect many organs such as eyes, kidneys, lungs, and the brain.
   - More than 40 genes have been reported to cause ciliopathies.

B. Etiologic Classification

1. Genetic:
   a. Single-gene disorders:
      - Autosomal recessive polycystic kidney disease (ARPKD).
      - Autosomal dominant polycystic kidney disease (ADPKD).
      - Nephronophthisis.
      - Autosomal dominant tubulointerstitial kidney disease (ADTKD).
      - Renal cysts and diabetes (RCAD) syndrome or Hepatocyte nuclear factor-1 beta (HNF1B)-related diseases.
      - Von Hippel–Lindau disease.
      - Tuberous sclerosis complex.

b. Syndromes associated with renal cysts:
   - Ciliopathies.
   - Non-ciliopathies.

2. Non-genetic:
   a. Developmental:
      - Multicystic dysplastic kidney.
      - Cystic dysplastic kidney.
      - Obstructive dysplasia.
   b. Non-developmental/acquired:
      - Simple renal cysts.
      - Multilocular complex renal cysts.
      - Cystic renal tumors.
      - Acquired cystic kidney disease.
      - Hypokalemia-related cysts.
3. Glomerulocystic kidney disease:
   a. Genetic:
      - Single-gene defects (autosomal dominant).
      - ADPKD glomerulocystic type.
      - Syndromic disorders.
   b. Non-genetic:
      - Urinary obstruction.
      - Sporadic/isolated caused by ischemia, drugs or post-hemolytic uremic syndrome.

C. Salient Clinical Features

1. Genetic
   a. Single-gene disorders:

Disease Gene Inheritance	Age of Presentation	Salient Kidney Features	Non-kidney Features
Autosomal recessive polycystic kidney disease (ARPKD): • Fibrocystin/polyductin (*PKHD1*). • DAZ interacting zinc finger protein 1-like protein *(DZIP1L)*. • Autosomal recessive.	• Prenatal, neonatal, infantile or childhood. • Perinatal onset typically has more kidney involvement. • Later onset variants have more liver involvement.	• Presentation: Abdominal masses. Polyuria, polydipsia. Urinary tract infection. Chronic kidney disease (CKD). • Complications: Oligohydramnios. Potter Sequence with pulmonary hypoplasia. Severe hypertension. Hyponatremia in infancy. • Microcysts increase with age. • Kidney size stabilizes or decreases with age.	• Caroli disease. • Caroli syndrome (congenital hepatic fibrosis). • Ascending cholangitis. • Portal hypertension. Note: Usually not present in-utero.
Autosomal dominant polycystic kidney disease (ADPKD): • Polycystin 1 (*PKD1*) (73%).	• Usually 20–40 years. • <1% in utero, neonatal or childhood.	• Presentation: ▪ Incidental finding of cysts. ▪ Positive family history.	• Rare in childhood. • Cysts in other organs (e.g., liver, pancreas). • Subarachnoid hemorrhage.

(*Continued*)

(*Continued*)

Disease Gene Inheritance	Age of Presentation	Salient Kidney Features	Non-kidney Features
• Polycystin 2 (*PKD2*) (14%). • Autosomal dominant with complete penetrance (5–10% de novo mutations).		• Complications (mainly in adults): ▪ Hematuria. ▪ Nephrolithiasis. ▪ Urinary tract infection. ▪ Flank pain. ▪ Hypertension (50% in 20–30 years). • Kidney failure (50% in the 5th to 6th decade). • Cyst number and size increase slowly with age.	• Coronary artery or aortic aneurysms. • Mitral valve prolapse. • Abdominal wall hernias. • Increased risk of renal cell carcinoma. Note: PKD2 have a less severe phenotype than those with PKD1.
Nephronophthisis: • *NPHP1–15.* • *AH11*, *CC2D2A, ATXN10, IFT43, IFT122, IFT140, CEP41* (causative genes unknown in ~30% of cases). • Autosomal recessive.	• Typically 4–6 years old. • Infantile: Median age 1 year. • Juvenile (most common): Median age 13 years. • Adolescent: Median age 19 years.	• Presentation: ▪ Polyuria, polydipsia, enuresis (decreased urinary concentrating ability and sodium reabsorption). ▪ Kidney failure. • Complications: ▪ Normocytic anemia before onset of kidney insufficiency. ▪ Growth retardation out of proportion to the degree of CKD.	• Isolated (no extrarenal). • Syndromic (10–20%): ▪ Hepatic fibrosis. ▪ Retinal defects. ▪ Cerebellar ataxia (cerebello-ocular-renal syndromes).

		▪ Severe hypertension. • Slow decline in kidney function, kidney failure generally before 20 years old. • Infantile variant: Hypertension and rapid progression to kidney failure before 5 years old. • Bland urinalysis.	
Autosomal dominant tubulointerstitial kidney disease (ADTKD):* • Uromodulin (*UMOD*). • Renin (*REN*). • Mucin-1 (*MUC1*). • Autosomal dominant.	• Teenage years to early adulthood.	• Presentation: ▪ Incidental. ▪ Polydipsia and polyuria. ▪ Usually no clinical findings in children. ▪ ESKD in adults. • Bland urinalysis with little or no proteinuria.	• *UMOD*: ▪ Hyperuricemia and gout in teenage years, with decreased fractional excretion of uric acid. • *REN*: ▪ Low or low-normal blood pressure. ▪ Anemia before CKD onset. ▪ Mild hyperkalemia. ▪ Hyperuricemia. • *MUC1*: ▪ Progressive CKD but no other distinguishing characteristics. ▪ Medullary cysts.

(*Continued*)

(Continued)

Disease Gene Inheritance	Age of Presentation	Salient Kidney Features	Non-kidney Features
*(ADTKD-*UMOD*): Uromodulin kidney disease (UKD), medullary cystic kidney disease type 2 (MCKD2), familial juvenile hyperuricemic nephropathy (FJHN) (ADTKD-*MOD*): Familial juvenile hyperuricemic nephropathy type 2 (FJHN2) (ADTKD-*MUC1*): Mucin-1 kidney disease (MKD), medullary cystic kidney disease type 1 (MCKD1)			
Renal cyst and diabetes syndrome (RCAD) or HNF1B-related diseases: • *HNF1B.* • Autosomal dominant (30–50% de novo mutations).	• Any age including prenatal.	• Highly variable: ▪ Large hyperechogenic kidneys. ▪ Multicystic kidney disease. ▪ Renal agenesis. ▪ Renal hypoplasia. ▪ Cystic dysplasia. ▪ Hyperuricemic tubulointerstitial ▪ Nephropathy. • During childhood, kidney size decreases while renal cysts increase in size. • Kidney failure during childhood in 50%. • Renal cell carcinoma later in life.	• Maturity onset diabetes of young type 5 (MODY 5) typical onset in adolescence. • Congenital anomalies of the urinary tract, genital malformations, e.g., uterine, hypoplastic testes. • Exocrine pancreas insufficiency. • Liver abnormalities. • Hyperuricemia and gout. • Hypomagnesemia. • Asymptomatic cholestasis.

Von Hippel–Lindau disease: • *VHL*. • Autosomal dominant.	• Childhood, adolescence or adulthood.	• Renal cysts. • Renal cell carcinoma. • Renal symptoms rare in childhood.	• Rare in children. • Central nervous system (CNS) and retinal hemangioblastomas. • Pheochromocytoma. • Pancreatic cysts.
Tuberous sclerosis complex: • *TSC1* • *TSC2* • Autosomal dominant (de novo mutations are common)	• Childhood.	• Rare in childhood. • Renal angiomyolipomas and angiofibroma. • Renal cysts. • Renal cell carcinoma.	• Facial angiofibromas. • Periungual fibroma. • Hypomelanotic macules. • Shagreen patch. • Retinal hamartoma. • CNS hamartomas. • Subependymal nodule. • Cardiac rhabdomyoma.
Hypoparathyroidism, sensorineural deafness and renal disease (HDR syndrome/Barakat syndrome): • *GATA3*. • Autosomal dominant.	• Childhood.	• Renal cysts. • Dysplasia/hypoplasia. • Nephrocalcinosis. • CKD.	• Hypoparathyroidism. • Hearing loss.

b. Syndromes associated with renal cysts:

i. Ciliopathies:

- A group of disorders associated with genetic mutations encoding defective proteins, which result in abnormal formation or function of cilia.
- Examples include ARPKD, ADPKD, Bardet–Biedl syndrome, Meckel syndrome, Joubert syndrome, nephronophthisis, Senior–Loken syndrome, Jeune asphyxiating thoracic dystrophy, oro-facial-digital syndrome type 1, Ellis–van Creveld syndrome, and Alström syndrome.
- Mutation in a gene can cause heterogeneous phenotypes, while mutations affecting different genes can cause similar phenotypes.
- Typical phenotypic features include kidney abnormalities, in particular nephronophthisis, liver disease, retinal degeneration, and skeletal dysplasias.

Syndrome Gene Inheritance	Kidney Anomalies	Non-kidney Manifestations (*Indicates Key Features)
Senior–Loken syndrome: • *NPHP1, INVS/NPHP2, NPHP3, NPHP4, IQCB1/NPHP5, CEP290/NPHP6, RPGRIP1L/NPHP8, NEK8/NPHP9, SDCCAG8/NPHP10,WDR19/NPHP13, CEP164/NPHP15, TRAF3IP1.* • Autosomal recessive.	• Renal cysts. • Juvenile nephronophthisis.	• Retinitis pigmentosa*. • Leber congenital amaurosis.

(*Continued*)

Syndrome Gene Inheritance	Kidney Anomalies	Non-kidney Manifestations (*Indicates Key Features)
Bardet–Biedl syndrome: • *BBS1, BBS2, ARL6/BBS3, BBS4, BBS5, MKKS/BBS6, BBS7, TTC8/BBS8, BBS9, BBS10, TRIM32/BBS11, BBS12, MKS1/BBS13, CEP290/BBS14, C2ORF86/BBS15, FRITZ, SDCCAG8, TTC21B, CEP164.* • Autosomal recessive.	• Renal dysplasia. • Nephronophthisis. • Renal medullary cysts. • Focal segmental glomerulosclerosis. • Abnormal kidney function.	• Obesity • Postaxial polydactyly*. • Rod-cone dystrophy*. • Learning disabilities. • Hypogonadism*.
Jeune asphyxiating thoracic dystrophy: • *DYN2CH1, IFT80, TTC21B, WDR19, IFT140.* • Autosomal recessive.	• Cystic kidney disease. • Glomerulosclerosis. • Nephronophthisis.	• Skeletal dysplasia (narrow thorax, short ribs*, hypoplastic iliac wings, rhizomelic limb shortening, polydactyly, brachydactyly). • Retinitis pigmentosa. • Fibrocystic disease of liver and pancreas.
Sensenbrenner Syndrome (Cranioectodermal dysplasia): • *IFT122, WDR35, IFT43, WDR19.* • Autosomal recessive.	• Renal cysts. • Nephronophthisis.	• Skeletal dysplasia*, (thoracic deformities, polydactyly). • Retinitis pigmentosa. • Hepatic fibrosis.

(*Continued*)

(*Continued*)

Syndrome Gene Inheritance	Kidney Anomalies	Non-kidney Manifestations (*Indicates Key Features)
Meckel-Gruber syndrome: • *MKS1, TMEM216, MKS3/TMEM67, CEP290, RPGRIP1L, CC2D2A, NPHP3.* • Autosomal recessive.	• Cystic dysplasia (mainly tubular cysts) • Nephronophthisis.	• Occipital encephalocele* and other posterior fossa defects. • Hepatic bile duct proliferation. • Postaxial polydactyly*. • Cleft palate. • Pulmonary hypoplasia.
Joubert syndrome: • *INPP5E, ARL13B, CC2D2A, RPGRIP1L, TMEM67, NPHP1, AH11, CEP290, CXORF5, TMEM216, TTC21B, ZNF423, CEP164, MKS2, ATXN10, CEP41.* • Autosomal recessive.	• Cystic dysplasia. • Nephronophthisis.	• Cerebellar vermis hypoplasia or aplasia*. • Polydactyly. • Hypotonia. • Developmental delay. • Irregular breathing pattern. • Oculomotor dyspraxia.
Cogan syndrome: • *NPHP1, NPHP4.* • Suspected autosomal recessive.	• Nephronophthisis.	• Congenital oculomotor apraxia* (absence or impairment of controlled, voluntary and purposeful horizontal eye movement).

(*Continued*)

Syndrome Gene Inheritance	Kidney Anomalies	Non-kidney Manifestations (*Indicates Key Features)
Oro-facial-digital syndrome type 1: • *OFD1.* • X-linked dominant.	• Renal cysts (majority glomerular cysts).	• Oral malformation (cleft palate, tongue-gingival frenula, abnormal dentition). • Craniofacial anomalies (facial asymmetry, hypertelorism, micrognathia, pseudocleft upper lip). • Coarse thin hair*. • CNS anomalies (intracerebral cysts, agenesis of the corpus callosum). • Digital malformations (brachydactyly, unilateral polysyndactyly*).
Saldino–Mainzer syndrome: • *IFT140.* • Autosomal recessive.	• CKD.	• Short stature. • Phalangeal cone-shaped epiphyses. • Femoral epiphyseal and metaphyseal anomalies. • Retinal pigmentary dystrophy. • Cerebellar ataxia. • Hepatic fibrosis.

ii. Non-Ciliopathies:

Syndrome Gene Inheritance	Kidney Anomalies	Non-kidney Manifestations
Beckwith–Wiedemann syndrome: • Deregulation of imprinting genes within the 11p15.5 region.	• Medullary dysplasia. • Renal cyst (tubular). • Nephrocalcinosis. • Duplicated collecting system. • Medullary sponge kidney. • Nephromegaly.	• Omphalocele. • Macroglossia. • Macrosomia. • Asymmetric overgrowth. • Tumors (Wilms tumor, hepatoblastoma, neuroblastoma or rhabdomyosarcoma).
Renal tubular dysgenesis: • *REN, AGT, ACE, AGTR1.* • Autosomal recessive.	• Renal tubular dysgenesis. • Severe oligohydramnios. • Hypotension.	• Pulmonary hypoplasia. • Skull ossification defects.
Renal-coloboma syndrome: • *PAX2.* • Autosomal dominant.	• Renal hypodysplasia. • Vesicoureteric reflux (VUR). • Multicystic dysplasia (less often). • Pelviureteric junction obstruction (PUJO) (less often).	• Optic nerve coloboma (optic disc split). • Optic nerve dysplasia. • Variable visual impairment. • Sensorineural hearing loss. • Arnold–Chiari malformation. • Seizures. • Joint laxity.
Brachio-oto-renal syndrome: • *EYA1, SIX1, SIX5.* • Autosomal dominant (incomplete penetrance).	• Renal aplasia or hypoplasia.	• Lateral cervical fistulas or cysts. • Periauricular pits. • Anomalies of the middle and external ear. • Hypoplasia of the cochlea. • Hearing loss.

(*Continued*)

Syndrome Gene Inheritance	Kidney Anomalies	Non-kidney Manifestations
Townes–Brocks syndrome: • *SALL1.* • Autosomal dominant.	• Unilateral or bilateral hypoplastic and/or dysplastic kidneys. • Renal agenesis. • Multicystic dysplastic kidney. • Horseshoe kidney. • VUR. • Posterior urethral valves.	• Imperforate anus. • Preaxial polydactyly and triphalangeal thumbs. • External ear anomalies. • Sensorineural hearing loss. • Cardiac anomalies. • Normal intelligence (majority).
Kallmann syndrome: • *KAL1, FGFR1, FGF8, CHD7, PROK2, PROKR2.*	• Unilateral renal agenesis. • Hydronephrosis or VUR (less frequent).	• Hypogonadotrophic hypogonadism. • Anosmia or hyposmia. • Cleft lip. • Heart defects. • Obesity. • Cognitive impairment.
Simpson–Golabi–Behmel syndrome: • *GPC3.* • X-linked.	• Duplicated collecting, megaureter, VUR, and UPJO. • Renal dysplasia and renal cysts, nephromegaly. • Wilms tumor.	• Prenatal and postnatal overgrowth. • Craniofacial anomalies. • Organomegaly. • Increased risk of tumors. • Moderate intellectual deficiency.
Fraser syndrome: • *FRAS1.* • *FREM2.* • Autosomal recessive.	• Bilateral renal agenesis, unilateral renal agenesis and/ or renal cystic dysplasia.	• Cryptophthalmos, coloboma, microphthalmia, or anophthalmia. • Cutaneous syndactyly. • Genital malformations with ambiguous genitalia. • Craniofacial anomalies. • Laryngeal malformations (stenosis or atresia).

(*Continued*)

(*Continued*)

Syndrome Gene Inheritance	Kidney Anomalies	Non-kidney Manifestations
Pallister–Hall syndrome: • *GLI3.* • Autosomal dominant.	• Renal dysplasia.	• Hypothalamic hamartoma. • Central and postaxial polydactyly. • Bifid epiglottis. • Imperforate anus.
Cenani–Lenz syndrome: • *LRP4.* • Autosomal recessive.	• Renal agenesis or hypodysplasia.	• Syndactyly and/or oligodactyly. • Facial dysmorphism.
CHARGE syndrome: • *CHD7.* • Autosomal dominant.	• Unilateral renal agenesis, renal hypoplasia. • Duplex kidneys, UPJO, or VUR.	• Coloboma of the retina or the iris. • Heart anomalies. • Choanal atresia. • Retardation of growth and development. • Genital anomalies. • Ear anomalies.

2. Non-genetic conditions:
   a. Congenital abnormalities of the kidney and urinary tract (CAKUT):

Kidney Anomaly	Salient Clinical Features
Multicystic dysplastic kidney: • Usually sporadic. • Can be familial (*PAX2*).	• Presentation: — Prenatal ultrasound finding. — Incidental abdominal mass at birth. — Urinary tract infection. • Affected kidney is non-functioning. • Bilateral multicystic dysplastic kidneys are not compatible with life due to severe oligohydramnios resulting in lung hypoplasia. • Compensatory hypertrophy of the contralateral kidney suggests a good prognosis.

(*Continued*)

Kidney Anomaly	Salient Clinical Features
	• Concomitant contralateral CAKUT can occur: — VUR (5–43%). — UPJO. • Involution of the affected kidney with time as the cysts shrink due to the absence of urine production: 60% will atrophy and disappear over a period of 5 years.
Renal hypoplasia and/or dysplasia: • Most are sporadic and isolated. • May be familial or syndromic.	• Presentation: — Antenatal ultrasound abnormality. — Incidental finding of unequal kidney sizes on ultrasound postnatally. — Urinary tract infection. — CKD (bilateral cases). • Most patients have both renal dysplasia and hypoplasia. • May be bilateral or unilateral. • Affected kidneys may have decreased or no function. • Concomitant ipsilateral or contralateral CAKUT anomalies may occur. • Look for extrarenal manifestations to decide if this is syndromic.
Obstructive dysplasia:	• Presentation: — Prenatal ultrasound finding. — Postnatal urinary obstruction with a poor urinary stream. — Urinary tract infection. • Due to fetal urinary obstruction such as posterior urethral valves. • Hydronephrosis and hydroureter varying with the degree of urinary obstruction. • Can progress to kidney failure in severe cases

b. Non-developmental or acquired conditions:

Disease	Salient Clinical Features
Simple cyst.	• Ultrasound finding, often incidental. • Rare before 20 years old, may be the first sign of ADPKD.
Multilocular cyst.	• Presentation: — Incidental finding. — Abdominal pain. — Hematuria. • Increased risk of malignancy, suggestive features: — Calcification. — Septa. — Loculation. — Wall thickening. — Contrast enhancement.
Cystic tumors: • Cystic nephroma (age ≤4 years). • Cystic Wilms tumor. • Adrenal hemorrhage. • Lymphangioma. • Clear cell sarcoma. • Cystic renal cell carcinoma.	• Presentation: — Incidental finding. — Painless abdominal mass. — Multilocular cyst comprising solid and cystic components. — Metastatic lesions such as hepatomegaly. • Perform contrast-ultrasound, contrast-enhanced computed tomography (CT), or magnetic resonance imaging (MRI) for better delineation.
Acquired cystic kidney disease: • Occurs in patients with kidney failure, especially dialysis (35–50%) or after liver transplantation.	• Presentation: — Surveillance scans or incidental finding. — Bleeding or infection of cysts. — Flank pain. • With time, cysts can increase in size and numbers. • Incidence increases with dialysis vintage (near 100% after 10 years). • Risk of malignancy: 6% (renal cell carcinoma). • After a kidney transplant, the cysts usually regress but patients continue to have an increased risk for malignancy in the native kidney.

(*Continued*)

Disease	Salient Clinical Features
Hypokalemia-related cyst: • Exclude medullary sponge kidney associated with distal renal tubular acidosis.	• Extent of cyst development correlated with lower potassium levels. • Increased renin and aldosterone levels in patients with chronic hypokalemia. • Normalization of serum potassium, renin or aldosterone can result in regression of the cysts.

D. Stepwise Approach to the Evaluation of Kidney Cystic Disease

I. Step 1: Identify patient with possible cystic kidney disease

1. Clinical presentation:
   a. Abnormal ultrasound findings noted antenatally or incidentally.
   b. Polyuria, polydipsia or secondary enuresis.
   c. Ballotable kidneys or abdominal masses.
   d. Extrarenal manifestations as part of a syndrome or single gene defect.
   e. CKD and/or its related complications (anemia, growth retardation, hypertension).
   f. Urinary tract obstruction.
   g. Urinary tract infection.
2. Consider the age of presentation:

Age	Hereditary Causes (More Likely Bilateral)	Nonhereditary Causes (More Likely Unilateral)
Antenatal and perinatal	• ARPKD. • ADPKD (rare <1%). • Nephronophthisis related ciliopathies. • Glomerulocystic kidney disease / *HNF1B* mutations.	• Dysplasia. • Cystic tumors.

(*Continued*)

(*Continued*)

Age	Hereditary Causes (More Likely Bilateral)	Nonhereditary Causes (More Likely Unilateral)
Childhood and adolescence	• Nephronophthisis-related ciliopathies. • ARPKD. • ADPKD (rare). • Glomerulocystic kidney disease.	• Dysplasia. • Simple/multilocular cysts. • Cystic tumors. • Acquired cystic kidney disease.
Adulthood	• ADTKD. • ADPKD (typical in adulthood). • Glomerulocystic kidney disease.	• Dysplasia. • Simple/multilocular cysts. • Cystic tumors. • Acquired cystic kidney disease.

3. Evaluate the family history:
   a. Consanguinity may suggest autosomal recessive conditions.
   b. Enquire for cystic renal conditions and renal impairment in the nuclear and extended family.
   c. Enquire for the presence of the following conditions in the nuclear and extended family:

Conditions in the Family	Possible Etiology
CAKUT, recurrent urinary tract infection	Monogenic causes of CAKUT such as *TCF2, HNF1B, PAX2*, uroplakins
Liver disease	*PKD1, PKD2, NPHP1–NPHP19*
Precocious gout or hyperuricemia	*UMOD, REN, HNF1B*
Early-onset hypertension	*PKD1, NPHP1–NPHP19*
Early-onset diabetes	*HNF1B*
Recurrent seizures, mental retardation, skin lesions	Tuberous sclerosis complex

   d. In the absence of family history, examine both parents for hypertension, and perform a urinalysis for hematuria and proteinuria, and consider renal ultrasound scans to look for autosomal dominant conditions, in particular, ADPKD.

- An absence of cysts in the parents, especially if they are >30 years old, suggests they do not have ADPKD.
- Affected parents with ADPKD below 25–30 years old may not have cysts detected on ultrasonography yet, and hence, ultrasonographic evaluation of the grandparents may be needed.
- 5–10% of ADPKD cases occur from spontaneous mutations.

e. Consider a postmortem examination and genetic testing of the fetus where applicable.

II. Step 2: Look for distinguishing features that could suggest etiology

1. Renal-related manifestations:
   a. Polydipsia, polyuria and enuresis suggest pathology in the collecting duct (nephronophthisis, ADTKD, ADPKD, ARPKD).
      - Polyhydramnios suggests polyuria.

   b. Hypertension:
      - Severe difficult-to-control hypertension is typical of ARPKD and nephronophthisis.
      - Patients with ADPKD may present with hypertension.

   c. Symptoms of urinary obstruction, such as dribbling and poor urinary stream suggest obstructive dysplasia.
   d. Urinary tract infection, consider:
      - CAKUT with kidney dysplasia.
      - Obstructive uropathy.
      - Cyst infection.

   e. Antenatal factors that predispose to renal hypodysplasia:
      - Teratogens during pregnancy, in particular, angiotensin-converting enzyme (ACE) inhibitors.
      - Intrauterine growth restriction.
      - Maternal vitamin A deficiency.
      - Infant of diabetic mother.

   f. Rapidity of the progression of CKD:
      i. Clinical presentation is dependent on the degree of kidney impairment:
         - Patients with a unilateral abnormality and normal contralateral kidney have normal kidney function.

- Patients with severe bilateral kidney involvement will present at a younger age.

ii. ADPKD can cause a progressive increase in the size and number of the renal cysts, distinguishing it from other etiologies where the increase in cyst size is not as phenomenal.

iii. Progression to kidney failure:
- Childhood/adolescence: ARPKD, nephronophthisis, ADPKD.
- Fifth to sixth decade of life: ADPKD, ADTKD.
- Variable: Glomerulocystic kidney disease.

g. Urine studies:
- Bland urine analysis (no/minimal proteinuria, minimal hematuria) in nephronophthisis and ADTKD.
- Early morning urine to measure urine osmolarity, as defective urinary concentration is seen in nephronophthisis, ADTKD, ADPKD and ARPKD.

h. Serum and urine electrolytes and creatinine to assess fractional excretion:
- Distal renal tubular acidosis suggests medullary sponge kidneys, which is a differential diagnosis for medullary hyperechogenicity.
- Hypercalciuria may be present in Dent disease and nephrocalcinosis.
- Hyperkalemia and propensity to prerenal azotemia suggest *REN* mutation (ADTKD).

2. Extrarenal manifestations:

a. Presence of classical extrarenal manifestations will help *rule in* the diagnosis.

i. The absence of extrarenal manifestations does not rule out a diagnosis as clinical presentations are variable, and some extrarenal manifestations do not manifest in early life.

ii. Extrarenal manifestations commonly affect the brain, eyes, ears, liver, skin, skeletal system.

iii. Liver involvement is common and can manifest as Caroli disease or syndrome:
- Caroli disease: Bile duct ectasia without other apparent hepatic abnormalities.

- Caroli syndrome (more common): Bile duct dilatation associated with congenital hepatic fibrosis.
- Rarely associated with other hepatorenal fibrocystic diseases including Nephronophthisis 13, Meckel–Gruber syndrome, Joubert syndrome and related disorders, Bardet–Biedl syndrome, and oro-facial-digital syndrome type 1.

b. Significant points in history:
   i. Antenatal: Fetal growth may be decreased in syndromic cases.
   ii. Visual anomalies including night blindness.
   iii. Precocious gout and/or hyperuricemia.
   iv. Recurrent seizures.
   v. Mental retardation.
   vi. Diabetes mellitus.

c. Physical examination:
   i. Dysmorphic features.
   ii. Growth retardation:
      - Syndromic patients with short stature due to skeletal dysplasia such as Jeune asphyxiating thoracic dystrophy.
      - Syndromic patients with short stature and obesity such as Bardet–Biedl syndrome.
      - Growth retardation out of proportion to the degree of renal impairment in non-dysmorphic patients suggests nephronophthisis.
   iii. Pubertal status:
      - Hypogonadism.
   iv. Skeletal:
      - Polydactyly, syndactyly, oligodactyly.
      - Small thoracic cage.
      - Joint involvement in gout.
   v. Congenital heart defects.
   vi. Gastrointestinal:
      - Liver involvement with or without portal hypertension.
      - Imperforate anus.
      - Abdominal organomegaly.

vii. Genital anomalies.
viii. Full neurological examination including cerebellar signs.
ix. Head and neck:
- Lateral cervical fistulas or cysts.
- Ear pits.
- Cleft lip/palate.

x. Eye:
- Visual acuity.
- Abnormal eye movements.
- Coloboma.
- Fundoscopy.

xi. Skin lesions suggestive of tuberous sclerosis.
xii. Left-right patterning defects:
- Situs ambiguus.
- Situs inversus.

xiii. Asymmetry or hemihypertrophy.

Ciliopathy Phenotype	Jeune	Senior–Loken	Meckel–Gruber	Bardet–Biedl	Joubert
Cerebellar hypoplasia				√	√
Encephalocele			√		
Hepatic disease	√	√	√	√	√
Mental retardation				√	√
Obesity				√	√
Postaxial polydactyly	√		√	√	√
Retinopathy		√		√	√
Situs inversus		√	√	√	√
Skeletal dysplasia	√		√		
Cleft palate			√		

d. Investigations:

i. Full blood count:
- Anemia with onset before CKD or out of proportion to CKD stage suggests nephronophthisis or *REN* mutations (ADTKD).

ii. Serum uric acid for hyperuricemia (RCAD, *UMOD*, *REN*).
    - Precocious gout (hyperuricemia with reduced fractional excretion of uric acid) with onset in adolescence, unexplained raised serum creatinine, positive family history, and bland urine analysis suggest *UMOD* or *REN* mutations (ADTKD).
    - Fractional excretion of uric acid <6%.

iii. Fasting glucose, HbA_1c for diabetes mellitus (RCAD).

iv. Liver function test:
    - Increased alkaline phosphatase and direct bilirubin seen in Caroli disease/syndrome.
    - Hepatic synthetic function (serum albumin, clotting studies) is preserved initially but can decrease with progressive liver damage due to recurrent cholangitis and biliary obstruction.

v. Renin levels:
    - In *REN* mutations, renin levels are usually in the low-normal range when obtained in a clinical setting that should increase renin levels (under periods of stress).

vi. Hepatobiliary imaging:
    - Hepatobiliary ultrasound to look for liver cysts, increased echogenicity, bile duct anomalies and portal hypertension (with Doppler).
    - Diagnosis of Caroli disease/syndrome can be established using ultrasonography, endoscopic retrograde cholangiopancreatography (ERCP), or magnetic resonance cholangiopancreatography (MRCP) to demonstrate bile duct ectasia and irregular, cystic dilation of the large proximal intrahepatic bile ducts with a normal common bile duct.

vii. Liver biopsy is rarely needed to confirm the type of hepatic lesion:
    - Features of cholangitis.
    - Caroli syndrome: Broad bands of mature fibrosis tissue and distorted bile duct structures characteristic of congenital hepatic fibrosis, hypoplasia of the portal vein branches.
    - Caroli disease: Only ectasia of the larger intrahepatic ducts.

viii. Abdominal and/or pelvic scans to look for:
- Pancreatic cysts.
- Angiomyolipoma.
- Urogenital anomalies (RCAD).

ix. MRI brain if there is cerebral involvement.
- Molar tooth sign suggests Joubert syndrome.

x. Formal ophthalmologic evaluation:
- Examine for minor degrees of coloboma, retinopathy, oculomotor apraxia.
- Consider visual evoked potential studies in newborns.
- Consider an electroretinogram from 8 months of age to detect retinitis pigmentosa.

xi. Formal otolaryngologic evaluation including audiometry.

III. Step 3: Look for distinguishing features on kidney imaging

1. Prenatal sonography:
   a. Sonographic anomalies may be noted as early as 15 weeks gestation.
   b. Severe oligohydramnios leading to Potter sequence and lung hypoplasia suggests a very early onset of bilateral renal involvement.
   c. Serial scans are helpful to assess amniotic fluid volume and appearance of kidneys.
      - In cases with ≥2 renal cysts and/or increased cortical echogenicity, monogenic disease may be found 50–70% of the time.
      - In isolated unilateral multicystic dysplastic kidney or cystic dysplastic kidney, or solitary cysts with normal echogenicity, genetic pathology is rare.
   d. In a fetus with large bilateral hyperechoic kidneys, consider ARPKD, ADPKD and RCAD:

	ADPKD*	ARPKD	RCAD
Fetal kidney sizes	• Moderately enlarged: 1–2 standard deviations (SD) above the mean. • Rarely, one kidney is larger. • Prenatal scans may be normal.	• Very massive: 4–15 SD above the mean. • Kidney sizes may be normal before the third trimester, with progressive enlargement subsequently.	• Small, normal or slightly enlarged: 2–8 SD above the mean.
Cysts	• Seen in ~15%, usually cortical.	• Isolated macroscopic cysts <10 mm in the medulla in 30%.	• Cortical or diffuse renal cysts.
Echogenicity and corticomedullary differentiation	• Hyperechoic cortex. • Relatively hypoechoic medulla causing "increased" corticomedullary differentiation.	• Hyperechoic including the medulla, causing "decreased" corticomedullary differentiation.	• Cortical hyperechogenicity.
Amniotic fluid	• Usually normal.	• Oligohydramnios. • Pulmonary hypoplasia.	• Normal or polyhydramnios.
Cyst progression	• May have rapid cyst progression in childhood.		• >90% have cysts in the postnatal period.

2. Ultrasound of the kidneys and bladder should be the first imaging modality in a child suspected of having cystic kidney disease.
   a. Unilateral or bilateral disease:
      i. Largely unequal kidney sizes or obvious unilateral kidney involvement suggest dysplasia or isolated cysts/tumors.
      ii. Oligohydramnios provides a clue to bilateral renal disease that results in a decreased production of fetal urine.
      iii. Bilateral disease may appear unilateral on renal imaging in the early stages.
   b. Features of cysts:
      i. Location: Cortex, medulla, corticomedullary junction or both.
      ii. Size, shape and number: Macrocysts versus microcysts, variably-sized cysts.
      iii. Shape: Round versus tubular shape.
      iv. Unilocular versus multilocular, presence of internal echoes and solid components.
      v. Differential diagnoses of medullary cysts or hyperechogenicity include non-cystic diseases involving the renal medulla such as Dent disease and medullary sponge kidney.
   c. Features of the kidneys:
      i. Size of the kidneys: Large, normal, or small.
      ii. Level of echogenicity of the cortex and medulla:
         - Normal: Cortex as echogenic as liver or spleen with relatively hypoechogenic medulla.
         - Hyperechogenic kidney: Cortex more echogenic than the liver and spleen.
         - Fetal kidneys are normally hyperechogenic in the first and early second trimesters.
         - Renal echogenicity is increased when there are microscopic cysts, dilated tubules, and/or interstitial fibrosis and inflammation.
      iii. Corticomedullary differentiation:
         - May be increased, reversed or absent.
         - In normal fetal kidneys, corticomedullary differentiation is visible after 20 weeks of gestation.
   d. Salient ultrasound findings:
      i. Genetic cystic kidney diseases:

Disease	Kidney Size	Cysts/Location	Parenchyma	Histology
Autosomal dominant polycystic kidney disease (ADPKD)	• Bilateral large, progressively massive over decades. • Cystic contour.	• Multiple variably sized *round* macrocysts. • Early: May be localized to the medulla. • Later stages: Both the cortex and the medulla. • Prenatal: Cysts are seen in ~15%, usually cortical.	• Hyperechoic cortex and relatively hypoechoic medulla; *increased* corticomedullary differentiation. • Less commonly hyperechogenic medulla with *absent* or *decreased* corticomedullary differentiation.	• Large spherical cystic dilatation in all parts of the nephron. • Focal areas of abnormal nephrons scattered among areas of normal nephrons. • Tubule wall expands and the cyst rapidly closes off from the nephron of origin.

Note Ultrasonographic criteria for ADPKD:

- Child <5 years old at 50% risk for ADPKD: Ultrasonography is less useful and screening is not recommended.
- Infancy: The finding of large echogenic kidneys with distinct macroscopic cysts is highly suggestive of ADPKD.

Pei–Ravine ultrasonographic criteria:

- Child, 0–15 years, at risk of ADPKD: Presence of one cyst adequate for diagnosis.
- Individual, 15–39 years, at risk of ADPKD with unknown PKD genotype or known to have *PKD2* mutations: Presence of at least 3 unilateral or bilateral kidney cysts is diagnostic.
- Individual, 15–39 years, at risk of ADPKD with known *PKD1* mutations: Presence of at least 2 unilateral or bilateral cysts is diagnostic.

Disease	Kidney Size	Cysts/Location	Parenchyma	Histology
Autosomal recessive polycystic kidney disease (ARPKD)	• Uniform, bilateral. • Massively large in fetus. • Less prominently enlarged in children. • Preservation of reniform shape.	• Many tiny microcysts up to 2 mm in diameter. • High-resolution ultrasound may detect tubular dilatations. • May have isolated macroscopic cysts <10 mm in the renal medulla. • Localized to the medulla. • May expand into the cortex in severe cases, but the outer cortex remains normal.	• Early: Hyperechoic medulla with a normal peripheral cortex (relatively hypoechoic). Corticomedullary differentiation *decreased* or *reversed* (pyramidal hyperechogenicity). • Later: Diffuse hyperechogenicity involving both the cortex and the medulla.	• Non-obstructive dilatation of the collecting tubules. • Cysts remain connected to the nephron of origin.
Nephronophthisis	• Normal or small. • Prenatal: Big kidneys.	• Numerous microcysts and small discrete cysts (mm to 2 cm). • Medulla and the corticomedullary junction.	• Hyperechoic. • Loss of corticomedullary differentiation.	• Tubular interstitial nephritis, normal-looking glomeruli. • Atrophic tubules with thickened basement membranes alternating with groups of dilated or collapsed tubules, normal-appearing glomeruli.

Autosomal dominant tubulointerstitial kidney disease (ADTKD)	• Normal to small.	• Medulla and the corticomedullary junction. • Cortical sparing. • Medullary cysts may be seen, but not present in most cases.	• Echogenic. • May be normal in the early stages with normal echogenicity and no cysts.	• Nonspecific diffuse tubular and interstitial fibrosis. • Tubular dilatations, which can enlarge to become tubular cysts.
Glomerulocystic kidney disease (may be non-genetic)	• Small, normal or moderately enlarged. • Hereditary cases: Small kidneys typically.	• Microcysts. • Cysts mainly in the cortical and subcapsular region. • Spares the medulla. • Subcapsular cysts are diagnostic, but not always present (may be more evident on MRI). • Cysts not always evident on ultrasound.	• Cortical hyperechogenicity may be seen instead of cysts. • Loss of corticomedullary differentiation.	• Uniform cystic dilatation of Bowman's space to more than 2–3 times of normal, involving at least 5% of the glomeruli.
Medullary sponge kidney (not cystic kidney disease, but an important differential diagnosis)		• Confined to the medullary pyramids. • Cortex is spared on CT or MRI.		• Tubular dilatation of the collecting ducts.

ii. Non-genetic cystic kidney diseases:

Disease	Kidney Size	Cyst/Location	Parenchyma
Multicystic dysplastic kidney	• Multiloculated kidney. • Reniform shape not preserved.	• Multiple variably-sized non-communicating cysts (complete septa in between cysts). • Thin-walled cysts. • Random distribution (early stages may be at the periphery).	• Intervening parenchyma is often hyperechogenic.
Severe hydro-nephrosis (not a renal cystic condition, but often confused with multicystic dysplastic kidneys)	• Large, preserved reniform shape.	• No complete septa in between “cysts”.	• Parenchyma of normal echogenicity may have cortical thinning.
Renal hypoplasia or dysplasia	• Normal, large or small. • An initially enlarged kidney may decrease in size with time.	• With or without small cortical cysts. • Cysts may be seen only later.	• Hyperechogenic. • Cortico-medullary differentiation may be preserved or lost.
Obstructive dysplasia	• Normal, large or small.	• With or without cortical cysts.	• Hyperechogenic.

Simple cyst	• Normal or large or small.	• Typically ≤1 cm. • Sharply defined thin smooth walls, no internal echoes, suggesting no internal debris or septa. • Cysts can increase slowly in size and numbers with time.	• Intervening parenchyma is usually normal.
Multilocular (complex) cyst	• Normal or large or small.	• Heterogeneous and/or thickened irregular wall or septa.	• Intervening parenchyma is usually normal.
Acquired cystic kidney disease	• Small bilateral kidneys, smooth contour.	• Multiple small bilateral simple or multilocular cysts (<0.5 cm to 2–3 cm). • Diagnostic if there are at least three cysts in each kidney.	• Hyperechoic, loss of corticomedullary differentiation.
Hypokalemia-associated renal cysts		• Cortical or medullary cysts, cysts of varying sizes.	• Cortical echogenicity or altered corticomedullary differentiation.

e. Algorithms following a renal ultrasound:

i. Evaluation of renal cysts:

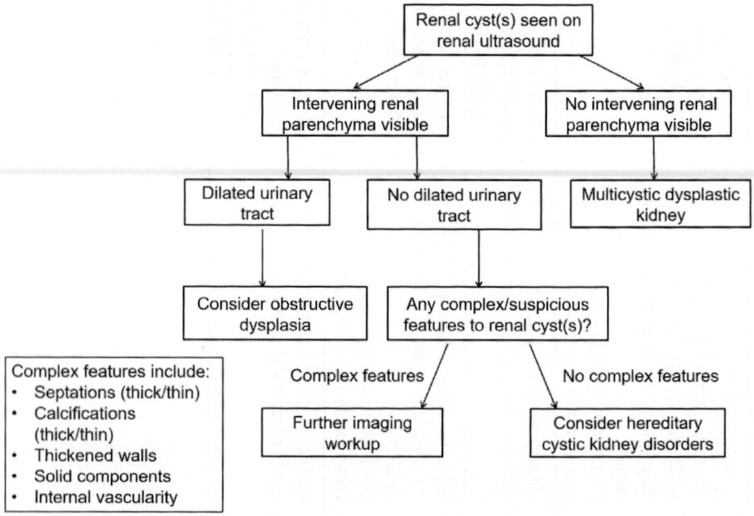

ii. Evaluation of hereditary cystic kidney disorders:

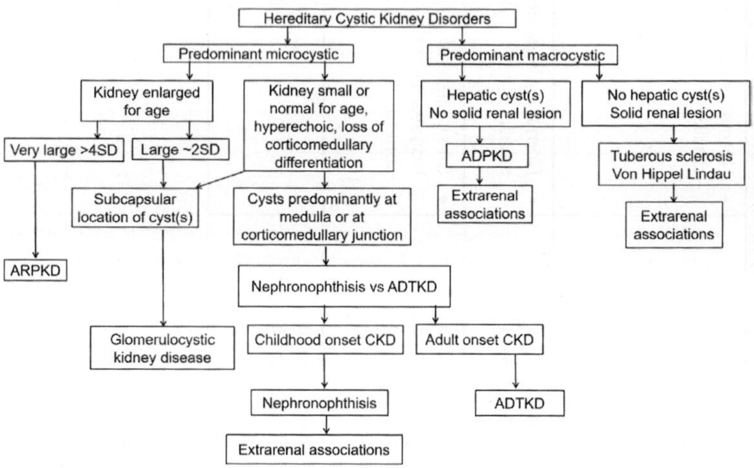

3. More sensitive imaging modalities:
   a. High-resolution ultrasound may detect tubular dilatations seen in ARPKD, which is different from the round cysts in ADPKD.
   b. Contrast-enhanced CT scanning:
      i. Able to pick up small cysts of 2 to 3 mm in diameter.
      ii. Morphologic findings evaluated:
         - Wall thickening.
         - Nodularity.
         - Septa.
         - Enhancement.
         - Calcification (not seen on MRI).
      iii. Refer to the Bosniak classification if there is a suspicion of malignancy.
   c. MRI with a 3-mm slice thickness or heavy-weighted unenhanced T2 MR images:
      i. Can help in the localization of pathology within the kidneys such as hyperintense lesions in the medullary region and/or sparing of the cortex (medullary sponge kidney).
      ii. Evaluates the same morphologic features as CT except for calcifications, which are not seen on MRI.
         - More sensitive than a CT or ultrasound in showing the enhancement of internal septations.
      iii. Most useful for evaluating the internal contents of cysts:
         - Heterogeneous composition of fluid due to blood or mucin is associated with a higher risk of malignancy.
4. Radionuclide scans:
   a. DMSA: Useful to determine the differential function in renal dysplasia.
   b. MAG3-diuretic renogram or MR urogram when urinary obstruction is suspected.
5. Micturating cystourethrogram may be performed in renal dysplasia as concurrent VUR can occur.

IV. Step 4: Consider other tests if the diagnosis is still unclear after imaging

1. Kidney biopsy is not routinely required.
   - May be performed in patients with unexplained CKD with hyperechogenic kidneys and no visible cysts, in the absence of genetic testing.

2. Gene analysis:
   a. Genetic tests:
      i. Useful in the following:
         - Diagnosis is not clear after careful evaluation, especially in atypical cases.
         - Planning for transplantation, especially living-related transplants.
         - Prenatal testing or preimplantation genetic testing for the next pregnancy.
      ii. Gene panels using next generation sequencing (NGS) may establish the diagnosis.
   b. Consider whole exome sequencing (WES) if the results from NGS are inconclusive. Polycystic kidney disease:
      i. ARPKD patients can be indistinguishable from early-onset ADPKD.
      ii. Gene analysis for mutations in both *PKHD1*, *PKD1* and *PKD2* should be performed.
      iii. In ADPKD where serial ultrasound scans over long periods are needed for diagnosis, genetic testing may be more cost-effective than repeated ultrasound scans.
   c. Glomerulocystic disease:
      i. Consider genetic testing if there is hyperuricemia or early-onset gout *(HNF1B, UMOD, REN*), or diabetes (*HNF1B)*.
   d. Nephronophthisis:
      i. ESKD onset <5 years: *NPHP2, NPHP3, NEK8.*
      ii. ESKD onset >5 years: Screen *NPHP1* first (25% of cases).
      iii. Retinitis pigmentosa: *NPHP5, NPHP6.*
      iv. Cerebellar ataxia/Joubert syndrome and related disorders: *NPHP6, RPGRIP1L, AHI1.*
      v. If the above are negative, then screen the rest of the genes.

E. Management

I. Problems associated with tubular dysfunction

1. Decreased urinary concentration ability with polyuria:
   a. Encourage fluid intake to match increased urine output.

2. Electrolyte abnormalities:
   a. Salt supplementation in patients with high urinary sodium losses due to distal nephron pathology.
   b. Potassium supplementation in patients with hypokalemia-related cysts.
   c. Correction of acidosis with Shohl's solution (sodium citrate) or sodium bicarbonate in patients with associated renal tubular acidosis.
   d. In type 4 renal tubular acidosis with hyperkalemia, add a loop diuretic such as furosemide.
   e. Patients with *REN* mutations have symptomatic low blood pressure and hyperkalemia.
      i. Start patient on a high salt diet.
      ii. If still symptomatic or hyperkalemic, treat with fludrocortisone.
         - Increase in blood pressure can improve the glomerular filtration rate, resulting in the lowering of the serum creatinine.

II. CKD complications and prevention of progression

1. Hypertension:
   a. Check blood pressure at every health care encounter.
   b. Maintain blood pressure at the 50th centile for height-centile, gender and age.
2. Proteinuria:
   a. Monitor early morning urine protein:creatinine ratio and urine albumin:creatinine ratio at least annually.
   b. Consider the use of ACE inhibitors and/or angiotensin receptor blockers (ARBs) if there is significant albuminuria and/or hypertension.
3. Hyperuricemia:
   a. Patients who develop gout should be treated with a xanthine oxidase inhibitor, either allopurinol or febuxostat.
4. Anemia:
   a. Anemia may occur early in nephronophthisis and in *REN* mutations, out of proportion to the CKD stage.
   b. Symptomatic anemia may be treated with erythropoietin.

III. Complications related to cysts

1. Recurrent or chronic flank pain:
   - Due to kidney enlargement in ADPKD (rare in children).
2. Infection:
   a. Urinary tract infection may occur in children with CAKUT.
   b. Cyst infection:
      i. Imaging studies:
         - Newly developed internal septations or layering material within the cyst may suggest the presence of infection.
         - Unreliable for diagnosing or excluding infection within a cyst.
      ii. Percutaneous aspirate with culture and Gram stain may be diagnostic.
      iii. Treatment:
         - Infected cysts are frequently refractory to antimicrobial therapy since many drugs do not readily penetrate the cyst.
         - Drugs that achieve therapeutic concentrations within the cyst and are active against gram-negative organisms include co-trimoxazole, ciprofloxacin, levofloxacin, and chloramphenicol.
         - Aminoglycosides and penicillins frequently do not penetrate cysts.
3. Rupture and hemorrhage:
   a. Characterized in simple cysts by high attenuation, non-enhancing internal debris on imaging.
   b. Presentation:
      i. Point tenderness: Cyst hemorrhage.
      ii. Diffuse flank pain: Rupture of a superficial cyst causing subcapsular hematoma.
      iii. Ipsilateral shoulder pain: Rupture of an upper pole cyst.
      iv. Acute abdominal pain: Rupture of a large renal cyst involving surrounding viscera.
   c. Supportive management:
      i. Intravenous volume repletion.
      ii. Analgesics.
   d. Surgical interventions may be needed when:
      i. Obstruction due to clots persists beyond 2 weeks.
      ii. There is prolonged and severe bleeding.

4. Nephrolithiasis:
   - Occurs in up to 25% of adults with ADPKD.
5. Malignancy:
   a. Risk of malignancy in multicystic dysplastic kidneys is minimal.
   b. High risk of malignancy in:
      - Multilocular complex cysts.
      - ADPKD.
      - Acquired cystic kidney disease in ESKD patients.
      - Cystic kidney diseases associated with Von Hippel–Lindau disease and tuberous sclerosis complex.
   c. The Bosniak classification system classifies renal cystic masses based on contrast-enhanced CT and helps to predict the risk of malignancy and guide management.
      - 40–60% of Bosniak Class III and 85–100% of Bosniak Class IV cysts turn out to be malignant.

Category/ Disease	Characteristics on CT	Management
Simple Cyst:		
Category I renal cyst	• Cyst with a hairline wall that does not contain septa, calcification or solid components.	• Typically does not require follow-up unless ≥3 cm
Category II renal cyst	• Cyst may contain few hairline thin septa. • Fine calcification may be present in the wall or septa.	• Must be distinguished from cystic kidney disease and a complex cyst.
Category IIF renal cyst	• Cyst may contain multiple hairline thin septa. • The wall or septa may contain calcifications that may be thick and nodular.	• Requires follow-up. • Consider imaging at 3, 6, and 12 months and then annually.

(Continued)

(*Continued*)

Category/ Disease	Characteristics on CT	Management
Multilocular Cyst:		
Category III renal cyst	• Cyst with thickened irregular walls or septa in which measurable enhancement is present.	• Close radiographic follow-up and/or surgical excision as the risk of malignancy is 33%.
Category IV renal cyst	• Cyst wall and septa with irregular thickening. • Thick, nodular, irregular calcifications are present. • There is an enhancement of the tissue and cyst.	• Surgical excision is recommended as the risk of malignancy is >92.5%.

IV. Nephrectomy

1. Routine removal of multicystic dysplastic kidney is not required:
   a. Low long-term risks of hypertension and infection.
   b. Risk of malignancy is not increased.
2. Nephrectomy or nephron-sparing surgery may be indicated in the following:
   a. Malignancy is strongly suspected.
   b. Large polycystic kidneys to create space before renal transplant.
   c. Recurrent urinary tract infections in a poorly functioning dysplastic kidney.

Recommended Reading

1. Guay-Woodford LM, Desmond RA. (2003) Autosomal recessive polycystic kidney disease: The clinical experience in North America. *Paediatrics* **111**:1072–1080.
2. Simms RJ, Eley L, Sayer JA. (2009) Nephronophthisis. *Eur J Hum Genet* **17**:406–416.
3. Waters AM, Beales PL. (2011) Ciliopathies: An expanding disease spectrum. *Pediatr Nephrol* **26**:1039–1056.
4. Loftus H, Ong AC. (2013) Cystic kidney diseases: Many ways to form a cyst. *Pediatr Nephrol* **28**:33–49.
5. Cramer MT, Guay-Woodford LM. (2015) Cystic kidney disease: A primer. *Adv Chronic Kidney Dis* **22**:297–305.
6. Frye TP, Abboud S. (2021) Cystic disease of the kidney. Edited by: Schwartz BF, Talavera F. *Medscape*. https://emedicine.medscape.com.
7. Bleyer A. (2020, updated) Autosomal dominant tubulointerstitial kidney disease (medullary cystic kidney disease). Edited by: Curhan GC, Perrone RD, Lam AQ. *UpToDateONLINE*. http://www.uptodateonline.com.
8. Ozcan T. (2021) Prenatal sonographic diagnosis of cystic renal disease. Edited by: Wilkins-Huang L, Levine D, Barss VA. *UpToDateONLINE*. http://www.uptodateonline.com.
9. Niaudet P. (2020, updated) Renal cystic diseases in children. Edited by Mattoo TK, Kim MS. *UpToDateONLINE*. http://www.uptodateonline.com.
10. Niaudet P. (2020, updated) Autosomal dominant polycystic kidney disease in children. Edited by Mattoo TK, Kim MS. U*pToDateONLINE*. http://www.uptodateonline.com.
11. Niaudet P. (2020, updated) Autosomal recessive polycystic kidney disease in children. Edited by Mattoo TK, Kim MS. *UpToDateONLINE*. http://www.uptodateonline.com.

1 Renal Tubular Acidosis

Lau PYW, Ambarsari CG, Chaturvedi S, Qader MA, Liu ID and Yap HK

A. Definition

1. Renal tubular acidosis (RTA) is a syndrome resulting from either a defect in proximal tubule bicarbonate (HCO_3^-) reabsorption or a defect in distal tubule hydrogen ion (H^+) secretion, or both.
2. This results in normal anion gap hyperchloremic metabolic acidosis (HCMA).

B. Physiology of Renal Acidification

1. Proximal HCO_3^- reabsorption:

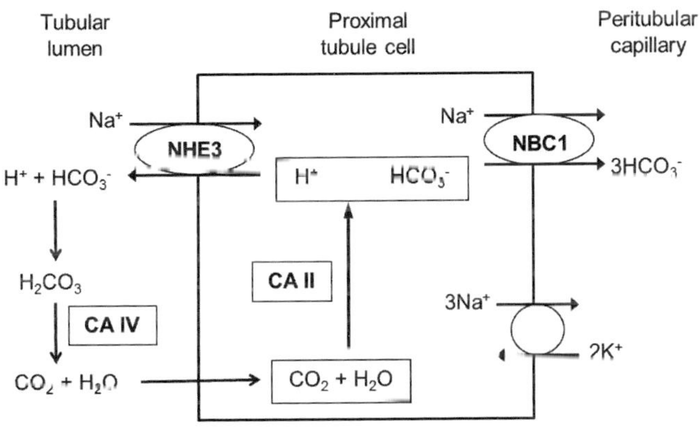

a. "HCO_3^- reclamation" occurs mainly in the proximal tubule (80%).
b. In the proximal tubule, HCO_3^- reabsorption occurs as follows:
   - Secretion of H^+ into HCO_3^- rich glomerular filtrate by the sodium (Na^+)-H^+ exchanger (NHE3) results in the formation of carbonic acid (H_2CO_3).
   - H_2CO_3 is rapidly converted, within the tubule lumen, by membrane-bound carbonic anhydrase (CA) type IV, to water (H_2O) and carbon dioxide (CO_2), which can freely diffuse into the proximal tubule.
   - H_2O and CO_2 are converted to intracellular H^+ and HCO_3^- by CA type II and the HCO_3^- exits the cell via the electrogenic Na^+-$3HCO_3^-$ symporter (NBC1), and H^+ is recycled via NHE3 into the lumen.

2. Distal urinary acidification in the distal nephron comprises 3 processes:
   a. Reclamation of filtered HCO_3^- that reaches the distal nephron (10–20%).
   b. Excretion of titratable acid.
   c. Generation of ammonia (NH_3) that buffers H^+ to form nondiffusible ammonium (NH_4^+).
3. Role of ammonia in distal urinary acidification:

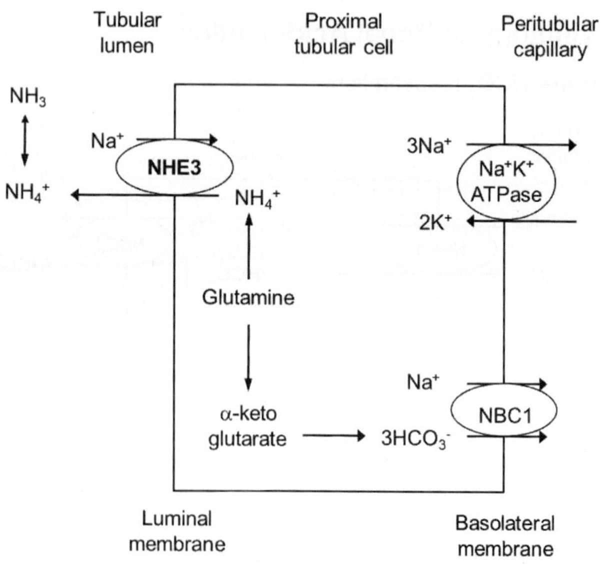

a. Ammoniagenesis occurs in the proximal tubule, chiefly by deamidation of filtered or secreted glutamine.
b. NH_3 is excreted into the proximal tubular lumen by NHE3, in the form of NH_4^+.
c. Accumulation of NH_3 in the medullary interstitium occurring due to NH_4^+ absorption with limited back diffusion of NH3 in the ascending loop of Henle results in an NH_4^+ medullary concentration gradient.
d. This medullary concentration gradient increases the driving force for diffusional entry of NH3 into the cortical collecting tubule.
e. This process is facilitated by binding to H^+ excreted by the α-intercalated cell in this region to form NH_4^+.

4. Titratable acid:
   a. Titratable acids are buffers include phosphate, sulfate and many other anions.
   b. Divalent basic phosphate (HPO_4^{2-}) is converted to the monovalent acid form ($H_2PO_4^-$) by accepting protons as they pass through the collecting duct where the pH is lower.

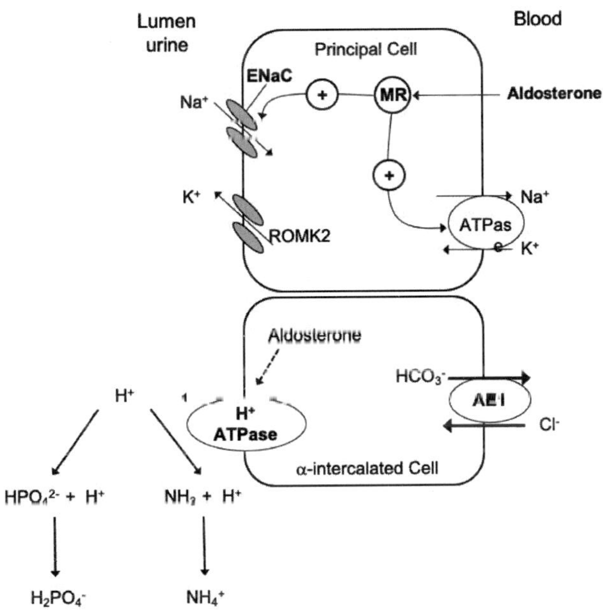

c. At the α-intercalated cell in the distal collecting duct, luminal H^+ secretion occurs via vacuolar H^+-ATPase, which is regulated by aldosterone.
d. The H^+ secretion is enhanced by luminal electronegativity generated by aldosterone-stimulation of active Na^+ transport via ENaC in the principal cells.
e. Intracellularly formed $HCO3^-$ leaves the cell by an electroneutral mechanism involving chloride (Cl^-)-$HCO3^-$ exchange, facilitated by anion-exchanger 1 (AE1).

C. Types of RTA

I. Hypokalemic RTA:

1. Type 1 or distal RTA:
   1. Due to impaired distal H^+ secretion.
   2. Incomplete distal RTA:
      - Milder form of classic distal RTA with defective distal H^+ secretion.
      - Plasma pH and $HCO3^-$ levels are normal but during induced acidosis, urine pH cannot be lowered below 5.3.
      - Hypercalciuria and hypocitraturia common, hence patients often present with nephrocalcinosis or nephrolithiasis.
2. Type 2 or proximal RTA:
   a. Due to impaired HCO_3^- reabsorption in the proximal tubule.
   b. Fanconi syndrome, which is a generalized proximal tubulopathy characterized by:
      - Tubular proteinuria.
      - Aminoaciduria.
      - Bicarbonaturia.
      - Phosphaturia resulting in hypophosphatemic rickets.
      - Sodium and potassium wasting.
      - Glycosuria.

3. Type 3 or mixed RTA:
   - Distal RTA with bicarbonate wasting.

II. Hyperkalemic RTA:

1. Type 4 RTA or hypoaldosteronism:
   - Due to a reduction in aldosterone secretion or responsiveness.
2. Voltage-dependent RTA (subtype of distal RTA).
   - Occurs with markedly reduced distal sodium delivery or with inherited or acquired defects in sodium reabsorption by principal cells (Na^+-K^+-ATPase pump).

D. Clinical Evaluation

I. Initial presentation:

1. Infancy:
   - Failure to thrive.
   - Vomiting and dehydration.
   - Urinary tract infection.
   - Circulatory collapse.
   - Obstructive uropathy.
2. Childhood:
   - Short stature and poor weight gain.
   - Polyuria and polydipsia.
   - Rickets with delayed walking, bowing of legs, and frontal bossing.
   - Urolithiasis.
3. Adolescence:
   - Urolithiasis.

II. *Etiological features*

1. Type 2 RTA (Proximal):
   a. Isolated genetic:

Inheritance	Non-Kidney Manifestation	Defective Protein	Gene
Autosomal recessive	• Ocular abnormalities (band keratopathy, cataract, glaucoma) • Defective dental enamel • Intellectual impairment • Basal ganglia calcification	Sodium bicarbonate cotransporter 1 (NBC1)	*SLC4A4*

b. Isolated sporadic (transient in infancy).
c. Multiple tubular dysfunction (Fanconi syndrome):
   i. Genetic:

Inheritance	Clinical Syndrome with Non-Kidney Manifestation	Defective Protein	Gene
X-linked recessive	• Dent disease	*CLCN5*	Renal chloride channel
	• Lowe syndrome	*OCRL1*	Phosphatidylinositol 4,5-bisphosphate-5 phosphatase
Autosomal dominant	• Fanconi renotubular syndrome type 1	*GATM*	Glycine amidinotransferase
	• Fanconi renotubular syndrome type 3 • Rickets	*EHHADH*	Enoyl-CoA hydratase / 3-hydroxyacyl CoA dehydrogenase
	• Fanconi renotubular syndrome type 4 • Maturity-onset diabetes of the young	*HNF4A*	Hepatocyte nuclear factor 4A
Autosomal recessive	• Cystinosis	*CTNS*	Cystinosin
	• Tyrosinemia type 1	*FAH*	Fumarylacetoacetate hydrolase

(*Continued*)

Inheritance	Clinical Syndrome with Non-Kidney Manifestation	Defective Protein	Gene
Autosomal recessive	• Fanconi-Bickel	*SLC2A2*	Glucose transporter GLUT2
	• Wilson disease	*ATP7B*	ATPase, Cu^{2+} transporting polypeptide
	Galactosemia	*GALT*	Galactose-1-phosphate uridylyltransferase
	Hereditary fructose intolerance	*ALDOB*	Fructose-1-phosphate aldolase
	Glycogen storage disease type 1a	*G6PC*	Glucose-6-phosphatase-α
	Glycogen storage disease type 1b	*SLC37A4*	Glucose-6-phosphate translocase
	Fanconi renotubular syndrome type 2	*SLC34A1*	Sodium-dependent phosphate transporter 2A
	Arthrogryposis-Renal dysfunction-Cholestasis (ARC) syndrome type 1	*VPS33B*	Class C vacuolar protein sorting protein
	Metachromatic leukodystrophy	*ARSA/ PSAP*	Aryl sulfatase A
	Mitochondrial disorders including Leigh syndrome	Multiple genes	Multiple genetic defects

ii. Acquired:
- Drug-induced:
  - Nucleotide reverse transcriptase inhibitors: Tenofovir, adefovir, cidofovir.
  - Nucleoside reverse transcriptase inhibitors: Didanosine, lamivudine, stavudine.
  - Diuretics: Acetazolamide.
  - Chemotherapeutic agents: Ifosfamide, oxaliplatin, cisplatin.

    - Anti-convulsants: Topiramate, valproic acid.
    - Antibiotics: Aminoglycosides, expired tetracyclines.
- Heavy metals: Lead, cadmium, mercury, copper.
- Disorders of calcium metabolism:
    - Vitamin D deficiency.
    - Hyperparathyroidism.
- Cyanotic congenital heart disease.
- Medullary cystic disease.
- Alport syndrome.
- Steroid-resistant nephrotic syndrome:
    - Focal segmental glomerulosclerosis.
    - Membranous nephropathy.
- Tubulointerstitial nephritis with uveitis (TINU).
- Paroxysmal nocturnal hemoglobinuria.
- Aristolochic acid (Chinese herb nephropathy).
- Kidney transplantation.

2. Type 1 RTA (Distal):
   a. Genetic:

Inheritance	Non-Kidney Manifestation	Defective Protein	Gene
Autosomal dominant	None	Anion exchanger-1 (AE1)	*SLC4A1*
Autosomal recessive	Hemolytic anemia (Southeast Asian ovalocytosis)	AE1	*SLC4A1*
	Early bilateral sensorineural hearing loss	β1 subunit of H^+-ATPase	*ATP6V1B1*
	Normal hearing/delayed hearing loss	α4 subunit of H^+-ATPase	*ATP6V0A4*
	Normal hearing	C2 subunit of H^+-ATPase	*ATP6V1C2*
	Early deafness	Forkhead transcription factor I1	*FOXI1*
	Dental enamel defects	Tryptophan-aspartate repeat domain 72	*WDR72*

b. Acquired:
   i. Autoimmune disease:
      - Systemic lupus erythematosus.
      - Sjögren's syndrome.
      - Chronic active hepatitis.
      - Primary biliary cirrhosis.
      - Rheumatoid arthritis.
      - Thyroiditis.
   ii. Associated with other genetic diseases:
      - Osteopetrosis.
      - Sickle-cell disease.
      - Ehlers-Danlos syndrome.
      - Wilson disease.
      - Hereditary fructose intolerance with nephrocalcinosis.
      - Primary hyperoxaluria type 1.
      - Carnitine palmitoyltyransferase I deficiency.
   iii. Disorders of calcium metabolism:
      - Primary hyperparathyroidism.
      - Hypercalcemic hyperthyroidism.
      - Vitamin D intoxication.
      - Idiopathic hypercalciuria with nephrocalcinosis.
      - Familial hypomagnesemia-hypercalciuria with nephrocalcinosis.
   iv. Obstructive and reflux nephropathy.
   v. Kidney transplant rejection.
   vi. Medullary sponge kidney.
   vii. Dysproteinemic syndromes.
   viii. Drug-induced:
      - Anti-fungal: Amphotericin B.
      - Anti-viral: Foscarnet.
      - Antibiotics: Trimethoprim, pentamidine.
      - Chemotherapeutic agents: Melphalan, ifosfamide.
      - Psychotropic agents: Lithium.
      - Toluene inhalation.

3. Type 3 RTA (Mixed):

	Non-Kidney Manifestation	Defective Protein	Gene
Autosomal recessive (Guibaud-Vainsel syndrome or marble brain disease)	• Osteopetrosis • Intellectual impairment • Cerebral calcification • Bone fractures • Facial dysmorphism • Conductive hearing loss • Blindness	Carbonic anhydrase II	*CA2*

4. Type 4 RTA (Hypoaldosteronism):
   a. Genetic:

	Clinical Syndrome with Non-Kidney Manifestation	Defective Protein	Gene
Autosomal recessive	• Congenital adrenal hyperplasia with hypertension	Aldosterone synthase (11-β hydroxylase)	*CYP11B2*
	• Congenital adrenal hyperplasia	21-hydroxylase	*CYP21*
Autosomal dominant	• Pseudohypoaldosteronism type 1	Mineralocorticoid receptor (MR)	*MR (NR3C2)*
Autosomal recessive	• Pseudohypoaldosteronism type 1 (involving kidney, colon and sweat glands)	Epithelial sodium channel (ENaC)	*SCNN1B*
	• Pseudohypoaldosteronism type 2 (Gordon syndrome)	WNK1 or WNK4	*PHA2B, PHA2C*

   b. Transient: Early childhood hyperkalemia.
   c. Acquired:
      i. Aldosterone deficiency without kidney disease:
         - Adrenal tuberculosis.
         - Adrenal necrosis.
      ii. Hyporeninemic hypoaldosteronism in chronic nephropathies:

- Diabetic nephropathy.
- Human immunodeficiency virus (HIV) nephropathy.
- Systemic lupus erythematosus.

iii. Aldosterone resistance in chronic interstitial nephropathies:
- Obstructive uropathy.
- Medullary cystic disease.
- Drug-induced interstitial nephritis.
- Kidney transplant rejection.
- Analgesia abuse nephropathy.
- HIV nephropathy.

iv. Drug-induced hyperkalemia
- Impaired renin-aldosterone production: Cyclo-oxygenase inhibitors, angiotensin-converting enzyme inhibitors, angiotensin receptor blockers, heparin.
- Inhibitors of renal potassium secretion: Potassium-retaining diuretics, trimethoprim, pentamidine, calcineurin inhibitors.
- Altered potassium distribution: Insulin antagonists, β-adrenergic antagonists, α-adrenergic agonists, digoxin, succinylcholine.

E. Stepwise Approach to the Diagnosis of RTA

I. Step 1: Determination of plasma anion gap and potassium

1. Blood urea, creatinine, sodium, potassium, chloride, and bicarbonate to determine the anion gap:
   a. RTA manifests as a normal anion gap hyperchloremic metabolic acidosis (NAGMA).
      - Plasma anion gap: $Na^+ - (Cl^- + HCO_3^-) \leq 12$
   b. Other causes of NAGMA include gastrointestinal losses of bicarbonate.
   c. Hypokalemia is associated with Type 1 and Type 2 RTA.
   d. Hyperkalemia is associated with Type 4 RTA and voltage-dependent Type 1 RTA.

II. *Step 2: Estimate urine pH, urine anion gap, and urine osmolal gap*

1. Urine pH:
   a. Should be measured electrometrically on a fresh voided, early morning urine specimen.
   b. Urine pH <5.5 suggests RTA type 2 or 4.
   c. Urine pH >5.5 in the presence of acidosis suggests distal RTA.
   d. Urine pH may be falsely elevated in:
      - Patients with chronic metabolic acidosis accompanied by hypokalemia.
      - Urinary tract infection with urease-splitting organisms.
      - Patients treated with alkali.
      - When the urine Na^+ concentration is <20 mmol/L as distal H^+ secretion is impaired with reduced-sodium delivery to distal tubule.
2. Urine sodium, potassium and chloride to determine the urine anion gap (UAG):
   a. $UAG = (Na^+ + K^+) - Cl^-$
   b. UAG reflects the rate of NH_4^+ excretion and becomes progressively negative as NH_4^+ excretion increases.
   c. Negative UAG indicates NH_4^+ excretion is adequate in ruling out a distal tubular acidification defect, that is, both RTA type 1 and 4.
   d. Positive UAG >40 mmol/L suggests RTA type 1 or 4.
   e. UAG may be falsely positive in patients with unmeasured urinary anions, including:
      - Beta-hydroxybutyrate and acetoacetate in ketoacidosis.
      - Hippurate following toluene inhalation (glue-sniffing).
      - Bicarbonate when proximal RTA is treated with alkali therapy.
      - D-lactate in D-lactic acidosis.
      - 5-oxoproline associated with chronic acetaminophen ingestion (especially in malnourished women).
      - Neonates who excrete unmeasured anions at relatively high rates.

3. Urine sodium, potassium, urea, and glucose to calculate the urine osmolal gap (UOG):
   a. UOG is a better indirect surrogate of the urine NH_4^+ excretion than UAG in conditions that disrupt the relationship between urine NH_4^+ concentration and UAG.
   b. Calculated urine osmolality = 2(Na^+ + K^+) + urea (mmol/L) + glucose (mmol/L)
   c. UOG = Measured urine osmolality – Calculated urine osmolality
   d. Normal UOG is approximately 10–100 mOsm/kg.
      - NH_4^+, together with other unmeasured anions, constitutes the UOG.
      - Urinary NH_4^+ excretion (5–50 mmol/L), estimated at half the urine osmolal gap, is considered appropriately increased if UOG >100 mOsm/kg.

III. Step 3: Look for associated defects

1. In suspected Type 1 RTA:
   a. Kidney ultrasound for medullary nephrocalcinosis.
      - Calcium-phosphate precipitation occurs in the presence of acidic urine and hypocitraturia.
   b. Urinary calcium excretion (urine calcium:creatinine ratio or 24-hour urine calcium) to look for hypercalciuria.
   c. Urinary citrate excretion (urine citrate:creatinine or 24-hour urine citrate) to look for hypocitraturia.
2. In suspected Type 2 RTA, look for Fanconi syndrome:
   a. Urinary amino acid quantification.
   b. Glycosuria on dipstick examination.
   c. Urine uric acid:creatinine ratio.
   d. Urine phosphate excretion (urine phosphate:creatinine ratio, tubular reabsorption of phosphate or tubular maximum for phosphate).
3. In suspected Type 4 RTA:
   a. Transtubular potassium concentration gradient (TTKG).
      - Estimates the action of aldosterone at the level of the late distal and cortical collecting tubules.

- TTKG <8 in the presence of hyperkalemia has been suggested to imply that potassium secretion is impaired, but this is not validated and should not be used in children.

b. Plasma renin and aldosterone:
   - Useful to differentiate aldosterone deficiency from aldosterone resistance states and hyporeninemic states.

4. Audiometry to detect hearing loss in subtypes of Type 1 RTA.

IV. *Step 4: Additional functional studies (optional)*

1. Bicarbonate loading test:
   a. Performed to calculate the fractional excretion of bicarbonate ($FEHCO_3$) and urine-to-blood CO_2 gradient (U-B pCO_2).
   b. Methodology:
      i. Administer IV 4.2% sodium bicarbonate infusion at the rate of 0.5–1 mmol/kg/hour.
      ii. During the sodium bicarbonate infusion, urine pH is measured in timed samples taken 30–60 minutes apart, with the urine collected under mineral oil, with the child voiding in the upright position.
      iii. A steady state is usually achieved after 3–4 hours from the start of the infusion, and the test is terminated when 3 samples of timed urine collections show urine pH >7.5 and serum bicarbonate is 18–20 mmol/L.
   c. Interpretation:
      i. $FEHCO_3$ is an important index of proximal tubular handling of bicarbonate.
      ii. $FEHCO_3 = (HCO^-_{3u} \times Cr_p)/(HCO^-_{3p} \times Cr_u) \times 100$,
      where HCO^-_{3u} = urine bicarbonate, HCO^-_{3p} = plasma bicarbonate, Cr_p = plasma creatinine, and Cr_u = urine creatinine.
         - In Type 2 RTA, serum bicarbonate is normal (>22 mmol/L), $FEHCO_3$ ≥15%.
         - In Type 1 RTA, serum bicarbonate is low, $FEHCO_3$ <5%.
      iii. U-B pCO_2 differentiates classical distal RTA from voltage-dependent distal RTA.
         - Measures distal H^+ secretion that reacts with luminal HCO_3^- to form carbonic acid, which dehydrates slowly in the

medullary collecting duct to form CO_2 that is trapped in the renal tubule, resulting in an increase in the U-B pCO_2.

- In classical distal RTA, urine pCO_2 <50 mmHg and U-B pCO_2 <10 mmHg as there is a failure of distal H^+ secretion.
- In voltage-dependent distal RTA, urine pCO_2 >70 mmHg and the U-B pCO_2 >20 mmHg because the ability to generate high urinary pCO_2 is retained, as the proton pump function is normal and the H^+ gradient does not favor back-diffusion during alkaline diuresis.

2. Ammonium chloride loading test:
   a. Performed to identify incomplete distal RTA, whereby impaired distal acidification exists but serum HCO_3^- is normal because the net acid excretion is maintained at a rate equal to acid generation.
   b. Methodology:
      i. Oral ammonium chloride 0.1 g/kg as a single dose or a 3-day modified acid load is given.
      ii. With the single dose acid load, urine pH (using pH meter) and serum bicarbonate concentration are measured at 2, 4 and 6 hours.
      iii. Adequate acidification is defined by a decrease in serum bicarbonate concentration by >3 mmol/L.
      iv. Problems include poor patient tolerance with nausea and vomiting due to gastric irritation.
   c. Interpretation:
      - Failure of the urine pH to fall to ≤5.3 is consistent with incomplete distal RTA.
3. Furosemide loading test:
   a. Performed to elucidate the possible site (cortical versus medullary) and mechanism of acidification defect in distal RTA.
   b. Methodology:
      i. Single oral dose of frusemide at 2 mg/kg (maximum 40 mg).
      ii. Urine pH is measured hourly for 8 hours.
      iii. Urine K^+ is measured at the end of 8 hours.
   c. Interpretation:
      i. Furosemide increases sodium delivery and reabsorption in the cortical collecting tubule, hence increasing luminal electronegativity.

ii. In hypokalemic type 1 or distal RTA, the urine pH does not fall, but the urine K^+ excretion increases.
iii. In voltage-dependent distal RTA, there is baseline hyperkalemia and no post-furosemide increase in H^+ or K^+ excretion since luminal electronegativity is not enhanced.

Defect	Site of Defect	Urine pH		K^+ Excretion	
		During Acidosis	After Furosemide	Baseline	After Furosemide
Normal	None	<5.5	Further decline	Normal	Increased
H^+-ATPase defect	Diffuse, cortical collecting tubule	>5.5	>5.5	Normal	Increased
H^+-ATPase defect	Medullary collecting tubule alone	>5.5	<5.5	Normal	Increased
Voltage defect	Cortical collecting tubule	>5.5	>5.5	Decreased	Unchanged

V. *Practical guide of investigations to differentiate types of RTA*

	Proximal RTA	Distal RTA		Type 4 RTA
		Classic	Hyperkalemic	
Plasma K^+	Normal/low	Normal/low	High	High
Urine pH	<5.5	>5.5	>5.5	<5.5
Urine anion gap	Negative	Positive	Positive	Positive
Urine NH_4^+	Normal	Low	Low	Low
Fractional HCO_3^- excretion	>10–15%	<5%	<5%	5–10%

(*Continued*)

	Proximal RTA	Distal RTA		Type 4 RTA
		Classic	Hyperkalemic	
U-B PCO_2 (mmHg)	>20	<20	>20	>20
Urine calcium	Normal	High	High	Normal/ low
Urine citrate	Normal	Decreased	Decreased	Normal
Other tubular defects	Often present	Absent	Absent	Absent
Nephrocalcinosis	Absent	Present	Present	Absent
Bone disease	Common	Often present	Uncommon	Absent

F. Management

1. Aims of treatment:
   a. Correction of biochemical abnormalities including acidosis, hypokalemia, hypercalciuria, hypophosphatemia, and hypocitraturia.
   b. Improvement of growth.
   c. Correction of bony abnormalities.
   d. Prevention of nephrocalcinosis.
2. Correction of metabolic acidosis:
   a. Bicarbonate requirements:
      i. Type 1 RTA:
         - Infants: 5–8 mmol/kg/day.
         - Children: 3–4 mmol/kg/day.
         - Adults: 1–2 mmol/kg/day.
      ii. Type 2 RTA:
         - 10–20 mmol/kg/day.
         - Larger doses are required, especially in infancy.
         - Requirement often decreases with age in isolated sporadic proximal RTA.
   b. Types of oral alkali:
      i. Sodium bicarbonate 500 mg tablet provides 6 mmol Na^+ and 6 mmol HCO_3^-.

ii. Sodium citrate/citric acid (Shohl's solution or Bicitra) provides 1 mmol Na^+ and 1 mmol citrate per ml.
iii. Potassium citrate:
- 30% Solution (per ml) = 2.8 mmol K^+ + 1.2 mmol citrate.
- Tablet (1080 mg) = 10 mmol K^+ + 3.3 mmol citrate.
- Polycitra (per ml) = 2 mmol K^+ + 2 mmol citrate.

c. Choice of alkali therapy:
i. Type 2 RTA:
- Mixture of sodium and potassium salts is required.

ii. Type 1 RTA:
- Potassium citrate is preferable as a high sodium load may enhance hypercalciuria and nephrocalcinosis.
- Citrate-containing solutions are preferable as hypocitraturia is a feature.

d. Dosing regimen:
i. Alkali therapy should be given in divided doses 6 hourly, especially in Type 2 RTA, to compensate for a rapid rate of urinary bicarbonate loss.
ii. A higher night-time dose for patients with Type 1 RTA and issues of non-compliance so as to optimize correction of metabolic acidosis during this period when maximal growth hormone secretion is occurring.

3. Correction of electrolyte abnormalities:
a. Hypokalemia:
- Potassium citrate rather than potassium chloride should be given unless the patient is alkalotic.

b. Hypophosphatemia:
i. Supplemental oral phosphate 1–3 g/day (0.3–0.1 mmol/day) given 4–5 times daily.
ii. Vitamin D supplementation should be added in children with rickets.

4. Prevention of nephrocalcinosis and urolithiasis:
a. Early diagnosis and adequate correction of acidosis in infancy are important to prevent the development of nephrocalcinosis in classical Type 1 RTA.
b. Correction of hypocitraturia preferably with potassium citrate:
- Avoid hypokalemia as this potentiates hypocitraturia by stimulating citrate reabsorption.

   c. Thiazide diuretics to reduce hypercalciuria may be required if this persists after a correction of acidosis.
      - Dose of hydrochlorothiazide: 1–1.5 mg/kg 12–24 hourly (maximum 50 mg/dose).
5. Treatment of hyperkalemia in hyperkalemic forms of RTA:
   a. Restrict potassium intake:
      i. Limit dietary intake of potassium.
      ii. Avoid potassium-retaining drugs.
   b. Correction of acidosis: 1.5–2 mmol/kg/day.
   c. Oral furosemide 0.5–1 mg/kg OM or BD if the correction of acidosis and restriction of potassium intake are unable to maintain serum K^+ <6 mmol/L.
   d. Cation-exchange resins may be indicated if frusemide is unable to reduce the serum K^+ <6 mmol/L.
      - Resonium 0.5–1 g/kg/dose (maximum 30 g) given 6–8 hourly.
   e. Indications for fludrocortisone (50–100 μg/m²/day):
      i. Hypoaldosteronism due to adrenal failure.
      ii. Pseudohypoaldosteronism:
         - In combination with a high salt intake.
         - Carbenoxolone is an alternative.
      iii. Hyporeninemic hypoaldosteronism:
         - Preferably in combination with a loop diuretic to reduce the risk of extracellular fluid volume expansion.

Recommended Reading

1. Soriano JR. (2002) Renal tubular acidosis: The clinical entity. *J Am Soc Nephrol* **13**:2160–2170.
2. Karet FE. (2009) Mechanisms in hyperkalemic renal tubular acidosis. *J Am Soc Nephrol* **20**:251–254.
3. Mattoo TK. (2010, updated) Etiology and clinical manifestations of renal tubular acidosis in infants and children. Edited by: Stapleton FB, Kim MS. *UpToDate ONLINE*. http://www.uptodateonline.com.
4. Emmet M, Palmer BF. (2020, updated) Etiology and diagnosis of distal (type 1) and proximal (type 2) renal tubular acidosis. Edited by: Sterns RH, Forman JP. *UpToDate ONLINE*. http://www.uptodateonline.com.
5. Emmet M, Palmer BF. (2021, updated) Urine anion and osmolal gaps in metabolic acidosis. Edited by: Sterns RH, Forman JP. UpToDate ONLINE. http://www.uptodateonline.com.
6. Lemaire M. (2021) Novel Fanconi renotubular syndromes provide insights in proximal tubule pathophysiology. *Am J Physiol Renal Physiol* **320**:F145–F160.

2 Urolithiasis and Nephrocalcinosis

Koh CT, Chaturvedi S, Liu ID, Ambarsari CG, K Prabhakaran and Yap HK

A. Definition

1. Urolithiasis: Presence of calculi in the urinary tract.
2. Nephrocalcinosis: Generalized deposition of calcium throughout the renal parenchyma (usually in the medullary region).

B. Etiology

1. The approximate frequency of kidney stone types in the pediatric age group is calcium with phosphate or oxalate (57%), struvite (24%), uric acid (8%), cystine (6%), endemic (2%), mixed (2%), and other types (1%).
2. Mechanisms of stone formation:
   a. Supersaturation of crystals due to solute excess.
   b. Decreased levels of inhibitors of crystallization:
      - Citrate.
      - Magnesium.
      - Pyrophosphate.
      - Macromolecules such as glycosaminoglycans, osteopontin, and urinary prothrombin fragment 1.
   c. Urine pH predisposes to certain stone formation:
      - Acid urine pH <7 favors uric acid precipitation.
      - Alkaline urine pH >8.5 promotes calcium phosphate stone formation.
3. Dietary considerations:
   a. Dietary oxalate excess such as spinach, starfruit, rhubarb, strawberries, beet, nuts, legumes, and vitamin C.

   b. Excessive vitamin D.
   c. Ketogenic diet:
      - Promotes enteric hyperoxaluria.
   d. Melamine-contaminated milk powder.
4. Enhanced enteric absorption of oxalate (enteric hyperoxaluria) related to fat malabsorption, bile salt injury to the colonic epithelium, or absence of oxalate-degrading bacteria following antibiotic treatment:
   a. Inflammatory bowel disease.
   b. Extensive bowel resection.
   c. Pancreatitis.
   d. Cystic fibrosis.
5. Environmental considerations:
   a. Dehydration due to environmental conditions.
   b. Immobilization with increased bone resorption.
6. Drugs:
   a. Steroids, loop diuretics and carbonic anhydrase inhibitors such as topiramate, zonisamide and acetazolamide:
      - Hypercalciuria.
   b. Tumor lysis syndrome:
      - Uric acid stones and calcium phosphate stones.
   c. Allopurinol:
      - Xanthine oxidase stones.
   d. Orlistat:
      - Inhibits gastrointestinal lipase causing secondary hyperoxaluria.
7. Urinary tract infections (20–25%):
   a. Struvite stones (magnesium ammonium phosphate) are associated with infection by a urea-splitting organism such as Proteus, Providencia, Klebsiella, Pseudomonas, and enterococci.
   b. Struvite stones tend to produce a staghorn appearance.
8. Structural abnormalities (10–25%):
   a. Medullary sponge kidney.
   b. Autosomal dominant polycystic kidney disease.
   c. Pelviureteric junction obstruction.
   d. Horseshoe kidney.
   e. Bladder exstrophy.
   f. Neurogenic bladder.
   g. Augmentation of the bladder.

9. **Genetic defects of metabolic pathways can lead to excessive excretion of calcium, oxalate, uric acid, cysteine, and xanthine.**

Type of Calculus	Disorders (Gene Mutation)	Gene *Mutation* Protein Product
Calcium oxalate	Primary hyperoxaluria, type I	*AGXT* alanine-glyoxylate-aminotransferase
	Primary hyperoxaluria, type II	*GRHPR* GR/HPR (glyoxylate reductase/hydroxylpyruvate reductase)
	Primary hyperoxaluria, type III	*HOGA1* 4-hydroxy-2-oxoglutarate aldolase
Calcium phosphate	Autosomal dominant renal tubular acidosis	*SLC4A1/AE1* basolateral chloride-bicarbonate anion exchanger-1
	Autosomal recessive distal renal tubular acidosis with hearing loss	*ATP6V1/B1* B1 subunit of vacuolar H+ ATPase
	Autosomal recessive distal renal tubular acidosis	*SLC4A1* A4 subunit of vacuolar H+ ATPase
	Autosomal dominant idiopathic hypercalciuria	*ADCY10* Adenylate cyclase 10 *VDR* Vitamin D receptor
	Autosomal dominant hypocalcemic hypercalciuria type 1	*CASR* Calcium sensing receptor
	Autosomal dominant hypocalcemic hypercalciuria type 2	*GNA11* G-protein subunit signaling partner Gα11

(*Continued*)

Type of Calculus	Disorders (Gene Mutation)	Gene *Mutation* Protein Product
Calcium phosphate	Familial hypomagnesemia with hypercalciuria and nephrocalcinosis	*CLDN16, CLDN19* Paracellulin (claudin 16, claudin 19)
	Dent's disease	*CLCN5* Chloride/proton antiporter CLC-5
	Lowe syndrome (Oculocerebrorenal syndrome)	*OCRL1* Phosphatidylinositol-4-5-biphosphate-5-phosphatase
	Bartter syndrome type 1	*SLC12A1/NKCC2* Bumetanide-sodium-potassium-chloride cotransporter
	Bartter syndrome type 2	*KCNJ/ROMK* Renal outer-medullary potassium channel
	Bartter syndrome type 3	*CLCNKB* CLC-Kb voltage-gated chloride channel
	Bartter syndrome type 4	*BSND* Barttin
	Bartter syndrome type 5	*CASR* (severe gain of function) Calcium sensing receptor
	Bartter syndrome type 6	*CLCN5* Chloride channel protein 5
	Williams–Beuren syndrome	Continuous gene deletion syndrome 7q11.23, including *ELN, LIMK1, RFC2* Elastin, LIM-kinase 1

(*Continued*)

(*Continued*)

Type of Calculus	Disorders (Gene Mutation)	Gene *Mutation* Protein Product
Calcium phosphate	Nephrolithiasis and osteopetrosis associated with hypophosphatemia	*NPT2a* Sodium-phosphate-cotransporter type 2a (SLC34A1)
	X-linked dominant hypophosphatemic rickets	*PHEX* phosphate regulating endo-peptidase homolog X-linked
	Hereditary hypophosphatemia with rickets and hypercalciuria	*NPT2c* Sodium-phosphate-cotransporter type 2c (SLC34A3)
	Infantile hypercalcaemia	*CYP24A1* Cytochrome P450 family 24 subfamily A member 1 *SLC34A1* Solute carrier family 34 member 1
Cystine	Cystinuria type A	Mutation of both alleles of *SLC3A1* rBAT
	Cystinuria type B	Mutation of both alleles of *SLC7A9* B^{o+}AT
	Cystinuria type A/B	*SLC3A1/SLC7A9* rBAT and B^{o+}AT
Uric acid	Lesch-Nyhan syndrome	*HPRT* Hypoxanthine-guanine-phosphoribosyltransferase
	Partial HPRT deficiency	*HPRT* Hypoxanthine-guanine-phosphoribosyltransferase

(*Continued*)

Type of Calculus	Disorders (Gene Mutation)	Gene *Mutation* Protein Product
	Glycogenosis type 1a	*G6PC* Glucose-6-phosphatase
	Glycogenosis type 1b	*SLC37A4* Glucose-6-phosphatase transporter
	Phosphoribosyl-phosphate synthetase I superactivity	*PRPS I* Phosphoribosyl-phosphate synthetase I
	Renal uric acid wasting	*SLC22A12* Solute carrier family 22 member 12 *SLC2A9* Solute carrier family 2 member 9
2,8-dihydroxyadenine	AR	*APRT* Adenine-phosphoribosyl-transferase
Xanthine stones	Hereditary xanthinuria type 1 (AR)	*XDH* Xanthine dehydrogenase
	Hereditary xanthinuria type 2 (AR)	*MOCOS* Molybdenum cofactor sulfurase
	Molybdenum cofactor deficiency	*MOCS1* Molybdenum cofactor biosynthesis protein 1 *MOCS2* Molybdopterin synthase sulfur carrier subunit *GPHN* Gephyrin

C. Diagnostic Evaluation

I. Clinical evaluation

1. Typical clinical presentations of stone disease in children:
   a. Sudden intense loin radiating towards the lower abdomen or groin.
   b. Gross hematuria with or without abdominal pain.
   c. Dysuria and urgency with or without urinary tract infection.
   d. Asymptomatic with an incidental finding on abdominal imaging.
2. History:
   a. Recurrent urinary tract infections.
   b. Frequent bouts of abdominal pain.
   c. Hematuria (gross or microscopic).
   d. Passage of previous calculus or sediments.
   e. Dietary intake:
      - Oxalate, purine, calcium, phosphate, fructose, animal protein, salt.
      - Fluid intake including habitual fluids such as cola drinks, milk, tea, sports drinks.
   f. Drug and vitamin intake.
   g. Underlying anatomical urinary tract abnormalities.
   h. Gastrointestinal disorders resulting in enhanced enteric absorption.
   i. Prolonged immobilization.
   j. History of prematurity including diuretic use.
   k. History of hearing loss.
   l. Family history of stone disease present in 40%.
3. Physical examination:
   a. Growth retardation or failure to thrive may indicate a congenital or metabolic disorder associated with nephrocalcinosis or urolithiasis.
   b. Dysmorphic features or signs of rickets suggestive of an associated metabolic disorder.
   c. Presence of an abdominal mass indicative of hydronephrosis or a neurogenic bladder.

II. Investigations

1. Prompt evaluation is important because urolithiasis can result in urinary tract obstruction.
2. Metabolic abnormalities occur in 42% to 84% of children with urolithiasis, therefore every child with urinary stone should have a complete metabolic evaluation.
3. To avoid erroneous results, a metabolic evaluation should ideally be performed in an outpatient setting where the patient is consuming a regular diet and is free of infections.
4. 24-hour urine biochemistry should be done at least 20 days after stone removal or expulsion.
5. Stepwise investigations should be carried out as follows:

Step	Investigations	
Step 1: Initial laboratory tests	• Urine microscopy for pyuria, hematuria. • Urine microscopy for crystals (calcium oxalate, calcium phosphate, struvite, uric acid, 2,8 dihydroxyadenine, cystine). • Early morning urine pH and specific gravity. • Urine culture. • Urine calcium:creatinine ratio. • Serum creatinine, urea, sodium, potassium, chloride, bicarbonate, calcium, phosphate, uric acid.	
Step 2a: Imaging	Modality	Limitations
	• Plain abdominal X-Ray of kidneys, ureters and bladder (KUB) to detect radiopaque stones (calcium, struvite, cystine). Note: Staghorn calculi are struvite stones.	• May miss 40% of stones: Radiolucent stones (uric acid, xanthine, 2,8-dihydroxy-adenine). Small stones. Stones overlying bony structures.
	• Kidney ultrasound to detect nephrocalcinosis and nephrolithiasis including radiolucent stones, hydronephrosis and hydroureter, bladder stones, and bladder wall abnormalities.	• Unable to detect small stones <5 mm, papillary or caliceal stones, or ureteral stones.

(Continued)

(*Continued*)

Step	Investigations	
	• Non-contrast helical computed tomography (CT) scan (most sensitive) to detect ureteral stones, radiolucent stones, and small stones (1 mm) not seen by other modalities, obstruction and other structural abnormalities.	
	• Diuretic renography with ^{99m}Technetium Mercaptoacetyltriglycine (MAG3) to detect obstruction and assess relative kidney function.	• Unable to detect stones.
Step 2b: Stone analysis	• Chemical analysis. • Infrared spectroscopy. • X–ray diffraction (amounts of <1 mg can be analyzed).	
Step 3a: Additional urine biochemistry (normal calcium diet)	• Spot urine:molar creatinine ratios of oxalate, uric acid, citrate, and magnesium. Note: Molar creatinine ratios may be erroneous if the patient has decreased muscle mass due to muscle disease. • Spot urine calcium:citrate ratio. • Cystine screening (nitroprusside test, quantitative cystine excretion). • 24-hour urine: Calcium, phosphorus, magnesium, oxalate, uric acid, citrate, cystine, protein, and creatinine.	
Step 3b: Blood/serum	Additional tests depend on the results of the initial evaluation: • Paired serum (with urine) calcium, phosphate, uric acid, and magnesium. • Parathyroid hormone (PTH) and vitamin D metabolites (if hypercalcemic). • Evaluate for renal tubular acidosis if initial results are indicative.	

6. Evaluation of hypercalciuria:
   a. Exclude causes of hypercalcemia.
   b. Distinguish between the types of hypercalciuria:
      - Absorptive hypercalciuria.

- Renal hypercalciuria.
- Resorptive hypercalciuria.

c. Repeat the 24-hour urine calcium excretion or urine calcium:creatinine ratio (first-morning specimen) after a 7-day low calcium diet (400 mg/day after infancy) to distinguish between absorptive and renal hypercalciuria or resorptive hypercalciuria.

7. Grading of nephrocalcinosis:

Grade of Nephrocalcinosis	Ultrasonographic Appearance
0	No abnormal echogenicity of the medullary pyramids.
I	Mild increase in echogenicity around the border of the medullary pyramids.
II	Mild diffuse increase in echogenicity of the entire medullary pyramid.
III	Greater, more homogeneous increase in the echogenicity of the entire medullary pyramid.

D. Management

I. Management of acute episode:

1. Pain relief:
   a. Non-steroidal anti-inflammatory agents if the kidney function is normal.
   b. Narcotic analgesics including intravenous morphine as needed.
2. Facilitating passage of stone.
   a. Majority of stones <5 mm in diameter will pass spontaneously, even in small children.
   b. Intravenous hydration at 1.5–2x the maintenance rate.
   c. Retrieval of stones should be attempted by using a urine strainer for several days in order to send for stone analysis.
   d. Monitor movement of stones by repeat kidney ultrasonography.
   e. Medical expulsive therapy with Tamsulosin:
      i. For children >2 years of age with symptomatic ureterovesical stones.

ii. Dose: 0.01 mg/kg (maximum 0.4 mg) in the evening before bedtime.
- 2–4 years: 0.2 mg.
- ≥5 years: 0.4 mg.

Note: Capsule can be broken and placed into food.

iii. Precautions:
- Main concern is orthostatic hypotension and may enhance the hypotensive effects of antihypertensives.
- Use with caution if there is a sulfonamide allergy, as there can be cross-reaction.
- Use with caution in children with enteral feeding tubes as it might cause blockage.

iv. To consider urological intervention if there is no spontaneous passage by 2–4 weeks.

3. Immediate urologic intervention is indicated in:
   a. Severe pain despite adequate analgesia (most often due to a pelviuretericor vesicoureteric junction stone or a stone >5 mm that is unable to pass spontaneously).
   b. Urosepsis in an obstructed system.
   c. Anuria with complete obstruction.
   d. Acute kidney injury secondary to partial obstruction by a stone in a solitary kidney or bilateral ureteric obstruction.

II. Prevention of recurrence:

1. Fluid intake:
   a. Should be at least 2L/1.73 m^2.
   b. Must be sufficient to maintain the following 24-hour urine volumes:
      - Infants: ≥750 ml.
      - Children <5 years: ≥1000 ml.
      - Children 5–10 years: ≥1500 ml.
      - Children >10 years: ≥2000 ml.
2. Metabolic control:
   a. Hypercalciuria:
      i. Dietary measures to reduce urinary calcium excretion include:
      - Avoid excessive animal protein intake, as this is associated with increased production of acids.

- Low-sodium diet as this enhances sodium and calcium renal tubular reabsorption.
- Ensure adequate potassium intake (fruits and vegetables) as low potassium intake enhances urinary calcium excretion.
- Maintain normal dietary calcium intake as low calcium intake results in increased oxalate absorption and secondary hyperoxaluria.
- Avoid vitamin D supplementation because elevated serum 1,25-dihydroxyvitamin D3 levels increase intestinal calcium absorption and promote bone resorption, resulting in hypercalciuria.

ii. Thiazide diuretics:
- Enhances sodium and calcium reabsorption in the distal renal tubule, reducing hypercalciuria.
- Should be considered if dietary measures fail to reduce urinary calcium levels over 3–6 months.
- Dose of hydrochlorothiazide: 1–1.5 mg/kg 12–24 hourly (maximum 50 mg/dose).
- Addition of amiloride increases calcium reabsorption in the cortical collecting tubule (avoid concomitant use of potassium citrate as this may result in hyperkalemia).
- Avoid hypokalemia as this results in intracellular acidosis, which enhances citrate metabolism, creating a more favorable gradient for citrate reabsorption.

iii. Other measures if there is persistent hypercalciuria:
- Potassium citrate: 2–3 mmol/kg (adult 30–80 mmol) daily as this raises the plasma bicarbonate concentration, increasing calcium reabsorption and decreasing calcium excretion.
- Neutral phosphate (orthophosphate). This may reduce calcium excretion and increase the excretion of inhibitors of crystallization such as pyrophosphate.
- Avoid sodium bicarbonate or sodium citrate as this will increase sodium and therefore calcium excretion and also increase the urinary excretion of citrate, a potent inhibitor of calcium stone formation.

b. Secondary hyperoxaluria:
   i. Low-fat diet in patients with fat malabsorption.
   ii. Adequate calcium intake as low calcium intake enhances enteric oxalate absorption.
   iii. Magnesium and pyrophosphate supplementation, which are inhibitors of calcium oxalate precipitation.
      - Magnesium 6 mg/kg/day (maximum 200–400 mg/day), to maintain a normal serum magnesium level and urinary magnesium excretion.
   iv. Cholestyramine in patients with fat malabsorption as this binds both intestinal bile acids and oxalate, but side effects may be limiting.

c. Hypocitraturia:
   i. Alkalinization of urine is recommended as alkalinization decreases the uptake of citrate by proximal tubular cells.
   ii. Potassium citrate at 2–3 mmol/kg (adult 30–80 mmol) daily is preferred as the alkalinization agent as there is also direct excretion of the administered citrate.
   iii. Precautions must be taken when providing alkali supplements in patients with calcium phosphate stones as alkali pH predisposes to calcium phosphate crystal formation.
      - Monitor the urine pH, urine calcium:creatinine ratio, 24-hour urine citrate excretion, and urine calcium:citrate ratio.
      - Optimal urinary citrate excretion should be closer to the 50th centile rather than the 5th centile.
      - Aim for a urinary calcium:citrate ratio <0.326 mg/mg (<0.0082 mmol/mg).
      - Discontinue supplemental alkali if the urine pH rises above 6.5 without a significant increase in urine citrate or decrease in urine calcium excretion.

d. Hyperuricosuria:
   i. Alkalinization of the urine to prevent uric acid precipitation and promote the dissolution of uric acid crystals and stones.
      - Use potassium citrate, not sodium citrate as sodium-induced volume expansion may result in hypercalciuria.
   ii. Restriction of dietary purine.
   iii. Dietary sodium restriction to decrease uric acid and calcium excretion.

iv. Allopurinol to decrease the production of uric acid.
- Generally indicated in children with a known disorder of uric acid metabolism.
- Dose: 5–10 mg/kg/day in divided doses (a maximum daily dose of 300 mg for uric acid stones, 600 mg in inborn errors of metabolism).
- Requires a dose adjustment in kidney failure: 50% of dose in those with a glomerular filtration rate of 10–50 ml/min/1.73m^2.
- Should not be taken with azathioprine or 6-mercaptopurine.
- Consider testing for HLA-B*5801 allele in patients with an increased risk of developing severe cutaneous adverse reactions, namely Koreans, Han Chinese and Thais.

v. Febuxostat can be used in those who are unable to tolerate allopurinol.
- Dose in adults: 40–120 mg daily.
- Should not be taken with azathioprine or 6-mercaptopurine.

e. Xanthinuria:
  i. High fluid intake.
  ii. Low purine diet.

f. 2,8-dihydroxyadenine crystalluria:
  i. High fluid intake.
  ii. Low purine diet.
  iii. Allopurinol in a dose of 5–10 mg/kg/day in divided doses (maximum 600–800 mg/day).
  iv. Febuxostat can be used in those with allopurinol hypersensitivity.

III. Interventional stone removal:

1. Indications for elective stone removal:
   a. Symptomatic children who fail to pass a stone after two weeks.
   b. Staghorn calculi (struvite stones).
   c. Stones >5 mm as they are less likely to pass spontaneously.
2. Choice of urological intervention depends on:
   a. Stone size.
   b. Location of stone.
   c. Composition of stone.
   d. Accompanying structural abnormalities.

3. Extracorporeal shockwave lithotripsy (ESWL):
   a. Good for stones <2 cm.
   b. Better for stones in the renal pelvis and upper ureter.
   c. Impacted stones, calcium oxalate monohydrate stones, cystine stones, and cases with unfavorable anatomy are less amenable to fragments.
   d. Struvite, calcium oxalate dihydrate, and uric acids fragment readily.
   e. Stent placement is recommended for stones >2 cm to reduce the risk of obstruction.
   f. Residual fragments <4 mm may pass without symptoms and may clear only after several months.
   g. Stone-free rates range from 70 to 90% after ESWL, depending on the experience of the clinician, complexity of the stones, and presence of an underlying structural abnormality.
   h. Monitoring with kidney ultrasound or X-Ray KUB should be performed at 1 year and, if negative, every 2–4 years thereafter.
4. Ureteroscopy with lithotomy or lithotripsy:
   a. Particularly effective for the treatment of proximal ureteral calculi, especially those (<1.5 cm) in the lower pole calyces.
   b. When ESWL, as the primary choice of treatment, fails to disintegrate the stones or when the stones are harder and not as amenable to ESWL.
   c. Especially useful for middle and lower-third ureteric stones.
5. Percutaneous nephrostolithotomy or lithotripsy:
   a. For renal pelvic and calyceal stones >2 cm.
   b. Preferred procedure if there is an accompanying calyceal dilatation or pelviureteric junction obstruction.
   c. When the stones are harder and therefore not as amenable to ESWL.
   d. Stone-free rates equivalent to ESWL.
6. Open nephrolithotomy:
   a. For children who have failed other urologic procedures or those with complex renal or ureteral anatomic abnormalities.
   b. Renal split in patients with staghorn calculi.

IV. Monitoring

1. Repeat metabolic studies 2–3 months after starting pharmacological interventions and subsequently 6-monthly to yearly if results have normalized.
2. Repeat kidney sonography should be done at 6 months, then yearly after stone removal or expulsion.

V. Management algorithm

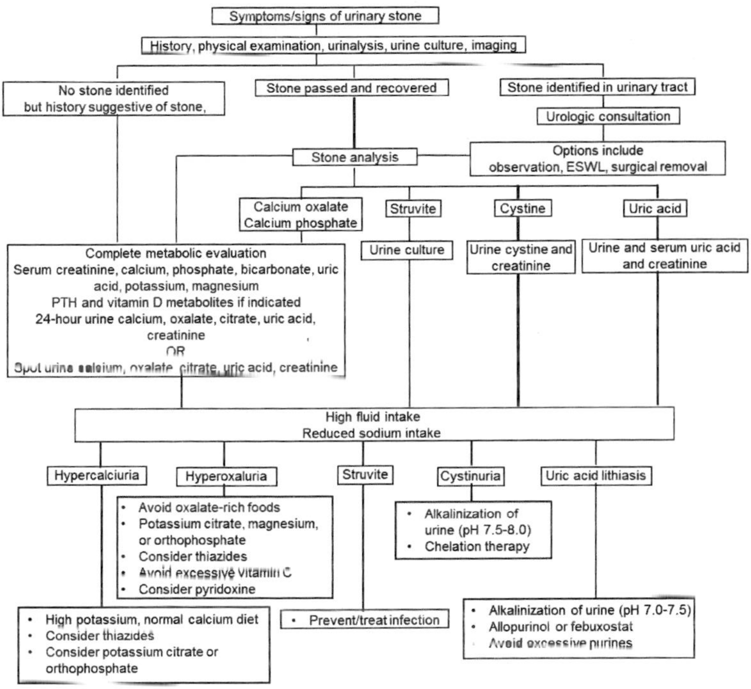

Recommended Reading

1. Dick PT, Shuckett BM, Tang B, Daneman A, Kooh SW. (1999) Observer reliability in grading nephrocalcinosis on ultrasound examinations in children. *Pediatr Radiol* **29**:68–72.
2. Habbig S, Beck BB, Hoppe BB. (2011) Nephrocalcinosis and urolithiasis in children. *Kidney Int* **80**:1278–1291.
3. Skolarikos A, Straub M, Knoll T, Sarica K, Seitz C, Petřík A, Türk C. (2015) Metabolic evaluation and recurrence prevention for urinary stone patients: EAU guidelines. *Eur Urol* **67**:750–763.
4. Türk C, Knoll T, Petrik A, Sarica K, Skolarikos A, Straub M, Seitz C. (2015) Management of urolithiasis in children. In: *2015 Guidelines on Urolithiasis. European Association of Urology*. pp. 34–35. http://uroweb.org/guideline/urolithiasis/.
5. Jackson EC, Avendt-Reeber M. (2016) Urolithiasis in children — Treatment and prevention. *Curr Treat Options Peds* **2**:10–22.
6. Smith J, Stapleton FB. (2019, updated) Prevention of recurrent nephrolithiasis in children. Edited by: Baskin LS, Kim MS. *UpToDate ONLINE*. http://www.uptodateonline.com.
7. Smith J, Stapleton FB. (2019, updated) Clinical features and diagnosis of nephrolithiasis in children. Edited by: Baskin LS, Kim MS. *UpToDate ONLINE*. http://www.uptodateonline.com.
8. Smith J, Stapleton FB. (2019, updated) Epidemiology and risk factors for nephrolithiasis in children. Edited by: Baskin LS, Kim MS. *UpToDate ONLINE*. http://www.uptodateonline.com.
9. Smith J, Stapleton FB. (2020, updated) Acute management of nephrolithiasis in children. Edited by: Baskin LS, Kim MS. *UpToDate ONLINE*. http://www.uptodateonline.com.
10. Howles SA, Thakker RV. (2020) Genetics of kidney stone disease. *Nat Rev Urol* **17**:407–421.

3 Management of Cystinuria

Lu L, Yap HK and Resontoc LP

A. Pathophysiology and Genetics

1. Pathophysiology:
   a. Amino acids are reabsorbed from the glomerular filtrate in the proximal tubule.
   b. Loss-of-function mutations in the dibasic amino acid transporter results in increased urinary excretion of cystine, ornithine, arginine, and lysine.
   c. Due to the low solubility of cystine, increased urinary concentration results in the formation of cystine uroliths.
   d. Mutations in *SLC3A1* and/or *SLC7A9*, which form the dibasic amino acid transporter, are present in 91% of patients with cystinuria.
   e. Inheritance is autosomal recessive or rarely digenic.
2. International Cystinuria Consortium Classification:

Classification	Type A	Type B	Type AB
Gene (locus)	*SLC3A1* encoding rBAT (Chromosome 2)	*SLC7A9* encoding $b^{0,+}$AT (Chromosome 19)	*SLC3A1/SLC7A9* (Chromosome 2 and 19)
Urinary excretion of cystine and dibasic aminoacids in heterozygotes	Normal	Elevated	Normal (rare, mild phenotype)

3. Hypotonia-cystinuria syndrome:
   - Occurs in patients with one mutant *SLC3A1* allele and a second mutant gene called prolyl endopeptidase-like (*PREPL*).
   - Presents with hypotonia and poor feeding during infancy.

4. 2p21 deletion syndrome with deletion of *PREPL* and two other genes:
   - Presents with severe developmental retardation, elevated serum lactate, hypotonia, poor feeding, and cystinuria.

B. Approach to Diagnosis

1. Clinical Presentation:
   a. Nephrolithiasis (usually in childhood or adolescence).
   b. Syndromic features (as above).
   c. Screening of:
      i. Asymptomatic sibling of the affected individual.
      ii. Infant with a hyperechoic colon on fetal ultrasound prior to 36 weeks of gestation.
2. Diagnosis:
   a. Stone analysis showing a cystine stone.
   b. Urine for hexagonal cystine crystals:
      - Detected in 20–25% of cases.
   c. Urine amino acid quantification:
      - Elevated urine cystine levels >1.7 mmol/day or >150 μmol/mmol creatinine.
      - Accompanied by elevated levels of the other dibasic amino acids (ornithine, arginine, lysine).
   d. Cyanide-nitroprusside test:
      - Screening test (urine cystine >312 μmol/L).
      - No longer recommended due to its low reproducibility and sensitivity.
3. Genetic testing:
   a. Not routinely performed due to limited genotype-phenotype correlation.
   b. Can still be considered in the first proband in the pedigree to confirm the diagnosis and genetic counseling of other family members.
   c. Next-generation sequencing-based methods, rather than Sanger sequencing, are preferred as a significant proportion of patients have large-scale rearrangements/copy number variants.

C. Theoretical Considerations in Medical Treatment

1. Aim of medical therapy is to maintain the cystine concentration in the urine below its solubility level.
2. The solubility of cystine in urine is pH-dependent, being higher at alkaline pH, and it is also affected by other urinary ions and macromolecules.
3. The limit of solubility of cystine in urine is about 1000 μmol/L (243 mg/L) at a urine pH of 7–7.5.
4. When cystine is present in concentrations above its solubility, the urine is supersaturated.
5. The degree of supersaturation may be expressed as the ratio between the actual concentration and the solubility limit, as shown here:

$$\text{Supersaturation of cystine} = \frac{\text{Measured cystine concentration}}{\text{Estimated cystine solubility}}$$

   - Cystine crystals will dissolve when the supersaturation is <1.0.
   - Supersaturation >1.0 is associated with an increased likelihood of stone formation.
   - Aim for a supersaturation level of 0.6 in a 24-hour urine specimen. This allows for variation in saturation over the course of the day, including the inevitable increase in supersaturation overnight when the urine volume drops.

D. Dietary Measures

1. Low protein diet in adolescents and adults (0.8–1 g protein/day): to reduce the methionine load.
   - Do not protein-restrict children, although food with high methionine content (i.e., dried cod, crayfish) can be avoided.
2. Low salt diet to reduce cystine excretion by decreasing natriuresis.
   - Adolescents and adults: ≤100 mmol/day.
   - Children: ≤1.5 mmol/kg/day.

E. Urine Dilution

1. Rate of cystine excretion can be used to estimate the optimal urine output to achieve a urine cystine concentration <1000 μmol/L.

- For example, if urine cystine excretion is 3000 μmol/day, then a urine output of at least 3 L/day will be needed to keep the urine cystine supersaturation <1.0 at a urine pH >7.0.

2. Typical urine output required:
   - Adolescents and adults: 4–5 L/day
   - Children: ≥2 L/m²/day
3. Drink throughout the day, and especially at night to ensure overnight diuresis, as urine cystine excretion is higher at night.
   - Drink before going to bed and when waking up at night to void.
   - Urine specific gravity can be monitored at home and should be ≤1.005.
   - Aim for early morning urine osmolality <500 mOsm/kg and urine cystine <1000 μmol/L.
4. Drink neutral and alkalinizing beverages such as herbal teas, citrus juices, and water.
5. Consider feeding via nasogastric tube or gastrostomy tube in children who are unable to meet required fluid targets.

F. Urine Alkalinization

1. Alkalinize urine: pH 7.5–8.0.
2. Use potassium citrate 20 mmol of citrate/dose 3–4 times a day.
   - Last dose should be taken at bedtime to provide round-the-clock urine alkalinization.
   - Further alkalinization can be achieved with orange juice, which contains potassium citrate.
3. Avoid the use of sodium bicarbonate, unless the patient has severe kidney insufficiency as sodium increases cystine excretion.
4. Urine pH should be monitored at least once a day at home at various times to ensure adequate round-the-clock urine alkalinization.
5. Avoid urine pH >8.5 due to the risk of calcium phosphate stones.
   - Avoid grapefruit juice as an increased incidence of calcium oxalate stones has been reported.

G. Medical Reduction of Cystine

1. Aim to reduce cystine to cysteine, which is 50x more soluble, especially in alkaline urine.

2. Chelation therapy with a thiol-containing drug may be used in conjunction with conservative measures if:
   a. Conservative measures fail after a 3-month trial defined by:
      - Failure to lower the urine cystine concentration to <1000 μmol/L.
      - Failure to raise the urine pH to >7.0 in a 24-hour urine.
      - Persistence of cystine crystals in the urine, which indicates supersaturation.
   b. Conservative measures are unrealistic, e.g., extremely high urine cystine excretion necessitating an impossibly high daily fluid intake.
   c. Tiopronin and d-penicillamine are the 2 common drugs in use.
      - Tiopronin and d-penicillamine have similar efficacy, but tiopronin is generally felt to have a better side-effect profile, although this is not supported by all studies.
   d. Captopril as a second-line agent if unable to tolerate.
3. Tiopronin (α-mercaptoproprionyl-glycine, MPG):
   a. Dose: 15–40 mg/kg/day (children) or 800–1500 mg/day (adults) in 3 divided doses.
      - A higher dose can be given at bedtime.
   b. Side effects:
      i. Dysgeusia (often transient).
      ii. Dermatological: Mucocutaneous lesions, exanthem, pemphigus, elastosis perforans serpiginosa.
      iii. Kidney: Proteinuria (Membranous nephropathy, minimal change disease).
      iv. Hematological: Neutropenia, thrombocytopenia, aplastic anemia
      v. Immune: Lupus-like drug reaction, myasthenia-gravis-like disease.
      vi. Others: Hepatotoxicity, zinc and copper deficiency.
   c. Starting with a lower dose and gradually up-titrating over 4 weeks may reduce side effects.
      - Particularly for mucocutaneous lesions developing soon after initiating treatment.

4. d-Penicillamine:
   a. Dose: 20–30 mg/kg/day (children) or 1–4 g/day (adults) in 3–4 divided doses.
      - A higher dose can be given at bedtime.
   b. Side effects:
      i. Similar to tiopronin, but also pyridoxine deficiency, and rarely crescentic glomerulonephritis.
      ii. Requires pyridoxine supplementation for those on long-term therapy.
         - Dose: 25–50 mg/day (not more than 2 mg/kg/day).
      iii. Although side effects are similar, adverse reactions of one drug do not preclude the use of the other.
5. Captopril:
   a. May be used if patient is unable to tolerate tiopronin or d-penicillamine, although its efficacy is limited.
   b. Dose: 0.1–0.3 mg/kg starting dose 8 hourly up to a maximum of 2 mg/kg 8 hourly (maximum adult dose: 50 mg 8 hourly).
   c. Dose limited by hyperkalemia and hypotension.

H. Monitoring

1. Urine cystine excretion:
   a. 24-hour urine cystine excretion (collect in preservative toluidine, or refrigerate) or urine cystine concentration: 3–6 months until the patient is stable, then 6–12 months, aiming for a urine cystine concentration <1000 μmol/L to prevent supersaturation.
   b. If stones still form, consider fractionated urine collection, e.g., separate collection of daytime and night-time urine to detect transient night-time supersaturation.
   c. For patients on thiol-containing drugs, this is not informative as most assays also detect drug-cysteine conjugates.
      - Monitor for crystalluria, and if available, urine supersaturation tests (urine cystine capacity).
2. Urine calcium, oxalate, uric acid, sodium, creatinine excretion either 24-hourly or a random urine solute:creatinine ratio: 6 monthly (3–12 monthly depending on the frequency of stone formation).
   - Advantage of a 24-hour collection is the estimation of urinary volume as a measure of fluid intake.

3. Ultrasound of the kidneys: 6 monthly (3–12 monthly depending on the frequency of stone formation).
4. For patients on tiopronin or d-penicillamine, the following should be monitored at least 3–6 monthly and more often after drug initiation or dose changes:
   a. Full blood count.
   b. Liver function test.
   c. Urine protein:creatinine ratio (UPCR).
   d. Consider measuring serum zinc and copper levels 6 monthly.
5. Monitoring for chronic kidney disease:
   a. From adolescence onward, or earlier if there are risk factors, e.g., nephron-reducing surgery.
   b. Blood pressure at every visit.
   c. Estimated glomerular filtration rate and UPCR at least annually.

I. Urological Interventions

1. Principles:
   a. Patients should be rendered stone-free whenever possible due to fast stone growth rates.
   b. Stones without urgent indication for removal, e.g., infection, obstruction, abnormal kidney function, can be observed for 4 weeks for spontaneous passage.
   c. Due to multiple stone passages, patients with cystinuria may be able to spontaneously pass larger stones than other patients with urolithiasis.
2. Interventions:
   a. Ureteroscopy is the main modality of removing ureteric stones and kidney stones <20 mm.
   b. Cystine stones are more resistant to extracorporeal shock wave lithotripsy (ESWL); however, it can be considered for stones <10 mm as it is non-invasive.
   c. Kidney stones >20 mm should be removed via percutaneous nephrolithotomy using miniaturized techniques, if possible.

   Consider staged ureteroscopic procedures if there is the necessary center-specific expertise.

Recommended Reading

1. Harvey E, Farhat WA. (2016) Renal Calculi. In: *Pediatric Kidney Disease*. Edited by: Geary DF, Schaefer F. Springer-Verlag Berlin Heidelberg. pp 1135–1191.
2. Goldfarb DS, Ferraro PM. (2020, updated) Cystine stones. Edited by: Goldfarb S, Lam AQ. *UpToDate ONLINE*. http://www.uptodate.com.
3. Servais A, Thomas K, Dello Strologo L, Sayer JA, Bekri S, Bertholet-Thomas A, Bultitude M, Capolongo G, Cerkauskiene R, Daudon M, Doizi S, Gillion V, Gràcia-Garcia S, Halbritter J, Heidet L, van den Heijkant M, Lemoine S, Knebelmann B, Emma F, Levtchenko E; Metabolic Nephropathy Workgroup of the European Reference Network for Rare Kidney Diseases (ERKNet) and eUROGEN. (2021) Cystinuria: Clinical practice recommendation. *Kidney Int* **99**:48–58.

4 Management of Primary Hyperoxaluria

Lu L, Ng KH, Teo S, Resontoc LP, Lau PYW, Liu ID and Yap HK

A. Genetics

1. Oxalate is a poorly soluble end product of the metabolism of amino acids and other compounds, where its immediate precursor is glyoxylate.
2. Primary hyperoxaluria (PH) results when enzymes involved in glyoxylate metabolism are deficient, resulting in the accumulation of glyoxylate, which is readily converted to oxalate by lactate dehydrogenase (LDH).

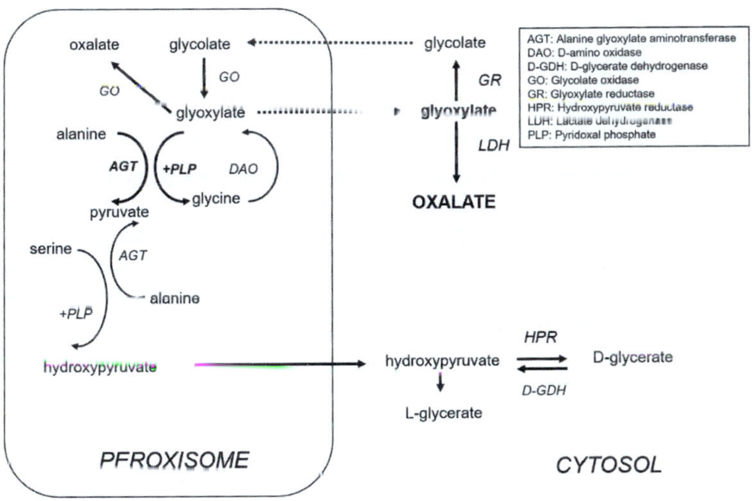

3. Primary hyperoxaluria type 1 (PH1) is the most common form of PH occurring in 70–80% (1:60000 to 1:120000 live births), whereas type 2 (PH2) occurs in 10% and type 3 (PH3) in 10–15%.

Classification	PH1	PH2	PH3
Inheritance	Autosomal recessive	Autosomal recessive	Autosomal recessive
Gene locus	Chromosome 2q37.3 (*AGXT*)	Chromosome 9q13-q21 (*GRHPR*)	Chromosome 10q24.2 (*HOGA1*)
Enzyme defect	Alanine:glyoxylate aminotransferase (AGT)	Glyoxylate reductase/hydroxyl-pyruvate reductase (GR/HPR)	4-hydroxy-2-oxoglutarate aldolase
Increased urinary excretion	Glycolate	L-glycerate	4-hydroxy-oxo-glutarate (HOG), dihydroxyglutarate (DHG), calcium
Kidney failure risk	50–100%	20%	Likely rare, with disease remission after infancy
Non-kidney manifestations (Systemic oxalosis)	++	Uncommon	Nil

4. Pyridoxine sensitivity is found in 10–30% of PH1 patients, as pyridoxal phosphate is a co-factor for AGT.
   - Patients with homozygous G170R and F152I mutations in *AGXT* have a high likelihood of responding to pharmacologic doses of pyridoxine, whereas the response remains unpredictable for other genotypes.

B. Clinical Manifestations

I. PH1:

1. Clinical presentations:
   a. Most common form with recurrent urolithiasis and progressive kidney failure, leading to a diagnosis during childhood or adolescence.
   b. Approximately similar proportion will only form stones occasionally in adulthood.
   c. Rare infantile form in 10–20% with early nephrocalcinosis and rapid kidney failure (infantile oxalosis).
   d. Rarely, PH1 is diagnosed after recurrence of disease after kidney transplantation.
   e. There is marked phenotypic variability, even within the same family.
2. Kidney involvement:
   a. Urinary tract symptoms: Loin pain, hematuria, urinary tract infection, passage of stones, nephrocalcinosis, uremia, metabolic acidosis, growth delay and failure to thrive, and anemia.
   b. Calculi are composed of calcium oxalate.
   c. Median age at presentation is 5 years, with kidney failure by 25 years of age in one-half of patients.
   d. The infantile form of PH1 often presents as a life-threatening condition due to a rapid progression to kidney failure in 80% by the age of 3.
3. Non-kidney involvement:
   a. Due to systemic oxalosis, that is, oxalate deposition in extrarenal organs when plasma oxalate concentration >30 µmol/L.
   b. Occurs when the glomerular filtration rate (GFR) falls below 40–50 ml/min/1.73m^2.
   c. Bone:
      - Oxalate osteopathy leads to pain, erythropoietin-resistant anemia, and spontaneous fractures, even in infancy.
      - Seen on radiographs as characteristic, dense supra-metaphyseal bands, with diffuse demineralization.

d. Joints:
  - Synovitis.
  - Chondrocalcinosis.

e. Heart:
  - Cardiomyopathy.
  - Arrhythmias: Heart block, even resulting in cardiac arrest.

f. Nerves:
  - Polyradiculo-neuropathy.
  - Mononeuritis multiplex.

g. Skin:
  - Ulcerating calcium oxalate nodules.
  - Calcinosis cutis.
  - Livedo reticularis.

h. Soft tissues:
  - Peripheral gangrene.

i. Retina:
  - Flecked retinopathy.
  - Choroidal neovascularization.

j. Others:
  - Intestinal infarction.
  - Hypothyroidism.
  - Dental problems (root resorption, pulp exposure).

II. PH2:

1. Recurrent episodes of urolithiasis in childhood.
2. Nephrocalcinosis is less common.
3. Generally less severe disease compared to PH1 with better preservation of kidney function.

III. PH3:

1. Early-onset urolithiasis (mean: 2 years old) that becomes more quiescent with age, with urolithiasis no longer occurring after 6 years of age.
2. Almost total absence of severe nephrocalcinosis.
3. May develop mild kidney impairment but do not typically progress to kidney failure.

4. Clinical remission with age (in spite of persisting hyperoxaluria) and presence of concomitant hypercalciuria are distinctive.

C. Diagnosis

1. Urine oxalate excretion:
   a. Urine oxalate:creatinine ratio (mmol/mmol).

Age (years)	Threshold Values for Diagnosis of PH
<6 months	<0.325–0.360
7 months to 2 years	<0.132–0.174
2–5 years	<0.098–0.101
6–14 years	<0.07–0.082
>16 years	<0.04

- To prevent alkaline conversion of ascorbate to oxalate in the urine, the sample must be strongly acidified to stabilize ascorbate and minimize the formation of calcium crystals, e.g., with 6N hydrochloric acid (HCl).
- Risk of false-negatives when GFR <30 ml/min/1.73m^2 as reduced GFR results in reduced oxalate excretion.
- In children younger than 1.5–2.0 years, rapidly changing GFR may make the interpretation of urine oxalate:creatinine ratio difficult.

   b. 24-hour urine oxalate excretion:

- Preferred method of diagnosis, as long as the kidney function is within normal limits.

Urinary Oxalate Excretion Rates (mmol/1.73m^2/day)						
Normal	PH1	PH2	PH3	Enteric Hyperoxaluria	Dietary Hyperoxaluria	Idiopathic Calcium Oxalate Urolithiasis
<0.5	>1	>0.7	>0.7	>1 (fluctuates with diet)	<0.6	<0.7

2. Urine metabolite excretion:
   a. Urine glycolic acid (glycolate):
      - Requires either reversed-phase high-pressure liquid chromatography or ion chromatography.
      - Hyperglycolic aciduria (>0.5 mmol/day/1.73m^2) suggests but does not confirm the diagnosis of PH1 in an individual with hyperoxaluria, as only 66% of individuals with PH1 have hyperglycolic aciduria.
      - Age-specific spot glycolate:creatinine ratios are also available.
   b. Urine L-glycerate:
      - Individuals with PH2 typically have elevated urine L-glycerate >28 mmol/mol creatinine or >5 μmol/L.
   c. Urine HOG:
      - Increased HOG (>40 μmol/day/1.73m^2) suggest PH3.
3. Plasma oxalate concentration:
   a. Useful in patients with GFR <30 ml/min/1.73m^2.
   b. Plasma oxalate concentration exceeding the upper limit of the normal range when corrected for kidney function is consistent with but not diagnostic of PH.
   c. Individuals with PH1 usually have plasma oxalate levels 2–5 times the upper limit of normal.
   d. Samples should be taken after fasting and pre-dialysis for patients on maintenance hemodialysis.
   e. Sample must be sent on ice, centrifugated to obtain plasma, and then acidified to a pH of 2.3–2.7 using 10 μl of 12M HCl (or 20 μl of 6M HCl) per ml of plasma.

	Individual with PH1 by Kidney Function			Individual Without PH1
	GFR >30 mL/min/1.73m^2	GFR <30 mL/min/1.73m^2	Maintenance Hemodialysis	Maintenance Hemodialysis
Plasma oxalate concentration	>2 μmol/L	>30–50 μmol/L	>80 μmol/L (pre-dialysis sample)	<60 μmol/L (pre-dialysis sample)

4. Molecular genetic testing:
   a. Confirming the diagnosis when biochemical indices are equivocal.
   b. Confirming the diagnosis of PH1 is important in terms of:
      - Applicability of PH1 specific therapy.
      - Organ transplant strategy (e.g., the need for liver transplantation in PH2 remains uncertain).
   c. If a single causative mutation is found on sequence analysis, copy number variants for *AGXT and GPHPR,* although rare, can be identified using multiplex ligation-dependent probe amplification assays (MLPA).
   d. Approximately 5% of patients do not have mutations in all 3 genes.

Gene Symbol	Tested Method	Mutations Detected	Mutation Detection Frequency For At Least One Mutation in a Proband by Test Method
AGXT	Targeted mutation analysis	Panel of more common mutations including p. Gly170Arg and c.33dupC (p.Lys12GinfsX156)	50–70%
	Sequence analysis	Sequence variants	100%
GRHPR	Targeted mutation analysis	Sequence analysis of exons 2 and 4, which contain the 2 most common mutations (c.103delG and c.403_405+2delAAGT)	56%
	Sequence analysis	Sequence variants	100%
HOGA1	Sequence analysis	Sequence variants	100%

5. AGT and/or GR/HPR catalytic activity
   a. Confirmation of the diagnosis of PH1 and PH2 can be made by enzymatic assay for AGT and GR/HPR activity, respectively, performed on liver tissue obtained by a biopsy.
      - Assay of enzymatic catalytic activity requires at least 2 mg of liver taken by a percutaneous needle biopsy or an autopsy.
   b. In patients with PH1:
      - Approximately 50–70% of affected individuals have undetectable levels of AGT catalytic activity.
      - About 30–50% of affected individuals have substantial residual AGT catalytic activity (2–48% of mean normal activity).
      - Most individuals with classic PH1 who have residual AGT enzymatic activity have a unique protein-targeting (or trafficking) defect in which functional AGT enzyme is synthesized in adequate amounts but about 90% of the enzyme produced is mislocalized to mitochondria and only about 10% is properly localized in the peroxisomes (where it catalyzes the glyoxylate substrate).
   c. This has been largely replaced by molecular genetic testing, except when *AGXT* or *GRHPR* mutations are not found in highly suspicious cases.
   d. There are no known HOGA1 enzymatic assays available for diagnostic purposes.
6. End organ evaluation for systemic oxalosis:
   a. History and physical examination to assess the risk of arterial insufficiency or ischemia based on vessel wall deposition.
   b. ECG to evaluate for an associated atrioventricular block.
   c. Full blood count to evaluate for anemia associated with either abnormal kidney function or marrow deposition of oxalate.
   d. Thyroid function testing.
   e. Bone X-Rays looking for radiodense metaphyseal bands and diffuse demineralization.
   f. Ophthalmologic evaluation for evidence of retinal oxalate deposition.

7. Algorithm for diagnosis of Primary hyperoxaluria:

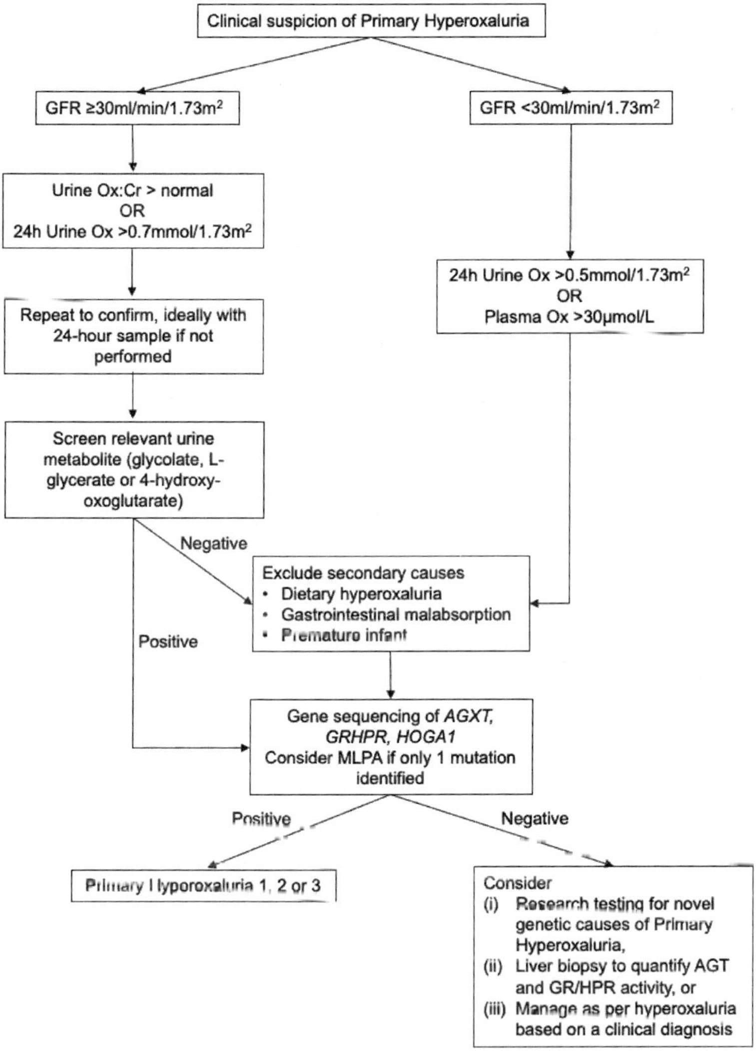

D. Treatment

I. Reduction of calcium oxalate supersaturation:

a. Urine dilution:
   - High fluid intake (>3 L/1.73m^2/day) orally, or enterally using a nasogastric or gastrostomy tube.
   - Drink throughout the day, and especially at night to ensure overnight diuresis.
   - Drink before going to bed and when waking up at night to void.
   - Low threshold for intravenous fluids when there is poor oral intake or fluid loss.

b. Calcium oxalate crystallization inhibitors:
   - Potassium citrate 0.3–0.5 mmol/kg/day (100–150 mg/kg/day) in 3–4 divided doses, to alkalinize urine pH to 6.5–7.0.
   - Phosphate 0.2–0.3 mmol/kg/day (20–30 mg/kg/day), up to 0.63 mmol/kg/day (60 mg/kg/day), in divided doses, can be added in patients with normal kidney function, as the pyrophosphate will complex with calcium and reduce calcium oxalate precipitation.
   - Consider magnesium oxide 500 mg/m^2/day in divided doses to further inhibit stone formation.
   - Avoid sodium preparations, including sodium bicarbonate and sodium phosphate, as the additional sodium load may increase hypercalciuria.

c. Thiazide diuretics can be given in patients with hypercalciuria, e.g., in PH3.
   - Hydrochlorothiazide 0.5–1 mg/kg/day in 1–2 divided doses (adult 25–50 mg/dose, maximum 200 mg/day).
   - Addition of amiloride in combination can be considered.

II. Reduce dietary oxalate:

1. Avoid foods high in oxalate, although this is of limited efficacy due to reduced intestinal absorption of oxalate in patients with PH:
   - Vegetables: Potato, celery, beans, spinach, eggplant, olives, pepper, summer squash, rhubarb, tempeh.

- Fruits: Blackberry, blueberry, grapes, kiwi, starfruit.
- Legumes, nuts and seeds: Almond, hazelnut, peanut, pistachio, sunflower seeds.
- Grains and starches: Cereal, oatmeal, whole-wheat flour, white corn, rye.
- Soy products.
- Dairy, meat and fish: Liver, sardines, yogurt.
- Miscellaneous: Chocolate, green tea, Graham crackers, peanut butter, oatmeal, popcorn, soya products.

2. Avoid excessive Vitamin C (oxalate precursor) or vitamin D (to avoid hypercalciuria).

III. Reduction of oxalate biosynthesis with pyridoxine:

1. A trial of pyridoxine or pyridoxal phosphate is recommended in all patients with PH1, even in kidney failure.
   a. Pyridoxal phosphate is a co-factor for AGT, while pyridoxine is its precursor.
   b. 10–30% of patients with PH1 are pyridoxine-responsive, defined as a ≥30% reduction in urine oxalate excretion following pyridoxine supplementation.
   c. There is an imperfect correlation between PH1 genotype and pyridoxine response, although it is known that patients homozygous for p.Gly170Arg mutation show normalization of plasma oxalate levels, while compound heterozygotes may demonstrate a partial reduction in plasma oxalate concentration by at least 30% of prior documented levels.
   d. Response to pyridoxine in advanced kidney failure can be evaluated by measuring plasma oxalate before and after the introduction of pyridoxine.
2. Dosage:
   a. Pyridoxine may be started at 5 mg/kg/day, increased in 5 mg/kg steps to 20 mg/kg/day over a period of 6 months if the patient is not responsive.
   b. Pyridoxine non-response should only be determined after 3 months at the maximum dose.
3. Paresthesia and sensory neuropathy is an uncommon but known complication of large doses of pyridoxine.

4. Individuals responsive to pyridoxine should continue this therapy after kidney transplantation to decrease the burden of oxalate on the kidney.

IV. Reduction of oxalate biosynthesis with lumasiran:

1. Approved by the European Medicines Agency (EMA) and Food and Drug Administration (FDA) in 2020 for patients of all ages with PH1.
2. Mechanism of action:
   a. Double-stranded small interfering RNA molecule reducing the expression of glycolate oxidase, which catalyzes the conversion of glycolate to glyoxylate.
      - Results in increased excretion of glycolate, which is highly soluble in urine.

   b. As glyoxylate is the immediate precursor of oxalate, preventing the accumulation of glyoxylate reduces oxalate production.
   c. Lumasiran is conjugated to N-acetylgalactosamine, which is selectively taken up by the liver, enabling preferential drug uptake in the liver.
3. Efficacy:
   a. ILLUMINATE-A: Phase 3 double-blind randomized control trial involving 39 patients above 6 years of age with genetic-proven PH1 and eGFR ≥30 ml/min/1.73m^2.
   b. 53.5% (95% CI: 44.8–62.3) or 0.98 (95% CI: 0.77–1.18) mmol/1.73m^2 reduction in 24-hour urinary oxalate excretion, resulting in 84% of patients with urinary oxalate excretion within 1.5x the upper limit of normal, and 52% of patients with urinary oxalate excretion within the normal range (≤0.514 mmol/1.73m^2).
   c. Significant reductions in urinary oxalate excretion even in patients already on pyridoxine therapy.
   d. Favorable interim data from ILLUMINATE-B, a similar trial conducted in patients ≤6 years of age.
4. Dosage:
   a. Subcutaneous administration.
   b. Loading dose: 3 mg/kg once a month × 3.

c. Maintenance dose: 3 mg/kg/dose every 3 months, beginning 1 month after completion of the loading dose.
5. Side effects:
a. Injection site reactions (32%) and abdominal pain (15.4%) were common, which were mild and transient.
b. No hepatic adverse events were noted, including transaminitis.
c. Inadequate data regarding use when eGFR <30 ml/min/1.73m^2.
- Theoretical risk of metabolic acidosis, due to impaired excretion of glycolate.

E. Monitoring

I. When GFR ≥30 ml/min/1.73m^2:

1. Monitoring for treatment efficacy 3 monthly:
a. 24-hour urine volume.
b. Urine pH.
c. 24-hour urine oxalate excretion or urine oxalate:creatinine ratio.
d. 24-hour urine citrate excretion or urine citrate:creatinine ratio.
e. 24-hour urine calcium excretion or urine calcium:creatinine ratio.
f. Urine magnesium:creatinine ratio.
g. Plasma oxalate concentration (if eGFR <60 ml/min/1.73m^2).
h. Plasma calcium-oxalate saturation $\{\beta_{CaOx}=(C_{Ca} \times C_{ox})/(K'_{sp.CaOx})\}$ where C_{Ca} is the calculated free calcium concentration, C_{ox} is the calculated oxalate concentration and $K'_{sp.CaOx}$ is the actual solubility product at the actual ionic strength of the plasma sample.
2. Kidney function monitoring 3 monthly:
a. Blood urea, creatinine, sodium, potassium, chloride, bicarbonate, calcium, phosphate.
b. Urine protein:creatinine ratio.
3. Ultrasound of the kidneys for nephrocalcinosis and stone formation 6 monthly.

II. When GFR <30 ml/min/1.73m²:

1. Plasma oxalate concentration monthly.
2. Kidney function monitoring monthly.
3. Screening for complications of systemic oxalosis 3–6 monthly.
   - More frequent screening should be done when plasma oxalate >30 μmol/L even when GFR ≥30 ml/min/1.73m².

F. Urologic Intervention

1. Intervention should only be performed when there is obstruction, infection, multiple uroliths, or other complications.
2. Avoid open and percutaneous surgery, and especially unilateral nephrectomy, because additional peri-operative kidney insults will exacerbate progressive kidney injury.
3. Where the necessary expertise is available, ureteroscopy is the preferred means of stone removal.
4. Shock-wave lithotripsy (SWL) is an available option with the advantage of being non-invasive but may harm the kidney due to the potential presence of nephrocalcinosis and microlithiasis.

G. Dialysis

1. Conventional dialysis is unsuitable for patients who have kidney failure because it cannot overcome the continuous excess production of oxalate.
   a. Maximum elimination of oxalate is 950–1440 mmol/day using standard maintenance hemodialysis or peritoneal dialysis.
   b. Oxalate production in PH1 is between 3500 and 7500 mmol/day.
   c. Long hemodialysis (6–8 hours) has only limited advantage as the maximum clearance of plasma oxalate is during the first 2 hours of hemodialysis.

2. Optimized regimens including combined daily high-flux hemodialysis (2–3 hours) and night intermittent peritoneal dialysis are preferred.
   a. Nevertheless, as no dialysis strategy can lead to net negative oxalate removal, period of dialysis dependence should be kept as short as possible.
   b. Aim for pre-HD plasma oxalate of <40 μmol/L to avoid systemic oxalosis, but even with optimized regimens, a pre-HD plasma oxalate of <100 μmol/L is often a more achievable target.
   c. Duration of HD can be individualized to the patient with hourly serum oxalate measurements during HD. High blood (Qb) and dialysate flow (Qd) may not be necessary.

H. Strategy for Organ Transplantation

Transplantation Strategy	Combined Simultaneous Liver-kidney Transplantation (LKT)	Sequential With Liver First, Kidney As Second Step	Isolated Kidney	Isolated Liver (Pre-emptive)
GFR >30–40 ml/min/1.73m^2	No	No	No	Consider
GFR <30 ml/min/1.73m^2	Yes	Yes	No	No
Infantile form (kidney failure <2 years)	Yes	Yes (emergency)	No	No
PH2	No	No	Yes	No
HD strategy	Peri-operative ± post-operative according to plasma oxalate concentration and GFR	Standard HD after liver transplant aiming at plasma oxalate <20–30 μmol/L	Pre-operative and peri-operative	Sometimes peri-operative

1. Considerations in PH1
   a. Isolated kidney transplantation is generally not recommended in children due to significant reductions in graft survival.
   b. Liver and kidney transplantation is thus required in advanced chronic kidney disease (eGFR <30ml/min/1.73m^2).
      - Should be performed before a prolonged period of systemic oxalosis.
      - If life-long Lumasiran is available, then liver transplant may not be required.
   c. A sequential approach enables an interim reduction of tissue oxalate burden with continued intensive dialysis before kidney transplantation, although this has to be weighed against the risks of re-operation for both the recipient and donor.
      - A sequential approach is accepted to be reasonable in infants, in which it is often indicated due to anatomic considerations and/or medical instability.
   d. Isolated liver transplantation is a consideration in those with eGFR >30 ml/min/1.73m^2, but the risks of liver transplantation need to be weighed against the variability of kidney prognosis between individuals.
   e. The suitability of a donor who is heterozygous for the *AGXT* mutation remains uncertain, as they have reduced hepatic AGT enzyme activity although their urine oxalate excretion and phenotype are normal.
   f. Immunosuppression requirements are typically milder in the presence of a liver allograft, compared to a kidney allograft.
2. Considerations in PH2 and PH3
   a. Isolated kidney transplantation is currently recommended in PH2:
      - *GRHPR* is also significantly expressed in non-hepatic tissues and thus liver transplantation does not fully reverse the metabolic defect.

- Systemic oxalate production and thus progression to kidney failure is less marked than in PH1.

b. Patients with PH3 are unlikely to require transplantation due to a milder clinical phenotype, which improves with age.

3. Bilateral nephrectomy may be considered at the time of kidney transplantation to limit the risk of further infections, stones and obstruction, as well as to reduce systemic oxalate stores.

I. Post-Combined Liver-Kidney Transplant Management

I. Immediate post-operative period

1. High-efficiency hemodiafiltration following simultaneous transplantation:
   a. Indicated in the following settings:
      - Any delay in achieving optimal kidney function of eGFR >40 ml/min/1.73m^2 due to acute tubular necrosis and delayed graft function (corresponding to a plasma oxalate concentration >50 μmol/L) with poor urine output <2 ml/kg/hour.
      - Small children (<2 years) with infantile oxalosis and those with significant systemic involvement.

   b. While this will provide a rapid drop in plasma oxalate concentrations and reduce the exposure of the transplanted kidney to high plasma oxalate concentrations, it may also increase the risk of calcium oxalate supersaturation due to the reduction in urine volume, especially if there is inappropriate fluid removal.
2. Pyridoxine supplementation in patients identified to be pyridoxine-responsive should be continued until the liver function recovers.
3. Post-operative anti-coagulation should be considered to attenuate the increased risk of graft vessel thrombosis related to oxalate deposition in the blood vessels (e.g., low molecular weight heparin).

II. Prevention of manifestations of recurrent oxalate deposition in the kidneys

1. Strategies for the reduction of calcium oxalate supersaturation should continue post-transplantation:
   a. Urine dilution, aiming for a urine oxalate concentration <0.25 mmol/L.
   b. Crystallization inhibitors, including potassium citrate, aiming for a urine pH 6.5–7.0.
   c. Use of loop diuretics to maintain dilute urine should be avoided as these can lead to hypercalciuria and the production of calcium oxalate stones.
   d. Urine glycolate returns to normal immediately post-transplantation, followed by plasma oxalate and finally urine oxalate excretion, which can take up to 2–5 years.
2. If serum calcium is low, start oral calcium with the following considerations:
   a. Keep serum ionized calcium at low normal levels (≈1.15 mmol/L) to reduce the plasma calcium-oxalate saturation.
   b. Calcium lactogluconate contains 300 mg elemental calcium in 15 ml.
   c. Give calcium supplements 2 hours apart from the neutral orthophosphate.
3. End-organ evaluation for systemic oxalosis should continue until the normalization of urine oxalate excretion and resolution of end-organ involvement.

III. Monitoring

	Urine pH	Urine Calcium: Creatinine Ratio	Urine Oxalate: Creatinine Ratio	Plasma Oxalate and Calcium-oxalate Saturation	Urine Glycolate	Kidney Ultrasound for Nephro-Calcinosis
Pre-transplant	1x	1x	1x	1x	1x	
Post-transplant D1	Hourly	12 hourly	12 hourly	Daily		Daily
D2	Hourly	12 hourly	12 hourly	Daily		Daily
D3 to D14	Hourly till serum creatinine is normal and urine pH is stable between 6–7, then 4–6 hourly	12 hourly till serum creatinine is normal, then daily	Daily	Daily till serum creatinine is normal	1x at D7	Daily if GFR <40 ml/min/1.73m², then weekly.
D15 to 3 months	Weekly	Weekly	Weekly	Weekly till plasma oxalate is normal, then monthly		Daily if GFR <40 ml/min/1.73m², then weekly.
>3 months to 1 year	Monthly	Monthly	Monthly	Monthly		Monthly

IV. Surveillance

Problem	Combined LKT (1st Year Post-transplant)	Pre-emptive Liver Transplantation
Kidney function	Monthly	6-monthly
Proteinuria	Monthly	6-monthly
Hypertension	Monthly	Yearly
Anemia	Monthly	Yearly
Kidney ultrasound for kidney stone burden and to exclude obstruction	Monthly for first 6 months, then 3–monthly	Yearly
Skin	3-monthly	Yearly
Bone: Radiograph of long bones	3-monthly	Yearly
Thyroid function test: Free T4, TSH	3-monthly	Yearly
Cardiac: ECG and 2-D echocardiography	6-monthly	Yearly
Ophthalmologic screen for crystals in retina	Yearly	Yearly

Recommended Reading

1. Cochat P, Fargue S, Harambat J. (2010) Primary hyperoxaluria type 1: Strategy for organ transplantation. *Curr Opin Organ Transplant* **15**:590–593.
2. Beck BB, Hoppe B. Primary Hyperoxaluria. (2016) In: *Pediatric Kidney Disease*. Edited by: Geary DF, Schaefer F. Springer-Verlag Berlin Heidelberg. pp 1037–1058.
3. Milliner DS, Harris PC, Cogal AG, *et al.* (2017) Primary Hyperoxaluria Type 1. In: *GeneReviews®*. Edited by: Adam MP, Ardinger HH, Pagon RA, *et al.* University of Washington, Seattle. https://www.ncbi.nlm.nih.gov/books/NBK1283/.
4. Mayo Clinic Laboratories. (2010) Hyperoxaluria diagnostic algorithm. Mayo Foundation for Medical Education and Research.
5. Scott LJ, Keam SJ. (2021) Lumasiran: First approval. *Drugs* **81**(2):277–282. doi: 10.1007/s40265-020-01463-0. PMID:33405070
6. Garrelfs SF, Frishberg Y, Hulton SA, Koren MJ, O'Riordan WD, Cochat P, Deschênes G, Shasha-Lavsky H, Saland JM, Van't Hoff WG, Fuster DG, Magen D, Moochhala SH, Schalk G, Simkova E, Groothoff JW, Sas DJ, Meliambro KA, Lu J, Sweetser MT, Garg PP, Vaishnaw AK, Gansner JM, McGregor TL, Lieske JC; ILLUMINATE-A Collaborators.

(2021) Lumasiran, an RNAi therapeutic for primary hyperoxaluria type 1. *N Engl J Med* **384**(13):1216–1226. doi:10.1056/NEJMoa2021712.

7. EMA. (n.d.) Alnylam Netherlands B.V. Oxlumo [package insert]. European Medicines Agency. https://www.ema.europa.eu/en/documents/product-information/oxlumo-epar-product-information_en.pdf.
8. Niaudet P. (2021, updated) Primary hyperoxaluria. Edited by: Mattoo TK, Kim MS. *UpToDate ONLINE*. http://www.uptodateonline.com.

5 X-Linked Hypophosphatemic Rickets

Lu L, Teo S, Loke KY and Yap HK

A. Genetics

1. X-linked hypophosphatemic rickets (XLH) is an X-linked dominant disorder.
2. It is due to inactivating mutations in the *PHEX* (**Ph**osphate regulating **E**ndopeptidase homolog **X**-linked) gene on chromosome Xp22.1.
3. *PHEX* encodes an endopeptidase, whose altered function results in excessive circulating levels of fibroblast growth factor 23 (FGF23).
4. FGF23, which is secreted by osteocytes, inhibits phosphate reabsorption by downregulating the sodium/phosphate cotransporter in the renal proximal tubule and also suppresses the renal 1,25 dihydroxy vitamin D_3 (calcitriol) production.
5. There are no obvious genotype-phenotype correlations.
   - XLH has complete penetrance, but its severity varies even among members of the same family.
   - No gender differences in disease severity.

B. Approach to the Evaluation of XLH

I. Step 1: Identify patients with possible XLH

1. The clinical presentation of XLH ranges from isolated hypophosphatemia to severe lower-extremity bowing.
   - Diagnosis is frequently made in the first 2 years of life when lower-extremity bowing becomes evident with the onset of weight-bearing.

2. Clinical presentation:
   a. Infants and children:
      - Poor growth and decreasing height velocity.
      - Delayed walking.
      - Lower limb deformities (valgus or varus deformities).
      - Craniosynostosis.
      - Dental abscesses.
   b. Adolescents and adults:
      - Short stature.
      - Bone pain.
      - Enthesopathy (calcification of tendons, ligaments and joint capsules).
      - Spinal stenosis.
      - Early osteoarthritis.
      - Periodontitis.
      - Sensorineural hearing loss.
3. Physical examination:
   a. Short stature.
      - In particular, reduced limb length, i.e., an elevated upper segment to lower segment ratio.
   b. Clinical signs of rickets:
      - Rachitic rosary.
      - Craniotabes.
      - Harrison's sulcus.
      - Epiphyseal swelling.
      - Valgus or varus knee deformities, tibial torsion.
      - Proximal muscular weakness, waddling gait.
   c. Craniosynostosis (in particular dolichocephaly).
4. Family history of XLH in the mother and siblings.
   - Approximately one-third of patients have a negative family history.
   - A history of male-male transmission in the pedigree suggests an alternative genetic form of rickets.

II. Step 2: Confirm radiographic evidence of rickets

1. X-Ray of limbs: Frayed, widened or cupped metaphyses.
   - Unlike calcipenic rickets, there can be cortical bone thickening in XLH and an absence of features of bone resorption.

2. X-Ray of hands: Delayed bone age.
3. X-Ray of axial skeleton: Dense appearance of axial skeleton.

III. Step 3: Assessment of biochemical parameters suggestive of XLH

1. Main biochemical findings characteristic of XLH:
   a. Low serum phosphate concentration.
   b. Reduced tubular resorption of phosphate (TRP) in the absence of glycosuria, bicarbonaturia, proteinuria, or aminoaciduria.
      - As TRP is affected by the glomerular filtration rate (GFR), a better index of tubular phosphate reabsorption is the ratio of the tubular maximum phosphate reabsorption to GFR (TMP/GFR).
      - TMP/GFR may be falsely low until serum phosphate levels are restored towards normal levels.

   c. Raised FGF23 levels (if available).
2. Other suggestive biochemical findings are:
   a. Normal serum calcium and 25-hydroxyvitamin D.
   b. Low 1,25 (OH) Vitamin D and urine calcium:creatinine ratio.
   c. Normal or mildly elevated parathyroid hormone (PTH) levels.
   d. Normal to high alkaline phosphatase (ALP) levels.

IV. Step 4: Establishing the diagnosis

1. Genetic testing for the *PHEX* mutation confirms the diagnosis.
   - A genetic diagnosis is recommended for the first proband in the pedigree.
2. Negative PHEX mutational analysis:
   a. May be due to test limitations (e.g., large deletions, mosaicism) OR
   b. Suggest an alternative genetic form of phosphopenic rickets, e.g., autosomal dominant hypophosphataemic rickets.

C. Management

I. Conventional drug treatment:

1. Conventional treatment:
   a. Oral phosphate (PO4) solution: 0.7–2.0 mmol/kg/day 4–6 times a day (maximum 66 mmol daily).
      Note:
      - 1 mmol (95 mg) of phosphate = 1 mmol (30 mg) of elemental phosphorus.
      - Sodium phosphate solution: 0.7 mmol phosphate per ml.
      - Phosphate Sandoz tablet: 16.1 mmol phosphate per tablet.
   b. Calcitriol 20 ng/kg/dose (maximum 1 µg) 2 times a day
      OR
      One-Alpha (alfacalcidol) 100 ng/kg daily for 3 months, then 50 ng/kg (maximum 2 µg) daily.
   c. Co-administration of active vitamin D with phosphate is required to facilitate intestinal absorption of phosphate and to prevent secondary hyperparathyroidism, which will worsen kidney phosphate wasting.
   d. Early treatment in children is associated with superior outcomes.
   e. Treatment should be considered in adults, in particular those who have skeletal complaints or dental issues.
2. Treatment-specific monitoring:
   a. Biochemical targets:
      i. Serum phosphate >1 mmol/L (2 hours after the dose of oral phosphate).
         - Normalization of serum phosphate levels is not a goal of conventional therapy.
         - Higher doses of phosphate supplementation may be associated with an increased risk of nephrocalcinosis.
      ii. Serum ALP <500 U/L.
      iii. PTH within normal range.
      iv. Serum calcium within age-specific normal range.
      v. Urine calcium:creatinine ratio within age-specific normal range.

   vi. Urine oxalate:creatinine ratio within age-specific normal range.
      - Dietary modification may be necessary to reduce intestinal oxalate absorption.
b. Frequency of monitoring of the above parameters: Monthly until biochemical parameters are stable, then 3–12 monthly depending on age.

3. Management of complications of treatment:
   a. Nephrocalcinosis:
      i. Due to hypercalcemia and hypercalciuria.
      ii. Reduce the dose of active Vitamin D.
      iii. Use potassium citrate with caution as urine alkalinization increases the risk of phosphate precipitation.
      iv. Consider thiazide diuretics if hypercalciuria is detected.
   b. Secondary hyperparathyroidism:
      i. Due to:
         - Complexing of calcium with phosphate, resulting in intermittent hypocalcemia.
         - Direct effect of FGF23 and phosphate on parathyroid cells.
      ii. Autonomous (tertiary) hyperparathyroidism can occur when secondary hyperparathyroidism is inadequately controlled, necessitating surgical intervention.
      iii. Increase active Vitamin D and reduce phosphate if possible.
      iv. If PTH is still elevated, add on a calcimimetic (Cinacalcet):
         - Start with 25 mg once daily.
         - Dose adjustments should not be made more frequently than every 2–4 weeks.
         - Titrate dose according to PTH levels measured 1–4 weeks after dose initiation or dosage adjustment.
         - Monitor serum calcium 2–4 weekly as hypocalcemia occurs commonly.

II. Burosumab:

1. Monoclonal antibody against FGF23.
2. Indications in children aged 1–18 years old:
   a. Failure of conventional therapy with phosphate supplementation and calcitriol.

b. Patients with complications related to conventional therapy.
c. Newly diagnosed patients with moderate-severe rickets:
   - In a randomized clinical trial, children with moderate-severe rickets on conventional therapy treated with burosumab had improvements in radiological rickets, lower limb deformities, linear growth velocity, and functional mobility, compared to children who continued on with conventional therapy.
d. No conclusive evidence for the use of burosumab in adults with XLH.

3. Contraindications:
   a. Children on oral phosphate supplementation or active Vitamin D analogs.
   b. Severe kidney impairment, i.e., eGFR <30 ml/min/1.73m^2.
4. Dosing:
   a. Discontinue phosphate supplementation and active Vitamin D one week prior to commencing burosumab.
   b. Demonstrate fasting hypophosphataemia before commencing burosumab injections.
   c. Initial subcutaneous dose:
      <10 kg: 1 mg/kg every 2 weeks.
      ≥10 kg: 0.8 mg/kg every 2 weeks (minimum starting dose 10 mg, maximum 90 mg).
      >18 years old: 1 mg/kg every 4 weeks (minimum starting dose 10 mg, maximum 90 mg).
   d. Titration phase:
      i. Monitor fasting phosphate levels and TMP/GFR 7–11 days after injection:
         - Every 2 weeks in the first month, then
         - Every 4 weeks during the following 2 months.
      ii. Escalate the dose every 4 weeks by 0.4 mg/kg each time to achieve **low-normal serum phosphate levels** to a maximum dose of 2 mg/kg or 90 mg absolute.
      Note: Average final dose is 1 mg/kg in pediatric trials.
      iii. If serum phosphate remains slightly low, but the TMP/GFR has normalized, maintain the current dose of burosumab as this may be transient due to high bone uptake with healing rickets.

iv. If serum phosphate >1.6 mmol/L, withhold burosumab and reassess serum phosphate in 4 weeks.
- When hypophosphataemia is observed, reinitiate burosumab at half the previous dose.

e. Steady state phase:
i. Defined as 3 months after a stable dosage is obtained.
ii. Monitor fasting phosphate levels prior to injection to identify hypophosphataemia and under-treatment.
iii. Adjust burosumab dose not more than once every 4 weeks and preferably every 2 months or longer.
iv. Recheck serum phosphate 4 weeks after dose adjustment.

5. Adverse reactions:
a. Injection site reactions are common and resolve after 1–3 days.
b. Headaches and pain in the extremities.
c. Dental abscesses and caries occur more commonly in the absence of vitamin D and phosphate supplementation.

6. Long-term monitoring (3 monthly):
a. Serum calcium, phosphate, creatinine, ALP and PTH.
b. TMP/GFR.
c. Urine calcium:creatinine and 1,25-OH Vitamin D (if available).
Note: Should be done fasting prior to injection.

III. Monitoring and management of complications:

1. A follow-up should be provided by a multi-disciplinary team comprising an expert in metabolic bone disease, orthopedic surgeons, otolaryngologists, dentists, and radiologists.
2. Frequency of follow-up should be tailored to individual patient requirements.
a. A higher frequency of monitoring is required during periods of rapid growth.
b. The following visit frequencies are a minimum:
- 0–5 years: 1–3 months.
- 5 years to the start of puberty: 3–6 months.
- Puberty: 3 months.
- Adulthood: 6–12 months.

Complication	Monitoring (Every Visit Unless Otherwise Stated)	Management
Poor linear growth	• Height and height velocity. • Bone age (as clinically indicated).	• Consider growth hormone therapy if there is short stature in spite of normalization of ALP and PTH.
Rickets	• Clinical signs of rickets, including deformity. • Intermalleolar and intercondylar distances. • Wrist, knee and ankle radiographs (at diagnosis, and as clinically indicated — consider EOS imaging for reduced radiation). • 6-minute walk test (1–2 yearly). • 25-OH Vitamin D (annually).	• Refer patients with substantial limb deformities to an orthopedic surgeon. • Consider early use of guided growth techniques (plates) if deformity persists after 1 year of optimized medical therapy. • If possible, definitive treatment of residual deformities via osteostomies should be delayed until skeletal maturity.
Craniosynostosis, Chiari type 1 malformation, spinal stenosis	• Head circumference, skull shape. • Neurological examination. • Consider brain MRI (<5 years old with signs of craniosynostosis, >5 years old with signs/symptoms of raised intracranial pressure).	• Refer to a neurosurgeon.

(Continued)

(*Continued*)

Complication	Monitoring (Every Visit Unless Otherwise Stated)	Management
Dental abscesses and periodontitis	• Frequency of dental abscesses and acute oral infections. • Dental evaluation after tooth eruption (twice yearly). • Orthopantomogram (5 years old, and subsequently as indicated). • Orthodontic evaluation (12 years old).	• Prophylactic sealing of occlusal surfaces of deciduous and permanent teeth using a flowable resin composite as soon as each tooth is sufficiently erupted.
Sensorineural hearing loss	• Hearing assessment (at diagnosis and subsequently as indicated).	• Supportive treatment for hearing loss: Hearing aids, prevent noise exposure and ototoxic drug use.
Nephrocalcinosis	• Kidney ultrasound (at diagnosis and every 1–2 years). • 24-hour urinary protein excretion and creatinine clearance if there is nephrocalcinosis (annually).	
Others	• Blood pressure (6 monthly). • Quality of life scores (2 yearly).	

IV. Screening of siblings:

1. Clinical and biochemical parameters can be evaluated at 3 and 6 months of age in younger siblings.

- Serum phosphate may still be normal within the first 3–4 months of life.

2. Genetic testing may enable an earlier diagnosis after birth, but it is not known if this improves clinical care.

Recommended Reading

1. Alon US, Levy-Olomucki R, Moore WV, Stubbs J, Liu S, Quarles LD. (2008) Calcimimetics as an adjuvant treatment for familial hypophosphatemic rickets. *Clin J Am Soc Nephrol* **3**:658–684.
2. Linglart A, Biosse-Duplan M, Briot K, Chaussain C, Esterle L, Guillaume-Czitrom S, Kamenicky P, Nevoux J, Prié D, Rothenbuhler A, Wicart P, Harvengt P. (2014) Therapeutic management of hypophosphatemic rickets from infancy to adulthood. *Endocr Connect* **3**:R13–R30.
3. Carpenter TO, Imel EA, Ruppe MD, Weber TJ, Klausner MA, Wooddell MM, Kawakami T, Ito T, Zhang X, Humphrey J, Insogna KL, Peacock M. (2014) Randomized trial of the anti-FGF23 antibody KRN23 in X-linked hypophosphatemia. *J Clin Invest* **124**:1587–1597.
4. Haffner D, Emma F, Eastwood DM, Duplan MB, Bacchetta J, Schnabel D, Wicart P, Bockenhauer D, Santos F, Levtchenko E, Harvengt P, Kirchhoff M, Di Rocco F, Chaussain C, Brandi ML, Savendahl L, Briot K, Kamenicky P, Rejnmark L, Linglart A. (2019) Clinical practice recommendations for the diagnosis and management of X-linked hypophosphataemia. *Nat Rev Nephrol* **15**:435–455.
5. Scheinman SJ, Carpenter T, Drezner MK. (2021, updated) Hereditary hypophosphatemic rickets and tumor-induced osteomalacia. Edited by: Sterns RH, Geffner ME, Hoppin AG. *UpToDate ONLINE*. http://www.uptodateonline.com.
6. Kyowa Kirin, Inc. (n.d.) Burosumab [package insert]. U.S. Food and Drug Administration website. https://www.accessdata.fda.gov/drugsatfda_docs/label/2019/761068s004lbl.pdf.

6 Management of Nephropathic Cystinosis

Lu L, Teo S and Yap HK

A. Genetics

1. Cystinosis is an autosomal recessive condition caused by bi-allelic mutations in the *CTNS* gene (17p13.2) encoding cystinosin.
   a. Cystinosin is a lysosomal transporter responsible for exporting cystine from lysosomes.
   b. Cystine is a product of protein degradation within the lysosomes of the cell and is normally transported to the cytosol where it is reutilized as cysteine.
   c. When cystinosin is defective, cystine accumulates in lysosomes forming crystals at low lysosomal pH.
   d. Cystinosin dysfunction results in the dysregulation of cell signaling, vesicle trafficking, and mitochondrial function, and increased oxidative stress and cell apoptosis.
2. Genotype-phenotype correlations:

Clinical Type	Genetics	Phenotype
Infantile nephropathic form (95%)	Severe truncating mutations of both alleles	Age of presentation: 6–12 months. Renal Fanconi syndrome with progressive loss of glomerular function leading to kidney failure.
Late onset juvenile form (5%)	At least one mild mutation in one allele	Age of presentation: 8 years. Varied presentation ranging from ocular symptoms, mild renal Fanconi syndrome, isolated proteinuria, or overt nephrotic syndrome. Progression to kidney failure after the age of 15 years.

(*Continued*)

Clinical Type	Genetics	Phenotype
Adult form or non-nephropathic ocular form	At least one mild mutation in one allele	Rarely presents before adulthood. Mainly photophobia from crystal deposits.

B. Clinical Manifestations

I. *Infantile nephropathic cystinosis*

1. Kidney involvement:
    a. Fanconi syndrome (tubular proteinuria with massive excretion of β2-microglobulin and lysozyme, glycosuria, phosphaturia, bicarbonaturia, and aminoaciduria) with sodium and potassium wasting.
        i. Polyuria and polydipsia, and severe dehydration.
        ii. Failure to thrive.
            - Normal weight and length parameters at birth dropping to the 3rd centile by 6–12 months of age.
        iii. Vomiting, constipation.
        iv. Electrolyte and metabolic imbalance:
            - Hypokalemia.
            - Metabolic acidosis.
            - Hypophosphatemia.
            - Hypocalcemia.
            - Hyponatremia.
            - Hypouricemia.
            - Decreased plasma carnitine.
        v. Vitamin D-resistant rickets.
        vi. Hypercalciuria with medullary nephrocalcinosis and nephrolithiasis.
    b. Glomerular proteinuria (urinary losses of albumin and high molecular weight proteins up to a nephrotic range).
2. Non-kidney involvement:
    a. Eyes:
        i. Corneal cysteine crystals not detectable at birth but are always present by the age of 18 months (100%):

- Blepharospasm.
- Photophobia.
- Watering.

ii. Mid-childhood and early adolescence (>10 years):
- Corneal erosions (20–40%).
- Superficial punctate keratopathy (3–18%).
- Retinopathy/retinal degeneration starting from the periphery (>5% from the first decade of life):
  - Pigmentary changes.
  - Nyctalopia.
  - Impaired color vision.
  - Visual field constriction.
  - Retinal blindness.

iii. Adolescence and adult (>15 years):
- Filamentary keratopathy (10–73%).
- Band keratopathy (8–40%).
- Peripheral corneal neovascularization primarily in adults (6%).
- Posterior synechiae associated with iris thickening (5–53%).
- Depigmentation of the peripheral retina.
- Phthisis (5–26.6%).
- Cataract.
- Retinopathy and visual impairment.

b. Endocrine:

i. Hypothyroidism (70% of untreated).
- Usually appears by the age of 8–12 years.

ii. Growth retardation (>70% from the first decade of life).
- Growth hormone deficiency (11%).

iii. Glucose intolerance and insulin-dependent diabetes (>30% from the second decade of life).

iv. Exocrine pancreatic insufficiency.

v. Primary hypogonadism.
- Occurs in 70% of boys who are usually azoospermic (100%).

vi. Delayed puberty.
- Mean age of puberty in girls is 15 years.
- Most girls are usually fertile.

c. Abdomen:
   i. Hepatomegaly:
      - Detected in one-third of patients by the age of 15.
      - Usually asymptomatic but rarely can cause cholestatic jaundice due to nodular hyperplasia.
   ii. Rarely portal hypertension and splenomegaly.
d. Muscle:
   i. Muscle weakness and wasting initially due to:
      - Hypokalemia.
      - Rickets.
      - Carnitine deficiency.
   ii. Progressive distal vacuolar myopathy:
      - Occurs generally in the second decade of life
      - Thenar and hypothenar muscle atrophy (>25%).
      - Dysarthria (>10%).
      - Swallowing dysfunction (>50%).
      - Restrictive lung disease (100% after the age of 20 if untreated).
      - Myopathic changes can be seen on electromyography in asymptomatic patients.
      - May also contribute to oromotor dysfunction in young children with feeding difficulties.
e. Neurologic (from the first decade of life):
   i. Chiari 1 malformation with tonsillar ectopia (18.9%).
   ii. Idiopathic intracranial hypertension.
   iii. Infancy:
      - Hypotonia.
      - Speech delay.
      - Gross and fine motor impairment.
   iv. Childhood:
      - Mild neurocognitive dysfunction with poor visual spatial and visual memory skills as well as higher-order executive functions (IQ within normal range).
      - Behavioral problems (22%) including social and attention problems and somatic complaints.
   v. Cystinotic encephalopathy (from the third decade of life, 5–10%).
      - Pyramidal and cerebellar signs, dementia, and pseudobulbar palsy.
      - Stroke-like episodes with ischemic lesions.

f. Bone deformities (from the first decade of life):
   i. Genu valgum.
   ii. Scoliosis.
   iii. Stress fractures.
   iv. Leg and joint pains.
   Note: Dual-energy X-Ray absorptiometry scans are not valuable in cystinosis, as bone cystine crystals will elevate the measured bone mineral density.
g. Skin:
   i. Congenital hypopigmentation.
   ii. Premature skin aging:
      - Subcutaneous infiltration of palpable amorphous material.
      - Telangiectasia.
      - Thinning of the epidermis.
   iii. Small erythematous macules and papules in sun-exposed areas.
   iv. Impaired sweating with heat intolerance (>60% after the age of 2).
   v. Impaired salivation.
   vi. Progressive coarse facial features.
   vii. Characteristic blond hair and white skin.
      - Seen in Caucasians as well as other ethnicities.

II. *Juvenile (late-onset) cystinosis*

1. Ocular discomfort and photophobia are common at presentation.
2. Proteinuria:
   a. Spectrum from asymptomatic isolated proteinuria to overt nephrotic syndrome.
   b. Kidney histology may reflect focal segmental glomerulosclerosis indistinguishable from the idiopathic form.
3. Fanconi syndrome: Mild or absent.
4. Slower progression rate to kidney failure.
5. Slower progression to non-kidney complications.
6. Growth retardation may not be a significant feature.

III. *Adult (ocular non-nephropathic) cystinosis*

1. Characterized by the presence of corneal crystals and photophobia.
2. Cystine crystals also present in the bone marrow.
3. Very rarely may have kidney complications.

C. Diagnosis

1. Detection of cystine crystals:
   a. Cystine corneal crystals by slit lamp examination.
      - Do not appear in the slit lamp examination until the second year of life.

   b. Cystine crystal laden macrophages on bone marrow examination.
2. Leukocyte (preferably isolated polymorphonuclear cells) cystine content by high-performance liquid chromatography or liquid chromatography-tandem mass spectrometry (LC-MS/MS):
   a. Definitive diagnosis if levels 3–20 nmol ½-cystine/mg protein.
      - Infantile form: >5 nmol ½-cystine/mg protein.
      - Intermediate form: 3–6 nmol ½-cystine/mg protein.

   b. Heterozygous carrier if levels <1.0 nmol ½-cystine/mg protein.
   c. Normal individual if levels <0.2 nmol ½-cystine/mg protein.
   d. Technical considerations:
      - Polymorphonuclear cells are preferred because cystine preferentially accumulates in these cells compared to lymphocytes and can lead to false negatives in infants who have higher proportions of lymphocytes.
      - Where available, local (laboratory-specific) reference levels should be used.
      - Conversion factor from ½ cystine per mg protein to cystine per mg protein is x2.
3. Mutation of the *CTNS* gene.
   - In a small percentage of patients (5–10%) with the clinical diagnosis of cystinosis, *CTNS* gene mutations cannot be identified because their pathogenic mutations might either be deeply intronic or in the promoter region.

D. Management

I. *Symptomatic therapy*

1. Fluid intake:
   a. Ensure adequate fluid intake commensurates with urine output.
   b. Increased fluid intake required in states of fever, diarrhea, vomiting, and external heat.
2. Nutrition:
   a. Calorie requirement: At least 100% of the suggested dietary intake.
   b. Nasogastric or gastrostomy tube feeding should be considered early in young infants with anorexia or frequent vomiting.
3. Correction of acidosis, hypokalemia and hyponatremia using either sodium bicarbonate or sodium/potassium citrate:
   a. Sodium loss:
      - 2–15 mmol/kg/day of sodium bicarbonate or citrate given in 4 divided doses.
   b. Bicarbonate loss:
      i. May need up to 10–15 mmol/kg/day of sodium bicarbonate or sodium/potassium citrate given in 4 divided doses.
      ii. Aim for a bicarbonate level of 21–24 mmol/L.
      iii. Use potassium citrate preferentially as high sodium intake may worsen hypercalciuria.
   c. Potassium loss:
      i. 2–10 mmol/kg/day of potassium citrate or potassium chloride given in 4 divided doses.
      ii. Aim for a potassium level >3.0 mmol/L.
4. Prevention of rickets:
   a. Phosphate supplementation:
      i. 0.6–2 mmol/kg/day (10–30 mmol/day) given in 4 divided doses to maintain normal age-related serum phosphate levels.
         - 1 mmol (95 mg) of phosphate = 1 mmol (30 mg) of elemental phosphorus.
         - Sodium phosphate solution: 0.7 mmol phosphate per ml.
         - Phosphate Sandoz tablet: 16.1 mmol phosphate per tablet.

ii. Measure trough levels before the next dose, aiming >1.2 mmol/L.
iii. High doses of phosphate can cause or aggravate nephrocalcinosis.

b. Vitamin D supplementation:
   - Calcidiol 400–1000 IU or 10–25 μg/day.
   - Active vitamin D (alfa-calcidol or calcitriol) 0.04–0.08 μg/kg/day (maximum starting dose of 0.25 mg/day).

5. L-Carnitine supplementation:
   a. Often given although there is no proven clinical benefit.
   b. Starting dose of 20–100 mg/kg/day divided into 3 doses.
   c. Titrate to maintain plasma carnitine levels in the normal range.
   d. If there are muscular complaints, cut the dose to 20–30 mg/kg/day.
6. Indomethacin:
   a. Reduces tubular losses of water, sodium and potassium.
   b. Also improves appetite and growth.
   c. Starting dose 0.5–3 mg/kg/day divided into 2–3 doses.
   d. Discontinue in conditions of dehydration.
   e. Concomitant use of angiotensin-converting enzyme inhibitors is contraindicated.
7. Hormone replacement therapy:
   a. Thyroxine replacement in hypothyroidism.
      i. Recommended dose:
         - 0–6 years: 3–4 μg/kg/day
         - 6–12 years: 2.5–3.5 μg/kg/day
         - >12 years: 1.5–2 μg/kg/day.
      ii. Start at 25% of the recommended dose, increasing to full dose in 4 weeks.
      iii. In some patients, TSH may still remain elevated despite the normalization of T4.
   b. Recombinant growth hormone therapy recommended in children with growth retardation after optimal cysteamine therapy and treatment of Fanconi syndrome.
8. Anti-proteinuric therapy:
   a. Angiotensin-converting enzyme inhibitors or angiotensin receptor blockers to reduce proteinuria.
   b. Dose at night to avoid hypotension.
   c. Generally not to be used in combination with indomethacin.

II. *Cystine-depleting therapy*

1. Cysteamine:
   a. Mechanism of action:
      - Reduces intracellular cystine content by entering the cell and concentrating within the lysosomes where it reacts with cystine to form both cysteine and a cystine-cysteamine complex that are able to leave the lysosomes.
   b. Immediate-release cysteamine bitartrate (IR-CYS): Cystagon®
      i. 1.3 $g/m^2/day$ (maximum dose: 1.95 $g/m^2/day$).
      ii. Start at a low dose (1/6 of the optimal dose) and gradually increase over 6–8 weeks to the maximum dose.
      iii. Dose should be given at 6-hourly intervals as leukocyte cystine content returns to its initial levels at 6 hours after administration.
   c. Delayed-release enteric-coated cysteamine bitartrate (DR-CYS): Procysbi™:
      i. Given at 12-hourly intervals.
      ii. If converting from immediate-release formulation, start at 100% of the current total daily dose.
      iii. If initiating therapy, similar maintenance dose of 1.3 $g/m^2/day$ (maximum dose 1.95 $g/m^2/day$).
         - Start at 1/6 to 1/4 the target dose.
         - Increase by 10% increments to the maintenance dose every 2 weeks (<6 years) or over a course of 4–6 weeks (>6 years).
   d. Monitoring:
      i. Measurement of leukocyte cystine levels:
         - Once the maintenance dose is reached
         - Followed by monthly for 3 months
         - Followed by quarterly for one year
         - Followed by twice a year.
      ii. Optimal target level <1 nmol ½-cystine/mg protein (or 90th centile of asymptomatic heterozygotes using specific laboratory's assay).
      iii. Blood sampling should be obtained 6 hours after dose of cysteamine.

e. Side effects:
   i. Gastrointestinal complaints (nausea, vomiting) due to increased gastric acid secretion.
   ii. Halitosis and bad sweat odor due to sulfur-containing metabolites of cysteamine (dimethylsulfide, methanethiol).
   iii. Skin striae with endothelial proliferative lesions on elbows (reactive angioendotheliomatosis on skin biopsy) seen with high cysteamine doses (>1.95 g/m²/day).
   iv. Bone pain and myalgia.
   v. Hyperthermia and lethargy.
   vi. Neutropenia.
   vii. Seizures.
   viii. Allergic rash.
f. Adjunctive therapy:
   i. Proton-pump inhibitors should be prescribed to prevent the gastric side effects of oral cysteamine.
   ii. Riboflavin supplementation or oral chlorophyll can be used to combat halitosis and bad sweat odor.

2. Cysteamine eye drops:
   a. Eye drops (0.55% Cysteamine or 0.44% cysteamine Cystaran®) should be prescribed, as oral formulation does not reach the cornea due to the absent corneal vascularization.
   b. May decrease the size of already present deposits.
   c. Given at least 6–10 times per day to be effective.
   d. May cause a burning sensation in the eyes due to low pH of formulation.
   e. An ophthalmic gel formulation 0.37% (Cystadrops®, Orphan Europe, Paris, France) can be used instead of eye drops and given 4 times a day.

III. *Kidney transplantation*

1. Kidney transplantation is the treatment of choice for cystinosis patients with kidney failure.
2. Kidney transplantation does not correct the basic metabolic defect in other tissues, and cystine continues to accumulate in other organs, causing organ damage.

- Oral and ophthalmic cysteamine should be continued after transplantation.

3. Fanconi Syndrome does not recur in the transplanted kidney but the native kidneys can still cause renal tubular disease if they produce urine.
4. Cystine crystals may be deposited within the interstitial tissue and glomeruli of the transplanted kidney as the crystals develop in the recipient mononuclear cells that infiltrate the transplant.

Recommended Reading

1. Emma F, Nesterova G, Langman C, Labbe A, Cherqui S, Goodyer P, Janssen MC, Greco M, Topaloglu R, Elenberg E, Dohil R, Trauner D, Antignac C, Cochat P, Kaskel F, Servais A, Whul E, Niaudet P, Van't Hoff W, Gahl W, Levtchenko E. (2014) Nephropathic cystinosis: An international consensus document. *Nephrol Dial Transplant* **29** Suppl 4:iv87–94.
2. Elmonem MA, Veys KR, Soliman NA, van Dyck M, van den Heuvel LP, Levtchenko E. (2016) Cystinosis: A review. *Orphanet J Rare Dis* **11**:47. doi:10.1186/s13023-016-0426-y.
3. Veys KR, Elmonem MA, Arcolino FO, van den Heuvel L, Levtchenko E. (2017) Nephropathic cystinosis: An update. *Curr Opin Pediatr* **29**:168–178.
4. Niaudet P. (2020, updated) Cystinosis. Edited by: Mattoo TK, Kim MS. *UpToDate ONLINE.* http://www.uptodateonline.com.

1 Approach to Hematuria in Children

Lau PYW, Yap HK and KML Nyein

A. Definition

Urine microscopic examination findings of:
- Red blood cells (RBCs) >5/μL in a fresh uncentrifuged midstream urine specimen.
- RBCs >3/hpf in centrifuged sediment from 10 ml of freshly voided midstream urine.

B. Differential Diagnosis of "Hematuria"

1. "Hematuria" may present as red or smoky dark brown or cola-colored urine.
2. Causes of colored urine:
   a. Dark yellow or orange urine:
      - Normal concentrated urine.
      - Drugs (rifampicin, warfarin, pyridium).
   b. Dark brown or black urine:
      - Bile pigments.
      - Methemoglobinemia.
      - Alanine.
      - Laxative (cascara).
      - Drugs (resorcinol, thymol).
      - Alkaptonuria (homogentesic acid), tyrosinosis.
   c. Red or pink urine:
      - Free hemoglobin (hemoglobinuria).

- Myoglobin (myoglobinuria).
- Porphyrins.
- Urates in high concentration (pinkish tinge).
- Foods (beetroot, blackberries, red dyes, dragonfruit).
- Drugs (benzene, chloroquine, desferoxamine, phenazopyridine, phenolphthalein).

C. Detection of Hematuria

1. Urine dipstick:
   a. Hemoglobin peroxidase activity converts the chromogen tetramethylbenzidine incorporated in the dipstick into an oxidized form, resulting in a green-blue color.
   b. Very sensitive test and can detect as little as 150 μg/L of free hemoglobin.
   c. Causes of false-positive results:
      - Hemoglobinuria.
      - Myoglobinuria.
      - Presence of oxidizing agents in the urine (hypochlorite and microbial peroxidases associated with urinary tract infection).
   d. Causes of false-negative results:
      - Presence of large amounts of reducing agents (ascorbic acid).
      - High urine specific gravity.
2. Urine microscopy:
   - Microscopic examination of the urine sediment is important in diagnosing and evaluating hematuria.

D. Etiology

1. Hematuria may originate from the glomeruli, renal tubules, and interstitium, or urinary tract (including collecting systems, ureters, bladder, and urethra).
2. A practical approach is to determine whether the hematuria is of glomerular or non-glomerular origin.

Glomerular	Non-glomerular

Familial hematuria syndromes
  Thin basement membrane nephropathy
  Alport syndrome
  Hereditary angiopathy, nephropathy, aneurysms, muscle cramps syndrome
  MYH9 syndromes (associated thrombocytopathies)
  C3 glomerulopathy
Glomerulonephritis (GN)
  Postinfectious GN
  Membranoproliferative GN
  Membranous nephropathy
  Crescentic GN
  IgA nephropathy
  IgA vasculitis nephritis
  Lupus nephritis
  Anti-neutrophil cytoplasmic antibodies (ANCA)-associated vasculitis
  Anti-glomerular basement membrane (GBM) antibody disease
Hemolytic uremic syndrome
Renal vein thrombosis
Interstitial nephritis
	Urinary tract infection
	Hypercalciuria
	Renal calculi
	Trauma
	Cystic kidney disease
	Exercise-induced
	Chemical cystitis (cyclophosphamide)
	Coagulopathy
	Vascular malformations
	Nutcracker syndrome
	Malignancies
	  Nephroblastoma
	  Renal cell carcinoma
	  Rhabdomyosarcoma of the bladder
	Renal vein thrombosis
	Menarche
	Factitious

E. Diagnostic Approach

1. Clinical evaluation:
   a. Macroscopic hematuria of glomerular origin is usually described as brown, tea or cola-colored, whereas that of lower urinary tract origin is usually pink or red.
   b. When bladder or urethral pathology is a consideration, initial hematuria suggests a urethral origin whereas terminal hematuria is indicative of a bladder cause.

c. History of menarche in peripubertal girls.
d. Accompanying edema and hypertension is suggestive of glomerulonephritis.
e. Accompanying voiding symptoms such as frequency, urgency, dysuria, and wetting suggest non-glomerular cause.
f. Preceding history of infection or synpharyngitic presentation.
g. Family history of kidney disease, hematuria, kidney calculi, deafness, intracerebral bleed, and coagulopathy.
h. History of drug ingestion.
i. History of sexual activity in pubertal adolescents.
j. Systemic symptoms and signs suggestive of secondary GN such as rashes, arthritis and fever.
k. Ballotable renal mass or palpable bladder on physical examination.
l. Asthenic habitus is associated with nutcracker syndrome.

2. Urine microscopic examination
   a. RBCs:
      - False-negative when urine is of low specific gravity or has an alkaline pH, as this results in RBC hemolyzing.
   b. White blood cells: Consider urinary tract infection and interstitial or glomerular inflammatory disorders.
      i. Neutrophils suggestive of urinary tract infection or post-infectious nephritis.
      ii. Eosinophils suggestive of interstitial nephritis.
   c. Casts:
      i. RBC casts suggestive of GN:
         - Should be done on fresh urine or acidic urine stored at 4°C.
         - RBC casts disintegrate readily in alkaline urine, taking on a granular appearance.
      ii. Hyaline casts:
         - Associated with proteinuria.
         - Found in concentrated early morning samples from healthy people.
      iii. Granular casts:
         - Finding associated with hematuria indicates glomerular origin.

   d. Crystals:
      i. Urate.
      ii. Calcium oxalate.
      iii. Cystine.
3. Urine phase contrast microscopy of freshly voided urine for RBC morphology:
   a. Non-glomerular: >90–95% isomorphic.
   b. Glomerular: >30% dysmorphic.
4. Urine protein estimation:
   a. Best done on early morning urine to exclude orthostatic proteinuria.
   b. Interpret with caution if the child has gross hematuria with isomorphic RBCs.
   c. Urine dipstick ≥2+ suggestive of glomerular hematuria.
   d. Urine protein:creatinine ratio (UPCR):
      - Indicated if urine dipstick is positive.
   e. 24-hour urine protein excretion:
      - Consider if UPCR ≥0.02 g/mmol.
5. Family screen:
   - Urine microscopy for family members to look for hematuria.
6. Hearing and eye assessment:
   a. Audiometry for high tone hearing loss.
   b. Ophthalmologic assessment for eye abnormalities including anterior lenticonus, subcapsular cataracts, and retinal and corneal changes.
7. Other investigations:
   a. Check kidney function:
      i. Serum creatinine and estimated glomerular filtration rate (eGFR).
      ii. Serum urea.
   b. Ultrasound of the kidneys and bladder.
      i. Indicated in non-glomerular hematuria to exclude congenital malformations, renal calculi, and tumors.
      ii. Indicated in glomerular hematuria to assess the size and echogenicity of kidneys to assess the chronicity of GN or if polycystic kidney disease is suspected.

c. Glomerular hematuria:
   i. Serum complements (C3, C4).
   ii. Serum IgA.
   iii. Anti-nuclear antibodies (ANA) or anti-dsDNA antibody.
   iv. Anti-streptolysin O titer (ASOT).
   v. ANCA: Anti-proteinase 3 and anti-myeloperoxidase antibodies.
   vi. Anti-GBM antibody if pulmonary hemorrhage is present.
   vii. Skin biopsy with immunostaining for α5(IV) chain (consider if suspicion of X-linked Alport syndrome is high).
   viii. Peripheral blood smear for macrothrombocytopenia and basophilic cytoplasmic leukocyte inclusion bodies (Döhle-like bodies) suggesting MYH9 syndromes.

d. Non-glomerular:
   i. Urine calcium:creatinine ratio.
   ii. Urine culture.
   iii. Urine adenovirus culture.
   iv. Screen for bleeding disorder:
      - Full blood count.
      - Prothrombin time (PT).
      - Activated partial thromboplastin time (aPTT).
   v. Plain abdominal X-Ray if ureteric calculi are suspected.
   vi. Doppler ultrasound of the left renal vein to exclude nut-cracker syndrome:
      - Anteroposterior diameter ratio between the distended and narrowed portions of the left renal vein is >4.0.
      - Peak velocity ratio between the narrowed and distended portions of the left renal vein >4.2.
      - Angle between the superior mesenteric artery and abdominal aorta <35°.
      - Left renal vein hilar to aorto-mesenteric diameter ratio >4.9.
   vii. Cystoscopy if bladder or urethral pathology is suspected or to lateralize the source of bleeding.

e. Genetic testing for familial hematuria syndromes.
   - Can contribute useful diagnostic and prognostic information and obviate the need for invasive kidney biopsy.

Etiology	Gene	Protein
Autosomal dominant Alport or thin basement membrane nephropathy (TBMN)	*COL4A3/A4* heterozygous	α3(IV) α4(IV)
X-linked Alport syndrome (males)	*COL4A5* hemizygous	α5(IV)
X-linked Alport syndrome (females)	*COL4A5* heterozygous	α5(IV)
Autosomal recessive Alport syndrome	*COL4A3* and *A4* mutations in trans or cis	α3(IV) α4(IV)
Digenic Alport syndrome	*COL4A3/A4* heterozygous	α3(IV) α4(IV)
Autosomal dominant HANAC syndrome	*COL4A1* heterozygous	α1(IV)
Autosomal dominant macrothrombocytopathies	*MYH9* heterozygous	Nonmuscle myosin heavy chain IIA
CFHR5 nephropathy	*CFHR5* heterozygous	Complement factor H-related protein 5
Glomerulopathy associated with fibronectin deposition	*FN1*	Fibronectin 1

F. Indications for Kidney Biopsy

1. Presence of significant proteinuria (>1 g/1.73m^2/day) except in post-infectious GN.
2. Persistently low serum complement C3.
3. Unexplained azotemia.
4. Systemic disease with significant proteinurias, such as systemic lupus erythematosus, IgA vasculitis, ANCA-associated vasculitis.
5. Family history of significant kidney disease suggestive of Alport syndrome.
6. Recurrent gross hematuria of unknown etiology.
7. Persistent glomerular hematuria and parental anxiety about diagnosis and prognosis.
   Note: A kidney biopsy is usually not indicated in isolated glomerular hematuria.

G. Algorithm for Investigating Hematuria

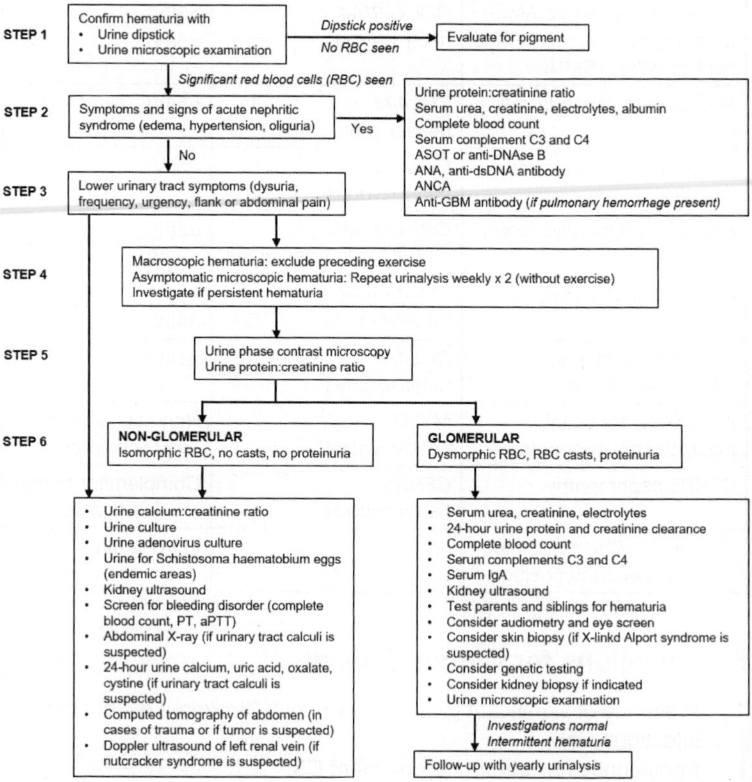

Recommended Reading

1. Yap HK, Lau PYW. (2008) Hematuria and proteinuria. In: *Comprehensive Pediatric Nephrology,* 1st edition. Edited by: Geary DF, Shaefer F. pp 179–194.
2. Deltas C, Pierides A, Voskarides K. (2013) Molecular genetics of familial hematuric diseases. *Nephrol Dial Transplant* **28**(12):2946–960.
3. Plevová P, Gut J, Janda J. (2017) Familial hematuria: A review. *Medicina (Kaunas)* **53**:1–10.

4. Ananthan K, Onida S, Davies AH. (2017) Nutcracker syndrome: An update on current diagnostic criteria and management guidelines. *Eur J Vasc Endovasc Surg* **53**:886–894.
5. Boyer OG. (2020, updated) Evaluation of gross hematuria in children. Edited by Niaudet P, Baskin LS, Kim MS. *UpToDate ONLINE*. http://www.uptodate.com.
6. Boyer OG. (2020, updated) Evaluation of microscopic hematuria in children. Edited by Niaudet P, Drutz JE, Kim MS. *UpToDate ONLINE*. http://www.uptodate.com.

2 Approach to Proteinuria in Children

Lau PYW, Ng KH, KML Nyein and Yap HK

A. Introduction

1. Significant proteinuria is associated with progressive kidney disease.
2. Proteinuria can also be a transient finding during times of stress, including exercise, fever and dehydration, and does not denote kidney disease.
3. Epidemiologic data in adults have demonstrated a strong graded relationship between albuminuria with both kidney and cardiovascular disease risk.
   a. KDIGO's (Kidney Disease Improving Global Outcomes) 2012 Clinical Practice Guideline for the Evaluation and Management of Chronic Kidney Disease has incorporated albuminuria in the criteria and classification of chronic kidney disease (CKD) in adults.
      - Urinary albumin excretion rate ≥30 mg/day sustained for >3 months is used to indicate CKD in adults.

   b. Urinary albumin excretion rates in children and adolescents vary with age:
      - Urinary albumin excretion is estimated to be lowest in children aged <6 years, followed by an increase through adolescent years, with a peak at 15–16 years.
      - Significance of albuminuria for conditions other than diabetic nephropathy in children and adolescents is less well defined.

B. Definitions

Urine Test	Normal Protein Excretion	Abnormal Protein Excretion	Nephrotic Range Proteinuria
Dipstick	Negative or trace	≥1+	≥3+ for 3 consecutive days
Sulfosalicylic acid test	Negative	≥1+	≥3+ for 3 consecutive days
Protein:creatinine ratio (g/mmol) Aged >2 years: Aged 6 months to 2 years:	 ≤0.02 ≤0.05	 >0.02 >0.05	 >0.22
24-hour protein excretion Aged >6 months old: (g/1.73m^2/day): (mg/m^2/hr): Aged <6 months old: (g/1.73m^2/day): (mg/m^2/hr):	 ≤0.15 ≤4 ≤0.3 ≤8	 >0.15 >4 >0.3 >8	 >3 >40 >3 >40
Albumin:creatinine ratio Aged >2 years: (g/mmol): (mg/g):	 ≤0.003 ≤30	 >0.003 >30	 >0.220 >2220
24-hour albumin excretion (mg/1.73m^2/day)	 ≤30	 >30	 >2200

1. Urinary protein excretion **<0.3 g/1.73m^2/day** is associated with regression of proteinuric chronic nephropathies, suggesting that investigations are only necessary above this level.
2. Exclude orthostatic proteinuria:
   a. Defined as early morning urine samples (supine) negative for protein, while evening urine samples (upright) may contain varying concentrations of protein.
   b. 24-hour urinary protein excretion rarely exceeds 1 g/1.73m^2/day.

C. Methods of Detection of Proteinuria

1. Urine dipstick:
   a. Excellent screening test for proteinuria.
   b. Able to detect protein concentrations as little as 0.1 to 0.15 g/L.
   c. Dipstick is impregnated with tetrabromophenol blue, buffered to pH 3.5, which after binding to protein results in the development of a blue color proportionate to the amount of protein present.
   d. False-positive results:
      - Dipstick left in urine for too long.
      - Presence of gross hematuria, pyuria and bacteriuria.
      - Contamination with antiseptics (such as chlorhexidine, benzalkonium).
      - Post-administration of radiographic contrast.
      - Drugs, e.g., penicillin or cephalosporin, tolbutamide or sulphonamides.
      - Urine specific gravity >1.025.
      - Very alkaline urine pH >8.0.
   e. False-negative results:
      - Urine specific gravity <1.002.
      - Very acidic urine pH <4.5.
      - Non-albumin proteinuria (such as globulins, mucoproteins, or Bence–Jones protein).
   f. Urine dipstick reading (Albustix® or Uristix®):

Dipstick Reading	Color	Urine Protein Concentration (g/L)
Negative	Yellow	Insignificant
Trace	Light yellow-green	<0.2
1+	Yellow-green	0.3
2+	Green	1.0
3+	Green-blue	3.0
4+	Blue	>20

2. Sulfosalicylic acid test:
   a. Based on sulfosalicylic acid precipitation of protein.
   b. Provides a more quantitative estimate of all the proteins present including albumin and low molecular weight proteins.
   c. False-positive with iodinated radiocontrast agents.
   d. Readings based on the turbidity of solution:

Grade	Appearance	Urine Protein Concentration (g/L)
0	No turbidity	0
Trace	Slight turbidity	0.01–0.1
1+	Turbidity through which print can be read	0.15–0.3
2+	White cloud without precipitate through which heavy black lines on a background can be seen	0.4–1
3+	White cloud with precipitate through which heavy black lines on a background cannot be seen	1.5–3.5
4+	Flocculent precipitate	>5

3. Quantification of protein:
   a. First morning urine specimen is recommended for spot urinary protein:creatinine ratio quantification.
   b. 24-hour urinary total protein quantification is the most precise way of protein quantification.
   c. 24-hour urinary total protein quantification may be difficult in very young patients or patients who have nocturnal enuresis.
   d. Urine creatinine in an accurately collected 24-hour urine specimen should be:
      - 0.13–0.20 mmol/kg ideal body weight for females.
      - 0.18–0.23 mmol/kg ideal body weight for males.

D. Causes of Proteinuria

Intermittent Proteinuria	Persistent Proteinuria	
	Glomerular	Tubular
Non-postural • Fever • Exercise • Dehydration • Emotional stress • No known cause ***Postural (Orthostatic)***	***Primary glomerulopathies*** • Minimal change disease • Focal segmental glomerulosclerosis • Mesangiocapillary glomerulonephritis • Rapidly progressive glomerulonephritis • Membranous nephropathy • Genetic glomerulopathies ***Secondary glomerulopathies*** • Post-infectious glomerulonephritis • Lupus nephritis • Immunoglobulin A (IgA) nephropathy • IgA vasculitis nephritis • Genetic glomerulopathies: Alport syndrome Genetic podocytopathies Mitochondrial diseases • Infections: Hepatitis B nephropathy Hepatitis C nephropathy Human immunodeficiency virus (HIV) nephropathy • Amyloidosis • Hemolytic-uremic syndrome • Diabetic nephropathy • Hypertension • Decreased nephron mass: Reflux nephropathy Congenital abnormalities of kidney and urinary tract (CAKUT)	***Hereditary*** • Proximal renal tubular acidosis • Dent's disease • Cystinosis • Galactosemia • Tyrosinemia type I • Hereditary fructose intolerance • Wilson disease • Lowe syndrome ***Acquired*** • Pyelonephritis • Tubulointerstitial nephritis • Acute kidney injury • Analgesic abuse • Drugs: Penicillamine • Heavy metal poisoning: Lead Cadmium Gold Mercury • Vitamin D intoxication

1. Glomerular proteinuria:
   a. May be due to the following factors:
      - Increase in glomerular permeability.
      - Loss of negative charge in the glomerular filtration barrier.
      - Direct injury to the glomerular filtration barrier.
      - Changes in glomerular capillary pressure.
   b. Selectivity of glomerular proteinuria:
      - Selective proteinuria defined by predominance of low molecular weight proteins (albumin or transferrin) compared to high molecular weight proteins (IgG).
      - Non-selective proteinuria defined by mixture of heavy and low molecular weight proteins.
      - Selectivity index defined by clearance ratio of IgG over albumin or transferrin:
        - Selectivity index <0.1 = highly selective proteinuria.
        - Selectivity index ≥ 0.1 = non-selective proteinuria or poorly selective proteinuria.
2. Non-glomerular proteinuria:
   a. Tubular proteinuria:
      - Occurs when there is damage to proximal convoluted tubules.
      - Amount of proteinuria usually <1 g/1.73m^2/day.
      - Distinguished from glomerular proteinuria by protein electrophoresis.
      - Markers used as the index for tubular proteinuria include β_2-microglobulin, α_1-microglobulin and retinol-binding protein.
   b. Overflow proteinuria:
      - Results when plasma concentration of filterable protein exceeds the renal threshold for that protein.
      - Can occur in normal kidney function.
      - Includes monoclonal gammopathy, hemoglobinuria, myoglobinuria, β_2-microglobulinemia, myelomonocytic leukemia, Bence–Jones proteinuria and sometimes following multiple transfusions of either albumin or whole blood.
   c. Secretory proteinuria:
      - Increased excretion of tissue proteins into the urine.

- Typical example is the excretion of Tamm–Horsfall protein in the neonatal period, accounting for the higher levels of protein excretion typically seen at this age.
- Occurs in urinary tract infection, analgesic nephropathy, and inflammation of accessory sex glands.

E. Clinical Approach

I. General principles:

1. When proteinuria is detected, it is important to determine whether it is transient, orthostatic or persistent in type.
2. It is important to exclude acute nephritic or nephrotic syndrome because these conditions demand urgent investigations and treatment.

II. History:

1. Symptoms of kidney failure or glomerulonephritis (edema, hematuria, polyuria, nocturia), and connective tissue disorders (including rashes and joint pain).
2. History of congenital kidney abnormalities or recurrent urinary tract infections.
3. Intake of drugs that may be associated with kidney injury such as non-steroidal anti-inflammatory medications or traditional medicines.
4. Family history of polycystic kidney disease, kidney failure or deafness.

III. Physical examination:

1. Evidence of chronic kidney failure such as growth failure, anemia and rickets.
2. Assess for hypertension as this is an important prognostic indicator in CKD.

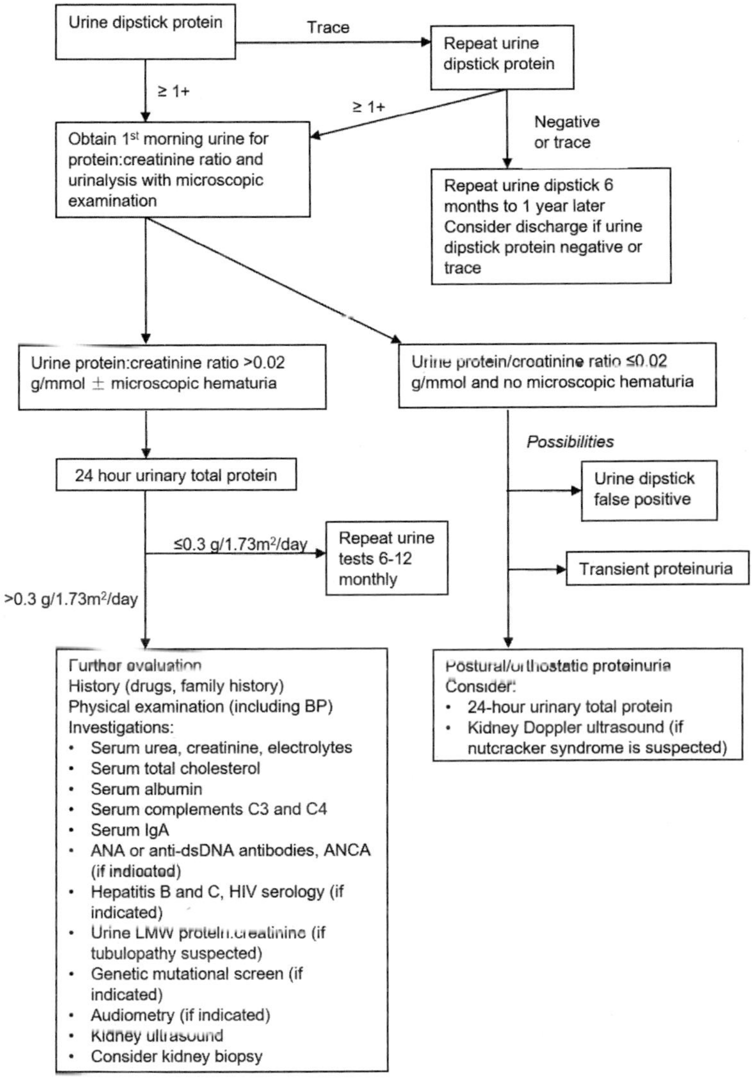
Urine dipstick protein
Trace
Repeat urine dipstick protein
≥ 1+
≥ 1+
Negative or trace
Obtain 1st morning urine for protein:creatinine ratio and urinalysis with microscopic examination
Repeat urine dipstick 6 months to 1 year later
Consider discharge if urine dipstick protein negative or trace
Urine protein:creatinine ratio >0.02 g/mmol ± microscopic hematuria
Urine protein/creatinine ratio ≤0.02 g/mmol and no microscopic hematuria
Possibilities
24 hour urinary total protein
Urine dipstick false positive
≤0.3 g/1.73m2/day
Repeat urine tests 6-12 monthly
Transient proteinuria
>0.3 g/1.73m2/day
Further evaluation
History (drugs, family history)
Physical examination (including BP)
Investigations:
• Serum urea, creatinine, electrolytes
• Serum total cholesterol
• Serum albumin
• Serum complements C3 and C4
• Serum IgA
• ANA or anti-dsDNA antibodies, ANCA (if indicated)
• Hepatitis B and C, HIV serology (if indicated)
• Urine LMW protein:creatinine (if tubulopathy suspected)
• Genetic mutational screen (if indicated)
• Audiometry (if indicated)
• Kidney ultrasound
• Consider kidney biopsy
Postural/orthostatic proteinuria
Consider:
• 24-hour urinary total protein
• Kidney Doppler ultrasound (if nutcracker syndrome is suspected)

3. Look for signs of fluid overload due to acute nephritic syndrome or kidney failure, such as raised jugular venous pressure, hepatomegaly and edema.
4. Signs of nephrotic syndrome such as generalized edema, ascites, pleural effusion, and scrotal edema (in boys).
5. Associated signs of systemic illnesses such as palpable purpuric rash on the lower limbs suggesting IgA vasculitis nephritis, and joint swelling suggesting connective tissue disorders.
6. Palpable flank masses may suggest hydronephrosis or polycystic kidney disease.

IV. Investigations:

1. Detailed investigations should be started early if:
   a. Child has signs and symptoms suggestive of kidney disease.
   b. Associated hematuria and proteinuria.
2. A step-by-step approach is recommended to evaluate isolated proteinuria in an asymptomatic child, as shown in the algorithm.
3. Measurement of urinary excretion of low-molecular-weight (LMW) proteins (tubular proteinuria) is helpful if a tubular disorder or interstitial nephritis is suspected from the history or urinary findings of eosinophils:
   - Urine β_2-microglobulin:creatinine ratio >0.04 mg/mmol (4×10^{-4} mg/mg).
   - Urine α1-microglobulin:creatinine ratio >2.2 mg/mmol (0.022 mg/mg).
   - Urine retinol-binding protein >0.024 mg/mmol (2.4×10^{-4} mg/mg).
4. Perform a kidney ultrasound to look for kidney scarring, CAKUT, cystic kidney disease, and medullary nephrocalcinosis.
   - Consider a kidney Doppler ultrasound to exclude nutcracker syndrome if there is orthostatic proteinuria.
5. Genetic testing
   a. Indications:
      i. Significant family history:
         - Parental consanguinity.

- Family members with nephrotic syndrome, proteinuria, hematuria, and kidney failure.
- Family members with relevant non-kidney manifestations, e.g., early-onset diabetes, sensorineural hearing defects, neurological disorders, and epilepsy.

ii. Significant non-kidney manifestations:
- Sensorineural hearing defects.
- Ophthalmologic abnormalities.
- Genitourinary malformations.
- Neurological or skeletal manifestations.

iii. Association with medullary nephrocalcinosis:
- ADCK4-related glomerulopathy.

b. Type of genetic test:
- Consider targeted gene panel consisting of podocytopathy genes.
- Consider whole exome or whole genome sequencing in atypical cases, or if the targeted gene panel is negative.

6. Indications for kidney biopsy:

a. Persistent significant proteinuria >1 g/1.73m^2/day or early morning urine protein:creatinine ratio of >0.05 g/mmol (>0.5 g/g) in a child aged >2 years old.
- An exception is a child who presents with typical steroid-sensitive nephrotic syndrome.

b. Proteinuria associated with urinary sediment abnormalities.

c. Decreased glomerular filtration rate (GFR) <60 ml/1.73m^2/min.
- An exception is a child who is recovering from acute glomerulonephritis, e.g., post-infectious glomerulonephritis, unless the child's GFR remains low at 1 month, a kidney biopsy should be considered.

d. Persistently low serum complement C3 levels >3 months.

e. Evidence of a collagen vascular disease or vasculitic (such as systemic lupus erythematosus, IgA vasculitis nephritis, ANCA-associated vasculitis), either clinically or serologically.

F. Treatment Options for Significant Proteinuria (Non-nephrotic)

1. Dietary protein recommendations:
   a. Avoid excess dietary protein.
   b. Suggested dietary intake (SDI) of protein for age.
2. Drugs with anti-proteinuric effects (see chapter "Adjunctive Therapy in Glomerular Disease").
3. High-dose coenzyme Q10 supplementation:
   a. Consider in children with genetic defects in coenzyme Q10 biosynthesis (*COQ2, PDSS2, COQ6, ADCK4*).
   b. Ubiquinol is the reduced, active form while ubiquinone is the oxidized form that needs to be converted in the body to the active form.
   c. Ubiquinol at the same dosage may yield more active compounds then ubiquinone.
   d. Starting dose: 30 mg/kg/day (at least three divided doses) and then increase to 50 mg/kg/day (maximum 2400 mg/day for adults).
   e. A decrease in proteinuria can be expected in 4–6 weeks.

Recommended Reading

1. Yap HK, Lau PYW. (2008) Hematuria and proteinuria. In: *Comprehensive Pediatric Nephrology*, 1st edition. Edited by: Geary DF, Shaefer F. Mosby, Elsevier. pp 179–194.
2. Kidney Disease: Improving Global Outcomes (KDIGO) CKD Work Group. (2013) KDIGO 2012 clinical practice guideline for the evaluation and management of chronic kidney disease. *Kidney Int Suppl* **3**:1–150.
3. Korkmaz E, Lipska-Ziętkiewicz BS, Boyer O, Gribouval O, Fourrage C, Tabatabaei M, Schnaidt S, Gucer S, Kaymaz F, Arici M, Dinckan A, Mir S, Bayazit AK, Emre S, Balat A, Rees L, Shroff R, Bergmann C, Mourani C, Antignac C, Ozaltin F, Schaefer F; PodoNet Consortium. (2016) ADCK4-associated glomerulopathy causes adolescence-onset FSGS. *J Am Soc Nephrol* **27**:63–68.
4. Boyer OG. (2020, updated) Evaluation of proteinuria in children. Edited by Niaudet P, Kim MS. *UpToDate ONLINE.* http://www.uptodate.com.

3 Acute Glomerulonephritis

Prasetyo RV, Teo S, Resontoc LP, Ng KH, Lau PYW and Yap HK

A. Definition

- Acute glomerulonephritis (acute nephritic syndrome):
  - Gross hematuria.
  - Edema.
  - Hypertension.
  - Oliguria.
  - ± Azotemia.

B. Etiology

I. Causes of acute glomerulonephritis

a. Infection-related glomerulonephritis:
   i. Bacterial infection-related glomerulonephritis:
      - Post-infectious glomerulonephritis.
      - Shunt nephritis.
      - Glomerulonephritis related to infective endocarditis.
      - IgA-dominant-infection-related glomerulonephritis (IgADIRGN).
   ii. Viral infection related glomerulonephritis.
   iii. Nephropathies due to infections with schistosomiasis, filariasis and malaria.

b. Systemic lupus erythematosus.

c. IgA vasculitis nephritis (Henoch–Schönlein purpura).

d. Anti-neutrophil cytoplasmic antibody (ANCA)-associated vasculitis.

e. Anti-glomerular basement membrane (GBM) disease.

f. C3 glomerulopathy.
g. Idiopathic crescentic glomerulonephritis.

II. Organisms associated with infection-related glomerulonephritis

Bacterial	Viral
Group A β-hemolytic streptococci[a] *Streptococcus viridans*[b] *Staphylococcus aureus*[b,c,d] *Staphylococcus albus*[b] *Staphylococcus epidermidis*[d] Leptospirosis *Salmonella typhi* *Escherichia coli* [c,d] *Pseudomonas sp.* [c] *Proteus mirabilis* [c] *Klebsiella sp.*[d] *Streptococcus pneumoniae* *Mycoplasma pneumoniae*	Hepatitis B Hepatitis C Cytomegalovirus Epstein–Barr virus Measles Mumps Varicella zoster Parvovirus B19 Coxsackie Human immunodeficiency virus (HIV)
Fungal and Rickettsial	**Parasitic**
Coccidioides immitis Scrub typhus	Malaria (*Plasmodium falciparum*) Filariasis Schistosomiasis *(Schistosoma mansoni, Schistosoma haematobium)*

[a]Peak incidence of post-streptococcal glomerulonephritis occurs in preschool and early school-age years (<5% in children aged <2 years and 5–10% in adults aged >40 years).
[b]Shunt nephritis should be excluded in patients with artificial vascular shunts.
[c]Visceral abscesses should be excluded.
[d]IgA-dominant-infection-related glomerulonephritis associated with skin infections, osteomyelitis, pneumonia, and bacteremia, in patients with underlying co-morbidities such as diabetes mellitus.

C. Approach to Diagnosis

I. History:

1. Gross hematuria (smoky, cola-colored).

2. Facial and leg swelling.
3. Weight gain.
4. Decreased urine output.
5. Headache and vomiting.
6. Preceding resolved streptococcal infection prior to the onset of symptoms:
   a. Pharyngitis: 7–14 days.
   b. Pyoderma or impetigo: 3–6 weeks.
7. Previous shunt operation.
8. Previous prosthetic heart valve or structural heart valve lesion.
9. History of blood product transfusion.
10. History of substance abuse.
11. History of immunocompromised status (diabetes mellitus, hypertension, heart disease, malignancy, kidney transplantation).
12. History of deafness.
13. History of hepatitis B, hepatitis C, HIV.
14. Hepatitis B immunization.
15. Symptoms of systemic disease:
    a. Fever.
    b. Rash ± photosensitivity.
    c. Mouth ulcers.
    d. Joint pains.
16. Family history of:
    a. Glomerulonephritis.
    b. Autoimmune diseases.
    c. Kidney failure.
    d. Hypertension.

II. Physical examination:

1. Blood pressure.
2. Evidence of fluid retention:
   a. Facial edema.
   b. Pedal edema.
   c. Ascites.
   d. Pleural effusion.
3. Evidence of circulatory congestion:
   a. Cardiomegaly.

   b. Raised jugular venous pressure.
   c. Pulmonary edema.
   d. Tender hepatomegaly.
4. Full neurological examination including fundoscopy.
5. Evidence of systemic disease:
   a. Lethargy.
   b. Fever.
   c. Clinical signs of bacteremia.
   d. Rashes.
   e. Oral ulcers.
   f. Joint swelling.
   g. Lymphadenopathy.
   h. Hepatosplenomegaly.
6. Evidence of active skin or tonsil infections.
7. Presence of ventriculo-atrial/prosthetic vascular shunts.
8. Presence of new or changed cardiac murmur.

III. Investigations

1. Urinalysis:
   a. Urine microscopy to look for red blood cells (RBCs), leukocytes and casts:
      - Presence of RBC casts suggest acute glomerulonephritis: Should be done on fresh urine or acidic urine stored at 4°C, as RBC casts disintegrate readily in alkaline urine, taking on a granular appearance.
      - Granular casts: Finding associated with hematuria indicates glomerular origin.
   b. Phase contrast study on fresh urine specimen to look for dysmorphic red blood cells (>30% indicates glomerular origin).
   c. Presence of proteinuria:
      - Urine protein:creatinine ratio or albumin:creatinine ratio.
      - 24-hour urine protein excretion or 24-hour urine albumin excretion.
2. Routine blood investigations:
   a. Full blood count.
   b. Erythrocyte sedimentation rate.

c. Urea, creatinine, sodium, potassium, chloride, bicarbonate.
d. Calcium, phosphate, alkaline phosphatase.
e. Uric acid.
f. Liver function test: Total protein, albumin, alanine aminotransaminase (ALT), aspartate aminotransferase (AST), bilirubin.
g. Serum complements C3 and C4.

> Low serum complement(s) are seen in:
> - Post-infectious glomerulonephritis (C3)
> - Lupus nephritis (C3 and/or C4)
> - C3 glomerulopathy (C3)

h. Anti-streptolysin O titer (ASOT) and/or anti-DNAase B titer and/or streptozyme test (ASOT, anti-DNAase B, anti-hyaluronidase).
i. Serum IgA.
j. Anti-nuclear antibodies or anti-double-stranded DNA antibody.
k. Anti-factor B antibody levels:
   - Autoantibody targeting factor B, a component of the alternative C3 convertase.
   - Present in >90% of children with acute post-infectious glomerulonephritis.
   - Highly specific for post-infectious glomerulonephritis, distinguishing it from C3 glomerulopathy.

3. Imaging:
   a. Chest radiograph.
   b. Echocardiography for cardiac valvular vegetations.
4. Specialized blood investigations:
   a. ANCA:
      - Anti-myeloperoxidase antibody (p-ANCA or MPO): Microscopic polyangiitis.
      - Anti-proteinase C antibody (c-ANCA or PR3): Granulomatosis with polyangiitis.
   b. Anti-GBM antibodies:
      - Anti-GBM disease.
      - Goodpasture's syndrome.
   c. Rheumatoid factor.
   d. Cryoglobulin.

e. Serological evidence of post-infectious etiology other than post-streptococcal, based on clinical suspicion:
   - Hepatitis B surface antigen.
   - Anti-hepatitis B surface antibody.
   - Anti-hepatitis C virus antibody.
   - Mycoplasma antibody.
   - Epstein–Barr virus serology.

5. Cultures:
   a. Post-infectious glomerulonephritis: Skin, tonsils.
   b. Shunt nephritis: Blood, cerebrospinal fluid, shunt tip (after removal).
   c. Endocarditis nephritis: Blood.
   d. IgADIRGN: Blood, tissues.

IV. Indications for kidney biopsy

1. Early stage:
   a. Synpharyngitic presentation.
   b. Severe anuria or rapidly progressive course.
   c. Hypertension >3 weeks.
   d. Depressed glomerular filtration rate >2 weeks.
   e. Normal serum complement levels.
   f. No evidence of prior streptococcal infection.
   g. Evidence of systemic disease.
2. Recovery phase:
   a. Hypocomplementemia >6 weeks.
   b. Persistent proteinuria >6 months.
   c. Persistent microscopic hematuria >18 months.

D. Medical Management

- Use of loop diuretics to remove excess fluid and sodium is the mainstay of treatment in acute glomerulonephritis.

I. General measures:

1. Fluid volume should be restricted to urine output plus insensible water loss calculated at 400 ml/m^2 per day or 30 ml/100 kcal.
2. Low salt diet: Sodium ≤1 mmol/kg/day or sodium chloride <2 g/day (adult).
   - 1 g sodium chloride = 393 mg sodium (17.1 mmol sodium).
3. Low potassium diet: 0–150 mg per serving (≤3.8 mmol per serving).
4. Daily monitoring of weight.
5. Strict input and output chart.
6. Close blood pressure monitoring:
   - Hourly blood pressure initially.
   - 2–4 hourly blood pressure monitoring if blood pressure is stable.

II. Management of complications:

1. Decrease fluid and sodium overload to prevent hypertensive encephalopathy:
   a. Use loop diuretics (oral or intravenous): Furosemide, 2–5 mg/kg/dose (maximum 240 mg single dose).
   b. Intravenous administration if the patient has severe fluid overload, and/or is hypertensive.
      - Should be administered over 5 to 30 minutes to minimize ototoxicity.
   c. Dose can be repeated in an hour and subsequently 4–6 hourly to achieve the desired diuresis.
   d. Diuretics should be continued until the patient is in the diuretic phase of the disease.
2. Treatment of hypertension:
   a. Intravenous furosemide to decrease fluid and salt overload.
   b. Anti-hypertensive medications should be started if blood pressure is still elevated after intravenous furosemide has been given.
   c. For treatment of hypertensive emergencies:
      - Oral nifedipine (2.5–10 mg, 4–6 hourly).
      - Intravenous glyceryl trinitrite infusion (1–10 µg/kg/min).
      - Intravenous labetalol infusion (0.4–3.0 mg/kg/hr).

d. Start a long-acting anti-hypertensive medication if blood pressure is persistently elevated.
   - Drug of choice: Calcium-channel blockers.
   - Avoid renin-angiotensin system blockers (RASBs) due to the risk of decreasing kidney function and hyperkalemia.

3. Treatment of hyperkalemia:
   a. Avoid high potassium-containing foods such as milk, tomatoes, fruits, and fruit juices.
   b. Intravenous furosemide, 2–5 mg/kg/dose.
   c. If serum potassium remains at 6–7 mmol/L despite 2 doses of furosemide, give oral resonium, 1 g/kg, to a maximum of 30 g.
   d. If serum potassium ≥7 mmol/L, accompanied by electrocardiographic changes such as peaked T waves, flattened P waves, increased PR interval, and widening of the QRS complex:
      - Intravenous 10% calcium gluconate, 0.5 ml/kg, up to a maximum of 20 ml given slowly over 15 minutes.
      - Nebulized salbutamol:
        Body weight <25 kg: 2.5 mg.
        Body weight ≥25 kg: 5 mg.
      - Intravenous salbutamol, 4 mg/kg.
      - Intravenous insulin, 1 IU/5 g dextrose and dextrose 0.5 g/kg.
      - Avoid sodium bicarbonate due to the risk of worsening of hypertension from the sodium load.
      - Prepare for dialysis.
4. Dialysis is indicated in a child with severe oliguria and is not responding to frusemide with the following criteria:
   a. Severe hyperkalemia ≥7 mmol/L.
   b. Severe acidosis.
   c. Uncontrolled hypertension and severe fluid overload.
   d. Pulmonary edema.

III. Antibiotics:

1. Antibiotics are indicated for underlying infections as per local guidelines.
2. Indicated in post-infectious glomerulonephritis if there are clinical features of streptococcal infection (pharyngitis or pyoderma), or serological or culture evidence of streptococcal infection.

a. Primarily done to prevent the spread of infection within communal sites where Group A streptococcus infection and scabies are highly prevalent.
b. Choice of antibiotics:
   - Oral penicillin V, 7.5–15 mg/kg, 6 hourly for 10 days.
   - Oral erythromycin, 10 mg/kg, 6 hourly in children with penicillin allergy.

E. Prognosis of Bacterial Infection-related Glomerulonephritis

1. Post-infectious glomerulonephritis:
   - Short-term prognosis in children is excellent in endemic regions.
   - Persistent albuminuria may occur and some adults develop abnormal kidney function.
2. Shunt nephritis:
   - Outcome is good with early diagnosis and treatment of infection.
   - Most patients recover some kidney function but are left with residual chronic kidney disease.
3. Endocarditis-related glomerulonephritis:
   - Immediate prognosis is good if the infection can be identified and promptly eradicated.
   - Some may require valve replacement.
4. IgADIRGN:
   - Dialysis is frequently required in the acute setting.
   - Recovery is guarded, with <20% returning to pre-morbid levels of kidney function.

Recommended Reading

1. Roy S 3rd, Murphy WM, Arant BS Jr. (1981) Poststreptococcal crescenteric glomerulonephritis in children: Comparison of quintuple therapy versus supportive care. *J Pediatr* **98**:403–410.
2. Johnston F, Carapetis J, Patel MS, Wallace T, Spillane P. (1999) Evaluating the use of penicillin to control outbreaks of acute post streptococcal glomerulonephritis. *Pediatr Infect Dis J* **18**:327–332.
3. Zaffanello M, Cataldi L, Franchini M, Fanos V. (2010) Evidence-based treatment limitations prevent any therapeutic recommendation for acute poststreptococcal glomerulonephritis in children. *Med Sci Monit* **16**:RA79–84.

4. Kidney Disease: Improving Global Outcomes (KDIGO). Glomerulonephritis Work Group. (2012) KDIGO Clinical Practice Guideline for Glomerulonephritis. *Kidney Int Suppl* **2**:218–221.
5. Chauvet S, Berthaud R, Devriese M, Mignotet M, Vieira Martins P, Robe-Rybkine T, Miteva MA, Gyulkhandanyan A, Ryckewaert A, Louillet F, Merieau E, Mestrallet G, Rousset-Rouvière C, Thervet E, Hogan J, Ulinski T, Villoutreix BO, Roumenina L, Boyer O, Frémeaux-Bacchi V. (2020) Anti-factor B antibodies and acute postinfectious GN in children. *J Am Soc Nephrol* **31**:829–840.

4 Childhood Nephrotic Syndrome

Ng KH and Yap HK

A. Useful Definitions

Nephrotic syndrome (NS)	Presence of heavy proteinuria defined as urine protein:creatinine ratio (UPCR) >0.2 g/mmol, urinary total protein excretion >3.0 g/day/1.73m^2 or >1,000 mg/m^2/day, hypoalbuminemia (<30 g/L), and generalized edema. Hypercholesterolemia (>5.2 mmol/L), invariably present, is not conventionally included as part of the diagnosis.
Complete remission	UPCR ≤0.02 g/mmol or the first morning urine dipstick is negative/trace for ≥3 consecutive days, and loss of edema.
Partial remission	UPCR >0.02 g/mmol but <0.2 g/mmol, and serum albumin ≥30 g/L.
Steroid sensitive NS (SSNS)	Complete remission achieved within 6 weeks of steroid therapy alone.
Steroid resistant NS (SRNS)	Failure to achieve complete remission after 6 weeks of daily high dose (60 mg/m^2/day) prednisolone therapy.
Relapse	In a child who had previously achieved remission, recurrence of nephrotic-range proteinuria defined (as defined as uPCR >0.2 g/mmol or 3 consecutive first morning urine dipstick >3+), with or without generalized edema or hypoalbuminaemia (<30 g/L).
Infrequent relapses	Relapses <2 episodes within the first 6 months, or <4 episodes within any subsequent one-year period.
Frequent relapses	Relapses ≥2 episodes within the first 6 months, or ≥4 episodes within any subsequent one-year period.

(*Continued*)

(*Continued*)

Steroid dependence	Frequent relapses with ≥2 consecutive relapses whilst on steroid therapy, or relapses occurring within 2 weeks of cessation of steroid therapy.
Secondary steroid-sensitive relapse	In a child with previous SRNS and treated with second-line immunosuppressive agents, and subsequent relapses that respond to standard steroid therapy.
Late onset steroid resistance	Children with initial SSNS who subsequently relapse and develop SRNS.

B. Diagnostic Approach

I. Causes of nephrotic syndrome:

1. Primary nephrotic syndrome:

	ISKDC (1978)*
Minimal change nephrotic syndrome (MCNS)	76%
Focal segmental glomerulosclerosis (FSGS)	7%
Focal global sclerosis (FGS)	2%
Mesangial proliferative glomerulonephritis	4%
Membranoproliferative glomerulonephritis (MPGN)	8%
Membranous nephropathy	2%
Chronic glomerulonephritis	1%

*International Study of Kidney Disease in Children

2. Genetic causes:
   a. Pathogenic genetic variants in podocyte genes, e.g., *NPHS1*, *NPHS2*, *TRPC6*, *ACTN4*, *COL4A4*, *COL4A5*.
   b. Mitochondrial diseases.
3. Secondary nephrotic syndrome:
   a. Immune diseases:
      - Systemic lupus erythematosus.
      - Immunoglobulin A (IgA) vasculitis nephritis.

- Anti-neutrophil cytoplasmic antibodies (ANCA)-associated vasculitis.
- IgA nephropathy.

b. Infections:
- Hepatitis B.
- Hepatitis C.
- Human immunodeficiency virus (HIV).
- Parvovirus.

c. Drugs:
- Heavy metals, e.g., mercury.
- Penicillamine.

d. Metabolic:
- Diabetic nephropathy.

II. Clinical evaluation:

1. Assess fluid status:
   a. Degree of edema including periorbital and pedal edema, scrotal edema, ascites, and pleural effusion.
   b. Blood pressure.
2. Look for features suggestive of secondary causes of nephrotic syndrome:
   a. History of chronic infections.
   b. History of drugs, in particular, traditional medicines.
   c. Features suggestive of possible autoimmune disease:
      i. Pallor, rash, petechiae, mouth ulcers.
      ii. Arthritis.
      iii. Hemoptysis, lung crepitations.
      iv. Hepatosplenomegaly.
   d. Features suggestive of genetic etiology:
      i. Family history:
         - Parental consanguinity.
         - Family members with nephrotic syndrome, proteinuria, hematuria, kidney failure (include the age of onset, response to medications, kidney function, kidney biopsy, and genetic tests).

- Family members with relevant non-kidney manifestations, e.g., early-onset diabetes, sensorineural hearing deficit, neurological disorders, and epilepsy.

ii. Sensorineural hearing deficit.
iii. Ophthalmologic abnormalities.
iv. Genitourinary malformations.
v. Neurological or skeletal manifestations.

III. Investigations to confirm nephrotic syndrome:

1. Early morning spot UPCR or timed (24-hour) urine protein excretion.
2. Urine microscopy.
3. Urea, creatinine, sodium, potassium, chloride, and bicarbonate.
4. Total corrected calcium, phosphate, and alkaline phosphatase.
5. Uric acid.
6. Liver function test: Total protein, albumin, alanine aminotransaminase (ALT), aspartate aminotransferase (AST), and bilirubin.
7. Lipid profile: Total cholesterol, triglycerides, low-density lipoprotein (LDL)-cholesterol, and high-density lipoprotein (HDL)-cholesterol.

IV. Investigations to evaluate etiology:

1. Step 1 (uncomplicated presentation):
   a. Full blood count.
   b. Serum complements (C3, C4).
   c. Anti-nuclear antibodies or anti-double-stranded DNA antibodies.
   d. Hepatitis B surface antigen.
2. Step 2 (atypical presentation):
   a. Anti-hepatitis C antibody (indicated in nephritic-nephrotic syndrome).
   b. ANCA (indicated in nephritic-nephrotic syndrome or if there is evidence of leukocytoclastic vasculitis):
      - Anti-myeloperoxidase antibody (p-ANCA or myeloperoxidase [MPO]).
      - Anti-proteinase-3 antibody (c-ANCA or PR3).

c. C3 nephritic factor (indicated in nephritic-nephrotic syndrome).
d. Serum immunoglobulins (IgG, IgM, IgA).
e. HIV antigen-antibody (steroid-resistant collapsing FSGS).
f. Parvovirus IgM, IgG and nucleic acid test (steroid-resistant collapsing FSGS).

3. Kidney biopsy:
   a. Indications:
      i. Steroid resistance (unless genetic tests are promptly available).
      ii. Features that suggest the etiology is not MCNS:
         - Aged <1 year.
         - Aged >12 years.
         - Hypertension.
         - Gross hematuria.
         - Hypocomplementemia.
         - Kidney failure (not related to intravascular volume depletion).
      iii. Steroid dependence with significant steroid toxicity.
      iv. Chronic kidney disease (CKD) prognostication:
         - Tubular atrophy, interstitial fibrosis, and glomerulosclerosis.
   b. Light microscopy, immunofluorescence and an electron microscopic examination should be performed.
4. Genetic testing:
   a. Indications:
      i. Initial steroid resistance.
      ii. Congenital or infantile onset.
      iii. Significant family history.
      iv. Significant non-kidney manifestations.
      v. Kidney biopsy suggestive of genetic etiology (e.g., Alport syndrome, diffuse mesangial sclerosis).
      vi. Prior to kidney transplantation.
   b. Type of genetic test:
      i. Consider targeted gene panel consisting of podocytopathy genes.
      ii. Consider whole exome or whole genome sequencing in atypical cases or if the targeted gene panel is negative.

V. Investigations for complications of refractory nephrotic syndrome:

1. Thyroid function test:
   - Free thyroxine.
   - Thyroid stimulating hormone.
2. Serum immunoglobulin G:
3. Thrombophilic screen:
   - Anti-thrombin III levels.

C. Treatment

I. Evaluation for risks of treatment:

1. Vaccination records, previous varicella infection, and varicella zoster IgG.
2. Growth charts and pubertal staging.
3. Diabetes mellitus:
   - Family history.
   - Fasting glucose.
   - Glycated hemoglobin (HbA1c).
4. 25-hydroxy Vitamin D.
5. Dental hygiene.
6. Tuberculosis (TB) (in endemic areas):
   a. Check family history of TB.
   b. Consider a chest X-Ray to exclude latent TB.
   c. TB screen if positive contact history or is living in high endemic area:
      i. Tuberculin skin test in patients aged <2 years.
      ii. Interferon-gamma release assay in patients aged ≥2 years:
         - TB T-spot test (preferred in immunocompromised patients).
         - TB Quantiferon (less sensitive in immunocompromised patients).

II. Prednisolone (PNL):

1. Indications:
   - First episode of nephrotic syndrome and subsequent relapses.
2. Titration of dose:
   a. PNL should be given as a single morning dose to minimize the side effects.
   b. First episode of nephrotic syndrome:
      i. 60 mg/m^2/day (maximum of 80 mg/day) for 4 weeks (extend by another 2 weeks if there is no complete remission).
      ii. If complete remission is achieved, taper to 40 mg/m^2 on alternate days for 4 weeks (extend by another 2 weeks if the child responds after 4 weeks of steroid treatment).
      iii. Taper off over 2–4 weeks (for <6 yrs) or stop (for ≥6 yrs).
      iv. About 50% of these children will relapse within 3–6 months.
   c. Relapse (infrequent relapsing):
      i. 60 mg/m^2/day (maximum 80 mg/day) for at least 14 days or until 3–5 days proteinuria-free.
      ii. If complete remission is achieved, 40 mg/m^2 on alternate days for 4 weeks, then discontinue.
   d. Relapse (while on steroids or when frequently relapsing):
      i. If the patient has proteinuria ≥2+ for more than 3 days without edema, increase alternate-day PNL to daily at the same or next higher dose until 3–5 days proteinuria-free, before reducing back to alternate day at the same dose for 14 days, and then tapering to the maintenance PNL dose.
      ii. If the patient has proteinuria ≥2+ and is mildly edematous, increase PNL to 0.5–1 mg/kg daily until 3–5 days proteinuria-free, before reducing to alternate day at the same dose for 14 days, and then tapering to the maintenance PNL dose.
      iii. If the patient has proteinuria ≥2+ and is grossly edematous, increase PNL to 60 mg/m^2/day daily until the patient is 3–5 days proteinuria-free, before reducing to 40 mg/m^2 on alternate day for 2 weeks, and then tapering to maintenance PNL dose.

e. Steroid-dependent nephrotic syndrome (SDNS):
   i. Taper PNL dose in accordance with the difficulty in attaining remission.
   ii. Suggested tapering protocols:

Protocol 1	Protocol 2	Protocol 3
40 mg EOD × 2 weeks	60 mg EOD × 2 weeks	Doses on alternate days: 60/55/60/50/60/45/60/40/60/35/60/30/60/25/60/20/60/15/60/10/60/5/60 mg
35 mg EOD × 2 weeks	55 mg EOD × 2 weeks	Continue with Protocol 2
30 mg EOD × 2 weeks	50 mg EOD × 2 weeks	
25 mg EOD × 2 weeks	45 mg EOD × 2 weeks	
20 mg EOD × 3 weeks	Continue with Protocol 1	
15 mg EOD × 4 weeks		
10 mg EOD × 6 weeks		
7.5 mg EOD × 8 weeks		
5 mg EOD × 12 weeks		
2.5 mg EOD until decision to discontinue		

Note: Alternate day dosing (EOD).

   iii. PNL dose should not be reduced unless the patient has been proteinuria-free (urine protein negative or trace) for at least 14 days.
   iv. Aim for maintenance PNL dose of 0.05–0.5 mg/kg on alternate days.
   v. Continue low dose maintenance therapy for at least 9–12 months.
      - Discontinue if the patient remains proteinuria-free during this period.
      - Consider a kidney biopsy and second-line immunosuppressive therapy if the patient has unacceptable steroid side effects.

vi. In patients who frequently relapse whilst on maintenance steroids, consider, when proteinuria is detected (urine protein ≥1+), increasing alternate day PNL to a daily dose or low daily dose PNL to 15 mg/m^2 until proteinuria-free for 3–5 days.

3. Surveillance for adverse effects (see chapter "Immunosuppressive Medications"):
   - Consider the use of deflazacort instead of PNL if there is significant steroid toxicity associated with PNL.

III. Calcineurin inhibitors (CNI):

1. General principles:
   a. Indications:
      i. Primary SRNS.
      ii. Primary SDNS with significant steroid toxicity.
   b. Use with caution in patients with reduced kidney function and/or uncontrolled hypertension.
   c. Response to treatment:
      i. 35% of those with genetic SRNS may respond fully or partially to CNI.
      ii. Patients with kidney biopsy findings of minimal change disease are more likely to achieve a complete remission with CNI therapy.
      iii. Patients who can achieve complete remission tend to have better kidney survival compared to partial or non-responders.
      iv. Remission rates are similar with the use of tacrolimus (Tac) or cyclosporine (CsA) in patients with SRNS.
2. CsA:
   a. Available as non-modified (Sandimmune) or microemulsion (Neoral).
      - Bioavailablity of Sandimmune is generally poor and unpredictable.
   b. Starting dose of 3–5 mg/kg/day (maximum starting dose 250 mg/day) given as 12-hourly doses to attain whole blood trough CsA levels at 80–150 μg/L.

- To maintain remission, keep at the lowest trough levels required.

c. Titration of dose up to 8 mg/kg/day may be required.
   - Levels of 250–300 μg/L may be targeted with careful monitoring of serum creatinine in patients who are unable to achieve remission at lower trough levels.

3. Tac:

a. Starting dose: 0.15 mg/kg 12 hourly (maximum starting dose, 3 mg 12 hourly).

b. Titrate dose to achieve trough Tac levels of 4–8 μg/L.
   - Levels of 12–15 μg/L may be targeted with careful monitoring of serum creatinine in patients who are unable to achieve remission at lower trough levels.

c. Monitor 3-monthly serum magnesium levels and fasting blood glucose levels and 6-monthly HbA1c levels.

4. Titration of CNI doses:

a. Monitor CNI levels and serum creatinine 2x for the first week, then once in 2 weeks for the first month, and then 4–6 weekly.

b. Use diltiazem 15–30 mg 12 hourly to increase CNI levels, increasing by 15 mg/dose until a maximum of 3 mg/kg/dose 8–12 hourly (maximum dose per day = 60 mg 8 hourly).
   - Effect of diltiazem should be seen by 3 weeks.
   - Stop diltiazem if the heart rate is ≤60 beats/min, as diltiazem has been associated with sinoatrial block.
   - Check electrocardiogram (ECG).

c. If serum creatinine is high:
   i. Consider if this is due to hypoalbuminemia and intravascular volume depletion.
   ii. Consider stopping renin-angiotensin system blockers or diuretics.
   iii. Aim for normoalbuminemia with albumin infusions to see if serum creatinine improves.

d. If CNI nephrotoxicity is suspected and serum creatinine increases by 25%, reduce CNI dose by 20% to determine if this is the cause.

e. Improvement in proteinuria should be seen in 2–6 weeks.

f. If complete remission is achieved, begin tapering off PNL.
   i. Keep CNI at the lowest dose that can maintain the patient in remission without steroids.
   ii. In MCNS, continue for 1–2 years before attempting to discontinue CNI.
      - If the patient relapses, re-start CNI with or without high dose oral PNL to achieve remission.
         - Consider adding mycophenolate in an attempt to taper off CNI.
   iii. In FSGS, continue for at least 2 years before adding mycophenolate in an attempt to taper off CNI.
      - If the patient relapses, re-start CNI with or without high dose oral PNL to achieve remission.
      - Consider IV rituximab and mycophenolate.
   iv. In those where CNI is continued beyond 2 years, a repeat kidney biopsy should be considered to assess for nephrotoxic effects.
      - If CNI-associated nephrotoxicity is present, consider IV rituximab with mycophenolate maintenance.
g. If complete remission is not achieved after 2 months:
   i. Consider changing CsA to Tac and/or add mycophenolate.
   ii. Consider giving IV rituximab and mycophenolate.
   iii If there is no response to CNI after 3–6 months of achieving therapeutic drug levels, taper off both CNI and PNL.
5. Adverse effects (see chapter "Immunosuppressive Medications").

IV. Mycophenolic acid (MPA):

1. Indications:
   a. SDNS with frequent nephrotic relapses and/or steroid toxicity.
   b. Alternative maintenance drug in those with CNI toxicity or reduced kidney function.
   c. Add-on maintenance therapy in patients who relapse while on PNL and CNI.
   d. MPA is good as maintenance therapy, but not as induction therapy.

2. Titration of dose:
   a. Mycophenolate mofetil (MMF):
      i. 600 mg/m^2/dose 12 hourly (15–23 mg/kg/dose 12 hourly).
      ii. Maximum adult dose: 1–1.5 g 12 hourly.
      iii. MMF + CsA: 600 mg/m^2/dose 12 hourly (15–23 mg/kg/dose 12 hourly).
      iv. MMF + Tac: 300 mg/m^2/dose 12 hourly (8–12 mg/kg/dose 12 hourly).
   b. Enteric-coated mycophenolate sodium (ECMS) (Myfortic®):
      i. 400 mg/m^2/dose 12 hourly.
      ii. Dose equivalence:
         - Myfortic® 180 mg = 250 mg MMF.
         - Myfortic® 360 mg = 500 mg MMF.
   c. In patients with severely decreased kidney function (eGFR <25 ml/min/1.73m^2), MPA dose should be adjusted based on AUC (area under the curve).
      - Drug is not removed by hemodialysis.
   d. If the disease is not well controlled or there are MPA side effects, measure MPA levels (see chapter "Immunosuppressive Medications").
      i. Aim AUC >50 mg L^{-1} hour.
      ii. MPA trough levels range from 2 to 4 mg/L.
         - Although less reliable than AUC, trough levels >3.5 μg/ml were 100% predictive of an AUC >50 mg L^{-1} hour.
         - If trough levels <3.5 μg/ml, increase the dose.
         - If trough levels >3.5 μg/ml, measure AUC and adjust accordingly.
3. Monitor for common adverse effects (see chapter "Immunosuppressive Medications"):
   a. Neutropenia (at 1–6 months of therapy):
      i. Full blood count (FBC) in 1 month and 3-monthly thereafter.
      ii. Omit if absolute neutrophil count is $<1.5 \times 10^9$/L.
   b. Gastritis, peptic ulceration, abdominal colic, diarrhea, gastrointestinal hemorrhage and perforation:

i. Start famotidine prophylactically at 0.5–1 mg/kg/dose daily or twice daily (maximum 40 mg/day).
ii. Dose adjustment for abnormal kidney function:
   - If eGFR = 30–50 ml/min/1.73m^2, 0.5 mg/kg/dose every 24 hours.
   - If eGFR = 10–29 ml/min/1.73m^2, 0.25 mg/kg/dose every 24 hours.
   - If eGFR <10 ml/min/1.73m^2, 0.125 mg/kg/dose every 24 hours.
iii. Consider changing to Myfortic® if gastrointestinal side effects persist.

V. Rituximab:

1. Indications:
   a. SRNS not responding well to conventional treatment.
   b. SDNS frequent relapses despite CNI treatment.
2. Titration of dose (see chapter "Anti-CD20 Monoclonal Antibody Therapy for Nephrotic Syndrome").
   a. Dosing:

Steroid-dependent	IV Rituximab, 375 mg/m^2 (maximum dose 1 g) once
Steroid-resistant and/or calcineurin inhibitor-resistant	IV Rituximab, 375 mg/m^2 (maximum dose 1 g) 2-weekly × 2 doses

   b. Rituximab should preferably be started during remission of nephrotic syndrome.
   c. Consider repeating the Rituximab course if there is a relapse of proteinuria, especially if CD19 counts have recovered.
3. Pneumocystis jirovecii pneumonia prophylaxis:
   a. Co-trimoxazole oral 3 mg/kg/dose on alternate days for 3 months.
   b. In glucose-6-phosphate dehydrogenase (G6PD)-deficient patients, use aerolized pentamidine 300 mg monthly (via a Respigard nebulizer).

c. In patients who are allergic to co-trimoxazole, use dapsone 2 mg/kg daily (maximum 100 mg) or atavaquone 30 mg/kg/day.

VI. Levamisole:

1. Indications:
   a. Frequently relapsing or steroid-dependent nephrotic syndrome with unacceptable steroid side effects, due to MCNS.
2. Treatment protocol:
   a. Start Levamisole 2.5 mg/kg alternate day for at least 6 months (maximum dose 150 mg).
   b. Taper PNL dose in accordance with the difficulty in attaining remission.
      i. PNL dose should not be reduced unless the patient has been proteinuria-free (urine protein negative or trace) for at least 14 days.
3. Adverse effects:
   a. Neutropenia and agranulocytosis: Neutropenia tends to occur in the first 3 months.
   b. ANCA-associated vasculitis: Reported in association with cocaine use.
4. Monitoring:
   a. Monitor total white count weekly for the first 4 weeks, then fortnightly for the next 12 weeks, then monthly.
   b. Stop drug if:
      i. Total white count <3.0 × 10^9/L or absolute neutrophil count (ANC) <1.0 × 10^9/L.
      ii. Purpuric rash develops (do not re-start).

VII. Cyclophosphamide (CYC):

1. Indications:
   a. SRNS with MCNS.
   b. SDNS with significant steroid toxicity.
   Note: Not used in many centers due to potential significant adverse effects.

2. Efficacy:
   a. Can induce sustained remission in children with frequently relapsing nephrotic syndrome and SDNS, especially in children aged >5 years of age.
   b. Similar remission rates have been noted in patients receiving intravenous or oral CYC.
3. Titration of dose:
   a. Start CYC 2.0–2.5 mg/kg/day preferably when the patient is in remission (maximum adult dose 125 mg daily).
   b. Duration of therapy:
      i. Frequent relapsing and SDNS: 8 weeks.
         - Start PNL taper while on CYC if the patient is in remission.
      ii. SRNS: 12 weeks.
         - Maintain PNL at 60 mg/m^2/day (maximum 60 mg) until proteinuria-free for at least 3 days before beginning PNL taper.
         - Wean Prednisolone to 40 mg/m^2/EOD and taper off over 8–12 weeks.
   c. If the patient is steroid-resistant and edematous, ensure good urine output using albumin or diuretics before starting CYC to prevent hemorrhagic cystitis.
4. Monitoring:
   a. Total white count weekly for the first 4 weeks, then fortnightly for the next 8 weeks.
   b. Stop drug if:
      i. Febrile illness.
      ii. Total white count <3.0 × 10^9/L or ANC <1.5 × 10^9/L.
      iii. Platelet count <100 × 10^9/L.
   c. Parents and patients should be informed of the potential risks of:
      i. Sterility, if the cumulative dose exceeds 168 mg/kg, especially in the post-pubertal patient.
         - Post-pubertal adolescent boys should be advised to consider sperm storage.
      ii. Malignancy (very low risk, unless the patient is given repeated courses for more than a year)

VIII. Comparison of steroid-sparing agents:

Drug	Indication	Remission Efficacy
CNI	SDNS	Excellent
MPA	FRNS/SDNS	Good
Rituximab	FRNS/SDNS	Good
Cyclophosphamide	FRNS/SDNS	Moderate Can induce sustained remission
Levamisole	FRNS	Moderate

D. General Management

1. Diet:
   a. Children with edema:
      - Salt restriction only if edema is present.
      - Avoid excessive fluid intake.
      - Avoid salt-containing intravenous fluids.

   b. Children on steroids:
      - Normal calories, low saturated fats, no refined sugars (10–14% protein, 40–50% poly- and mono-unsaturated fats, and 40–50% carbohydrates).

   c. Protein requirements:
      - High protein intake: No evidence of benefit unless there is massive loss preventing growth.

2. Control of edema:
   a. Albumin infusion 20% 1 g/kg over 4–6 hours, followed by IV frusemide 0.5–2 mg/kg at the end of infusion and midway if the patient is grossly fluid-overloaded.
   b. Consider chronic diuretic therapy in patients with intractable edema, using a combination of:
      i. Furosemide: 1–2 mg/kg OM or BD
      ii. Spironolactone:
      0–10 kg: 6.25 mg BD
      11–20 kg: 12.5 mg BD
      21–40 kg: 25 mg BD
      >40 kg: 25 mg 8 hourly

iii. Bumetanide: 25–50 μg/kg (maximum 3 mg) daily, increasing to 8–12 hourly.
iv. Metolazone: Starting dose 0.1–0.2 mg/kg daily up to 0.5 mg/kg (maximum 30 mg).

3. Renin-angiotensin system blockers (RASBs) (see chapter "Adjunctive Therapy in Glomerular Disease"):
   a. RASBs should be started in patients with SRNS unless there is unstable kidney function or intravascular volume depletion.
      - Use with caution in eGFR <30ml/min/1.73m^2.
   b. Start at a low dose and aim to increase gradually according to response.
      - Aim for maximum dosages, as antiproteinuric effects are dose-dependent.
      - Start with the shorter-acting drugs first to minimize side effects, especially in smaller children.
   c. Consider giving the dose nightly if patient's blood pressure is low and patient has dizziness during the day.
   d. Stop the drugs if there are side effects of:
      - Intravascular volume depletion.
      - Acute kidney injury.
      - Hyperkalemia.
   e. Combined use of angiotensin-converting enzyme inhibitors (ACEi) and angiotensin II receptor blockers (ARB) has not been shown to be beneficial in nephrotic syndrome and may lead to acute kidney injury and hyperkalemia.
4. Control hypercholesterolemia (see chapter "Adjunctive Therapy in Glomerular Disease"):
   a. Dietary restriction: Avoid saturated fats (<7% of calories) and high cholesterol foods.
   b. Statins: 3-hydroxy-3-methylglutaryl coenzyme A (HMG CoA) reductase inhibitors are more effective at correcting the lipid profile than the use of dietary restriction of fats and cholesterol alone, in patients with nephrotic syndrome.
      - Avoid simvastatin due to increased risk of rhabdomyolysis, especially with the concomitant use of CNI.
      - Rosuvastatin in combination with CNI has the lowest risk of rhabdomyolysis
      - Monitor serum AST, ALT and serum creatine kinase monthly for first 3 months, then 3-monthly.

5. Decrease hypercoagulopathy:
   a. Avoid hypovolemia.
   b. Consider prophylactic warfarin therapy in relapsing nephrotic children with:
      i. Previous thromboembolic events.
      ii. High risk of thrombosis:
         - Serum albumin <20 g/L and
         - Serum fibrinogen level >6 g/L OR antithrombin III level <70% of normal.
   c. Anticoagulant therapy if there is a thrombotic event:
      i. Initiate therapy with low molecular weight heparin (LMWH) for 5–10 days followed by either LMWH or vitamin K antagonist for 3 months.
      ii. Dosing of LMWH:
         - Enoxaparin subcutaneously 1 mg/kg 12 hourly.
         - Reduce dose to 1 mg/kg daily if eGFR <30 ml/min/1.73m^2 with close monitoring.
         - Monitor with anti-factor Xa assay with a sample taken 4–6 hours after the last injection: therapeutic range 0.5–1 U/ml.
      iii. Warfarin:
         - Initial dose: 0.1–0.2 mg/kg daily (maximum 5 mg).
         - Adjust dose to keep international normalized ratio (INR) between 2 and 2.5 for prophylaxis and 2–3 for treatment.
         - Check INR daily till levels are in the target range for ≥2 consecutive days, then 1–2 weekly until stable.
         - Vitamin K 0.5–1 mg daily starting dose, increasing up to 2–5 mg, to normalize INR.
   d. Stop LMWH or warfarin at least one week prior to kidney biopsy. Ensure that the prothrombin time and partial thromboplastin time are normal before proceeding with the procedure
6. Medical nephrectomy:
   - Consider the use of non-steroidal anti-inflammatory drugs (NSAIDs) if the patient remains nephrotic and preservation of the kidney function is not an issue.

E. Treatment Algorithms

I. SSNS:

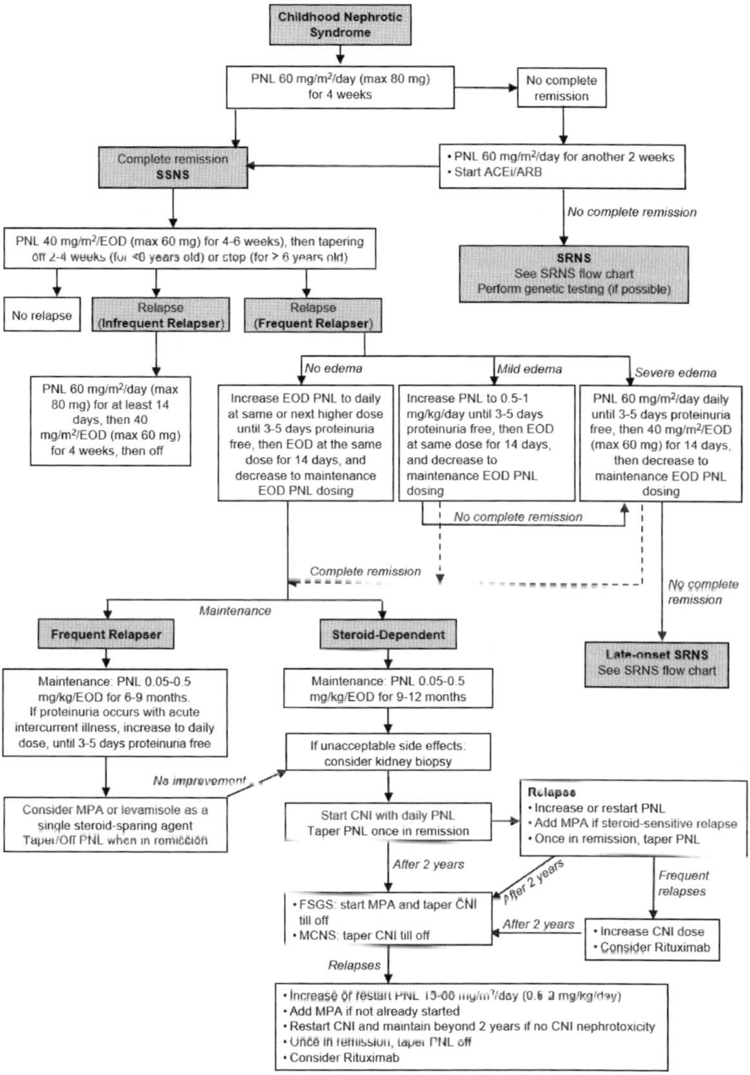

II. SRNS:

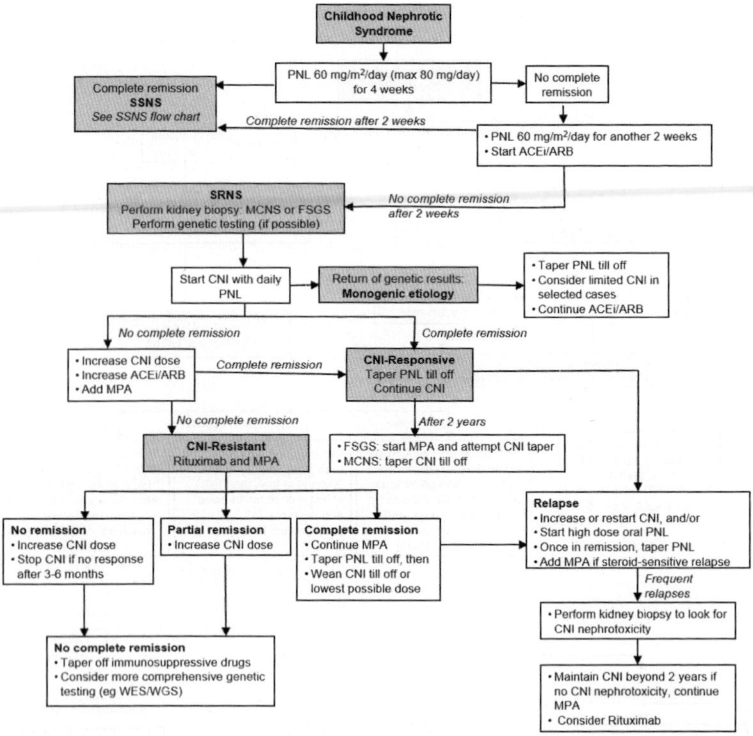

Recommended Reading

1. British Association for Paediatric Nephrology. (1991) Levamisole for corticosteroid-dependent nephrotic syndrome in childhood. *Lancet* **337**:1555–1557.
2. Hahn D, Hodson EM, Willis NS, Craig JC. (2015) Corticosteroid therapy for nephrotic syndrome in children. *Cochrane Database Syst Rev 2015* CD001533. doi: 10.1002/14651858.CD001533.pub5.
3. Larkins NG, Liu ID, Willis NS, Craig JC, Hodson EM. (2020) Non-corticosteroid immunosuppressive medications for steroid-sensitive nephrotic syndrome in children. *Cochrane Database Syst Rev 2020* **4**:CD002290. doi:10.1002/14651858.CD002290.pub5.

4. Niaudet P. (2020, updated) Etiology, clinical manifestations, and diagnosis of nephrotic syndrome in children. Edited by Mattoo TK, Kim MS. *UpToDate ONLINE*. http://www.uptodate.com.
5. Trautmann A, Vivarelli M, Samuel S, Gipson D, Sinha A, Schaefer F, Hui NK, Boyer O, Saleem MA, Feltran L, Müller-Deile J, Becker JU, Cano F, Xu H, Lim YN, Smoyer W, Anochie I, Nakanishi K, Hodson E, Haffner D; International Pediatric Nephrology Association. (2020) IPNA clinical practice recommendations for the diagnosis and management of children with steroid-resistant nephrotic syndrome. *Pediatr Nephrol* **35**:1529–1561.
6. Niaudet P. (2021, updated) Treatment of idiopathic nephrotic syndrome in children. Edited by Mattoo TK, Kim MS. *UpToDate ONLINE*. http://www.uptodate.com.
7. Christian MT, Maxted AP. (2021) Optimizing the corticosteroid dose in steroid-sensitive nephrotic syndrome. *Pediatr Nephrol* **20**:1–11.

5 Congenital Nephrotic Syndrome

Ng KH, Teo S and Yap HK

A. Definition

1. Congenital nephrotic syndrome (CNS):
   - Nephrotic syndrome with onset in utero or within the first 3 months of life.
2. Infantile nephrotic syndrome:
   - Nephrotic syndrome with onset between 4 and 12 months.

B. Etiology

1. Primary (genetic) causes:
   a. Syndromic (with non-kidney manifestations):
      - Denys–Drash syndrome: *WT1* (Wilms tumor 1).
      - Pierson syndrome: *LAMB2* (laminin-β2).
      - Herlitz junctional epidermolysis bullosa, e.g., *LAMB3* (laminin-β3).
      - Galloway–Mowat syndrome, e.g., *WDR73* (WD repeat domain 73).
      - Mitochondrial myopathies, e.g., Leigh syndrome: *PDSS2* (Decaprenyldiphosphate synthase subunit 2).
      - Nail-patella syndrome: *LMX1B* (LIM homeobox transcription factor 1 beta).
      - *SGPL1* (sphingosine-1-phosphate lyase 1).

   b. Kidney-limited manifestations:
      - *NPHS1* (nephrin).
      - *NPHS2* (podocin).
      - *NPHS3/PLCE1* (phospholipase C, epsilon 1).

- *WT1*.
- *LAMB2*.
- *ARHGDIA* (Rho GDP-dissociation inhibitor alpha).
- *MAGI-2* (Membrane-associated guanylate kinase inverted 2).

2. Secondary causes:
   a. Congenital infections:
      - Cytomegalovirus (CMV).
      - Toxoplasmosis.
      - Syphilis.
      - Rubella.
      - Human immunodeficiency virus (HIV).
      - Hepatitis B.
      - Hepatitis C.
      - Herpes simplex viruses (HSV1 and HSV2).
      - Varicella zoster (VZ).
      - Parvovirus.
      - Malaria.

   b. Immune-related:
      - Neonatal lupus erythematosus secondary to maternal alloantibodies.
      - Neonatal antibodies against neutral endopeptidase (NEP).

   c. Others:
      - Pertussis.
      - Mercury exposure.
      - Maternal steroid-chlorpheniramine treatment.

C. Pathogenic Genetic Variants

1. More than 80% of primary CNS are caused by (likely) pathogenic variants in 1 of 5 genes: *NPHS1, NPHS2, WT1, LAMB2, PLCE1*.
2. *NPHS2* and *NPHS1* genetic variants account for approximately 95% of primary nephrotic syndrome with congenital and infantile onset.
   - *NPHS1* mutations are the most common in CNS.
3. While *WT1* and *PLCE1* cause Denys–Drash and Pierson syndromes, respectively, mutations in these genes can also be present in non-syndromic cases.

4. WT1-associated glomerulopathy is the only autosomal dominant disorder with variable expressivity and incomplete penetrance that can manifest as CNS.
5. Concurrent mutations in different genes can occur.

D. Clinical Approach

1. CNS is suggested antenatally or perinatally by:
   a. High alpha-fetoprotein in amniotic fluid and maternal serum.
   b. Hydrops fetalis.
   c. Enlarged placenta (>25% of total birth weight).
   d. Growth retardation, meconium-stained liquor, prematurity, and being small for gestational age.
2. Confirm diagnosis of CNS:
   a. Presence of proteinuria:
      - Nephrotic-range proteinuria, hypoalbuminemia and severe edema may be present right after birth in severe CNS.
      - In less severe cases, the degree of proteinuria varies and clinical signs may not be present in the first weeks of life.
      - Proteinuria may only become severe after a partial correction of hypoalbuminemia with albumin infusions.
   b. Microscopic hematuria or leukocyturia may be present.
   c. Patients with *NPHS1* mutations generally have normal kidney function in the first few months, whereas in other genetic causes like *WT1*, rapid deterioration of the kidney function may occur.
3. Look for congenital infections:
   a. Antenatal history of maternal infections.
   b. Clinical examination of infant:
      - Dysmorphic features including microcephaly.
      - Eye anomalies including cataracts and retinopathy.
      - Rash or cutaneous scars.
      - Cardiac anomalies.
      - Jaundice or hepatosplenomegaly.
   c. Initial investigations showing evidence of:
      - Anemia.
      - Thrombocytopenia.
      - Hepatitis.

d. Confirmatory investigations:
   - Patient or maternal serology looking for specific IgM antibody titers.
   - Nucleic acid testing.
4. Look for maternal disorders:
   a. Maternal drug ingestion during pregnancy.
   b. Maternal history of systemic lupus erythematosus.
5. Exclude acquired infections and toxins:
   a. *Bordetella pertussis* infection.
   b. Mercury exposure.
   c. Traditional medicines.
6. Look for genetic causes:
   a. Take a detailed family history:
      i. Parental consanguinity.
      ii. Previous fetal or early infantile deaths.
      iii. CNS or heavy proteinuria.
      iv. Unresolved neurological or kidney diseases of infancy.
      v. Relevant non-kidney manifestations.
   b. Look for non-kidney features suggestive of genetic causes:
      - Primarily neurological, skeletal, eye, genitourinary anomalies, dysmorphic features, and sensorineural hearing loss.

Gene (Syndrome) Mode of Inheritance	Salient Clinical Findings
WT1 (Denys–Drash syndrome) • Autosomal dominant	• Wilms tumor. • Gonadal dysgenesis (male pseudohermaphroditism): XY patients have ambiguous or complete female genitalia. • Risk of gonadoblastoma in dysgenetic gonads.
LAMB2 (Pierson syndrome) • Autosomal recessive	• Eye anomalies: Microcoria (small pupils not responsive to light) — the most distinctive feature. Iris hypoplasia. Lens opacities. Retinopathy. • Congenital neuromuscular disease or neurodevelopmental abnormalities.

(*Continued*)

(*Continued*)

Gene (Syndrome) Mode of Inheritance	Salient Clinical Findings
LAMB3 (Herlitz junctional epidermolysis bullosa) • Autosomal recessive	• Epidermolysis bullosa. • Joint deformities (contractures).
WDR73 (Galloway-Mowat syndrome) • Autosomal recessive	• Microcephaly and other brain anomalies. • Severe mental retardation. • Hiatus hernia.
LMX1B (Nail-patella syndrome) • Autosomal dominant	• Limb and pelvic skeletal abnormalities: Hypoplastic or absent patella. Dysplasia of elbows and iliac horns. • Nail and distal digital abnormalities: Nail hypoplasia. Nail dystrophic changes. • Sensorineural hearing loss.
Mitochondrial disease (Leigh syndrome) • Autosomal recessive • Mitochondrial pattern • X-linked recessive	• Developmental delay or psychomotor regression. • Ataxia. • Dystonia. • External ophthalmoplegia. • Myopathy and peripheral neuropathy. • Lactic acidosis.
SGPL1 • Autosomal recessive	• Primary adrenal insufficiency. • Ichthyosis. • Immunodeficiency. • Neurological abnormalities including sensorineural hearing loss.

c. Karyotyping in phenotypic females or infants with ambiguous genitalia to look for male pseudohermaphroditism with a 46 XY genotype (*WT1*).
d. Abdominal and pelvic ultrasound scans to look for Wilms tumor or gonadal dysgenesis (*WT1*).
e. Genetic testing is highly recommended in primary CNS.
   i. Genetic testing can help in directing:
      - Immunosuppressive strategies.
      - Kidney prognostication.

- Targeted surveillance of non-kidney manifestations.
- Genetic counseling for the family.

ii. A gene panel that includes at least *NPHS1*, *NPHS2*, *WT1*, *LAMB2* and *PLCE1* is recommended.
- If this is negative, more comprehensive screening using either an expanded gene panel or whole exome sequencing is recommended.
- If clinical features strongly suggest a single genetic etiology, then sequencing of the likely single gene can be performed.

iii. If genetic results are available, a kidney biopsy is generally not necessary.

7. Kidney biopsy:
   a. Not routinely recommended.
   b. Kidney biopsy findings are generally nonspecific and often do not correlate with genotypes.
   c. Kidney biopsy may be considered in sporadic non-syndromic cases for the following indications:
      i. Genetic testing cannot be performed, or no genetic cause is identified found on comprehensive genetic testing.
      ii. Congenital membranous nephropathy due to anti-NEP antibodies or other glomerulopathies are possible etiologies.
      iii. For kidney prognostication:
      - Degree of interstitial fibrosis or glomerular sclerosis can help in prognostication

      Note: Errors in focal sampling.
   d. Specific kidney histology may be suggestive of certain etiologies:

Histology	Gene(s)
Diffuse mesangial sclerosis*	• *WT1* • *PLCE1* • *LAMB2*
Irregular microcystic dilatation of proximal tubules	• *NPHS1* (CNS of the Finnish type)
Membranous nephropathy	• Congenital infections • Neonatal lupus nephritis • Nephropathy due to anti-NEP antibodies

* Diffuse mesangial sclerosis:
- Seen exclusively in infancy and is associated with rapid progression to kidney failure.
- Can be isolated in kidneys or as part of Denys–Drash or Pierson syndrome.

8. Assess for complications:
   a. Growth parameters:
      - Height or length.
      - Weight.
      - Head circumference if aged <2 years.
      - Body mass index.
      - Annual height velocity.
   b. Blood pressure.
   c. Degree of fluid overload:
      - Ascites.
      - Pericardial effusion.
      - Pleural effusion.
   d. Blood biochemistry:
      - Urea, creatinine, sodium, chloride, potassium, bicarbonate, magnesium, and uric acid.
      - Albumin, glucose, cholesterol, and triglycerides.
   e. Thyroid function:
      - Free thyroxine, thyroid-stimulating hormone (TSH).
   f. Serum IgG level.
   g. Mineral bone metabolism:
      - Ionized calcium, phosphate, alkaline phosphatase, parathyroid hormone (PTH), and 25-hydroxyvitamin D.
   h. Ultrasound of abdomen and pleural space:
      - Kidney size, echogenicity and tumor mass (*WT1* gene).
      - Effusions, ascites and thrombosis.
   i. 2-D echocardiogram:
      - Pericardial effusion and left ventricular mass.

E. Management

I. Control edema:

1. Albumin infusion:
   a. Administer when clinically indicated (not based on serum albumin levels):
      i. Intravascular hypovolemia:
         - Tachycardia.

- Hypotension.
- Prolonged capillary time.
- Oliguria.
- Abdominal discomfort.

ii. Acute kidney injury (AKI) related to intravascular hypovolemia.

iii. Complications of severe edema:

- Thrombosis.
- Recurrent infections.
- Poor nutrition and growth.
- Unstable hemodynamics.

b. Dose and frequency should be adjusted according to clinical severity:

i. Intravenous (IV) 20% albumin 1–4 g/kg/day.

ii. Albumin infusions can be given daily in patients with severe CNS.

iii. Initiation of therapy:

- Divide into 3 infusions a day, each infusion 0.2–1 g/kg over 2 hours.
- Give 1–2 boluses of intravenous furosemide (0.5–2 mg/kg) with each albumin infusion (end of infusion and/or midway).

iv. Maintenance after a few weeks:

- 20% albumin may be given at night as one infusion (3–4 g/kg) over 6–8 hours.
- When the maximum albumin dose of 4 g/kg/day has been reached, additional furosemide boluses can be given during the day.
- Consider home albumin infusions.

v. Urinary protein losses may decrease with time, even in the absence of kidney impairment, allowing the decrease or discontinuation of albumin infusions.

c. Vascular access:

i. Indwelling deep-vein catheters may be needed if regular albumin infusions are needed.

- Thrombosis and infection risks are high.
- Give prophylactic anticoagulation when central lines are used.

ii. Where possible, preserve central veins and peripheral arteries and veins for future dialysis access.

iii. Avoid peripherally inserted catheters and unnecessary venepunctures.

2. Chronic diuretic therapy:
   a. Use with caution, especially in patients not receiving albumin, to avoid intravascular volume depletion.
   b. Furosemide:
      i. In very edematous patients, IV furosemide is preferred but in more stable patients, oral furosemide may be given.
      ii. Intravenously or oral dose: 0.5–2 mg/kg per dose up to six times daily (maximum 10 mg/kg per day).
         - High doses >6 mg/kg/day should not be given for periods longer than 1 week.
      iii. Infusions should be administered over 5–30 minutes to avoid hearing loss.
   c. In stable patients, oral furosemide (2–5 mg/kg per day) may be combined with a thiazide or potassium-sparing diuretic.
      - Epithelial sodium channel (ENaC) inhibitors like amiloride are preferred over mineralocorticoid inhibitors like spironolactone.
      - Amiloride dose: 0.2 mg/kg 12–24 hourly (maximum 5 mg).
   d. Monitor blood pressure, urine output, electrolytes, and kidney function.
3. Anti-proteinuric measures:
   a. Renin-angiotensin-aldosterone system (RAAS) blockade:
      i. Start only after a post-term age of 4 weeks, to minimize effects on physiological RAAS functions in early life, and avoid severe hypotension and AKI.
      ii. Start at a very low dose and gradually increase to the maximal effective and tolerated dose.
         - Monitor proteinuria, urine output, serum creatinine, and potassium frequently.
      iii. First anti-proteinuric drug of choice is captopril because of its shorter half-life.
         - Infants <3 months old: Start at 0.01–0.5 mg/kg/dose and increase slowly to maximal daily dose of 2 mg/kg.

- Infants ≥3 months old: Start at 0.15–3 mg/kg/dose and increase slowly to maximal daily dose of 6 mg/kg.

iv. If stable, consider switching to a long-acting angiotensin-converting enzyme inhibitor (ACEi) or angiotensin receptor blocker (ARB).
- ARB should not be combined with ACEi due to increased adverse effects.

b. Non-steroidal anti-inflammatory drugs (NSAIDs):

i. May be added to RAAS blockade in refractory cases, though the evidence is limited.

ii. Start after post-term age of 4 weeks to avoid oliguric AKI and erosive gastritis.

iii. Indomethacin (non-selective Cyclooxygenase [COX] inhibitor): Start at 0.5 mg/kg/day and increase gradually to a maximum of 3 mg/kg/day.
- Gastric protection with histamine H_2-receptor antagonists and/or proton pump inhibitors is recommended.

iv. Celecoxib, a selective COX-2 inhibitor, may be used to minimize gastrointestinal adverse effects.

v. Stop if there is no increase in serum albumin levels and/or reduction in edema after 2–4 weeks.

vi. Do not administer in advanced CKD G4-5.

c. Precautions:
- Chronic diuretics, RAAS inhibitors and NSAIDs should be stopped if there is a risk of non-kidney volume losses (e.g., vomiting, diarrhea, worsening hypoalbuminemia) because of the risk of AKI and thrombosis.

d. Unilateral or preemptive bilateral nephrectomies may be considered only in patients with refractory edema-related complications despite maximal conservative therapy.

II. Nutrition:

1. Nutritional intake should be higher to promote catch-up growth:

a. Calories: 130–150 kcal/kg/day.

   b. Protein: 3–4 g/kg/day.
   c. Composition: 40–50% carbohydrate, 10–14% protein, 40–50% fat (poly- and mono-unsaturated fats).
   d. High-calorie milk formulas, feed fortification, and tube feeding are usually required.
2. Vitamin supplementation:
   a. Complete multivitamin supplementation according to the recommended age-specific dietary allowances for healthy children.
   b. Vitamin D2 or D3 (400–2000 IU/day) if deficient.
   c. Alphacalcidol or calcitriol if parathyroid hormone level is increased.
3. Mineral supplementation to keep serum levels within normal range:
   a. Magnesium: 40–60 mg/day
   b. Calcium (monitor ionized calcium):
      - <6 months: 500 mg/day
      - 6–12 months: 750 mg/day
      - >1 year: 1000 mg/day
4. Nutritional intake may be modified with declining kidney function.
5. Growth hormone may be considered in children >6 months old with growth failure and no treatable factors like malnutrition and metabolic acidosis.

III. Fluid and salt intake

1. Avoid unnecessary intravenous salt-containing fluids and salt supplements.
2. Fluid restriction may be required in severe hyponatremia and very severe edema, but care should be taken to avoid intravascular volume depletion.
3. Fluid prescription should allow adequate nutrition.
4. Provide a low-salt diet:
   a. Infants <6 months: <0.5 g/day.
   b. Infants 7–12 months: <1 g/day.

c. Children 1–3 years: <2 g/day.
d. Children >3 years: <3 g/day.

IV. Manage nephrotic complications:

1. Hypothyroidism:
   a. Check serum TSH 1–3 monthly, as it may initially be normal but increase in subsequent months.
   b. Replace with thyroxine if TSH is high.
2. Thrombosis:
   a. Consider preventive anticoagulation in CNS patients with:
      - Deep vein catheters.
      - Thrombocytosis >750 × 10^9/L.
      - Prior thrombosis.
      - Risk of dehydration.
   b. Warfarin:
      - Recommended drug.
      - Keep international normalized ratio (INR) between 2 and 2.5 for prophylaxis and 2–3 for treatment.
   c. Low molecular weight heparin:
      - May be ineffective due to reduced anti-thrombin III in CNS.
   d. Anti-platelet therapy:
      - Low-dose aspirin or dipyridamole may be used in patients with thrombocytosis.
      - Aspirin might induce AKI, especially in high doses.
   e. Anti-thrombin III:
      - Before surgical or vascular procedures, administer anti-thrombin III (50 IU/kg) 1 hour before the procedure.
   f. Severe hypocalcemia and hypomagnesemia may promote thrombosis.
3. Infections:
   a. Prophylactic antibiotics are generally not indicated.
   b. Give prophylactic intravenous gammaglobulin (IVIG) 500 mg/kg if:
      - Serum IgG is low and
      - Presence of recurrent and/or severe infections.

c. Consider early empirical parenteral broad-spectrum antibiotics to target nosocomial infections.
   - C-reactive protein levels and blood leukocyte levels may be falsely low.
   - A high index of suspicion for infection is important.

d. Prophylaxis for VZ infections:
   i. Consider in patients:
      - Not immunized previously.
      - No previous history of VZ infection.

   ii. Consider giving VZ immunoglobulin within 10 days of exposure OR
   iii. Oral acyclovir 10 mg/kg (maximum 800 mg) 4x/day or valacyclovir 20 mg/kg (maximum dose 1 g) 8 hourly for 7 days.

4. Hypercholesterolemia:
   - Consider 3-hydroxy-3-methylglutaryl coenzyme A (HMG-CoA) reductase inhibitors (statins) when fasting, low-density lipoprotein (LDL) cholesterol is persistently >4.1 mmol/L or >3.4 mmol/L in patients with additional cardiovascular risk factors such as hypertension and obesity.

5. Anemia:
   a. Transferrin saturation and ferritin levels are unreliable in CNS.
   b. Erythropoietin deficiency:
      i. Urinary losses of erythropoietin can occur in CNS.
      ii. A trial of erythropoietin therapy should be considered in patients with anemia after correction of iron deficiency.
      iii. Increased doses of erythropoietin may be required.
      iv. Subcutaneous route might be more efficacious than intravenous route.
      v. Monitor response to therapy by using reticulocyte count.

   c. Consider copper, ceruloplasmin or vitamin B12 deficiency in anemia refractory to iron and erythropoietin therapy.

V. Immunizations:

1. Immunizations against encapsulated organisms should be given:
   - Conjugated pneumococcal vaccine.

- Haemophilus influenzae type B (HiB) vaccine.
- Meningococcal vaccine.

2. Continue Hepatitis B immunization.
3. Primary and booster doses of vaccines should be given according to the immunization schedule, including:
   - Diphtheria, tetanus, acellular pertussis (DTaP) vaccines.
   - Inactivated polio vaccine.
4. Live attenuated vaccines should only be given at least 6 months after the last dose of IVIG.
   - Measles, mumps, rubella vaccines.
   - VZ vaccine.
5. Annual influenza vaccines should be given.

VI. Treatment specific to etiology:

1. Immunosuppression:
   a. Immunosuppression is generally not recommended in genetic cases.
   b. Consider a trial of immunosuppression if all the following criteria are satisfied:
      - No detectable genetic diagnosis on comprehensive genetic testing.
      - No evidence of secondary CNS.
      - Absence of significant sclerosis or diffuse mesangial sclerosis on kidney biopsy.
2. Coenzyme Q10 (CoQ10) supplementation in patients with CoQ10-related genetic defects may decrease proteinuria and slow CKD progression.
   a. Initial dose: 30 mg/kg/day in three divided doses.
   b. May increase to 50 mg/kg/day (maximum 1500 mg/day for adolescents and 2400 mg/day for adults).
   c. Ubiquinol is the reduced, active form while ubiquinone is the oxidized form that needs to be converted in the body to the active form.
      - Ubiquinol at the same dosage may yield a more active compound than ubiquinone.
   d. May be given as a therapeutic trial whilst waiting for, or in the absence of, genetic results.

e. Discontinue therapy if there is no improvement in kidney function or proteinuria is noted after 4–6 weeks.

3. In secondary CNS due to infections, consider specific anti-microbial therapy.

VII. Renal replacement therapy:

1. Most CNS patients progress to kidney failure within a few years.
2. Preemptive nephrectomies before kidney failure are not required in stable patients with no refractory edema-related complications.
3. Peritoneal dialysis is the modality of choice as it preserves vascular access.
4. Considerations prior to kidney transplant:
   a. Patients should not be in a nephrotic state and serum albumin should be normal to minimize thrombotic risk to the new graft.
      - In persistently nephrotic patients with kidney failure, consider bilateral nephrectomies to induce resolution of the nephrotic state.

   b. Genetic testing of the living-related donor should be performed if the recipient has a proven genetic diagnosis, especially for dominant genes.
   c. Post-transplant recurrence of nephrotic syndrome rarely occurs in patients with certain *NPHS1* or *NPHS2* mutations.

VIII. Malignancy risk in Denys–Drash syndrome:

1. Risk of Wilms tumor in patients with exonic *WT1* variants:
   a. Prophylactic bilateral nephrectomies should be performed after the onset of kidney failure and initiation of dialysis.
   b. If nephrectomies have not been performed, routine ultrasound surveillance for Wilms tumor should be carried out every 3 months until 7 years old.
2. Risk of gonadoblastoma:
   a. Risk of gonadoblastoma is significantly increased in 46XY male to female sex reversal.

b. Gonadal function should be assessed by a pediatric endocrinologist.
   i. Perform an ultrasound of the gonads and measure tumor markers (human chorionic gonadotrophin and alpha-fetoprotein) 6-monthly in the presence of streak gonads.
   ii. The need and timing for gonadectomy should be discussed, based on the karyotype.

Recommended Reading

1. Hölttä T, Jalanko H. (2020) Congenital nephrotic syndrome: Is early aggressive treatment needed? Yes. *Pediatr Nephrol* **35**:1985–1990.
2. Niaudet P. (2021, updated) Congenital and infantile nephrotic syndrome. Edited by: Mattoo TK, Kim MS. *UpToDate ONLINE*. http://www.uptodateonline.com.
3. Boyer O, Schaefer F, Haffner D, Bockenhauer D, Hölttä T, Bérody S, Webb H, Heselden M, Lipska-Zie Tkiewicz BS, Ozaltin F, Levtchenko E, Vivarelli M. (2021) Management of congenital nephrotic syndrome: Consensus recommendations of the ERKNet-ESPN Working Group. *Nat Rev Nephrol* **17**:277–289.

6 Management of Lupus Nephritis in Children

Resontoc LP, Teo S, Lau PYW, Ng KH and Yap HK

A. Introduction

a. Systemic lupus erythematosus (SLE) has an estimated mean annual incidence in children of 0.36 to 0.9 per 100000.
b. SLE is a chronic autoimmune disease characterized by multisystem inflammation and the presence of circulating autoantibodies directed against self-antigens.
c. The onset of disease tends to be more acute and severe in children, with high rates of organ involvement, especially lupus nephritis (LN).
d. 60–80% of these children will exhibit kidney involvement at the onset of disease.

B. Clinical Presentation

1. Known SLE patient with evidence of kidney involvement:

Clinical Presentation	Prevalence
Nephrotic syndrome: Urinary protein excretion ≥3 g/day/1.73m^2 Urine protein:creatinine ratio ≥0.2 g/mmol)	55%
Non-nephrotic range proteinuria: Urinary protein excretion ≥0.3 g/day/1.73m^2 Urine protein:creatinine ratio ≥0.02 g/mmol)	43%
Macroscopic hematuria	1.4%
Active urinary sediment: >5 red blood cells (RBC)/high-power field (hpf) >5 white blood cells (WBC)/hpf in the absence of infection Cellular casts limited to RBC or WBC casts	79%

(*Continued*)

Hypertension	40%
Reduced estimated glomerular filtration rate (eGFR <80 ml/min/ 1.73 m^2)	50%
Acute kidney injury	1.4%

2. Suspect LN in a patient with an isolated presentation of glomerular disease with or without serological evidence of SLE, but with a kidney biopsy sample demonstrating immune complex-mediated glomerulonephritis with "full-house" immunoglobulin deposition on immunofluorescence (IMF).

C. 2019 EULAR/ACR Classification Criteria for Systemic Lupus Erythematosus

Entry Criterion

Antinuclear antibodies (ANA) at a titer of ≥1:80 on Hep-2 cells or an equivalent positive test (ever)

↓

If absent, do not classify as SLE, If present, apply additive criteria

↓

Additive Criteria

Do not count a criterion if there is more likely explanation than SLE. Occurrence of a criterion on at least one occasion is sufficient.
SLE classification requires at least one clinical criterion and ≥ 10 points. Criteria need not occur simultaneously.
Within each domain, only the highest weighted criterion is counted toward the total scores

Clinical domains and criteria	Weight
Constitutional	
Fever	2
Hematologic	
Leukopenia	3
Thrombocytopenia	4
Autoimmue hemolysis	4
Neuropsychiatric	
Delirium	2
Psychosis	3
Seizure	5
Mucocutaneous	
Non-scarring alopecia	2
Oral ulcers	2
Subacute cutaneous OR discoid lupus	4
Acute cutanaeous lupus	6
Serosal	
Pleural or pericardial effusion	5
Acute pericarditis	6
Musculoskeletal	
Joint involvement	6
Renal	
Proteinuria > 0.5 g/24h	4
Renal biopsy Class II or V LN	8
Renal biopsy Class III or IV LN	10

Immunologic domains and criteria	Weight
Antiphospholipid antibodies	
Anti-cardiolipin antibodies OR	
Anti-β2GP1 antibodies OR	
Lupus anticoagulant	2
Complement proteins	
Low C3 OR Low C4	3
Low C3 AND Low C4	4
SLE-specific antibodies	
Anti-ds-DNA antibody* OR	
Anti-Smith antibody	6

Total score

↓

Classify as Systemic Lupus Erythematosus with a score of 10 or more if entry criterion fulfilled.

*https://www.ncbi.nlm.nih.gov/pmc/articles/PMC6827566/pdf/nihms-1029532.pdf for the SLE classification criteria.

D. Initial Investigations

I. Objectives:

1. Establish diagnosis.
2. Assess degree of systemic involvement.

II. Investigations:

1. Diagnostic:
   a. SLE panel:
      i. Complement C3.
      ii. Complement C4.
      iii. Anti-double-stranded (ds) DNA antibody.
         - Highly specific 95%, sensitivity 75%.
         - Association with LN.
   b. Anti-nuclear antibodies (ANAs)
      - Best diagnostic test where the risk of SLE is <0.14 if ANA is negative.
   c. Anti-phospholipid screen:
      i. Prothrombin time (PT).
      ii. Partial thromboplastin time (aPTT).
      iii. Lupus anti-coagulant.
      iv. Anti-cardiolipin IgG and IgM.
      v. Anti-β2 glycoprotein-1 IgG and IgM.
   d. Anti-ENA (extractable nuclear antigens) panel:
      i. Anti-Ro (SSA):
         - Found in Sjögren's syndrome and 10–60% of SLE patients.
         - Associated with lymphopenia, photosensitivity, subacute cutaneous lupus, cutaneous vasculitis (palpable purpura), interstitial lung disease, neonatal lupus, and congenital heart block.
      ii. Anti-La (SSB):
         - Found in Sjögren's syndrome and 10–35% of SLE.
      iii. Anti-Smith or Sm:
         - Highly specific 55–100%, sensitivity 25%.

- Remains high when anti-dsDNA antibody levels have returned to normal.

iv. Anti-RNP (U1 RNP) or ribonuclear protein:
- Found mainly in mixed connective tissue disease (MCTD), and only in 3–69% of SLE.
- Association with myositis, Raynaud's phenomenon, and less severe lupus.

v. Anti-SCL70 (anti-topoisomerase-1):
- Seen in systemic sclerosis.
- Associated with lung fibrosis.

vi. Anti-Jo1:
- Myositis-specific antibody seen in dermatomyositis or polymyositis.
- Associated with interstitial lung disease, arthritis, Raynaud's phenomenon, and mechanic's hand (anti-synthetase syndrome).

2. Systemic involvement:
- Full blood count.
- Reticulocyte count.
- Peripheral blood film.
- Direct Coomb's test.
- Erythrocyte sedimentation rate.
- C-reactive protein.
- Urine microscopy.
- Urine protein:creatinine ratio or 24-hour urine protein excretion.
- Creatinine clearance
- Blood urea, creatinine, sodium, potassium, chloride, bicarbonate
- Calcium, phosphate, alkaline phosphatase
- Uric acid.
- Liver function test: Total protein, albumin, alanine aminotransaminase (ALT), aspartate aminotransferase (AST), bilirubin.
- Serum cholesterol, triglycerides, low-density lipoprotein (LDL)-cholesterol, high-density lipoprotein (HDL)-cholesterol.
- Chest radiograph if indicated.
- 2-D echocardiography.
- Kidney biopsy.

E. Assessment of Activity of Lupus Nephritis

I. Clinical assessment of activity of SLE: Systemic Lupus Erythematosus Disease Activity Index (SLEDAI) — Selena Modification:

Weight	Descriptor	Definition
8	Seizure	Recent onset, exclude metabolic, infectious or drug causes.
8	Psychosis	Altered ability to function in normal activity due to severe disturbance in the perception of reality. Includes hallucinations, incoherence, marked loose associations, impoverished thought content, marked illogical thinking, or bizarre, disorganized, or catatonic behavior. Exclude uremia and drug causes.
8	Organic brain syndrome	Altered mental function with impaired orientation, memory, or other intellectual function, with rapid onset and fluctuating clinical features, inability to sustain attention to the environment, plus at least 2 of the following: Perceptual disturbances, incoherent speech, insomnia or daytime drowsiness, or increased or decreased psychomotor activity. Exclude metabolic, infectious, or drug causes.
8	Visual disturbance	Retinal changes of SLE: Includes cytoid bodies, retinal hemorrhages, serous exudate or hemorrhages in the choroid, or optic neuritis. Exclude hypertension, infection, or drug causes.
8	Cranial nerve disorder	New onset of sensory or motor neuropathy involving cranial nerves.
8	Lupus headache	Severe, persistent headache, may be migrainous, but must be nonresponsive to narcotic analgesia.
8	Cerebrovascular accident	New onset cerebrovascular accident(s). Exclude arteriosclerosis.

(*Continued*)

Weight	Descriptor	Definition
8	Vasculitis	Ulceration, gangrene, tender finger nodules, periungual infarction, splinter hemorrhages, or biopsy or angiogram proof of vasculitis.
4	Arthritis	≥2 joints with pain and signs of inflammation: Tenderness, swelling or effusion.
4	Myositis	Proximal muscle aching/weakness, associated with elevated creatine phosphokinase or aldolase or electromyogram changes or a biopsy showing myositis.
4	Urinary casts	Heme-granular or red blood cell casts.
4	Hematuria	>5 RBC/hpf. Exclude stones, infection or other causes.
4	Proteinuria	>0.5 g/24 hours.
4	Pyuria	>5 WBC/hpf. Exclude infection.
2	Rash	Inflammatory type rash.
2	Alopecia	Abnormal, patchy, or diffuse loss of hair.
2	Mucosal ulcers	Oral or nasal ulcerations.
2	Pleurisy	Pleuritic chest pain with pleural rub or effusion, or pleural thickening.
2	Pericarditis	Pericardial pain with at least 1 of the following: Rub, effusion, or electrocardiogram or echocardiogram confirmation.
2	Low complement	Decrease in CH50, C3, or C4 below the lower limit of normal for testing laboratory.
2	Increased DNA binding	Increased DNA binding by Farr Assay above the normal range.
1	Fever	>38°C. Exclude infectious causes.
1	Thrombocytopenia	Platelets <100 × 10^9/L. Exclude drug causes.
1	Leukopenia	WBC <3 × 10^9/L. Exclude drug causes.

II. Assessment of activity of glomerulonephritis

1. Clinical disease manifestations:
   - Presence of nephrotic syndrome.
   - Blood pressure control.
2. Presence of active urine sediment on urine microscopy:
   - Hematuria >5 RBC/hpf.
   - Pyuria in the absence of infection >5 WBC/hpf.
   - RBC or WBC (granular) casts.
3. Degree of proteinuria:
   - Urine protein:creatinine ratio.
   - 24-hour urine protein excretion.
4. Kidney function:
   - Estimation of glomerular filtration rate.

III. Kidney biopsy

1. Aims:
   a. Classify the glomerular disease to guide therapy and assess prognosis.
   b. Evaluate for activity and chronicity, and tubular and vascular changes.
   c. Identify additional or alternative causes of kidney disease, such as tubular necrosis related to medications, hypovolemia or hypotension.
2. Indications:
   a. All previously untreated patients with clinical evidence of active LN should undergo a kidney biopsy unless strongly contraindicated:
      - Increasing serum creatinine without compelling alternative causes such as sepsis, hypovolemia or medication.
      - Confirmed proteinuria of ≥1.0 g/day/1.73m^2.
      - Confirmed proteinuria of ≥0.5 g/day/1.73m^2 and ≥5 RBC/hpf or cellular casts.

   b. Persistent proteinuria of >0.3 to 1 g/day/1.73m^2 after starting treatment for active SLE.

3. Modified National Institutes of Health (NIH) activity and chronicity index (2018):

Activity Index	Definition (According to % Glomerular or Cortical Involvement)			Score
	<25%	25–50%	>50%	
Endocapillary hypercellularity	1	2	3	0–3
Neutrophils/Karyorrhexis	1	2	3	0–3
Fibrinoid necrosis	1	2	3	(0–3) × 2
Hyaline deposits (wireloop lesions and/ or hyaline thrombi)	1	2	2	0–3
Cellular/fibrocellular crescents	1	2	3	(0–3) × 2
Interstitial inflammation	1	2	3	0–3
Total				**0–24**
Chronicity Index				
Total glomerulosclerosis score (global and/or segmental sclerosis	1	2	3	0–3
Fibrous crescents	1	2	3	0–3
Tubular atrophy	1	2	3	0–3
Interstitial fibrosis	1	2	3	0–3
Total				**0–12**

4. 2018 Revised International Society of Nephrology/Renal Pathology Society (ISN/RPS) classification of LN:

Class I	**Minimal mesangial LN** Normal glomeruli by LM, but mesangial immune deposits by IMF.
Class II	**Mesangial proliferative LN** The presence of >4 nuclei fully surrounded by matrix in the mesangial area not including the hilar region. May be a few isolated subepithelial or subendothelial deposits visible by IMF or EM, but not by LM.

(Continued)

(*Continued*)

Class III	**Focal LN**	• Endocapillary hypercellularity (increase in cells in mesangial, endocapillary, and/or extracapillary locations).
		• Crescent is used for a lesion consisting of extracapillary hypercellularity, composed of a variable mixture of cells. Fibrin and fibrous matrix may be present; 10% or more of the circumference of Bowman's capsule should be involved.
		  ▪ Cellular crescent: More than 75% cells and fibrin and less than 25% fibrous matrix.
		  ▪ Fibrous crescent: More than 75% fibrous matrix and less than 25% cells and fibrin.
		  ▪ Fibrocellular crescent: 25–75% cells and fibrin and the remainder fibrous matrix.
		• Adhesion: An area of isolated continuity of extracellular matrix material between the tuft and capsule even when the underlying segment does not have overt sclerosis.
		• Fibrinoid necrosis: Fibrin associated with glomerular basement membrane disruption and/or lysis of the mesangial matrix; this lesion does not require the presence of karyorrhexis.
		• Membranoproliferative glomerulonephritis (MPGN) pattern is subsumed in Class III and IV LN as a form of endocapillary injury.
		• Subendothelial deposits that can be seen by light microscopy (i.e., wire loops) and hyaline masses within capillary lumens caused by immune complexes (i.e., hyaline thrombi) as lesions indicative of Class III or IV.

Class IV	**Diffuse LN**	
Class V	**Membranous LN** Global or segmental subepithelial immune deposits or their morphologic sequelae by LM and by IMF or EM, ± mesangial alterations. May occur in combination with Class III or IV, in which case both will be diagnosed. May show advanced sclerosis.	
Class VI	**Advanced sclerosing LN** ≥90% of glomeruli globally sclerosed without residual activity.	

- LM: light microscopy; IMF: immunofluorescence; EM: electron microscopy.
- Indicate and grade (mild, moderate, severe) tubular atrophy, interstitial inflammation and fibrosis, the severity of arteriosclerosis or other vascular lesions.

5. Other histological subtypes:
   a. Lupus podocytopathy:
      - Features of minimal change disease with podocyte foot process effacement and the absence of major immune complex deposition.

   b. Thrombotic microangiopathy (TMA):
      - Presence of glomerular and vascular thrombi.
      - Associated with antiphospholipid antibodies or antibodies against the von Willebrand factor convertase.

   c. Interstitial nephritis:
      - Presents with a rising plasma creatinine concentration and benign urinalysis or with minimal red and/or white cells.
      - Associated signs of tubular dysfunction such as Type 1 renal tubular acidosis, hyperkalemia due to impaired distal potassium secretion, or hypokalemia due to salt wasting and secondary hyperaldosteronism.
      - Associated autoantibodies directed against the acid-secreting intercalated cells in the collecting tubule.

F. Immunosuppressive Therapy in LN

I. Principles of immunosuppressive therapy in LN

1. Induction phase:
   - Administration of potent immunosuppressive drug combinations to achieve clinical and immunologic kidney response leading to the restoration of kidney function.

2. Maintenance phase:
   - Less aggressive immunosuppressive therapy for a prolonged duration to prevent relapse of the systemic autoimmunity and reduce proteinuria to prevent the progression of CKD.

II. Therapy of ISN/RPS Class I

1. Glucocorticoids (GC):
   - Low dose prednisolone (PNL) <0.5 mg/kg/day can be considered.
2. If other organ systems are involved, treatment choice should be guided by these other clinical features.

III. Therapy for ISN/RPS Class II (see chapter "Immunosuppressive Medications"):

1. GC:
   a. Starting PNL dose of 0.25–0.5 mg/kg/day, with a maximum of 30 mg/day.
   b. Tapering over a total duration of 3–6 months.
2. Mycophenolic acid (MPA) or Azathioprine (AZA):
   a. Can be considered if proteinuria is persistent and/or prednisolone is unable to be weaned in 3 months.
   b. May be added to control extrarenal involvement.
   c. Drug dosing:
      i. Mycophenolate mofetil (MMF): 600 mg/m^2/dose 12 hourly (15–23 mg/kg/dose 12 hourly).
         - Maximum adult dose: 1–1.5 g 12 hourly.
      ii. Myfortic®: 400 mg/m^2/dose 12 hourly
         - Maximum adult dose: 720 mg 12 hourly.
      iii. AZA: 2 mg/kg/day.
         - To identify patients at risk for toxicity: Check for thiopurine methyltransferase (TPMT).
   d. Monitor full blood count monthly.
      - Omit if absolute neutrophil count is <1.5 × 10^9/L.

IV. Therapy of ISN/RPS Class III/IV and V:

1. Multi-targeted MPA-calcineurin inhibitor (CNI) protocol:
   a. GC:
      i. Intravenous (IV) monthly pulse methylprednisolone (MP) 10–30 mg/kg/dose (maximum 1 g) for 3 days × 6 courses.

ii. Oral PNL starting at 0.5–1.0 mg/kg (maximum 30 mg) daily, and tapering by 5 mg/day on a monthly basis following each MP pulse, depending on the disease activity.
iii. Tapering of oral PNL therapy should be continued monthly over 6–12 months, and can be changed to alternate day therapy once proteinuria decreases to <0.3 g/day/1.73m^2 and serological remission is attained (defined as the normalization of serum complement C3 and C4 levels).

b. Mycophenolate mofetil (MMF):
  i. Oral MMF is started together with IV pulse methylprednisolone at induction.
  ii. MMF Dose: 600 mg/m^2/dose 12 hourly (15–23 mg/kg/dose 12 hourly). Maximum dose: 1g 12 hourly.
  iii. Monitor full blood count monthly.
    • Omit if absolute neutrophil count <1.5 × 10^9/L.
  iv. Serum MPA levels when side effects present.
    • Trough levels range from 2 to 4 mg/L.
  v. Estimation of MPA area under the time-concentration curve (AUC):
    • Target MPA AUC 30–60 mg*h/L.
  vi. Due to gastrointestinal side effects, start famotidine prophylactically at 0.5–1 mg/kg/day once nightly or a divided dose 12 hourly (maximum 40 mg), or rabeprazole 0.5–1.0 mg/kg once nightly or a divided dose 12 hourly (maximum 40 mg).
  vii. Consider changing to Myfortic® if gastrointestinal side effects persist. Myfortic®: 180 mg = 250 mg (dose equivalent of Cellcept®).
  360 mg = 500 mg (dose equivalent of Cellcept®).

c. CNI:
  I. Types of CNI:
    • Cyclosporine (CsA).
    • Tacrolimus (Tac).
  ii. Add oral CNI if there is persistent moderate proteinuria (defined as urine protein excretion >1g/day/1.73m^2) after 3 months of treatment, provided the serum creatinine or eGFR is normal.
  III. Dose:
    • CsA: 3–6 mg/kg/day in 2 divided doses to achieve whole blood trough CsA levels of 150–200 µg/L.

- Tac: 0.2 mg/kg/day in 2 divided doses to achieve whole blood trough Tac levels of 8–10 μg/L.

iv. Use diltiazem 15–30 mg 8–12 hourly to increase CNI levels, increasing by 15 mg/dose until a maximum of 60 mg 8–12 hourly.

v. Monitor:
- CNI trough levels 4–6 weekly after the target level has been achieved.
- Serum creatinine levels 4–6 weekly, and if this increases by 25%, reduce CNI dose by 20% to determine if CNI nephrotoxicity is the cause.
- Blood glucose levels at 4–6 weeks, then 3-monthly if on Tac.
- HbA1c levels 6-monthly if on Tac.

vi. CNI is continued for 3–6 months and discontinued once complete remission is achieved.

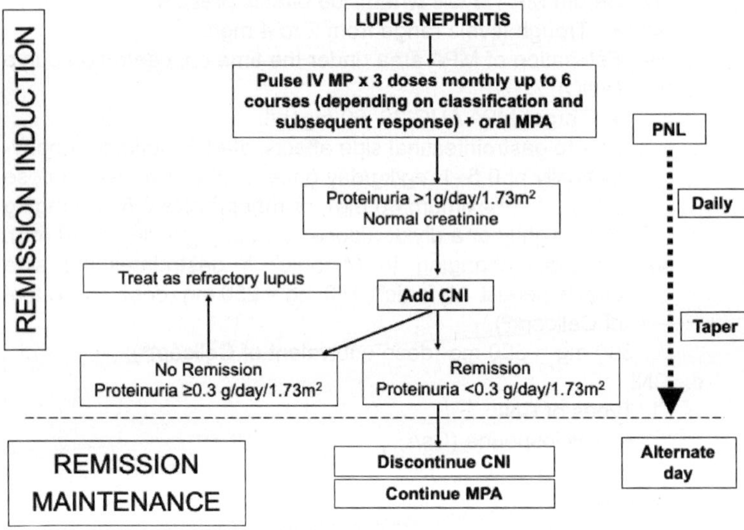

2. Low-dose IV cyclophosphamide (CYC) protocol:
   a. GC:
      i. IV pulse MP 10–30 mg/kg/dose (maximum 1 g) for 3 days.
      ii. Oral PNL starting at 0.5–1.0 mg/kg (maximum 60 mg) daily after the MP pulse, and tapering by 5 mg/day on a monthly basis depending on disease activity, and subsequently tapering to a minimal amount necessary to control the disease.
   b. IV CYC 500 mg/m^2 once every 2 weeks for 6 doses followed by:
      i. Oral AZA 2 mg/kg daily OR
      ii. Oral MMF 600 mg/m^2/dose 12 hourly (maximum dose 1 g 12 hourly).

V. Therapy of lupus podocytopathy:

1. GC:
   a. Intravenous (IV) monthly pulse MP 10–30 mg/kg/dose (maximum 1 g) for 3 days up to a maximum of 3 courses.
   b. Oral PNL starting at 0.5–1.0 mg/kg (maximum 30 mg) daily, and tapering by 5 mg/day after each monthly pulse OR on a 2-weekly basis if the patient has gone into remission, that is, proteinuria decreases to <0.3 g/day/1.73m^2 and serological remission is attained (defined as the normalization of serum complement C3 and C4 levels).
2. Continue MMF at 600 mg/m^2/dose 12 hourly.
3. CNI:
   a. Consider adding CNI if the patient is unable to attain complete remission or continues to relapse after 1–3 months, aiming for therapeutic levels:
      - CsA 150–200 μg/L.
      - Tac 8–10 μg/L.
   b. Taper off CNI once PNL has been tapered off or reached baseline and the patient has remained in remission.
4. Consider IV rituximab (2–4 doses) 375 mg/m^2 if the patient has recurrent relapses of nephrotic syndrome.

VI. *Criteria for response:*

1. Complete remission: Defined by the presence of all of the following criteria in at least two determinations one month apart:
   a. SLEDAI ≤2.
   b. Normalization of serum C3 and C4 levels.
   c. Normalization of kidney function (eGFR ≥90 ml/min/1.73m^2).
   d. Absence of hematuria (≤5 RBC/hpf).
   e. Urinary protein excretion ≤0.3 g/day/1.73m^2.
2. Partial remission:
   a. 50% improvement in serum creatinine level and/or urinary protein excretion.
   b. Improvement in serum complement levels.
   c. Improvement in SLEDAI.

VII. *Refractory lupus nephritis:*

1. Definition:
   a. Worsening nephritis by 3 months AND/OR
   b. Failure to attain complete clinical remission after the appropriate induction immunosuppressive therapy at 6 months.
   c. Rule out:
      i. Non-immunologic cause of kidney injury: TMA and secondary FSGS.
      ii. Medication non-adherence.
      iii. Insufficient dosing: Check drug levels.
2. Anti-CD20 monoclonal antibody therapy (Rituximab®):
   a. Dose: IV 375 mg/m^2 weekly for 4 doses or 750 mg/m^2 2-weekly for 2 doses.
   b. Prophylaxis for Pneumocystis jirovecii (see chapter "Anti-CD20 Monoclonal Antibody Therapy for Nephrotic Syndrome").
3. Plasmapheresis:
   a. Indicated in patients with features of TMA or pulmonary hemorrhage.
   b. Dose: 5–10 exchanges depending on response in terms of:
      - Hematological remission of microangiopathic hemolytic anemia (MAHA).

- Activity of SLE.
- Recovery of kidney function.

c. Plasmapheresis should be carried out concurrently with the selected immunosuppressive protocol.

G. Adjunctive Therapy in LN

1. Hydroxychloroquine:
   a. Dose: 6.5 mg/kg/day (maximum 400 mg).
   b. Avoid in patients with glucose-6-phosphate dehydrogenase (G6PD) deficiency due to the risk of acute hemolysis.
   c. Benefits as shown in randomized controlled trials:
      - Lower lupus flare rates.
      - Lower damage accrual including kidney damage.
      - Reduce the risk of thrombotic events in patients with antiphospholipid syndrome.
   d. Requires annual ophthalmologic screen for hydroxychloroquine-induced retinopathy:
      - Presents with abnormal color vision, visual disturbances, blurred vision, photophobia, and scotoma.
      - Pigmentary retinopathy may be reversible if detected early.
2. Control of proteinuria (see chapter "Adjunctive Therapy in Glomerular Disease"):
   a. Patients with proteinuria ≥0.5 g/day/1.73m^2 should be treated with angiotensin-converting enzyme (ACE) inhibitors and/or angiotensin receptor blockers (ARBs).
   b. Benefits of blockade of the renin-angiotensin system:
      - Reduces proteinuria by 30%.
      - Significantly delays doubling of serum creatinine and progression to kidney failure.
      - Contraindicated in pregnancy.
3. Control of hypertension.
   a. Good blood pressure control is essential to delay the progression of chronic kidney disease (CKD).
   b. Target for blood pressure control:
      - Age <13 years: <90th percentile (clinic BP)
      - Age ≥13 years: <130/80 mmHg (clinic BP)

- 24-hour mean arterial pressure (MAP) <50th percentile by ambulatory BP monitoring.

4. Hyperlipidemia (see chapter "Adjunctive Therapy in Glomerular Disease"):
   a. SLE and CKD stage 3 are independent risk factors for accelerated atherosclerosis.
   b. Statin therapy should be initiated in patients with LDL-cholesterol >3.36 mmol/L.
5. Management of anti-phospholipid syndrome:
   a. Diagnosis:
      - Presence of at least one type of anti-phospholipid antibody in the serum AND
      - Occurrence of venous or arterial thrombosis and/or pregnancy morbidity.
   b. Treatment:
      i. For acute thrombotic events, the first therapy is either unfractionated heparin or low molecular weight (LMW) heparin.
      ii. Unfractionated heparin is preferred to LMW heparin in the setting of hemorrhage, which occurs rarely, when antibodies to prothrombin are present.
      iii. Advantage of unfractionated heparin is that it is quickly reversible with protamine.
      iv. Warfarin is the standard of care for the chronic management of anti-phospholipid syndrome in non-pregnant patients.
         - Warfarin is contraindicated in pregnancy.
      v. Warfarin should be started 4–5 days prior to the discontinuation of heparin, aiming for an International Normalized Ratio (INR) between 2.0 and 3.0 for 2 consecutive days.
         - Loading dose:
           Day 1: 0.2 mg/kg (maximum dose 10 mg).
           Days 2–4: If INR = 1.1–1.3, repeat the initial loading dose.
           If INR = 1.4–1.9, give 50% of the initial loading dose.
           If INR = 2–3, give 50% of the initial loading dose.
           If INR = 3.1–3.5, give 25% of the initial loading dose.
           If INR >3.5, hold warfarin and check INR daily until INR <3.5, then restart at 50% of the previous dose.
         - Maintenance dose (Day 5 and beyond):

If INR = 1.1–1.4, increase the dose by 20% of the previous dose.
If INR = 1.5–1.9, increase the dose by 10% of the previous dose.
If INR = 2–3, do not change the dose.
If INR = 3.1–3.5, decrease the dose by 10% of the previous dose.
If INR >3, hold warfarin and check warfarin until INR <3.5, then restart at 50% of the previous dose.

vi. If there is difficulty in maintaining a therapeutic INR, then patients can be treated with either LMW heparin, or with a lower dose of warfarin plus aspirin.

c. Prophylaxis with anti-platelet agents:
   i. Aspirin (5 mg/kg/dose, maximum 100 mg) should be given as prophylaxis to reduce the risk of thrombosis in patients with anti-phospholipid antibodies.
   ii. Consider changing from warfarin to aspirin in patients with a previous history of thrombosis, who have become negative for anti-phospholipid antibodies.

d. Advise against oral contraceptives, especially those with high estrogen content in patients with anti-phospholipid antibodies.

6. Avoid non-steroidal anti-inflammatory agents (NSAIDs) if the kidney function is decreased (eGFR <80 ml/min/1.73m^2).

Recommended Reading

1. Kamanamool N, McEvoy M, Attia J, Ingsathit A, Ngamjanyaporn P, Thakkinstian A. (2010) Efficacy and adverse effects of mycophenolate mofetil versus cyclophosphamide for induction therapy of lupus nephritis. Systematic review and meta-analysis. *Medicine* **89**:227–235.
2. Aragon E, Chan YH, Ng KH, Lau YW, Tan PH, Yap HK. (2010) Good outcomes with mycophenolate-cyclosporine-based induction protocol in children with severe proliferative lupus nephritis. *Lupus* **19**:965–973.
3. Groot N, de Graeff N, Marks SD, Brogan P, Avcin T, Bader-Meunier B, Dolezalova P, Feldman BM, Kone-Paut I, Lahdenne P, McCann L, Özen S, Pilkington CA, Ravelli A, Royen-Kerkhof AV, Uziel Y, Vastert BJ, Wulffraat NM, Ceresford MW, Kamphuis S. (2017) European evidence-based recommendations for the diagnosis and treatment of childhood-onset lupus nephritis: the SHARE initiative. *Ann Rheum Dis* **76**:1965–1973.
4. Bajema IM, Wilhelmus S, Alpers CE, Bruijn JA, Colvin RB, Cook HT, D'Agati VD, Ferrario F, Haas M, Jennette JC, Joh K, Nast CC, Noël LH, Rijnink EC, Roberts ISD,

Seshan SV, Sethi S, Fogo AB. (2018) Revision of the International Society of Nephrology/Renal Pathology Society classification for lupus nephritis: Clarification of definitions, and modified National Institutes of Health activity and chronicity indices. *Kidney Int* **93**:789–796.

5. Erkan D, Ortel TL. (2018, updated) Treatment of antiphospholipid syndrome. Edited by Pisetsky DS, Curtis MR, Tirnauer JS. *UpToDate ONLINE.* http://www.uptodateonline.com.
6. Yo JH, Barbour TD, Nicholls K. (2019) Management of refractory lupus nephritis: Challenges and solutions. *Open Access Rheumatol* **11**:179–188.
7. Aringer M, Costenbader KH, Daikh D. *et al.* (2019) 2019 EULAR/ACR Classification criteria for systemic lupus erythematosus. *Arthritis Rheumatol* **71**:1400–1412.
8. Klein-Gitelman M. (2019, updated) Systemic lupus erythematosus in children: Treatment, complications, and prognosis. Edited by Sundel R, TePas E. UpToDate ONLINE. http://www.uptodateonline.com.
9. Levy DM. (2020, updated) Childhood-onset systemic lupus erythematosus (SLE): Children: Clinical manifestations and diagnosis. Edited by Klein-Gitelman M, TePas E. UpToDate ONLINE. http://www.uptodateonline.com.

7 Management of Primary Immunoglobulin A (IgA) Nephropathy in Children

Resontoc LP, Liu ID and Yap HK

A. Diagnostic Approach

I. Clinical presentation

1. Disease manifestations:
   a. Microscopic hematuria ± proteinuria.
   b. Recurrent gross hematuria.
   c. Nephrotic syndrome.
   d. Acute nephritic syndrome.
   e. Crescentic glomerulonephritis with rapidly deteriorating kidney function.
   f. Acute kidney injury associated with macroscopic hematuria.
2. Exclude secondary causes of IgA nephropathy, such as:
   a. Liver disease.
   b. Inflammatory bowel disease.
   c. Celiac disease.
   d. HIV infection.
   e. Ankylosing spondylitis.
   f. Dermatitis herpetiformis.
   g. Bronchiolitis obliterans.
   h. Disseminated tuberculosis.
   i. Lymphomas.
3. Serum IgA may be raised in 8–16% of children with IgA nephropathy.

II. Kidney biopsy

1. Indications:
   a. If a histological diagnosis is necessary.
   b. If considering starting immunosuppressive therapy:
      i. Proteinuria ≥1 g/day/1.73 m^2 or urine protein:creatinine ratio (UPCR) ≥0.1 g/mmol.
      ii. Chronic kidney disease (CKD) with decreased glomerular filtration rate (GFR).
      iii. Hypertension.
      iv. Acute worsening of kidney function, to distinguish acute tubular necrosis from crescentic IgA nephropathy.
2. The Oxford Classification of IgA Nephropathy (IgAN) 2016 Update (Revised MEST-C score):

Variable	Definition	Score
Mesangial hypercellularity	0 = <4 mesangial cells/mesangial area 1 = 4–5 mesangial cells/mesangial area 2 = 6–7 mesangial cells/mesangial area 3 = >8 mesangial cells/mesangial area (The mesangial hypercellularity score is the mean score for all glomeruli).	M0 ≤0.5 M1 >0.5
Segmental glomerulosclerosis	Any amount of the tuft involved in sclerosis, but not involving the whole tuft or the presence of an adhesion. Note the presence or absence of podocytopathic features (podocyte hypertrophy/tip lesions).	S0: absent S1: present
Endocapillary hypercellularity	Hypercellularity due to the increased number of cells within the glomerular capillary lumina causing narrowing of the lumina.	E0: absent E1: present
Tubular atrophy/ interstitial fibrosis	Percentage of cortical area involved by the tubular atrophy or interstitial fibrosis, whichever is greater.	T0: 0–25% T1: 26–50% T2: >50%
Crescent	No crescents. Crescents in <25% of glomeruli. Crescents in >25% of glomeruli.	C0 C1 C2

B. Treatment

I. General guidelines

1. Immunosuppressive therapy should not be employed for:
   a. Patients who are at low risk of developing progressive kidney disease:
      - Asymptomatic microscopic hematuria.
      - Recurrent gross hematuria.
      - Proteinuria <0.5 g/day/1.73m^2 or UPCR <0.05 g/mmol.

   b. Patients who have progressed to chronic kidney disease (CKD) stages 3–5 where the inexorable progression is assessed to be irreversible.
2. Supportive therapy of IgA nephropathy to retard the progression of chronic kidney disease should be instituted, especially strict control of blood pressure.
   a. Renin-angiotensin system blockers (RASBs):
      i. Angiotensin-converting enzyme inhibitors (ACEi) and angiotensin-receptor blockers (ARB) should be used for the control of blood pressure (BP) and proteinuria.
      ii. In children, expert opinion suggests a favorable outcome when time-averaged proteinuria is reduced to <0.5 g/day/1.73m^2 or urine protein:creatinine ratio (UPCR) <0.05 g/mmol.
      iii. Consider using ACEi and ARB in combination if the proteinuria goal of <0.5 g/day/1.73m^2 or UPCR <0.05 g/mmol is not reached with monotherapy at the maximum recommended dose.
         - Use with caution as combination therapy is associated with increased risk of AKI and hyperkalemia if the patient is hypovolemic.

   b. Fish oil: Eicosapentaenoic acid (EPA) and docosahexanoic acid (DHA)
      i. There is no clear evidence that fish oil improves outcomes in IgA nephropathy.
      ii. Used as adjunctive therapy in patients with mild disease, in conjunction with ACEi and ARB.
      iii. Dose: 3 g/day.
      iv. Side effects: Mild gastrointestinal intolerance.

c. Statins:
   - Statin therapy should be introduced in patients with low-density lipoprotein (LDL)-cholesterol >3.36 mmol/L.

II. Patients with severe disease

1. Indications for immunosuppressive therapy:
   a. Proteinuria ≥1 g/day/1.73m^2 or UPCR ≥0.1 g/mmol (including nephrotic syndrome with poorly selective proteinuria).
   b. Acute worsening of kidney function not due to acute tubular necrosis.
   c. Presence of crescents on kidney biopsy and histologic evidence of active inflammation (e.g., proliferative or necrotizing glomerular changes).
   d. Patients with an acute onset of nephrotic syndrome and diffuse foot process fusion on kidney biopsy are treated as if they have minimal change disease.
2. Multi-targeted immunosuppressive protocol:
   a. Corticosteroids:
      i. Intravenous monthly pulse methylprednisolone 10–30 mg/kg/dose (maximum 1 g) for 3 days up to a maximum of 6 courses.
      ii. Following pulse methylprednisolone course, oral prednisolone is started at 0.5–1.0 mg/kg (maximum 30 mg) daily. This is tapered by 5 mg/day on a monthly basis following each methylprednisolone pulse.
      iii. Pulse therapy is discontinued when:
         - Proteinuria decreases to <0.3 g/day/1.73m^2 or UPCR <0.03 g/mmol AND
         - Recovery of kidney function occurs.
      iv. Tapering of oral prednisolone therapy should be continued monthly over 6–12 months and can be changed to alternate day therapy once proteinuria decreases to <1 g/day/1.73m^2 or UPCR <0.1 g/mmol.
      v. Alternatively, daily oral prednisolone at 1–2 mg/kg (maximum 60 mg/day) can be used as an initiation therapy for 3 months.

b. Mycophenolate mofetil (MMF):
   i. MMF may be started at the time of steroid therapy, except in patients with nephrotic syndrome (minor abnormalities on histology) with highly selective proteinuria and no hematuria.
   ii. MMF Dose: 600 mg/m^2/dose 12 hourly (15–23 mg/kg/dose 12 hourly). Maximum dose: 1 g 12 hourly.
   iii. Monitor full blood count (FBC) monthly.
      - Omit if absolute neutrophil count $<1.5 \times 10^9$/L.
   iv. Consider monitoring serum mycophenolate (MPA) levels if necessary (target 2–4 mg/L).
   v. Estimation of MPA area under the time-concentration curve (AUC):
      - Target MPA AUC 30–60 mg*h/L.
   vi. In view of gastrointestinal side effects, start famotidine prophylactically at 0.5–1 mg/kg/day once nightly or divided dose 12 hourly (maximum 40 mg), or rabeprazole 0.5–1.0 mg/kg once nightly or divided dose 12 hourly (maximum 40 mg).
   vii. Consider changing to Myfortic® if gastrointestinal side effects persist.
   Myfortic®: 180 mg = 250 mg (dose equivalent of Cellcept®).
   360 mg = 500 mg (dose equivalent of Cellcept®).

c. Agents to reduce proteinuria
   i. Calcineurin inhibitors (either cyclosporine or tacrolimus) may be added in patients with persistent proteinuria in the nephrotic range.
   ii. Angiotensin-converting enzyme inhibitors (ACEi) and angiotensin receptor blockers (ARB).

3. High-dose intravenous cyclophosphamide protocol:

a. Corticosteroids:
   i. Intravenous pulse methylprednisolone 10 mg/kg/dose (maximum 1 g) for 3 days.
   ii. Oral prednisolone starting at 0.5–1.0 mg/kg (maximum 60 mg) daily after the methylprednisolone pulse, and tapering by 5 mg/day on a monthly basis depending on disease activity, and subsequently tapering to a minimal amount necessary to control the disease.

b. IV cyclophosphamide 500–1000 mg/m^2 monthly for 6 doses followed by:
   i. 3-monthly IV cyclophosphamide for 24 months OR
   ii. Oral azathioprine 2 mg/kg daily OR
   iii. Oral MMF 600 mg/m^2/dose 12 hourly (maximum dose 1 g 12 hourly).

III. Patients with mild to moderate proteinuria

1. There is moderate quality evidence suggesting a favorable outcome when time-averaged proteinuria is reduced to <1 g/day in adults.
   - In children, expert opinion suggests a goal of <0.5 g/day/1.73m^2 or UPCR <0.05 g/mmol.
2. Start ACEi or ARB when proteinuria >0.3 g/day/1.73m^2 or UPCR >0.02 g/mmol.
3. Immunosuppression:
   a. Consider using immunosuppression in patients with persistent proteinuria >0.5 g/day/1.73m^2 or UPCR >0.05 g/mmol despite 3–6 months of optimized supportive care.
   b. Trial of corticosteroids and/or MMF for 6–12 months.

IV. Patients with recurrent gross hematuria

1. Patients with only recurrent gross hematuria, without proteinuria, may be treated conservatively.
2. Close monitoring for proteinuria should be performed 6 monthly or after recurrence of gross hematuria.
3. There is insufficient evidence to recommend tonsillectomy for the treatment of recurrent gross hematuria.

V. Patients with CKD stage G2–G4

1. ACEi and ARB are used to delay the progression of kidney disease.
2. Consider Sodium-glucose-cotransporter-2 (SGLT2) inhibitors in emerging adults to delay the progression of kidney disease.

3. Start adjunctive therapy for patients with CKD stage G2–G4, including:
    a. Control blood pressure.
    b. Control each component of the metabolic syndrome.
    c. Control fluid intake.
    d. Salt restriction and diuretic therapy.
    e. Consideration of aldosterone antagonist for anti-fibrotic effect and reduction of proteinuria when used in combination with ACEi or ARB.
    f. Avoidance of smoking.
    g. Consideration of allopurinol or febuxostat to decrease pro-inflammatory effect of hyperuricemia.
    h. Avoidance of nephrotoxic agents including non-steroidal anti-inflammatory drugs.
    i. Avoidance of prolonged severe hypokalemia.
    j. Avoidance of phosphate cathartics.
    k. Treat vitamin D deficiency.
    l. Treat mineral bone disease and control hyperphosphatemia.

VI. Algorithm

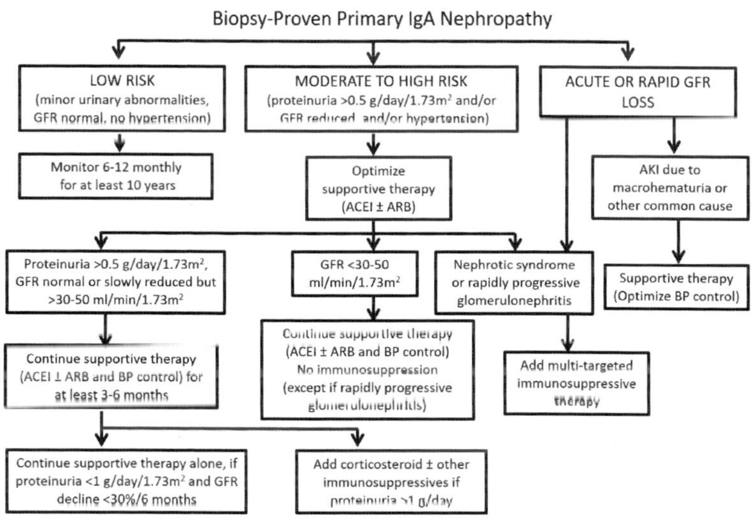

Recommended Reading

1. Hogg RJ. (2010) Idiopathic immunoglobulin A nephropathy in children and adolescents. *Pediatr Nephrol* **25**:823–829.
2. Floege J, Eitner F. (2011) Current therapy for IgA nephropathy. *J Am Soc Nephrol* **22**:1785–1794.
3. Cattran DC, Appel GB, Hunder G. (2021, updated) Treatment and prognosis of IgA nephropathy. Edited by Glassock RJ, Fervenza FC, Forman JP. *UpToDate ONLINE*. http://www.uptodate.com.
4. Trimarchi H, Barratt J, Cattran DC, Cook HT, Coppo R, Haas M, Liu ZH, Roberts IS, Yuzawa Y, Zhang H, Feehally J; IgAN Classification Working Group of the International IgA Nephropathy Network and the Renal Pathology Society, Conference Participants. (2017) Oxford classification of IgA nephropathy 2016: An update from the IgA Nephropathy classification working group. *Kidney Int* **91**:1014–1021.
5. Natale P, Palmer SC, Ruospo M, Saglimbene VM, Craig JC, Vecchio M, Samuels JA, Molony DA, Schena FP, Strippoli GF. (2020) Immunosuppressive agents for treating IgA nephropathy. *Cochrane Database Syst Rev* **3**:CD003965. doi: 10.1002/14651858.CD003965.pub3.

8 Management of IgA Vasculitis Nephritis

Resontoc LP and Yap HK

A. Diagnostic Approach

I. Clinical presentation:

1. The 2010 European League Against Rheumatism (EULAR), Pediatric Rheumatology International Trials (PRINTO) and Pediatric Rheumatology European Society (PReS) consensus criteria for the classification of Henoch–Schönlein purpura, now known as IgA vasculitis (IgAV) (2012 Revised International Chapel Hill Consensus Conference Nomenclature of Vasculitides) include the following:
   a. Palpable purpura (mandatory).
      - Typically over the extensor surfaces of the lower limbs and buttocks.
      - Can also involve the arms, face and ears but usually spares the trunk.
        (Note: Absence of rash at presentation does not rule out IgAVN, as the rash may be evolving.)

      + AT LEAST 1 of the following 4 features:

   b. Diffuse abdominal pain.
   c. Arthritis (acute) or arthralgia.
      - Usually affects the large joints of the lower limbs.
   d. Kidney involvement (any haematuria and/or proteinuria).
   e. Any biopsy showing predominant IgA deposition.
2. Other manifestations include:
   a. Gastrointestinal: Vomiting, gastrointestinal hemorrhage, intussusception, ischemic bowel.
   b. Neurological: Nonspecific headache, subtle encephalopathy, seizures.

   c. Pulmonary (rare and severe): Diffuse alveolar hemorrhage.
   d. Genitourinary: Orchitis.
3. Specific renal manifestations and clinical prognostication:

Initial Renal Symptoms	Progression to Chronic Kidney Disease (%)
Nephrotic-nephritic syndrome	>50
Nephrotic syndrome	40
Nephritic syndrome	15
Heavy non-nephrotic proteinuria	15
Hematuria and/or minimal proteinuria	<5
Severely impaired glomerular filtration rate	Relative risk of progression = 3.83

II. Investigations:

1. Urinalysis:
   a. Urine microscopy to look for red blood cells RBCs, leukocytes and casts.
   b. Phase contrast study on fresh urine specimens to look for dysmorphic red blood cells (>30% indicates glomerular origin).
   c. Urine protein:creatinine ratio (UPCR) or a 24-hour urine protein excretion.
2. Blood investigations:
   a. Full blood count.
   b. Erythrocyte sedimentation rate.
   c. Urea, creatinine, sodium, potassium, chloride, bicarbonate.
   d. Calcium, phosphate, alkaline phosphatase.
   e. Uric acid.
   f. Liver function test: Total protein, albumin, alanine aminotransaminase (ALT), aspartate aminotransferase (AST), and bilirubin.
   g. Serum IgA.
3. Ultrasonography of the abdomen:
   - Exclude intussusception in a patient with severe abdominal pain ± bloody stools.

4. Specialized investigations to exclude other causes of leukocytoclastic vasculitis and systemic lupus erythematosus, especially if the presentation is atypical or severe:
   a. Blood investigations:
      i. Serum complements C3 and C4.
      ii. Anti-nuclear antibodies or anti-double stranded DNA antibody.
      iii. Anti-streptolysin O titer (ASOT) and/or anti-DNAase B titer and/or streptozyme test (ASOT, anti-DNAase B, anti-hyaluronidase).
      iv. Anti-neutrophil cytoplasmic antibodies (ANCA).
         - Anti-myeloperoxidase antibody.
         - Anti-proteinase C antibody.
   b. Skin biopsy of purpuric lesion for IgA deposits on immunofluorescence.

III. Kidney biopsy:

1. Indications:
   a. If confirmation of the diagnosis is required.
   b. If considering starting immunosuppressive therapy:
      i. Persistent proteinuria ≥1 g/day/1.73m^2 or UPCR ≥0.1 g/mmol.
      ii. Decreased glomerular filtration rate (GFR).
      iii. Nephritic and/or nephrotic syndrome.
      iv. Acute worsening of kidney function, to distinguish acute tubular necrosis from crescentic disease.
2. International Study of Kidney Disease in Children (ISKDC) Classification:
   - Based primarily on the presence and number of crescents.

Grade	Histology
Group I	Minimal changes
Group II	Pure mesangial proliferation without crescents
Group III	Mesangial proliferative glomerulonephritis with $<50\%$ crescents IIIa. Focal IIIb. Diffuse

(Continued)

(*Continued*)

Grade	Histology
Group IV	Mesangial proliferative glomerulonephritis with 50–75% crescents IVa. Focal IVb. Diffuse
Group V	Mesangial proliferative glomerulonephritis with >75% crescents Va. Focal Vb. Diffuse
Group VI	Membranoproliferative (mesangiocapillary) glomerulonephritis

B. Treatment

I. General guidelines:

1. Immunosuppressive therapy should not be employed for:
   a. Prevention of the development of kidney disease.
   b. Patients who are at low risk of developing progressive kidney disease:
      - Asymptomatic microscopic hematuria.
      - Proteinuria <0.3 g/day/1.73m^2.
   c. Patients who have progressed to chronic kidney disease (CKD) stages 3–5 where the inexorable progression is assessed to be irreversible.
2. Supportive therapy to retard the progression of CKD should be instituted in particular, strict control of blood pressure.
3. Caution should be exercised in the use of non-steroidal anti-inflammatory drugs (NSAIDs) for the treatment of arthralgia/arthritis.
4. Outcome is favorable when time-averaged proteinuria is reduced to:
   - <1 g/day in adults (moderate quality evidence).
   - <0.5 g/day/1.73m^2 in children (expert opinion).

II. Definition of the severity of IgAVN in accordance with SHARE (Single Hub and Access Point for Pediatric Rheumatology in Europe) recommendations:

Severity of IgAVN	Definition
Mild	Normal GFR and mild (UPCR <0.1 g/mmol) or moderate proteinuria (UPCR 0.1–0.25 g/mmol)
Moderate	<50% crescents on kidney biopsy, and impaired GFR (<80 ml/min/1.73m^2) or severe persistent proteinuria (>0.25 g/mmol for at least 4 weeks)
Severe	>50% crescents on kidney biopsy, and impaired GFR (<80 ml/min/1.73m^2) or severe persistent proteinuria (>0.25 g/mmol for at least 4 weeks)
Persistent proteinuria	UPCR >0.25 g/mmol for 4 weeks UPCR >0.1 g/mmol for 3 months UPCR >0.05 g/mmol for 6 months

III. Patients with severe disease:

1. Immunosuppressive therapy is indicated in patients who present with:
   a. Nephritic-nephrotic syndrome.
   b. Acute worsening of kidney function not due to acute tubular necrosis.
   c. Presence of crescents on kidney biopsy.
2. Multi-targeted immunosuppressive protocol:
   a. Glucocorticoids (GC):
      i. Intravenous monthly pulse methylprednisolone (MP) 10–30 mg/kg/dose or 1 g/1.73 m^2 (maximum 1 g) for 3 days up to a maximum of 6 courses.
      ii. Following pulse MP course, oral prednisolone is started at 0.5–1.0 mg/kg or 20–30 mg/m^2 (maximum 30 mg) daily.
         - This is tapered by 5 mg/day on a monthly basis following each methylprednisolone pulse.
      iii. Pulse therapy is discontinued when:
         - Proteinuria decreases to <0.3 g/day/1.73m^2 and
         - Recovery of kidney function occurs.

iv. Tapering of oral prednisolone therapy should be continued monthly over 6–12 months and can be changed to alternate day therapy once proteinuria decreases to <1 g/day/1.73m^2.
v. Alternatively, daily oral prednisolone at 1–2 mg/kg or 40–60 mg/m^2 (maximum 60 mg/day) can be used as initiation therapy for 3 months.

b. Mycophenolate mofetil (MMF):
   i. MMF should be started at the time of steroid therapy.
   ii. MMF dose: 600 mg/m^2/dose 12 hourly (15–23 mg/kg/dose 12 hourly). Maximum dose: 1 g 12 hourly.
   iii. Monitor full blood count monthly.
      - Omit if absolute neutrophil count <1.5 × 10^9/L.
   iv. Serum mycophenolate (MPA) levels when side effects present.
      - Trough levels range from 2–4 mg/L.
   v. Estimation of MPA area under the time–concentration curve (AUC):
      - Target MPA AUC 30–60 mg*h/L.
   vi. Due to gastrointestinal side effects, start famotidine prophylactically at 0.5–1 mg/kg/day once nightly or a divided dose 12 hourly (maximum 40 mg), or rabeprazole 0.5–1.0 mg/kg once nightly or a divided dose 12 hourly (maximum 40 mg).
   vii. Consider changing to Myfortic® if gastrointestinal side effects persist.
   Myfortic®: 180 mg = 250 mg (dose equivalent of Cellcept®).
   360 mg = 500 mg (dose equivalent of Cellcept®).

c. Agents to reduce proteinuria:
   i. Calcineurin inhibitors may be added in patients with persistent proteinuria in the nephrotic range:
      - Cyclosporine (CsA): 3–5 mg/kg/day targeting trough levels of 150–200 μg/L.
      - Tacrolimus (Tac): 0.2 mg/kg/day in 2 divided doses to achieve whole blood trough Tac levels of 8–10 μg/L.
   ii. Angiotensin-converting enzyme inhibitors (ACEi) and angiotensin receptor blockers (ARB).

3. High-dose intravenous cyclophosphamide (CYC) protocol:
   a. GC:
      i. Intravenous pulse MP 10 mg/kg/dose (maximum 1 g) for 3 days.

ii. Oral prednisolone starting at 0.5–1.0 mg/kg (maximum 60 mg) daily after the MP pulse, and tapering by 5 mg/day on a monthly basis depending on disease activity, and subsequently tapering to a minimal amount necessary to control the disease.

b. IV CYC 500–1000 mg/m^2 monthly for 6 doses followed by:
   i. Oral azathioprine (AZA) 2 mg/kg once daily, OR
   ii. Oral MPA 600 mg/m^2/dose 12 hourly (maximum dose 1 g 12 hourly).

IV. Patients with mild to moderate proteinuria:

1. ACEI and/or ARB (see chapter "Adjunctive Therapy in Glomerular Disease").
2. Immunosuppression:
   a. Consider using immunosuppressive drugs in patients with the following features:
      - Proteinuria ≥1g/day/1.73m^2 or UPCR >0.1 g/mmol at presentation.
      - Nephrotic syndrome.
      - Persistent proteinuria between 0.5 and <1 g/day/1.73m^2 or UPCR >0.05 g/mmol despite 3–6 months of optimized supportive care.

      ESPECIALLY if one of the following are present:
      - Severe abdominal pain.
      - Recurrent rash.
      - Recurrent gross hematuria.
   b. GC ± MMF as a steroid-sparing agent for 3–6 months.
      i. Oral prednisolone 1–2 mg/kg/day in divided doses for at least 2 weeks until the rashes and abdominal pain resolve, before decreasing to a daily dose.
      ii. Dose should be gradually tapered by 5 mg/day every 2 weeks, depending on daily urine dipstick results.
      iii. Dose can be changed to alternate day therapy once proteinuria decreases to <0.3 g/day/1.73m^2 or UPCR ≤0.02 g/mmol and subsequently tapered off.
      iv. MMF can be added at 600 mg/m^2/dose 12 hourly as a steroid-sparing agent.

V. Patients with persistent isolated microscopic hematuria OR systemic manifestations without nephritis:

1. There is moderate quality evidence to recommend that corticosteroids not be given at presentation if there is no evidence of nephritis, since they do not appear to influence the development of persistent kidney involvement.
2. Non-steroidal anti-inflammatory agents (NSAIDs) and/or paracetamol:
   a. Indications:
      - Arthralgia and/or acute arthritis in the absence of nephritis, or with microscopic hematuria as the only manifestation of IgAVN.
      - Diffuse abdominal pain.

   b. Contraindicated in the presence of active gastrointestinal bleeding.
   c. Ensure adequate hydration (oral fluid intake) when giving NSAIDs.
3. GC may be given in the following situations:
   a. Severe abdominal pain: Intravenous hydrocortisone converting to oral prednisolone once the pain has resolved.
   b. Joint pains severe enough to limit ambulation or activities of daily living.
   c. Recurrent arthritis.
   d. Recurrent purpura.
   e. Orchitis.
   f. Cerebral vasculitis.
   g. Pulmonary hemorrhage.
   h. Persistent hematuria.
   i. Other severe organ or life-threatening vasculitis manifestations.

VI. Algorithm for management of IgA vasculitis nephritis

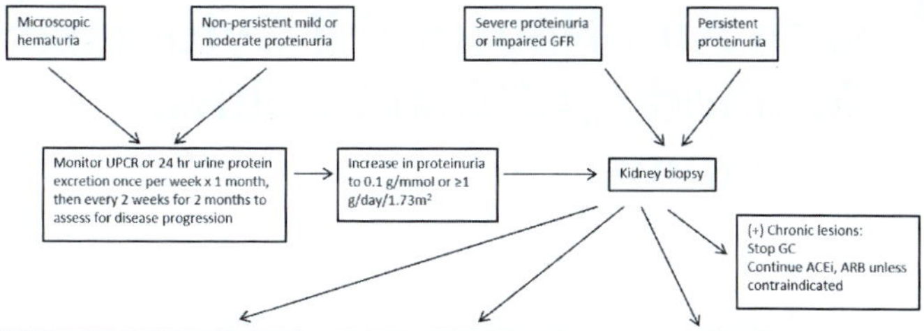

Treatment	Mild nephritis	Moderate nephritis	Severe nephritis
First line	• GC	• Oral GC and/or IV MP + MMF or AZA or IV CYC	• IV MP and oral GC + MMF ± CsA or Tac if eGFR >60 ml/min/1.73m² OR • IV MP and oral GC + IV CYC
Second line (if response is not satisfactory)	• Add IV MP or AZA or MMF or CsA	• Add CsA or Tac if eGFR >60 ml/min/1.73m²	• If poor response to IV CYC protocol, switch to IV MP and oral GC + MMF ± CsA or Tac
+ ACEi and/or ARB			

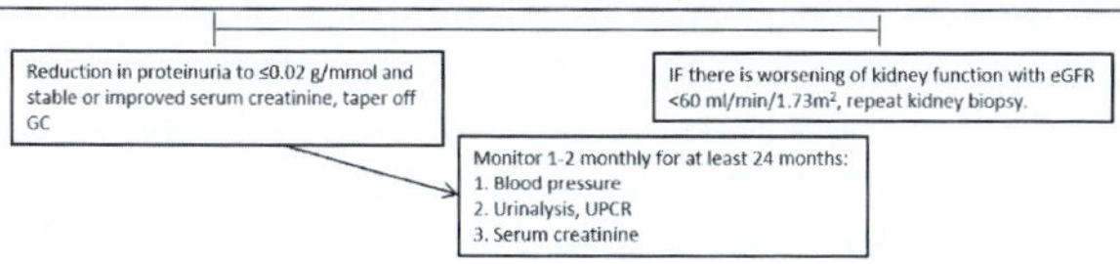

Recommended Reading

1. Davin JC. (2011) Henoch-Schönlein purpura nephritis: Pathophysiology, treatment, and future strategy. *Clin J Am Soc Nephrol* **6**:679–689.
2. Kidney Disease: Improving Global Outcomes (KDIGO) Glomerulonephritis Work Group. (2012) KDIGO clinical practice guideline for glomerulonephritis. *Kidney Int Suppl* **2**:218–221.
3. Kidney Disease: Improving Global Outcomes (KDIGO) Glomerulonephritis Work Group. (2018) KDIGO GN Guideline update — Evidence summary. IgA nephropathy and IgA vasculitis — Henoch-schönlein purpura (HSP) nephritis.
4. Ozen S, Marks SD, Brogan P, Groot N, de Graeff N, Avcin T, Bader-Meunier B, Dolezalova P, Feldman BM, Kone-Paut I, Lahdenne P, McCann L, Pilkington C, Ravelli A, van Royen A, Uziel Y, Vastert B, Wulffraat N, Kamphuis S, Beresford MW. (2019) European consensus-based recommendations for diagnosis and treatment of immunoglobulin A vasculitis-the SHARE initiative. *Rheumatology (Oxford)* **58**:1607–1616.
5. Dedeoglu F, Kim S. (2019, updated) IgA vasculitis (Henoch-Schönlein purpura): Clinical manifestations and diagnosis. Edited by: Sundel R, TePas E. *UpToDate ONLINE.* http://www.uptodateonline.com.

9 Glomerulonephritis Associated with Anti-Neutrophil Cytoplasmic Antibody (ANCA) Positive Vasculitis

Aragon EE, Resontoc LP, Koh CT and Yap HK

A. Definition

1. ANCA-positive vasculitis (AAV): Heterogeneous group of autoimmune conditions characterized by necrotizing inflammation of the small to medium vessels in association with autoantibodies against the cytoplasmic region of the neutrophil, namely, proteinase 3 (PR3) in cytoplasmic pattern (cANCA), and myeloperoxidase (MPO) in perinuclear pattern (pANCA).
2. Includes 3 main diseases (Chapel Hill Consensus Conference 2012):
   a. Granulomatosis with polyangiitis (GPA).
   b. Microscopic polyangiitis (MPA).
   c. Eosinophilic granulomatosis with polyangiitis (EGPA)
      - No reported renal involvement in children.
3. Renal-limited vasculitis (RLV) is considered part of the GPA/MPA spectrum with similar histopawthologic findings as approximately 80% is ANCA-positive, predominantly MPO.

B. Approach to Diagnosis

I. Kidney manifestations in AAV:

1. Kidney involvement is more common and severe at presentation in pediatric MPA (75–90%) as compared to GPA (75%).
2. Clinical presentation:

a. Acute glomerulonephritis to rapidly progressive glomerulonephritis spectrum with hematuria, hypertension and edema associated with a rapidly rising serum creatinine.
b. Significant proteinuria and nephrotic range proteinuria.
c. Recurrent asymptomatic hematuria.

II. Look for extrarenal manifestations that may suggest a systemic vasculitic syndrome:

1. GPA:
   a. Constitutional symptoms such as fever, malaise, anorexia, and weight loss heralding other symptoms are common in children.
   b. Upper airway involvement (70–100%):
      - Chronic or recurrent purulent or bloody nasal discharge or crusting.
      - Recurrent epistaxis.
      - Nasal septum perforation or saddle nose deformity.
      - Chronic or recurrent sinus inflammation.
   c. Laryngotracheobronchial involvement (50%):
      - Subglottic, tracheal or bronchial stenosis presenting as hoarseness or stridor.
   d. Pulmonary involvement (80%):
      - Dyspnea, chronic cough, and hemoptysis.
      - Chest X-Ray or computerized tomography (CT) scan showing nodules, cavities or fixed infiltrates.
      - Pulmonary hemorrhage.
   e. Ocular symptoms (37–53%):
      - Proptosis.
      - Conjunctivitis.
      - Episcleritis.
      - Uveitis.
   f. Cutaneous symptoms (35–53%):
      - Palpable purpura.
      - Petechiae.
      - Nodules.
   g. Musculoskeletal (57%)

- Arthralgia.
- Myalgia.
- Arthritis.

h. Gastrointestinal (42%):
- Chronic nausea.
- Diarrhea.
- Non-specific abdominal pain.

i. Neurologic (3.5–25%):
- Headache.
- Dizziness.
- Acute mononeuritis.
- Cerebellar involvement.
- Seizures.
- Upper motor neuron signs.

2. MPA:

a. Constitutional symptoms such as fever, malaise and weight loss.

b. Upper airway involvement (3–10.5%):

c. Pulmonary involvement (26–62%):
- Chronic cough.
- Hemoptysis.
- Nodules.
- Pulmonary hemorrhage/capillaritis.
- Pulmonary infiltrates.

d. Ocular symptoms (5–31%):
- Scleritis.
- Conjunctivitis.

e. Cutaneous symptoms (35–53%):
- Purpuric rash.
- Necrotizing vasculitis.
- Lesions that mimic pyoderma gangrenosum.

f. Musculoskeletal (10–52%):
- Arthralgia.
- Myalgia.
- Arthritis.

g. Gastrointestinal (9–58%):

h. Neurologic (5–21%):

- Headache.
- Seizures.
- Optic neuritis.
- Peripheral neuropathy.

III. Steps in investigation:

1. Confirm the presence of glomerulonephritis:
   a. Urine microscopy and red cell morphology.
   b. Urine protein:creatinine ratio or a 24-hour urine protein excretion.
   c. Renal function test:
      - Urea, creatinine, sodium, potassium, chloride, bicarbonate, calcium, phosphate, and uric acid.
      - Creatinine clearance.
      - Estimated glomerular filtration rate (eGFR).
2. Determine the cause of the vasculitis:
   a. Serum complements C3 and C4.
   b. Serum immunoglobulins including IgG, IgM, IgA, and IgE.
   c. Antinuclear antibodies (ANA).
   d. Anti-double-stranded (ds) DNA antibody.
   e. ANCA:

	PR3-ANCA	MPO-ANCA	Other
GPA	75%	20%	5% ANCA negative
MPA	30%	60%	10% ANCA negative
RLV	10%	80%	10% ANCA negative

   f. Anti-glomerular basement membrane (GBM) antibody.
      - 5–14% of patients with AAV, primarily MPA, have circulating anti-GBM antibody.
   g. Anti-phospholipid antibody screen:
      - Prothrombin time (PT).
      - Partial thromboplastin time (aPTT).
      - Lupus anticoagulant.
      - Anti-cardiolipin IgG and IgM.
      - Anti β2 glycoprotein-1 IgG and IgM.
   h. Anti-ENA (extractable nuclear antigens) panel.
   i. Rheumatoid factor (if nephritis or interstitial lung disease).

3. Kidney biopsy is the gold standard for the diagnosis of AAV-associated glomerulonephritis:
   a. Should be done early in patients with kidney involvement.
   b. Characteristic pauci-immune crescentic necrotizing glomerulonephritis.
   c. Light microscopy:
      - Acute lesions: Glomerular crescents or tubular intraepithelial infiltrates.
      - Chronic inflammation: Glomerulosclerosis, interstitial fibrosis or tubular atrophy.
      - Arteritis is occasionally seen.
      - Patients with GPA, but not MPA, may have granulomatous changes.
      - Glomerulosclerosis is more prominent in MPA whereas GPA has a greater proportion of normal glomeruli.
   d. Electron microscopy:
      - Subendothelial edema.
      - Microthrombi.
      - Degranulation of neutrophils.
   e. Immunofluorescence shows a pauci-immune pattern of immune deposits.
      - Evidence of immune complex deposition is found in 50% of biopsies and is associated with a higher percentage of crescents.
   f. Histopathologic classification:

Class	
Focal	≥50% normal glomeruli
Crescentic	≥50% glomeruli with crescents
Mixed	<50% normal, <50% crescentic, <50% globally sclerotic glomeruli
Sclerotic	≥50% globally sclerotic glomeruli

4. Exclude infectious diseases:
   a. Blood culture.
   b. Anti-streptolysin O antibody titer (ASOT) and/or anti-DNase B.
   c. Mycoplasma serology.
   d. Varicella zoster IgG.

e. Hepatitis B surface (HBs) antigen and anti-HBs antibody.
f. Anti-hepatitis C virus antibody.
g. Human immunodeficiency virus antibody.
h. Parvovirus B19 nucleic acid testing.
i. Epstein–Barr virus, cytomegalovirus, adenovirus, and BK virus nucleic acid testing.
j. Stool or rectal swab for enterovirus nucleic acid testing.
k. Mantoux and/or tuberculosis quantiferon testing.

5. Assess the degree of systemic involvement:
   a. Hematology and acute phase reactants:
      - Full blood count.
      - Erythrocyte sedimentation rate.
      - C-reactive protein.
   b. Basic biochemistry:
      - Liver function test: Total protein, albumin, alanine aminotransaminase (ALT), aspartate aminotransferase (AST), and bilirubin
      - Lactate dehydrogenase.
      - Creatine kinase.
      - Thyroid function test: Free thyroxine (T3 and T4) and thyroid-stimulating hormone (TSH).
      - Amylase and lipase (if there is abdominal pain).
   c. Imaging:
      - X-Ray and/or CT scan and/or magnetic resonance imaging (MRI) of the chest and/or paranasal sinuses.
      - 2D-echocardiography.
      - Cranial MRI/MR angiography.
   d. Others:
      - Ambulatory blood pressure monitoring.
      - Electrocardiogram (ECG).
      - Digital clinical photography of lesions.
      - Nerve conduction studies (if neurological symptoms present).
      - Lung biopsy:

	Histology
GPA	Evidence of vasculitis and necrotizing granuloma formation
MPA	Capillaritis without granuloma formation

6. Exclude malignancy if clinical suspicion:
   a. Lymph node excision biopsy.
   b. Bone marrow analysis.
   c. Positron emission tomography (PET-CT).

C. Assessment of Disease Activity and Damage

1. Pediatric Vasculitis Activity Score (PVAS)
   a. PVAS is scored from 0 to 63, based on the presence or absence of clinical items attributable to active vasculitis after the exclusion of other causes such as infection.
      - A higher PVAS score indicates higher disease activity.
   b. Should be performed at diagnosis and ongoing follow-up to assess disease activity.

1. General	**4. Ear, Nose and Throat**	**7. Abdominal**
Myalgia	Nasal discharge / crusts / ulcers / granuloma	Abdominal pain
Arthralgia or arthritis	Paranasal sinus involvement	Peritonitis
Fever ≥38.0°C	Subglottic stenosis / hoarseness/stridor	Blood in stools or bloody diarrhoea
Weight loss ≥5% body weight	Conductive hearing loss	Bowel ischemia
2. Cutaneous	Sensorineural loss	**8. Renal**
Polymorphous exanthema	**5. Chest**	Hypertension >95th centile (for age, sex and height)
Livedo	Wheeze or expiratory dyspnea	Proteinuria >0.3g/24h; >20 mg/mmol creatinine
Panniculitis	Endobronchial / endotracheal involvement	Hematuria ≥2+ or 5 rbc/hpf or red cell casts
Purpura	Nodules or cavities	eGFR 50–80 ml/min/1.73m^2
Skin nodules	Pleural effusion / pleurisy	eGFR 15–49 ml/min/1.73m^2

(*Continued*)

Infarct (nail edge lesion, splinter hemorrhage)	Infiltrate	eGFR <15 ml/min/1.73m^2
Ulcer (full-thickness necrosis)	Massive hemoptysis / aveolar hemorrhage	Rise in creatinine > 10% or creatinine clearance (eGFR) fall >25%
Gangrene (extensive necrosis)	Respiratory failure	**9. Nervous system**
Other skin vasculitis (specify below)	**6. Cardiovascular**	Headache
3. Mucous Membranes/Eyes	Loss of pulses	Meningitis / encephalitis
Mouth ulcers/ granulomata	Bruits over accessible arteries	Organic confusion / cognitive dysfunction
Genital ulcers	Blood pressure discrepancy	Seizures (not hypertensive)
Adnexal inflammation	Claudication of extremities	Stroke
Significant proptosis	Ischemic cardiac pain	Cord lesion
Rod oye (epi) scleritis	Cardiomyopathy	Cranial nerve palsy
Red eye conjunctivitis / blepharitis/keratitis)	Congestive heart failure	Sensory peripheral neuropathy
Uveitis	Valvular heart disease	Motor mononeuritis multiplex
Blurred vision	Pericarditis	10. Other
Sudden visual loss		Persistent disease only
Retinal vasculitis / retinitis vessel thrombosis / retinal exudates / hemorrhages		

2. Pediatric Vasculitis Damage Index (PVDI)
   a. The PVDI is a standardized clinical assessment tool for damage in pediatric systemic vasculitides: http://www.mypan.org.uk/Training.html.
   b. Validation studies are ongoing.
3. Clinical AAV subgroups modified from the European Vasculitis Study group (EUVAS):

Category	Description
Localized	Upper and/or lower respiratory symptoms without other system involvement or constitutional symptoms.
Early systemic	Disease without threatened organ function or life-threatening disease (also known as "non-organ or life-threatening").
Generalized	Renal or other organ-threatening disease.
Severe	Renal or other organ failure (eGFR <15 ml/min/1.73m^2). Also known as "immediately life threatening".
Refractory	Disease unresponsive to glucocorticoids or cyclophosphamide.

D. Medical Management

I. Definitions:

Outcome of Therapy	Features
Complete remission	• Absence of any clinical manifestations that are deemed secondary to ongoing active vasculitis. • Does **not** mean that all parameters have returned to baseline, because persistent abnormalities may reflect irreversible injury induced during the period of active inflammation.
Partial remission	• Persistence of glomerular hematuria (dysmorphic red blood cells) ± red blood cell casts despite improvement in or stabilization of the serum creatinine and disappearance of extrarenal signs of active disease.

(*Continued*)

Outcome of Therapy	Features
Refractory disease	• Worsening disease or persisting disease activity with limited improvement after a period of appropriate therapy.
Relapse	• Recurrence of signs or symptoms of active vasculitis in any organ system after remission is achieved.

II. Remission induction:

1. Glucocorticoids (GC):
   a. IV Methylprednisolone 10–30 mg/kg (maximum 1 g/day) for 3 consecutive days followed by oral prednisolone.
   b. Oral prednisolone:
      i. 1 mg/kg/day (maximum 30 mg/day) for 1 week
      ii. Then 0.5 mg/kg/day for 1 week
      iii. Then taper by 2.5–5 mg monthly until 0.2 mg/kg/day or 5 mg/day, whichever is the lower by 16 weeks.
2. Cyclophosphamide (CYC):
   a. IV 350–750 mg/m^2 (maximum 1.2 g) monthly (with mesna to prevent hemorrhagic cystitis) for 6 months.
   b. Reduce dose if:
      i. Kidney or hepatic failure.
      ii. Persistent severe lymphopenia/neutropenia.
      iii. Presence of infections.
   c. Alternatively, oral CYC dosing 2–3 mg/kg (maximum 200 mg) once daily for 2–3 months.
3. Rituximab (RTX):
   a. IV 750 mg/m^2/dose IV (maximum 1000 mg), 2 doses 2 weeks apart OR
   b. IV 375 mg/m^2, once a week for 4 weeks.
   c. Considerable removal of RTX with therapeutic plasma exchange (TPE):
      • Hold TPE for 48 hours after RTX.
   d. Superior to CYC for remission-induction in patients with PR3-positive ANCA.

4. Mycophenolate mofetil (MMF):
   a. Dose: 600 mg/m^2 12 hourly (15–23 mg/kg 12 hourly) (maximum dose 1 g 12 hourly).
   b. Target trough level: 1.2–2.4 mg/L.
   c. Start on famotidine 0.5 mg/kg/dose 12 hourly.
      - Renal adjustment dose required if eGFR <50 ml/min/1.73m^2.
   d. Non-inferior to IV CYC in terms of long-term kidney and patient outcomes; however, relapses are more common with MMF.
   e. Consider changing to Myfortic® if gastrointestinal side effects persist.
      - Myfortic®: 180 mg = 250 mg (dose equivalent of Cellcept®)
      - Myfortic®: 360 mg = 500 mg (dose equivalent of Cellcept®)
5. Therapeutic plasma exchange:
   a. Indications:
      i. Diffuse pulmonary hemorrhage.
      ii. Overlap of ANCA vasculitis and anti-GBM disease.
      iii. Consider in severe acute kidney injury where eGFR <30 ml/min/1.73m^2 without significant interstitial fibrosis.
   b. Protocol:
      i. Plasma exchanges: 1.5–2x plasma volume.
      ii. Frequency:
         - Diffuse pulmonary hemorrhage: Daily until bleeding stops, then every other day for a total of 7–10 treatments.
         - Vasculitis in association with anti-GBM antibodies: Daily for 14 days or until anti-GBM antibodies are undetectable.
      iii. Replacement fluid:
         - 5% albumin solution in patients without bleeding or a recent biopsy.
         - Fresh frozen plasma for patients with risk of bleeding and with active hemorrhage.
      iv. Give IV immunoglobulin (IVIG) 0.5 g/kg after 5–10 treatments depending on serum IgG levels.

III. Refractory disease/Failed primary induction therapy/ Major relapse:

1. Exclude alternative diagnoses:
   a. Permanent tissue damage due to a previous injury.
   b. Non-adherence to therapy.
   c. Inadequate initial immunosuppression.
   d. Medication toxicity.
   e. Infection.
   f. Incorrect original diagnosis.
   g. Unresponsive disease manifestations:
      i. Residual orbital pseudotumor (retrobulbar inflammatory masses) with compression symptoms.
      ii. Subglottic stenosis from scarring.
2. Change current disease-modifying anti-rheumatic drugs (DMARD):
   a. Patients resistant to induction with CYC: Treat with Rituximab.
   b. Patients resistant to induction with Rituximab: Treat with CYC.
   c. Patients resistant to induction with CYC and Rituximab: Treat with MPA.
3. Repeat pulse methylprednisolone followed by a higher oral dose of GC:
   a. IV Methylprednisolone 10–30 mg/kg (maximum 1 g/day) for 3 consecutive days followed by oral prednisolone.
   b. Oral prednisolone:
      - Increase prednisolone to 1 mg/kg/day (maximum 60 mg/day), gradually reducing to 0.25 mg/kg/day by 4 weeks, further tapering will depend on the clinical situation then.
4. Consider biological agents in select cases to induce remission:
   - C5a receptor inhibitor (Avacopan) is currently undergoing clinical trials.

IV. Remission maintenance:

1. Glucocorticoids (GC):
   a. Aim to wean prednisolone to alternate-day dosing.
   b. Consider discontinuing prednisolone if stable.

2. Azathioprine (AZA):
   a. Dose: 0.5–2.5 mg/kg once daily PO for 1 year or more (maximum 200 mg).
      - Start at 0.5 mg/kg/day (maximum 50 mg) for 1 week and gradually increase the dose after 1 week if it is tolerated well.
   b. Start at least 14 days after the last CYC dose.
   c. Monitor:
      i. Full blood count 2 weekly for the first month then monthly for the first year.
         - Omit if absolute neutrophil count $<1.5 \times 10^9$/L.
      ii. Liver function test monthly for the first year.
   d. Consider genotyping thiopurine methyltransferase (TPMT) and nucleoside diphosphate linked moiety X-type motif 15 (NUDT15) first before starting AZA, as these 2 genes encode enzymes involved in AZA metabolism.
3. Mycophenolate mofetil (MMF):
   a. Dose: 600 mg/m^2 12 hourly.
   b. More useful in MPO-ANCA positive patients as PR3-ANCA positive patients tend to have more relapses.
   c. Monitor full blood count monthly.
      - Omit if absolute neutrophil count $<1.5 \times 10^9$/L.
   d. Serum mycophenolate levels when side effects present.
      i. Trough levels range from 2 to 4 mg/L.
      ii. Estimation of mycophenolate area under the time–concentration curve (AUC):
         - Target AUC 30–60 mg*h/L.
4. Rituximab:
   a. IV 375 mg/m^2 (adult 500–1000 mg) every 4–6 months OR
   b. "On-demand" dosing strategy:
      i. Monitor peripheral B lymphocyte (CD19-positive cells) counts and ANCA titers.
      ii. Re-dose when B lymphocytes reconstitute and the ANCA titer becomes positive.
   c. Monitor serum IgG levels monthly for 3 months after RTX dosing:
      - Give IVIG 0.5 g/kg if there is associated hypogammaglobulinemia, especially with recurrent infections.

V. Treatment algorithm:

1. Generalized disease with mild to moderate kidney failure:

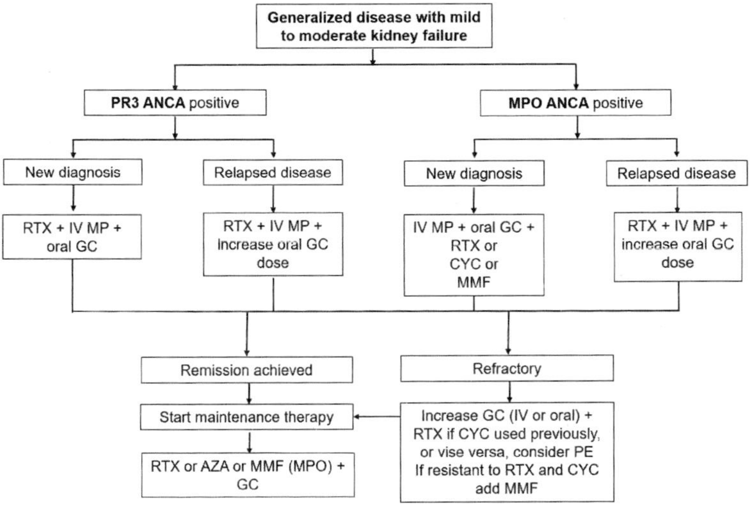

2. Severe kidney failure:

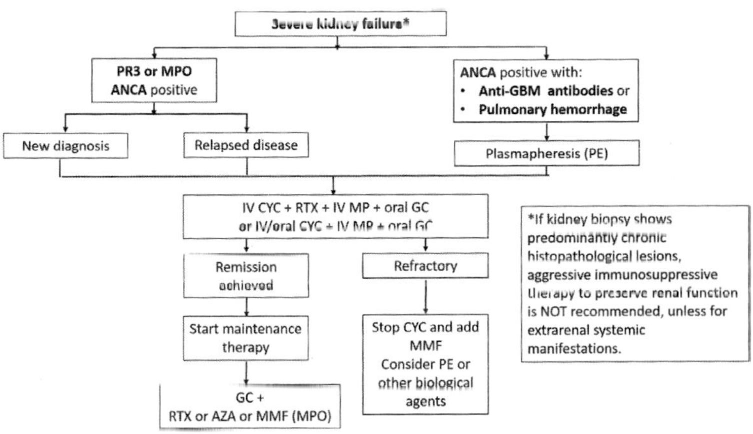

VI. Duration of maintenance therapy:

1. Risk factors for relapse:
   a. Clinical:
      i. GPA (PR3-ANCA disease).
      ii. Lung, upper respiratory tract, and cardiac involvement.
      iii. Preserved kidney function.
      iv. Prior relapses.
   b. Laboratory:
      i. Persistence of ANCA after induction therapy.
      ii. Increase in ANCA titers (more predictive of a renal relapse).
   c. Treatment-related:
      i. Short duration of immunosuppressive treatment.
      ii. Lower cumulative dose of CYC.
      iii. Discontinuation of GC.
      iv. Use of MMF for maintenance therapy.
      v. B-cell reconstitution post-rituximab therapy.
   d. Chronic nasal carriage of *Staphylococcus aureus*.
   e. HLA-DP1*04 allele (PR3-ANCA disease).
2. Maintenance therapy duration:
   a. Patients with MPO-ANCA negative at the end of induction: Careful monitoring without any maintenance therapy.
   b. Patients at low risk of relapse defined as MPO-ANCA seropositive but with no respiratory tract involvement prior to remission: 6–12 months maintenance therapy.
   c. Patients in complete remission: 12–24 months maintenance therapy.
   d. Patients with multiple risk factors for relapse (PR3-ANCA seropositivity, pulmonary involvement, and upper respiratory tract involvement): 24–36 months maintenance therapy.
   e. Patients with ≥1 relapses and/or sustained significant organ damage such as limited residual kidney function: Indefinite maintenance therapy.

VII. Immunization and infection prophylaxis:

1. Vaccination:
   a. Including pneumococcal, influenza, hepatitis B, and COVID-19 vaccines.
   b. Avoid live vaccines during immunosuppressive therapy.
2. Infection prophylaxis during induction therapy and for 6 months after the last dose of rituximab:
   a. *Pneumocystis jirovecii*:
      i. Co-trimoxazole 3 mg/kg on alternate days.
      ii. Dapsone 2 mg/kg daily (maximum 100 mg) for patients who are allergic to co-trimoxazole.
      iii. Aerosolized pentamidine 300 mg monthly (via Respigard nebulizer) if allergic to co-trimoxazole or glucose-6-phosphate dehydrogenase deficient.
   b. Latent tuberculosis:
      i. Isoniazid 10–15 mg/kg (maximum 300 mg) once daily for 6 months OR
      ii. Weekly high dose isoniazid for 12 weeks:
      Aged 2–11 years: 25 mg/kg/dose (maximum 900 mg).
      Aged ≥12 year: 15 mg/kg/dose (maximum 900 mg).
      iii. Pyridoxine: 0.5–1 mg/kg daily (maximum 50 mg).
      Infants: 5–10 mg daily.
      Children and adolescents: 10–50 mg daily

Recommended Reading

1. Dolezalova P, Price-Kuehne FE, Özen S, Benseler SM, Cabral DA, Anton J, Brunner J, Cimaz R, O'Neil KM, Wallace CA, Wilkinson N, Eleftheriou D, Demirkaya E, Böhm M, Krol P, Luqmani RA, Brogan PA. (2013) Disease activity assessment in childhood vasculitis: Development and preliminary validation of the Paediatric Vasculitis Activity Score (PVAS). *Ann Rheum Dis* **72**:1628–1633.
2. Plumb LA, Oni L, Marks SD, Tullus K. (2018) Paediatric anti-neutrophil cytoplasmic antibody (ANCA)-associated vasculitis: An update on renal management. *Pediatr Nephrol* **33**:25–39.
3. Relling MV, Schwab M, Whirl-Carrillo M, Suarez-Kurtz G, Pui CH, Stein CM, Moyer AM, Evans WE, Klein TE, Antillon-Klussmann FG, Caudle KE, Kato M, Yeoh AEJ, Schmiegelow K, Yang JJ. (2019) Clinical pharmacogenetics implementation consortium guideline for thiopurine dosing based on TPMT and NUDT15 genotypes: 2018 update. *Clin Pharmacol Ther* **105**:1095–1105.

4. de Graeff N, Groot N, Brogan P, Ozen S, Avcin T, Bader-Meunier B, Dolezalova P, Feldman BM, Kone-Paut I, Lahdenne P, Marks SD, McCann L, Pilkington C, Ravelli A, van Royen A, Uziel Y, Vastert B, Wulffraat N, Kamphuis S, Beresford MW. (2019) European consensus-based recommendations for the diagnosis and treatment of rare paediatric vasculitides — the SHARE initiative. *Rheumatology (Oxford)* **58**:656–671.
5. Geetha D, Jefferson JA. (2020) ANCA-associated vasculitis: Core curriculum 2020. *Am J Kidney Dis* **75**:124–137.
6. Jariwala M, Laxer RM. (2020) Childhood GPA, EGPA, and MPA. *Clin Immunol* **211**:108325. doi: 10.1016/j.clim.2019.108325.
7. Walsh M, Merkel PA, Peh CA, Szpirt WM, Puéchal X, Fujimoto S, Hawley CM, Khalidi N, Flo mann O, Wald R, Girard LP, Levin A, Gregorini G, Harper L, Clark WF, Pagnoux C, Specks U, Smyth L, Tesar V, Ito-Ihara T, de Zoysa JR, Szczeklik W, Flores-Suárez LF, Carette S, Guillevin L, Pusey CD, Casian AL, Brezina B, Mazzetti A, McAlear CA, Broadhurst E, Reidlinger D, Mehta S, Ives N, Jayne DRW; PEXIVAS Investigators. (2020) Plasma exchange and glucocorticoids in severe ANCA-associated vasculitis. *N Engl J Med* **382**:622–631.
8. Bellos I, Michelakis I, Nikolopoulos D. (2021) The role of plasma exchange in antineutrophil cytoplasmic antibody-associated vasculitis: A meta-analysis. *Clin Rheumatol* **40**:1447–1456.
9. Merkel PA, Kaplan AA, Falk RJ. (2020, updated) Granulomatosis with polyangiitis and microscopic polyangiitis: Induction and maintenance therapy. Edited by Appel GB, Fervanza, FC. *UpToDate ONLINE.* http://www.uptodate.com.
10. Jayne DRW, Merkel PA, Schall TJ, Bekker P; ADVOCATE Study Group. (2021) Avacopan for the treatment of ANCA-associated vasculitis. *N Engl J Med* **384**:599–609.

10 Membranous Nephropathy

Teo S, Resontoc LP, Aragon EE and Yap HK

A. Definition

1. Membranous nephropathy (MN) is immune-mediated and refers to a histologic pattern characterized by the thickening of the glomerular basement membrane (GBM) due to the deposition of subepithelial immune complexes.
2. MN can be classified as:
   a. Primary MN (PMN): When the disease is associated serologically with antibodies to known antigens.
      - Idiopathic MN is a term reserved for when the target antigen is unknown and the disease does not appear to be associated with other systemic disease or potential secondary causes.

   b. Secondary MN: When the disease is associated with other systemic illnesses or exposure.

B. Etiology

1. PMN:
   a. May have autoantibodies to podocyte antigens:
      i. M-type phospholipase A2 receptors (PLA2R).
         - PLA2R-associated MN. Either positive immunofluorescence staining for PLA2R antigen on kidney biopsy or detectable anti-PLA2R antibodies.

      ii. Thrombospondin type-1 domain-containing 7A (THSD7A).
         - Several reports of concurrent malignancy and THSD7A-associated MN in which the cancer tissues overexpress THSD7A.

   iii. Neural epidermal growth factor-like 1 (NELL 1).
   iv. Semaphorin-3B (SEMA3B).
   v. Protocadherin 7 (PCDH7).
  b. Negative serologies do not exclude PMN, as up to 20% of cases may be seronegative at presentation.

2. Secondary MN:
  a. Autoimmune diseases:
   i. Lupus nephritis (ISN/RPS Class V).
   ii. Autoimmune thyroiditis.
   iii. Mixed connective tissue disease.
  b. Alloimmune MN:
   i. Cationic bovine serum albumin (BSA).
   ii. Neural endopeptidase (NEP): Placental transmission from genetically deficient mothers who have been alloimmunized during a miscarriage.
   iii. Hematopoietic stem-cell transplant.
   iv. Post kidney transplantation.
    - *De novo* MN.
  c. Infections:
   i. Hepatitis B virus (HBV).
   ii. Hepatitis C virus (HCV).
   iii. Epstein–Barr virus (EBV).
   iv. Cytomegalovirus (CMV).
   v. Varicella zoster virus (VZV).
   vi. Syphilis (secondary or congenital).
   vii. Tuberculosis.
   viii. Malaria.
   ix. Schistosomiasis.
  d. Medications:
   i. Captopril.
   ii. Clopidogrel.
   iii. Penicillamine.
   iv. Non-steroidal anti-inflammatory drugs (NSAIDs).
   v. Lithium.
   vi. Mercury.
  e. Malignancy
   i. Solid tumors — bladder, breast.
   ii. Hematologic — lymphoma, chronic lymphocytic leukemia.

C. Natural History

1. A common cause of nephrotic syndrome in adults but is less frequent in children.
   a. Accounts for less than 5% of all pediatric nephrotic syndrome cases.
   b. Secondary causes tend to be more common in children (35–75%) compared to adults (25%).
2. Spontaneous complete remission is seen in up to 20% of patients with PMN and partial remission is seen in up to 15–20%.
   a. Mean time to remission is 14.7 ± 11.4 months from presentation.
   b. Children with MN have a much higher rate of spontaneous remission and almost always have normal kidney function compared to adults.
   c. Risk factors for progressive decline in kidney function:
      - Older age of onset.
      - Male gender.
      - Persistent heavy proteinuria.
      - Elevated serum creatinine at diagnosis.

D. Approach to Diagnosis

I. Establish the diagnosis of membranous nephropathy:

1. Clinical presentation:
   a. Varying degrees of proteinuria, ranging from asymptomatic proteinuria to nephrotic syndrome.
      - Nephrotic patients tend to be steroid-resistant.
   b. Microscopic hematuria.
   c. Hypertension.
2. Findings on kidney biopsy:
   a. Light microscopy (LM):
      i. Diffusely thickened glomerular basement membrane (GBM) throughout all glomeruli.
      ii. Early stages may have no alterations visible by light microscopy.
      iii. "Spike" appearance on Jones silver stain resulting from projections of the basement membrane matrix as a reaction to deposits.

b. Immunofluorescence (IMF):
   - Diffuse granular staining for IgG and complement 3 along the capillary wall.

c. Electron microscopy (EM):
   - Finely granular, electron-dense deposits along the subepithelial surface of the glomerular capillary wall between podocyte foot processes.

d. Histological differences between PMN and secondary MN:

Histopathology	Primary MN	Secondary MN
LM	Uniform thickening of the GBM diffuse to all glomeruli with no proliferation.	Endocapillary hypercellularity may be seen in SLE or cancer. Mesangial proliferation seen in SLE.
Target Antigen (examples)	Intrinsic podocytes (PLA2R, THSD7A).	Planted antigen, immune complexes or alloantibodies (HBV, SLE, tumors, drugs).
IMF	Predominant IgG, C3. Typically IgG4 predominant. Subepithelial deposits (global). Often stains for relevant auto-antigen.	May also have IgA, IgM and C1q ("full house" pattern). Non-IgG4 subclasses predominant. Deposits can be segmental. EXT1/2* staining in Class V lupus.
EM	Paramesangial deposits allowed.	Additional mesangial and/or subendothelial deposits. Tubuloreticular inclusions in endothelial cells.

*EXT1/2 = Exostosin 1/2

II. Assessment of kidney function and baseline investigations:

1. Baseline investigations:
   a. Full blood count.
   b. Urea, creatinine, sodium, potassium, chloride, and bicarbonate.

c. Calcium, phosphate, alkaline phosphatase, and uric acid.
d. Liver function test: Total protein, albumin, alanine aminotransaminase (ALT), aspartate aminotransferase (AST), and bilirubin.

2. Quantify the degree of proteinuria and hematuria:
   a. Urine protein:creatinine ratio (UPCR) or a 24-hour urine protein excretion.
   b. Urine microscopy to look for red blood cells (RBCs), oval fat bodies, lipid droplets, and fatty casts.

III. Exclude secondary MN:

1. History and examination:
   a. Systemic symptoms: Rash, joint pain, and fever.
   b. Antenatal and birth history.
   c. Medications including traditional medications.
   d. Travel history.
2. Clinical features:
   a. Skin: Purpura, petechiae, and vasculitis.
   b. Arthritis.
   c. Features of hyper- and hypothyroidism and goitre.
   d. Hepatosplenomegaly and lymphadenopathy.
3. Investigations:
   a. Serum complements C3 and C4.
   b. Anti-nuclear antibody (ANA).
   c. Anti-double-stranded DNA antibody (anti-dsDNA).
   d. Thyroid function test (TFT).
   e. Infection screen:
      i. Hepatitis Bs antigen (HBsAg).
      ii. Hepatitis Be antigen (HBeAg).
      iii. Hepatitis B virus serology (anti-HBs, anti-HBc total).
      iv. Hepatitis C virus serology (anti-HCV).
      v. Human immunodeficiency virus serology (HIV Ag/Ab combo test).
      vi. Syphilis screen (Treponemal test to be done if non-treponemal test is positive).
      vii. EBV polymerase chain reaction (PCR).
      viii. CMV PCR.
      ix. Tuberculin skin test and/or interferon-gamma release assay.

IV. Serological testing for PMN:

1. If no secondary causes of MN can be found, look for autoantibodies associated with PMN.
2. Plasma anti-PLA2R antibody:
   a. Enzyme-linked immunosorbent assay (ELISA):
      - <14 RU/ml = Negative.
      - ≥14 to <20 RU/ml = Borderline.
      - ≥ 20 RU/ml = Positive.

   b. Indirect immunofluorescence: Yields only semiquantitative titers (e.g., 1:10, 1:100).
3. Serum anti-THSD7A antibody:
   - Indirect immunofluorescence assay.
   - If THSD7A-associated MN is diagnosed, an aggressive screening for cancer to diagnose secondary MN should be performed.
4. Biopsy tissue staining for antigens such as PLA2R and THSD7A.

E. Treatment of MN

I. General guidelines:

1. All patients with MN should receive supportive therapy with renin-angiotensin system blockers (RASBs) to prevent the progression of kidney disease (see chapter "Adjunctive Therapy in Glomerular Disease").
2. For patients with secondary MN:
   a. Treat the underlying disease or stop the offending agent.
   b. For malignancy-associated MN, treatment of malignancy is paramount and MN can initially be treated supportively.
      - If the patient subsequently does not show remission of proteinuria, a trial of immunosuppression is recommended.
3. Immunosuppressive therapy should not be employed in:
   a. Patients who are at low risk of developing progressive kidney disease:
      - Proteinuria <0.5 g/day/1.73m^2 or UPCR <0.05 g/mmol AND serum albumin >30 g/L.
      - Normal kidney function.
      - Proteinuria that normalizes in response to RASBs.

b. Patients who have progressed to CKD stages 3–5 where the inexorable progression is assessed to be irreversible.

II. Evaluation for risks of treatment:

1. Vaccination records, previous varicella infection, and varicella zoster IgG.
2. Tuberculosis (TB) (in endemic areas):
   a. Check family history of TB.
   b. Consider chest X-Ray to exclude latent TB.
   c. TB screen if positive contact history or living in a high endemic area:
      i. Tuberculin skin test in patients aged <2 years.
      ii. Interferon-gamma release assay in patients aged ≥2 years:
         - TB T-spot test (preferred in immunocompromised patients).
         - TB Quantiferon (less sensitive in immunocompromised patients).
3. Risk of developing diabetes mellitus:
   - Family history.
   - Fasting glucose.
   - Glycated hemoglobin (HbA1c).

III. Immunosuppressive therapy:

1. Wait-and-see strategy with supportive therapy alone is usually not adopted in pediatrics.
2. Immunosuppressive therapy is indicated in patients who present with:
   a. Nephrotic syndrome.
   b. PLA2R-associated MN.
   c. Abnormal kidney function.
   d. Persistent non-nephrotic range proteinuria >0.5 g/day/1.73m^2 or UPCR >0.05 g/mmol despite 6 months of optimized supportive care.
3. Non-PLA2R-associated MN: Combination therapy with glucocorticoid (GC) and a calcineurin inhibitor (CNI).

a. Oral prednisolone (PNL) of 60 mg/m^2 or 2 mg/kg (maximum 60 mg) daily for 4–8 weeks.
   - Prior to the diagnosis, most would have received at least 4 weeks of daily PNL as treatment for childhood nephrotic syndrome before kidney biopsy.

b. Start CNI if the kidney function is normal:
   i. Cyclosporine (CsA): 3–5 mg/kg/day targeting trough levels of 125–225 μg/L.
   ii. Tacrolimus (Tac): 0.05–0.1 mg/kg/day in 2 divided doses to achieve whole blood trough Tac levels of 3–8 μg/L.

c. Once remission of proteinuria (UPCR ≤0.02 g/mmol) is achieved, oral PNL is then changed to alternate day therapy at the same dose, gradually tapering off over 3–6 months depending on response.

d. Continue CNI for 1–2 years before attempting to taper off the treatment.

e. If proteinuria recurs, re-induce with CNI ± PNL, and consider adding mycophenolate (MPA) with an attempt to taper off CNI.
   i. Dose of mycophenolate mofetil (MMF): 600 mg/m^2/dose 12 hourly (15–23 mg/kg/dose 12 hourly).
      - Maximum adult dose: 1–1.5 gm 12 hourly.
   ii. MMF + CsA: 600 mg/m^2/dose 12 hourly (15–23 mg/kg/dose 12 hourly).
   iii. MMF + Tac: 300 mg/m^2/dose 12 hourly (8–12 mg/kg/dose 12 hourly).
   iv. Enteric-coated mycophenolate sodium (Myfortic®): 400 mg/m^2/dose 12 hourly.
   v. Dose equivalence:
      - Myfortic® 180 mg = 250 mg MMF.
      - Myfortic® 360 mg = 500 mg MMF.

f. Continue MPA for 1–2 years before attempting to taper it off.

g. If the patient continues to relapse, consider IV Rituximab followed by MPA maintenance.

4. PLA2R-associated MN:
   a. Induction with IV Rituximab (RTX):
      i. IV RTX 375 mg/m^2 once a week for 2–4 weeks OR
      ii. IV RTX 750 mg/m^2/dose (maximum 1000 mg) 2 doses 2 weeks apart.

b. Maintenance therapy:
   i. Oral MPA targeting trough levels of 2–4 mg/L or MPA AUC 30–60 mg*h/L OR
   ii. RTX maintenance dosing: IV 375 mg/m^2 (adult 500–1000 mg) every 4–6 months OR "on-demand" dosing strategy:
      - Monitor peripheral B lymphocyte (CD19-positive cells) counts and anti-PLA2R antibodies.
      - Re-dose when B lymphocytes reconstitute or the anti-PLA2R antibody titer becomes positive >2–3 RU/ml.

c. Monitor serum IgG levels monthly for 3 months after RTX dosing:
   - Give IVIG 0.5 g/kg if there is associated hypogammaglobulinemia, especially with recurrent infections.

5. Monitoring of the patient's response to therapy:
   a. Serum creatinine, albumin and urine protein excretion (UPCR or a 24-hour urine protein excretion) 1–3 monthly.
   b. Serial assessment of anti-PLA2R antibodies in PLA2R-associated MN patients.
      i. Risk of progressive loss of kidney function based on anti-PLAR2R antibody levels:
         - Low risk: <50 RU/ml.
         - High risk: >150 RU/ml.
      ii. Disappearance of anti-PLA2R antibodies precedes clinical remission.
         - Wait 6–12 months after antibody disappearance before evaluating the treatment response.

6. In patients who do not respond to IV RTX and remain clinically nephrotic, consider:
   a. Adding CNI if the kidney function is normal.
   b. Alternate anti-CD20 antibody therapy such as Obinutuzumab (see chapter "Anti-CD20 Monoclonal Antibody for Nephrotic Syndrome").
   c. Modified Ponticelli regimen: Cyclophosphamide (CYC) and GC alternating months for 6 months.
      i. Months 1, 3 and 5: IV methylprednisolone 10–30 mg/kg/dose (maximum 1 g) for 3 days followed by oral PNL 0.5 mg/kg for 28 days.

ii. Months 2, 4 and 6: Oral cyclophosphamide (CYC) 2 mg/kg/day (maximum cumulative dose 175 mg/kg).
iii. Titrate the CYC dose to achieve a peripheral lymphocyte count of $<0.7 \times 10^9$/L while keeping the white blood cell count $>3.5 \times 10^9$/L.

IV. *Algorithm for management of membranous nephropathy*

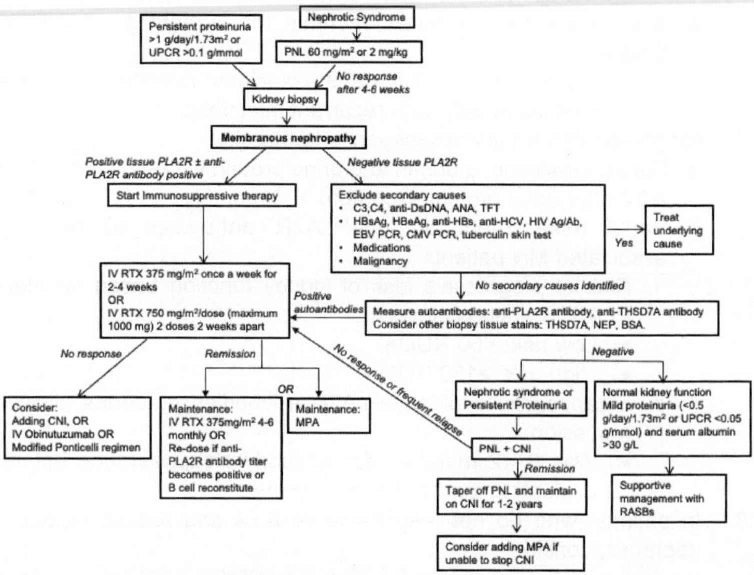

Recommended Reading

1. Menon S, Valentini RP. (2010) Membranous nephropathy in children: Clinical presentation and therapeutic approach. *Pediatr Nephrol* **25**:1419–1428.
2. Kidney Disease: Improving Global Outcomes (KDIGO) Glomerulonephritis Work Group. (2012) KDIGO clinical practice guideline for glomerulonephritis. *Kidney Int Suppl* **2**:218–221.

3. Safar-Boueri L, Piya A, Beck LH Jr, Ayalon R. (2021) Membranous nephropathy: Diagnosis, treatment, and monitoring in the post-PLA2R era. *Pediatr Nephrol* **36**(1):19–30
4. Alsharhan L, Beck LH Jr. (2021) Membranous nephropathy: Core curriculum 2021. *Am J Kidney Dis* **77**(3):440–453.
5. De Vriese AS, Wetzels J, Cattran DC. (2021, updated) Membranous nephropathy: Treatment and prognosis. Edited by: Glassock RJ, Fervenza FC, Lam AQ. *UpToDate ONLINE*. http://www.uptodateonline.com.

11 Hemolytic-Uremic Syndrome

Lu L, Resontoc LP, Qader MA, Patil M, Liu ID and Yap HK

A. Overview and Definitions

1. Thrombotic microangiopathy (TMA):
   a. Describes a specific pathologic lesion in which abnormalities in the vessel wall of arterioles and capillaries lead to microvascular thrombosis.
   b. TMAs are characterized by:
      - Systemic or intrarenal aggregation of platelets.
      - Thrombocytopenia.
      - Mechanical injury to erythrocytes.
2. Types of TMA:
   a. Hemolytic-uremic syndrome (HUS):
      i. Characterized by the simultaneous occurrence of:
         - Acute kidney injury (AKI) of varying severity.
         - Microangiopathic hemolytic anemia (MAHA).
         - Thrombocytopenia.
      ii. Etiology is heterogeneous, which dictates management.
   b. Thrombotic thrombocytopenic purpura (TTP):
      i. Characterized by:
         - MAHA.
         - Thrombocytopenia.
         - Ischemic organ injury with a predilection for the involvement of the central nervous system and/or gastrointestinal tract.
      ii. In contrast to HUS, the lungs are spared and there are minimal abnormalities for kidney function despite the presence of microthrombi in the kidney.

iii. Caused by severely reduced activity of the von Willebrand factor-cleaving protease ADAMTS13, typically <10%, either due to congenital absence of functional protein or acquired anti-ADAMTS13 antibodies.

iv. Rare in children.

c. Other forms of TMA occur in specific clinical contexts and include:

i. Disseminated intravascular coagulation (DIC).

ii. Malignant hypertension.

iii. Pre-eclampsia/HELLP syndrome (hemolysis, elevated liver enzymes, and low platelets).

B. Complement Regulation

1. Alternative complement pathway (ACP):

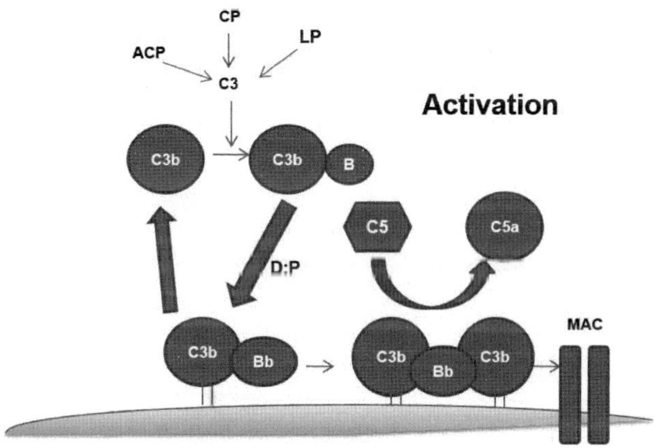

a. Positive feedback amplification loop providing rapid antibody-independent defense against microorganisms.

b. Continuously activated through spontaneous hydrolysis of C3 to C3b that combines with complement factor B (CFB), which is then cleaved by factor D to form the C3 convertase (C3bBb).

c. This enzyme complex is stabilized by properdin (P) and is bound to the target covalently by C3b while Bb is the catalytic serine protease unit.

d. C3b is an opsonin that assists effective phagocytosis and clearance of microbial components and triggers the formation of the terminal products of complement activation, C5a and C5b-9, the membrane attack complex (MAC).
e. The MAC is a pore-like structure that inserts into cell membranes, resulting in cell lysis of invading pathogens.
f. Host cells exposed to sub-lytic doses of the MAC undergo cell activation.

2. Regulation of ACP:
   a. To limit damage to host cells, the alternative pathway is down-regulated by cofactor activity (CA) that leads to the permanent inactivation of C3b to iC3b, and decay-accelerating activity (DAA) that increases the rate of C3 convertase dissociation.

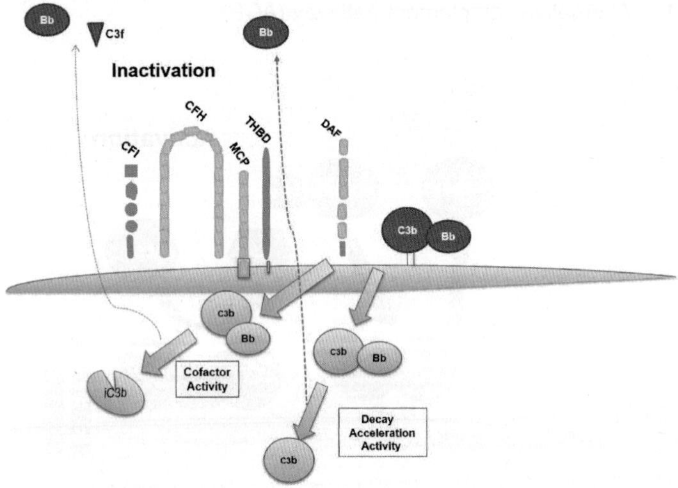

- CA requires both a cofactor protein, complement factor H (CFH), or membrane cofactor protein (MCP also known as CD46), and a serine protease, complement factor I (CFI), and is also enhanced by thrombomodulin (THBD).
- DAA is mediated by the decay-accelerating factor (DAF, CD55).

C. Etiological Classification

I. Primary or genetic causes:

1. Complement mediated HUS:
   a. Gain of function mutations in proteins involved in the alternative pathway:
      - *C3, CFB*.
   b. Loss of function mutations in complement regulatory proteins involved in CA or DAA:
      - *CFH*, *CD46* (*MCP*), *CFI*, and *THBD*.
   c. Acquired complement dysregulation due to antibodies against CFH:
      - Often associated with mutations in CFH-related proteins (*CFHR1*, *CFHR3*, *CFHR4*).
      - These genes are composed of short consensus repeats (SCRs) that share different degrees of identity with SCRs in CFH.
      - Up to 90–95% of patients with anti-CFH antibodies have a homozygous deletion of *CFHR1–CFHR3*, resulting in a complete deficiency of the CFHR1 and CFHR3 protein.
2. Mutations in non-complement genes:
   a. Coagulation pathway:
      i. Diacylgylcerol kinase epsilon (*DGKE*):
         - *DGKE* inactivates arachidonic acid-containing diacylglycerols (DAG), an activator of protein kinase C that promotes thrombosis.
         - Recessive mutations in *DGKE* are associated with HUS.
      ii. Plasminogen (*PLG*):
         - Plasminogen deficiency results in decreased degradation of thrombi.
      iii. Thrombomodulin (*THBD*).
         - Thrombomodulin enhances CA and is also involved in initiating the protein C anticoagulant pathway.
   b. Cobalamin C (*MMACHC*):
      - Mutations in methylmalonic aciduria and homocystinuria type C (*MMACHC*) gene result in functional Cobalamin C deficiency, as Cobalamin C is a co-factor for methylmalonyl-CoA

mutase and methionine synthase (transforms homocysteine to methionine).

3. Genetic epidemiology:

Complement Abnormality	Prevalence (%)
Complement mediated:	53–64.7
CFH	21.3–25.6
Homozygous	4.2–4.4
Heterozygous	16.8–21.1
MCP	9.2–13.5
Homozygous	5.6
Heterozygous	7.8
CFI	2.6–6.7
C3	3.9–7.8
CFB	0.4–1
THBD	0–7.8
Anti-CFH	3.9–11
Combined (Digenic)	3–3.4
DGKE	7.9
Unknown	27.4–47

- Mutations are generally low penetrance (~50%).

II. Secondary causes:

1. Infection-induced:
   a. Shiga and Shiga-like toxin (STx)-producing bacteria (>90% of HUS):
      i. Shiga toxin-producing enterohemorrhagic Escherichia coli (STEC):
         - Common serotypes: O157:H7 (North America and Northwest Europe), O26 (Southern Europe), O111:H8 (Australia), O103:H2, O123.
         - Risk of HUS is 8–15% during infection with O157:H7, with a lower risk amongst non-O157:H7 strains.
         - Increased risk may be related to the production of Stx2 (Shiga-like toxin type 2) compared to Stx1.

ii. *Shigella dysenteriae* type 1 (SD1):
- Entero-invasive unlike STEC, i.e., hematogenous spread.
- Pathogenesis of HUS is related to a combination of Stx1 and bacterial lipopolysaccharide, and thus unlike STEC-HUS, patients with Shigella-associated HUS can have concomitant DIC.
- Risk of HUS is estimated at 8% during SD1 infection.
- Though uncommon, HUS can also be caused by non-SD1 shigellosis (risk of HUS ~1%), e.g., S. flexneri, S. boydii and S. sonnei.

iii. *Citrobacter freundii:*
- A commensal of the gastrointestinal tract, but can infrequently cause diarrhea upon the acquisition of virulence factors.
- Some strains are able to produce Shiga-like toxins, including *Stx2*.

b. *Streptococcus pneumoniae:*

i. Reported in 5–15% of all childhood cases of HUS, and 40% of non-STEC HUS cases.

ii. Occurs mainly in infants and young children, and rarely affects adults.

iii. Pathogenesis remains unclear, with proposed mechanisms including:
- Classically, neuraminidase is thought to be produced by HUS-inducing pneumococci, leading to cleavage of sialic acid and exposure of Thomsen–Friedenreich antigen (T-antigen) on erythrocytes, platelets and glomeruli, resulting in binding and cell lysis by normally circulating anti-T antibodies.
- However, anti-T antibodies are IgM, i.e., low-affinity at body temperature, and erythrocyte desialylation can also occur in pneumococcal disease not progressing to HUS.
- An alternative hypothesis is that pneumococcal neuraminidase may disrupt CFH binding sites, resulting in unregulated alternative pathway activation similar to complement-mediated primary HUS.

c. Human immunodeficiency virus.
- Uncommon with effective anti-retroviral therapy.

d. Other infections:
  - Influenza A (H1N1/H3N2)-associated HUS.
  - *Entamoeba histolytica* intestinal infection.
  - *Mycoplasma pneumoniae* infection.
  - Hepatitis A (HAV).
  - Hepatitis B (HBV).
  - Cytomegalovirus (CMV).
  - Epstein–Barr virus (EBV).

2. Non-infectious secondary causes of HUS
   a. Systemic lupus erythematosus (SLE) and anti-phospholipid antibody syndrome:
      - May be associated with decreased ADAMTS13 levels or vWF-cleaving protease inhibitor.
      - May be due to direct endothelial injury with the production of anti-endothelial cell antibodies.
   b. Organ transplantation:
      - Associated with high-dose calcineurin inhibitors (CNIs) in solid organ transplantation.
      - Also associated with bone marrow transplantation.
   c. Drug-induced:
      - Quinine-induced HUS has been associated with antibodies against platelet glycoproteins.
   d. Pregnancy:
      - Typically in the post-partum period.
   e. Malignancy.
   f. May be associated with predisposing mutations in complement genes:

	Complement Abnormality	Prevalence (%)
a. Organ transplantation	Mutations in *CFH* Mutations in *CFI*	15 16
b. Drugs • Cytotoxic agents • Ionizing radiation • CNIs • Oral contraceptives	Rare *CFH* mutations	
c. Pregnancy	Mutations in *CFH* Mutations in *CFI*	20 15

D. Diagnostic Approach

I. Diagnosis of HUS:

1. Clinical features:
   a. Pallor and oliguria following the onset of infection in typical HUS.
   b. Purpura and bruising are usually mild or absent.
   c. Mild jaundice occurs in about a third of the cases and there is often a mild and transient elevation of liver enzymes, and less often hepatomegaly.
   d. Hypertension often appears transiently later in the course of AKI.
   e. Non-kidney manifestations:
      i. Central nervous system (CNS) disturbances usually present early in the course of the illness:
         - Irritability, confusion, hallucination, and seizures.
         - Cranial nerve palsy, dysphasia, diplopia, retinal injury, or cortical blindness.
         - Diffuse massive cerebral edema can induce hindbrain compression leading to brainstem death.
      ii. Pancreatic involvement leading to overt diabetes mellitus.
      iii. Cardiomyopathy and myocarditis may occur several weeks later.
2. Laboratory investigations:
   a. Full blood count (FBC) and reticulocytes:
      i. Hemoglobin <10 g/dL.
      ii. Platelet count $<150 \times 10^9$/L.
      iii. Reticulocytosis.
   b. Peripheral blood film for evidence of MAHA:
      i. Red blood cells (RBCs) fragmentation, e.g., schistocytes, helmet cells.
      ii. Decreased platelets.
   c. Liver function test and haptoglobin.
      i. Elevated lactate dehydrogenase (LDH) as an index of hemolysis.
      ii. Unconjugated hyperbilirubinemia.
      iii. Decreased serum haptoglobin.
   d. Assessment of kidney function:
      i. Urea, creatinine, sodium, potassium, chloride, bicarbonate, calcium, phosphate, alkaline phosphatase, and uric acid.

- Raised urea and creatinine with a decreased glomerular filtration rate (GFR).

ii. Urine protein:creatinine ratio or a 24-hour urine protein excretion for evidence of significant proteinuria.

iii. Urinalysis, urine microscopy and phase contrast study on a fresh urine specimen for evidence of hematuria.

e. Coagulopathy screen:
   - Normal coagulopathy screen in the absence of fulminant sepsis.

II. Differentiate infection-induced HUS from other causes:

1. Shiga toxin associated-HUS:
   a. Children >6 months.
      - Greatest risk at ages 3–5 years.

   b. STEC-endemic region or Shigella endemic region.
      - Risk factors for infection with STEC include salads and vegetables from contaminated surface soil, bathing in contaminated water, and direct contact with animals.

   c. History of bloody diarrhea in the 2 weeks prior to the onset of HUS.

   d. Subclinical infection in close contacts.

   e. Investigation for STEC-HUS should be routine in all patients unless another cause is apparent.
      - STEC can often result in mild diarrhea without hematochezia and approximately 5% of STEC-HUS cases have no prodromal diarrhea.
      - 30% of complement-mediated HUS cases have concurrent diarrhea or gastroenteritis.

2. *Streptococcus pneumoniae*-associated HUS:
   a. Generally restricted to infants and toddlers.

   b. Invasive *Streptococcus pneumoniae* infection.
      - Generally pneumonia (70–80%), with two-thirds complicated by empyema.
      - Remaining cases are due to meningitis or acute otitis media, which may be complicated by a subdural abscess.
      - 80% of patients are bacteremic.

   c. Onset of HUS usually 1–2 weeks after the onset of illness.

3. When to suspect primary (atypical) HUS:
   a. No recent diarrhea OR
   b. Recent diarrhea with any one of the following:
      i. Age <6 months.
      ii. Insidious onset: No thrombocytosis (15%) or anemia (6%), with preserved kidney function initially (17%) in spite of heavy proteinuria.
      iii. Relapse of HUS.
      iv. Suspected previous HUS.
      v. Previous unexplained anemia.
      vi. HUS post-solid organ transplantation.
      vii. Asynchronous family history of HUS.
   c. Suggestive clinical features:
      i. Disorders of complement proteins.
         - Insidious onset precipitated by relatively minor illnesses such as upper respiratory tract infections or gastroenteritis.
         - Consistent finding at the onset is severe hypertension, which can lead to heart failure and encephalopathy.
         - Heavy proteinuria and hematuria occur in those with preserved urine production.
         - Non-kidney manifestations are less frequent than in STEC-induced HUS.
         - Retinal thrombotic microangiopathy with pain in the eye and visual loss occurs mainly with *CFH* mutations.
         - Hematological relapse is common.
         - Patients presenting in early infancy have a high risk of progression to kidney failure in the first episode, and once this has occurred, the MAHA and thrombocytopenia tend to resolve.
      ii. Congenital cobalamin-C mutations:
         - Predominance of neurocognitive symptoms, i.e., hypotonia, lethargy, seizures, anorexia, failure to thrive in the neonatal period, or neuropsychiatric manifestations and myelopathy in later-onset forms.
         - Leukopenia and megaloblastic anemia.

	STEC	Shigella	Streptococcus Pneumoniae	Primary HUS
Age	1–5 years	Median age: 3 years	<2 years	<6 months or >5 years
Onset of HUS	3–10 days after onset of bloody diarrhea (range: 1–14 days)	Median time to onset: 7 days	7–9 days (range: 3–13 days)	Can be rapid but usually subacute (>10 days) following minor illnesses
Non-kidney manifestations	Neurological complications frequent (25%)	Neurological complications frequent	Empyema common; Neurological complications rare	Neurological complications rare
Presence of coagulopathy at onset	Nil	Yes, if septicemic	Yes, if septicemic	Nil
Further investigations	• Stool culture and enhancement and selection techniques such as sorbitol MacConkey agar enriched with tellurite • Stx immunoassay and real-time PCR for Stx and other virulence vectors (from fresh stool and overnight broth culture) • Serological response to locally relevant O serotypes (Serum IgM or saliva IgA/IgM) • Stool culture from household contacts if negative from the patient	• Stool culture	• Chest X-ray • Blood cultures • Respiratory cultures, pleural tap OR cerebrospinal fluid cultures • Direct Coomb's test (positive in 90%)	Requires • Full investigation for alternative causes of HUS • Investigation for STEC infection including urine microscopy and culture as unusual presentations can occur

III. Exclude TTP and investigate for other causes of HUS:

1. Inherited or acquired ADAMTS13 deficiency:
   a. Plasma vWF protease (ADAMTS13) activity.
      - Measure in the acute phase of illness.
      - Significant if activity <10% of normal.

   b. Test for inhibitor if ADAMTS13 activity is persistently decreased even in remission.
      - Presence of inhibitor suggests an acquired antibody inhibitor.
      - Absence of inhibitor suggests inherited ADAMTS13 deficiency.
2. Human immunodeficiency virus (HIV) infection:
   - HIV antigen and antibody screen.
3. Systemic lupus erythematosus and anti-phospholipid syndrome:
   a. Direct Coombs' test.
   b. Serum complements C3 and C4.
   c. Anti-nuclear antibodies (ANA).
   d. Anti-double stranded DNA antibody.
   e. Lupus anti-coagulant.
   f. Anti-cardiolipin antibody (ACA).
   g. Anti-β2-glycoprotein-1 antibody.
4. Disorders of cobalamin metabolism:
   a. Homocysteine and methylmalonic acid (MMA) (plasma and urine).
      - Vital to test regardless of clinical suspicion as potentially treatable with hydroxycobalamin.

   b. Mutation analysis in the *MMACHC* gene.
5. Disorders of complement regulation (should be done before the commencement of plasma infusions or plasmapheresis):
   a. Serum complement C3:
      - Low C3 in 30% of patients with complement-associated HUS, including 40–60% in patients with anti-CFH antibodies.
      - Not specific, as low C3 levels can transiently occur in STEC-associated and Streptococcus pneumoniae-associated HUS, as well as patients with *DGKE* mutations.

   b. Plasma/serum CFH, CFI and CFB concentrations:
      - Caution in interpretation as CFH and CFI concentrations may be normal in mutations that do not affect secretion.

- CFH <60% suggests deficiency.
- CFI <60% suggests deficiency.
- Low CFB levels suggest an alternate pathway activation.

c. CD46 (MCP) on peripheral blood mononuclear cells by flow cytometry.
- Time from venesection to analysis should be <4 days because the expression of MCP is stable at room temperature for up to this duration.
- No expression: Homozygous deficiency.
- MFI is 50% in heterozygous individuals.

d. CFH autoantibody (enzyme-linked immunosorbent assay).
- Using standardized assay.

6. Gene mutation analysis for *CFH*, *CFI*, *MCP*, *CFB*, *CFHR1-5*, *THBD*, *C3*, and *MMACHC*.
   a. Considerations:
      i. Normal levels or expression of CFH, CFI and CD46 do not rule out the possibility of a normally expressed but functionally impaired mutant.
      ii. *DGKE* should also be included in the testing panel for patients aged <2 years.
      iii. Blood for genetic studies should be taken only after 2 weeks following blood transfusions.
   b. Indications:
      i. After confirmation that there is no causative disease, no STEC infection, and no severe ADAMTS13 deficiency.
      ii. Start genetic screening without delay if:
         - Relapse of HUS.
         - Familial history of non-synchronous HUS.
         - Pregnancy/post-partum HUS.
         - *De novo* post-transplant HUS.
      iii. Genetic screening required before kidney transplantation for primary HUS.
         - Not recommended before transplantation for infection-induced HUS, unless this diagnosis was uncertain or unproven.

IV. Diagnostic algorithm:

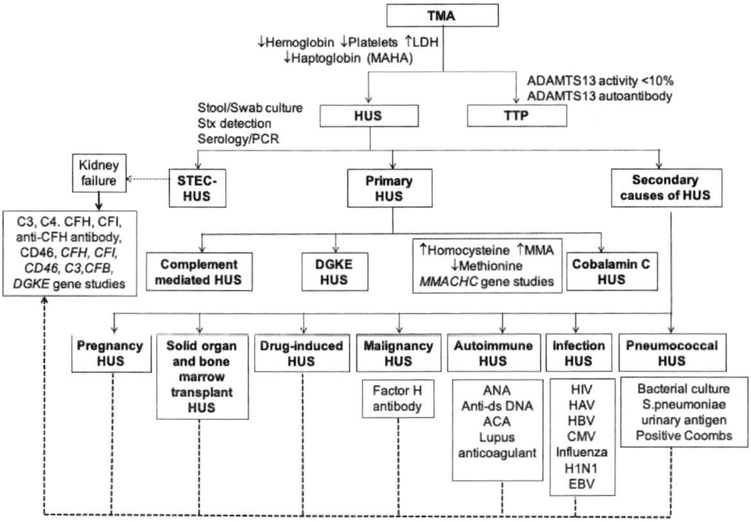

E. Therapy of HUS

I. Supportive therapy:

1. Fluid resuscitation and correction of electrolyte abnormalities and acidosis:
   a. Early and generous volume expansion in STEC-HUS may attenuate the disease course.
      i. Aim for a volume expansion of 10% of working weight by infusion with 0.9% normal saline of 10 to 15 ml/kg per hour.
      ii. Avoid fluid overload >10%.
      iii. Restrict fluids at the first sign of hypertension or cardiopulmonary overload.
   b. In all other cases, aim for clinical euvolaemia to maintain tissue perfusion.

c. Plasma potassium should be closely monitored as it can rise steeply in the presence of red cell fragmentation or with blood transfusion.
d. Consider dialysis when:
   i. Symptomatic uremia.
   ii. Blood urea ≥30–35 mmol/L
   iii. Hyperkalemia.
   iv. Acidosis.
   v. Diuretic-refractory fluid overload.
   vi. Need for nutritional support in a child requiring fluid restriction.

2. Transfusion of blood products:
   a. Packed RBC transfusions:
      i. Consider transfusion if hemoglobin is <6 g/dL or hematocrit <18% to avoid cardiovascular and pulmonary compromise.
      ii. Post-transfusion goal of hemoglobin level between 8–9 g/dL is recommended.
         - Restoring the hemoglobin level to normal may cause heart failure, pulmonary edema, and hypertension.
      iii. Transfusion of packed RBCs should be given slowly and cautiously at a total volume of 10 ml/kg over 3–4 hours, with frequent monitoring of the patient's vital signs, which typically produces an increase in hemoglobin of 1 g/dL.
      iv. Blood products should be volume-reduced and preferably depleted of leukocytes and platelets to avoid alloimmunization in the event transplantation is subsequently required.
      v. Monitor potassium levels closely in the presence of AKI.
      vi. If the patient is undergoing hemodialysis, transfusions should be given during dialysis to minimize the risks of hypervolemia and hyperkalemia.
      vii. No indication for the routine use of erythropoietin-stimulating agents.
   b. Platelet transfusions:
      i. Should be avoided in HUS, so as to prevent alloimmunization and concerns about fueling further thrombosis.
      ii. Consider platelet transfusions if:
         - Clinical bleeding (rare).
         - Platelet count $<10 \times 10^9$/L (uncommon).

- Invasive procedures are planned, although increased bleeding complications have not been demonstrated in HUS patients who are not transfused.

c. Transfusions in *Streptococcus pneumoniae*-associated HUS:
   i. Consider using washed RBCs to prevent additional administration of anti-T antibodies.
   ii. Consider avoiding plasma infusions (or select plasma with low anti-T titers), due to concerns about driving anti-T mediated hemolysis.
   iii. These are expert recommendations, although there is limited evidence in support.

3. Antibiotics and antimotility agents:
   a. Antibiotics and antimotility drugs (such as anticholinergic agents and narcotics) should be avoided in patients with confirmed or suspected STEC-HUS.
      - Antibiotics may injure the bacterial membrane, causing an acute release of preformed Shiga toxin, and may induce the bacteriophage carrying the Stx gene, resulting in further toxin production.
   b. Antibiotics are indicated in:
      - HUS caused by *Shigella dysenteriae* as it is enteroinvasive.
      - *Streptococcus pneumoniae*-associated HUS.
4. Other measures:
   a. Antihypertensive therapy.
      i. Calcium channel blockers are recommended as the initial choice of antihypertensive agents in the acute phase of the illness.
      ii. After the acute phase of HUS, angiotensin-converting enzyme (ACE) inhibitors may be given to patients who have renal sequelae.
   b. Neuroprotective measures and anti-seizure treatment for patients with neurological features.
   c. Respiratory support including pleural tap in *Streptococcus pneumoniae*-associated HUS, as clinically indicated.
   d. Discontinuing nephrotoxic drugs, especially those that may be implicated in drug-associated HUS.
   e. Parenteral nutrition can be given for those who cannot tolerate enteral feeding.

II. C5 inhibitor:

1. Pharmacology:
   a. Mechanism of action:
      - Recombinant humanized monoclonal IgG antibody that inhibits the cleavage of C5 to C5a and C5b, thus preventing the formation of the MAC C5b-9.
      - Eculizumab is currently in clinical use with a plasma $T_{½}$ of 11 days.
      - Ravulizumab is a longer-acting form currently undergoing clinical trials.

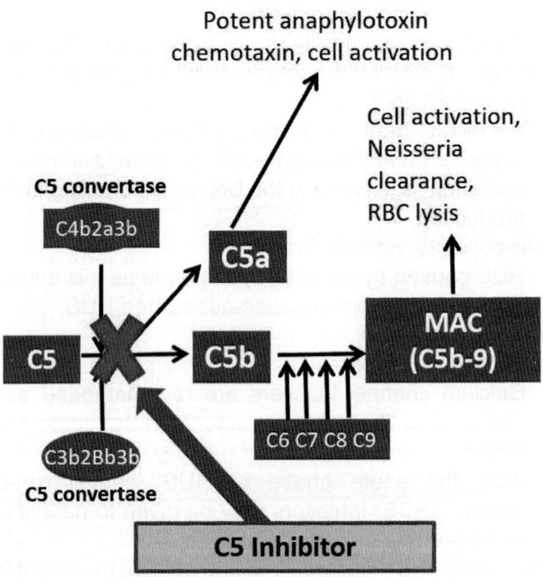

2. Indications:
   a. First-line therapy for cases of complement-mediated HUS, including the anti-CFH antibody disease.
      - To be started within 24–48 hours of onset/admission.
      - In anti-CFH antibody disease, add plasmapheresis if severe non-kidney manifestations or high anti-CFH titer (>2000 AU/ml).
   b. Consider in STEC-HUS with neurological complications.

3. Efficacy:
   a. Normalization of hematological parameters and improvement of kidney function in 82% and 64% respectively at 6 months, and 88% and 76% respectively at 2 years.
   b. Effective complement blockade may be assessed through CH_{50} prior to the 2nd dose, aiming <10%.
      - CH_{50} cannot be measured in those with complete CFH deficiency.
      - Eculizumab blood levels should be measured in complete CFH deficiency aiming levels ≥100 μg/ml.
   c. Failure of Eculizumab to prevent complement activation may occur in some *C5* variants, which have been described in Japanese and Asian-origin patients with paroxysmal nocturnal hemoglobinuria (PNH).
   d. Not effective in patients with primary HUS due to *DGKE* mutations.
4. Main side effect is increased susceptibility to infections with encapsulated bacteria, in particular, *Neisseria meningitidis*, *Streptococcus pneumoniae*, and *Hemophilus influenzae*.
5. Dosage regimen; see chapter "Eculizumab (Anti-C5 Monoclonal Antibody) Therapy for Complement-Mediated Injury".
6. Eculizumab maintenance therapy:
   a. Current paradigm is for life-long therapy to prevent disease recurrence, with doses repeated at 2-weekly Intervals.
   b. Consider stretching dosing interval based on pre-dose CH_{50}, aiming ≤10%.
   c. Discontinuation may be considered as data emerges regarding the risk, severity and sequelae of relapses of specific mutations:
      i. In patients with no mutations identified due to a lower risk of relapse.
         - Should be performed after 3–5 years when viral infections decline in frequency.
      ii. In patients with isolated CD46 mutations due to relatively favorable prognosis, even in pre-Eculizumab era despite a relapsing course.
7. Frequent monitoring is required for early detection of relapse and re-initiating therapy, including twice-weekly urine dipstick and FBC weekly for 2 months and, subsequently, monthly.

III. Plasma therapy:

1. Plasma infusion:
   a. Replaces defective complement components and regulators with functional proteins.
   b. In complement-mediated HUS, plasma infusion may be considered in the absence of eculizumab if there is:
      - Mild kidney involvement with conserved urine output.
      - A family member who has responded to plasma infusion.
   c. Dose:
      - 20–30 ml/kg daily initially.
      - May be limited because of abnormal kidney function and hypertension.
   d. If plasma infusion appears successful with the reversal of MAHA, the dose and frequency can be reduced to weekly or biweekly intervals.
2. Plasmapheresis or plasma exchange (PE):
   a. Offers additional advantage of the removal of mutant CFH, CFI, CFB, C3, and CFH autoantibodies while restoring functional complement regulators (except CD46, which is membrane-bound).
   b. Indications:
      i. First-line therapy for severe complement-mediated HUS when eculizumab is not available, except when caused by CD46 mutations.
      ii. Definitive therapy for anti-CFH antibody disease with concomitant immunosuppression.
   c. PE should be initiated as soon as possible, within 24 hours, to preserve kidney function.
   d. Prescription:
      i. Schedule: Daily for 5 days, then 5 sessions per week for 2 weeks, then 3 sessions per week for 2 weeks.
      ii. Volume of exchange: 1.5 times plasma volume or 60–75 ml/kg in young children.
      iii. Fresh frozen plasma should be used as the replacement.
   e. PE may be discontinued when the patient enters hematological remission.

IV. Anti-CFH antibody disease:

1. Principle:
   a. Aim of therapy is to:
      - Block anti-CFH antibody action, through PE or Eculizumab AND
      - Inhibit anti-CFH antibody production, through immunosuppression.

   b. If long-term Eculizumab therapy is available, consider Eculizumab monotherapy to achieve and maintain remission, especially in the presence of concomitant pathogenic mutations in other complement genes.
2. Treatment algorithm:

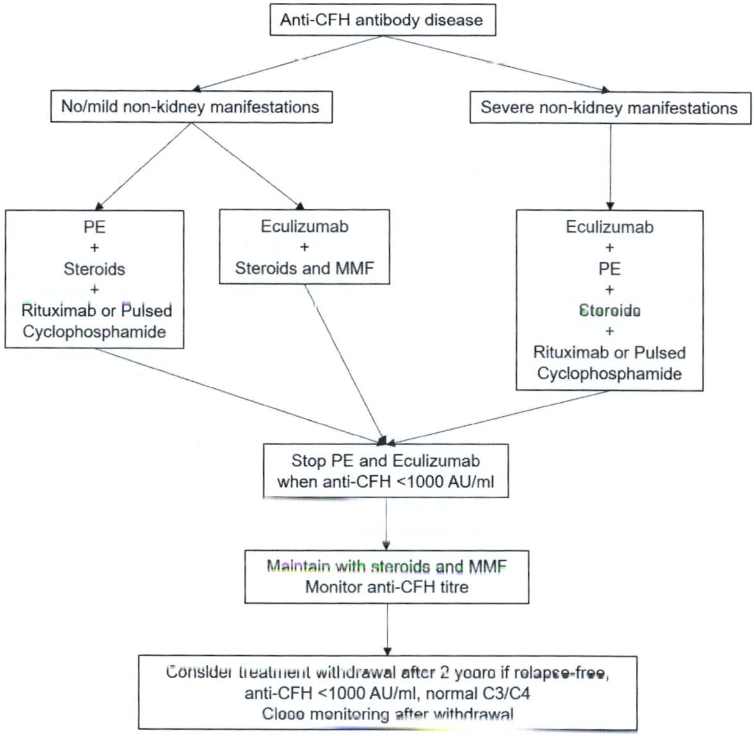

3. Dosing:
   a. Eculizumab (see chapter "Eculizumab (Anti-C5 Monoclonal Antibody) Therapy for Complement-Mediated Injury").
   b. PE:
      i. Daily exchanges (1.5 times plasma volume, 60 ml/kg) with plasma as the replacement fluid for at least 5 days, or until hematological remission is achieved.
      ii. If disease is still active after 7 exchanges, i.e., schistocytes >2% AND platelets <100 × 10^9/L within the last 2 days, consider addition of Eculizumab.
      iii. Subsequently, reduce PE to alternate days (1-time plasma volume, 40 ml/kg) for 6 sessions, then twice weekly for 6 sessions or until anti-CFH <1000 AU/ml.
   c. Prednisolone:
      - 1 mg/kg per day × 4 weeks, then
      - 1 mg/kg alternate day for 4 weeks, then
      - Taper by 0.25 mg/kg every 2 weeks to 0.1–0.2 mg/kg on alternate days.
   d. Rituximab:
      i. 375 mg/m^2 × 2 doses 1 week apart following hematological remission.
      ii. Avoid PE for 48–72 hours following infusion.
      iii. Consider re-induction with cyclophosphamide-based regime if relapse occurs while CD19+ population is still suppressed.
   e. Cyclophosphamide:
      i. IV 500 mg/m^2 for 2–5 doses every 3–4 weeks following hematological remission.
      ii. Avoid PE for 48–72 hours following infusion.
   f. Mycophenolate mofetil (MMF):
      i. 250–375 mg/m^2/dose twice daily if cyclophosphamide-based induction regime is used.
      ii. 600 mg/m^2/dose twice daily if non-cyclophosphamide-based induction regime is used.

V. Long-term follow-up of primary HUS:

1. Follow-up monthly, and subsequently 3-monthly if stable.
2. Hematology:
   a. Hematological remission is defined as:
      i. Platelet count >150 × 10^9/L for 2 weeks
      ii. No signs of hemolysis as determined by:
         - Presence of fragmented RBCs.
         - Raised lactate dehydrogenase.
         - Decreased haptoglobin level.
   b. Hematological relapse is defined as the return of MAHA and thrombocytopenia after these parameters have normalized for a period of at least 2 weeks.
      - Recurrence of HUS should lead the clinician to consider primary or genetic HUS if not previously suspected.
3. Kidney:
   a. Serum creatinine and estimated GFR.
   b. Blood pressure.
   c. Urine protein:creatinine ratio and albumin:creatinine ratio.
4. Other end-organ follow-up depending on the type of non-kidney involvement during the acute phase of the disease.

VI. Treatment summary:

Disease	Causes	Treatment
Infection	STEC-HUS	• Supportive • No antibiotics • Consider Eculizumab for severe neurological manifestations
	Shigella-associated HUS	• Supportive • Antibiotics
	Streptococcus pneumoniae associated HUS	• Supportive • Antibiotics • Consider avoiding plasma infusions, and using washed RBCs for transfusions

(*Continued*)

(Continued)

Disease	Causes	Treatment
Disorders of Complement Regulation	Anti-CFH antibodies	• PE and/or Eculizumab • Immunosuppressive therapy
	Without anti-CFH antibodies	• Eculizumab • Consider discontinuation in those with no mutation identified, or *CD46* mutations
DGKE Associated HUS	Mutations in *DGKE*	• Eculizumab discontinuation, especially after 5 years • Close monitoring
Cobalamin C Associated HUS	Mutations in *MMACHC*	• Parenteral hydroxocobalamin • Betaine • Methionine • Leucovorin calcium • Carnitine supplements • Genetics referral
Secondary Causes	Drugs	• Drug withdrawal • Consider Eculizumab if it is a severe and refractory disease. • Consider N-acetylcysteine if there is evidence of TTP
	SLE ± antiphospholipid syndrome	• Immunosuppressive therapy • PE • ± Anticoagulants
	Viral	• Supportive • Anti-viral therapy • If features suggestive of viral-triggered complement-mediated HUS, consider Eculizumab, or alternatively PE or plasma infusion

F. Transplantation

1. Principle:
   a. Determining the risk of relapse and *de novo* disease by screening for complement gene mutations in the recipient and living-related donor, respectively.

   b. Perioperative and post-operative prophylaxis will be determined by the risk of relapse.
   c. Eculizumab must be available as rescue therapy, as PE is not effective in recurrent disease in the graft.
   d. Avoid endothelial damage.
2. Donor selection
   a. Consider a living donor if possible.
   b. A living-related donor is suitable if a pathological mutation is found in the recipient, and this mutation is absent in the donor.
   c. For deceased donor transplant, avoid prolonged cold ischemia time and non-heart-beating donors.
3. Perioperative and post-operative prophylaxis:
   a. Prophylactic Eculizumab in those at high risk of recurrent HUS:
      - Mutations in *CFH*, *CFI*, *C3*, and *CFB*.
      - Previous post-transplant recurrence.
   b. Prophylactic Eculizumab can be considered in those at moderate risk:
      - Combined *CD46* mutation.
   c. No prophylaxis is required for those at low risk:
      - Isolated *CD46* mutations.
      - *DGKE* mutations.
      - No mutations identified.
      - Low anti-CFH titer in anti-CFH antibody disease.
   d. Consider adding Rituximab to transplant immunosuppressive regime in those with anti-CFH antibody disease.
   e. If Eculizumab is not available, consider PE for responsive patients a few hours before transplantation, followed initially by daily PE post-transplantation, and subsequently with gradual reduction in frequency.
4. Avoiding endothelial damage:
   a. Antibody-mediated rejection: Avoid transplantation across preformed donor-specific antibody or positive cross-match.
   b. Infections: CMV prophylaxis.
   c. Immunosuppression: Careful monitoring of CNI levels to avoid over-dosing with consideration for low-dose regimes.
      - CNI-free mTORi-based regimes should be avoided.
   d. Hypertension: Strict blood pressure control.

5. Role of liver transplantation:
   a. Many (but not all) complement components and regulatory proteins are synthesized in the liver.
   b. Combined liver-kidney transplant or pre-emptive liver transplant is potentially curative in those with high-risk mutations, i.e., *CFH*, *CFI*, *C3*, and *CFB*, or otherwise at high risk of recurrence.
   c. May be an alternative to long-term post-kidney transplant Eculizumab prophylaxis, but there is currently limited experience.
   d. These patients will still require perioperative prophylaxis (possibly including PE), without which perioperative mortality may be 100%.

Recommended Reading

1. Waters AM, Kerecuk L, Luk D, Haq MR, Fitzpatrick MM, Gilbert RD, Inward C, Jones C, Pichon B, Reid C, Slack MP, Van't Hoff W, Dillon MJ, Taylor CM, Tullus K. (2007) Hemolytic uremic syndrome associated with invasive pneumococcal disease: The United Kingdom experience. *J Pediatr* **151**:140–144.
2. Legendre CM, Licht C, Muus P, Greenbaum LA, Babu S, Bedrosian C, Bingham C, Cohen DJ, Delmas Y, Douglas K, Eitner F, Feldkamp T, Fouque D, Furman RR, Gaber O, Herthelius M, Hourmant M, Karpman D, Lebranchu Y, Mariat C, Menne J, Moulin B, Nürnberger J, Ogawa M, Remuzzi G, Richard T, Sberro-Soussan R, Severino B, Sheerin NS, Trivelli A, Zimmerhackl LB, Goodship T, Loirat C. (2013) Terminal complement inhibitor eculizumab in atypical hemolytic-uremic syndrome. *N Engl J Med* **368**:2169–2181.
3. Saland J. (2014) Liver-kidney transplantation to cure atypical HUS: Still an option post-eculizumab? *Pediatr Nephrol* **29**:329–332.
4. Ardissino G, Tel F, Possenti I, Testa S, Consonni D, Paglialonga F, Salardi S, Borsa-Ghiringhelli N, Salice P, Tedeschi S, Castorina P, Colombo RM, Arghittu M, Daprai L, Monzani A, Tozzoli R, Brigotti M, Torresani E. (2016) Early volume expansion and outcomes of hemolytic uremic syndrome. *Pediatrics* **137**. doi:10.1542/peds.2015–2153.
5. Loirat C, Fakhouri F, Ariceta G, Besbas N, Bitzan M, Bjerre A, Coppo R, Emma F, Johnson S, Karpman D, Landau D, Langman CB, Lapeyraque AL, Licht C, Nester C, Pecoraro C, Riedl M, van de Kar NC, Van de Walle J, Vivarelli M, Frémeaux-Bacchi V; HUS International. (2016) An international consensus approach to the management of atypical hemolytic uremic syndrome in children. *Pediatr Nephrol* **31**:15–39.
6. Durey MA, Sinha A, Togarsimalemath SK, Bagga A. (2016) Anti-complement-factor H-associated glomerulopathies. *Nat Rev Nephrol* **12**:563–578.
7. Goodship TH, Cook HT, Fakhouri F, Fervenza FC, Frémeaux-Bacchi V, Kavanagh D, Nester CM, Noris M, Pickering MC, Rodríguez de Córdoba S, Roumenina LT, Sethi S, Smith RJ; Conference Participants. (2017) Atypical hemolytic uremic syndrome and C3

glomerulopathy: Conclusions from a "Kidney Disease: Improving Global Outcomes" (KDIGO) Controversies Conference. *Kidney Int* **91**:539–551.

8. Brocklebank V, Johnson S, Sheerin TP, Marks SD, Gilbert RD, Tyerman K, Kinoshita M, Awan A, Kaur A, Webb N, Hegde S, Finlay E, Fitzpatrick M, Walsh PR, Wong EKS, Booth C, Kerecuk L, Salama AD, Almond M, Inward C, Goodship TH, Sheerin NS, Marchbank KJ, Kavanagh D. (2017) Factor H autoantibody is associated with atypical hemolytic uremic syndrome in children in the United Kingdom and Ireland. *Kidney Int* **92**:1261–1271.
9. Percheron L, Gramada R, Tellier S, Salomon R, Harambat J, Llanas B, Fila M, Allain-Launay E, Lapeyraque AL, Leroy V, Adra AL, Bérard E, Bourdat-Michel G, Chehade H, Eckart P, Merieau E, Piètrement C, Sellier-Leclerc AL, Frémeaux-Bacchi V, Dimeglio C, Garnier A. (2018) Eculizumab treatment in severe pediatric STEC-HUS: A multicenter retrospective study. *Pediatr Nephrol* **33**:1385–1394.
10. Brocklebank V, Kumar G, Howie AJ, Chandar J, Milford DV, Craze J, Evans J, Finlay E, Freundlich M, Gale DP, Inward C, Mraz M, Jones C, Wong W, Marks SD, Connolly J, Corner BM, Smith-Jackson K, Walsh PR, Marchbank KJ, Harris CL, Wilson V, Wong EKS, Malina M, Johnson S, Sheerin NS, Kavanagh D. (2020) Long-term outcomes and response to treatment in diacylglycerol kinase epsilon nephropathy. *Kidney Int* **97**:1260–1274.
11. Niaudet P, Boyer OG. (2020, updated) Clinical manifestations and diagnosis of Shiga toxin-producing Escherichia coli (STEC) hemolytic uremic syndrome (HUS) in children. Edited by: Kaplan SL, Mattoo TK, Kim MA. *UpToDate ONLINE*. http://www.uptodateonline.com.
12. Niaudet P, Boyer OG. (2021, updated) Overview of hemolytic uremic syndrome in children. Edited by: Mattoo TK, Kim MA. *UpToDate ONLINE*. http://www.uptodateonline.com.
13. Niaudet P, Boyer OG. (2021, updated) Treatment and prognosis of Shiga toxin-producing Escherichia coli (STEC) hemolytic uremic syndrome (HUS) in children. Edited by: Mattoo TK, Kim MA. *UpToDate ONLINE*. http://www.uptodateonline.com.
14. Niaudet P, Boyer OG. (2021, updated) Complement-mediated hemolytic uremic syndrome in children Edited by: Mattoo TK, Kim MA. *UpToDate ONLINE*. http://www.uptodateonline.com.
15. Fakhouri F, Fila M, Hummel A, Ribes D, Sellier-Leclerc AL, Ville S, Pouteil-Noble C, Coindre JP, Le Quintrec M, Rondeau E, Boyer O, Provôt F, Djeddi D, Hanf W, Delmas Y, Louillet F, Lahoche A, Favre G, Châtelet V, Launay EA, Presne C, Zaloszyc A, Caillard S, Bally S, Raimbourg Q, Tricot L, Mousson C, Le Thuaut A, Loirat C, Frémeaux-Bacchi V. (2021) Eculizumab discontinuation in children and adults with atypical hemolytic-uremic syndrome: A prospective multicenter study. *Blood* **137**:2438–2449.

12 Immunosuppressive Medications

Teo S, Resontoc LP, Lu L, Ng KH and Yap HK

A. Glucocorticoids (GCs)

1. Mechanism of action:
   a. Binds to intracellular GC receptor and translocates to the nucleus where the complex interacts with glucocorticoid responsive elements (GRE) and other transcription factors.
   b. Anti-inflammatory effects of GCs result from:
      - Binding to and blocking promotor sites of proinflammatory genes such as interleukin (IL)-1α and IL-1β.
      - Recruiting of transcription factors to promoter sequences of genes coding for anti-inflammatory gene products including I-κ-Bα, IL-10, IL-1R-II, annexin 1, α-2 macroglobulin, and secretory leukocyte-protease inhibitor.
      - Inhibition of synthesis of inflammatory cytokines.
   c. Effect of GCs on the immune system:
      - Lymphopenia affecting mainly T-cells.
      - Marked reduction in circulating dendritic cells.
      - Inhibition of cytokine production and degranulation by mast cells.
      - Decrease in IgG and IgA levels.

2. Formulation:

GC	Side Group*	Equivalent Doses (mg)	Anti-inflammatory Activity Relative to Hydro-cortisone	Mineralo-corticoid Activity Relative to Hydro-cortisone
Short acting (8–12 hours):				
Hydrocortisone (cortisol)		20	1	1
Cortisone acetate		25	0.8	0.8
Intermediate acting (12–36 hours):				
Prednisone		5	4	0.8
Prednisolone (PNL)		5	4	0.8
Methylprednisolone (MP)	Methylated	4	5	Minimal
Deflazacort	Methyl-oxazine at positions 16,17	6	4	
Triamcinolone	Fluorinated	4	5	0
Long acting (36–72 hours):				
Dexamethasone (Dexa)	Fluorinated	0.75	30	Minimal
Betamethasone	Fluorinated	0.6	30	Nil
Mineralocorticoid (12–36 hours)				
Fludrocortisone	Fluorinated	#	10–15	125–150

*GC fluorinated at the 6α- or 9α-position or methylated at the 6α-position or methyloxazoline at position 16,17 are protected from oxidation inactivation by the 11-β-hydroxysteorid dehydrogenase type 2 isoenzyme found mainly in mineralocorticoid target tissues, explaining their salt-retaining properties.

#GC doses providing mineralocorticoid effect equivalent to 0.1 mg fludrocortisone are: Prednisone (or PNL) 50 mg and hydrocortisone 20 mg.

3. Drug interactions:
   a. GCs are metabolized by cytochrome P450 3A4 (CYP3A4), and Dexa, MP and PNL are also substrates of P-glycoprotein membrane (P-gp) efflux transporters.
   b. Increased GC concentration:
      i. Estrogen derivatives (oral contraceptives).
      ii. Strong inhibitors of CYP3A4 (in particular, MP and Dexa):
         - Macrolide antibiotics, e.g., clarithromycin.
         - Antifungals, e.g., posaconazole, voriconazole, itraconazole, ketoconazole.
         - Antivirals, e.g., ritonavir, atazanavir, boceprevir, darunavir, fosamprenavir, indinavir, lopinavir, nelfinavir, saquinavir, telaprevir.
         - Calcineurin inhibitors (CNIs).
         - mTOR inhibitors.
   c. Decreased GC concentration:
      i. Decreased oral absorption:
         - Aluminium/magnesium containing antiacids.
      ii. Strong inducers of CYP34A and/or P-gp (in particular, MP):
         - Anti-epileptic drugs: Carbamazepine, phenobarbitone, phenytoin, primidone.
         - Anti-microbials:
            - Anti-tuberculous drugs: Rifampin, rifabutin, rifapentine.
            - Antibiotics: Nafcillin.
            - Antiviral: Efavirenz, etravirine.
   d. Altered CsA concentrations (increased or decreased) with Dexa.
   e. Decreased everolimus concentrations with Dexa (avoid if possible).
   f. Increased anticoagulant effect of warfarin.
      - Monitor international normalized ratio (INR) within 3–7 days after initiating GC.
   g. GC potentiates the potassium-wasting effect of diuretics.
      - Check serum potassium levels if on concomitant diuretics.
   h. Increased risk of tendinopathy with the use of fluoroquinolones, e.g., ciprofloxacin, levofloxacin.
   i. Glucose dysregulation in patients on hypoglycemic agents.

   j. Increased risk of peptic ulcer disease with concomitant use of non-steroidal anti-inflammatory drugs (NSAIDs).

4. Adverse effects associated with systemic use:
   a. Appearance and skin:
      - Skin thinning, purpura, ecchymoses, acne, hirsutism, facial erythema, striae.
      - Cushingoid appearance.
      - Weight gain with truncal obesity.
   b. Ophthalmology:
      - Posterior subcapsular cataract.
      - Glaucoma, elevated intraocular pressure.
      - Exophthalmos.
   c. Cardiovascular:
      - Hypertension.
      - Fluid retention.
      - Arrhythmias.
   d. Gastrointestinal:
      - Gastritis, peptic ulcer disease, gastrointestinal bleeding.
   e. Musculoskeletal:
      - Growth failure.
      - Osteoporosis.
      - Proximal myopathy.
      - Avascular necrosis of bone.
   f. Metabolic:
      - Hyperglycemia.
      - Dyslipidemia.
      - Hypothalamic-pituitary-adrenal insufficiency.
   g. Neuropsychiatric:
      - Insomnia.
      - Mood disorders.
      - Memory impairment.
      - Psychosis.
      - Pseudotumor cerebri may be related to rapid tapering of high dose GC.
   h. Immune system:
      - Increased risk of infection.
   i. Hematological:
      - Leukocytosis.

5. Baseline assessment before initiation of GC therapy:
   a. Assess for underlying conditions that may be exacerbated by GC therapy:
      i. History including family history and physical examination for diabetes mellitus, dyslipidemia, behavioral disorders, infections such as tuberculosis, and varicella-zoster immune status.
      ii. Concomitant medications that may interact with GCs.
   b. Baseline height, weight, body mass index (BMI), pubertal assessment, nutritional status, and blood pressure.
   c. Investigations:
      i. Full blood count (FBC).
      ii. Glucose (urine or random/fasting/2-hour post-prandial blood glucose or HbA1c).
      iii. Lipid profile (total cholesterol, LDL-cholesterol, HDL-cholesterol, triglycerides).
      iv. Tuberculin skin test and/or chest X-ray to exclude tuberculosis in adolescents with a positive family history or from high endemic countries.
6. Monitoring for long-term GC use:
   a. Weight and blood pressure at every clinic visit (1–3 monthly).
   b. Height, growth charting, height velocity, body mass index (3–6 monthly).
   c. Pubertal assessment (6–12 monthly).
   d. Metabolic screen:
      i. Glucose:
         - Urine or blood glucose (fasting or 2-hour post-prandial) at least annually.
         - Consider oral glucose tolerance test (OGTT) if the child is obese or has multiple risk factors for diabetes.
      ii. Cholesterol and triglycerides at least annually.
   e. Ophthalmologic screen for intraocular pressure and cataracts at least annually.
   f. Bone health:
      i. Consider baseline spine bone mineral density (BMD) and lateral spine X-ray in children receiving >3 months GC.
      ii. Consider repeating 1–2 yearly if risk factors persist:
         - Low trauma extremity fractures.
         - Back pain.

- Decline in spine BMD Z-scores.
- Growth deceleration.
- Cushingnoid features.

g. Screening for adrenal suppression:
   i. Risk for adrenal suppression:
      - If the patient has been on systemic supraphysiological doses of GC for >2 consecutive weeks or >3 cumulative weeks in 6 months
   ii. Suspect in patients with the following features suggestive of adrenal insufficiency:
      - Weakness, fatigue, malaise.
      - Nausea, vomiting, diarrhea, abdominal pain.
      - Morning headache
      - Poor weight gain and/or growth.
      - Myalgia and arthralgia.
      - Hypotension.
      - Hypoglycemia.
   iii. Early morning cortisol.
      - Short and intermediate-acting GC dose should be tapered to the physiologic dose before the test, while long-acting GCs should be switched to hydrocortisone before the test.
      - Hold dose evening and morning prior to the test.
      - Complete the test by 8 am.
      - Diagnostic if early morning cortisol <85 nmol/L.
   iv. Low dose adrenocorticotropic hormone (ACTH) test:
      - Indicated if early morning cortisol is normal, but the patient has features suggestive of adrenal suppression.
      - Give 1 mcg IV cosyntropin (Synacthen), then measure cortisol levels at 0, 15 and 30 minutes.
      - Diagnostic if peak cortisol <500 nmol/L.

B. Cyclophosphamide (CYC)

1. Mechanism of action:
   a. Alkylating agent of the nitrogen mustard type.
      - Metabolized primarily in the liver to 4-hydroxy CYC and aldophosphamide, which is then converted to the active

metabolite phosphoramide mustard and the highly reactive aldehyde, acrolein.

b. Activated form binds to DNA, resulting in cross-linking of strands of DNA and RNA and inhibition of protein synthesis.

c. Cytotoxic agent resulting in absolute lymphopenia and inhibition of immune function.

d. Acrolein is responsible for bladder and cardiac toxicity.

2. Drug dosing:

a. Oral: 2–2.5 mg/kg/day (maximum adult dose 200 mg).

- Adjustment of oral dose in kidney function impairment:

Estimated Glomerular Filtration Rate (eGFR) ml/min/1.73m²	CYC Dose (mg/kg/day)
≥90	2.0
50–89	1.5
25–49	1.2
15–24	1.0
<15 or dialysis	0.8

- Administer CYC tablets in the morning and encourage liberal fluid intake of 2 L/1.73m² (at least 8 glasses) throughout the day.
- Empty the bladder before sleeping so as to decrease exposure time to the toxic metabolite acrolein.

b. Intravenous: 500 mg/m², 750 mg/m² and 1000 mg/m² depending on indications. (See chapter "Intermittent Intravenous Cyclophosphamide Therapy for Glomerulonephritis".)

3. Drug interactions:

a. Drugs that induce hepatic microsomal enzymes, in particular, CYP2B6, resulting in increased metabolism of CYC into its active metabolites:

- Anti-epileptic drugs: Carbamazepine, phenobarbitone, phenytoin.
- Anti-tuberculous drugs: Rifampin.

b. Drugs that inhibit hepatic microsomal enzymes, decreasing conversion of CYC to active metabolites:

- Antiplatelet agent: Clopidogrel.
- Tricyclic antidepressant: Desipramine.
- Serotonin reuptake inhibitor: Sertraline, paroxetine.

c. CYC prolongs succinylcholine effect on neuromuscular blockade due to the reduction of plasma pseudocholinesterase activity.
d. Allopurinol increases systemic exposure to toxic metabolites of CYC by altering liver metabolism or kidney excretion.
e. Anticholinergic agents delay bladder emptying while prolonging bladder exposure to acrolein.
   - Oxybutinin, detrussitol, tricyclic antidepressants.
f. Thiazide diuretics may potentiate neutropenia.

4. Adverse effects:
   a. Hematologic toxicity:
      - Neutropenia (absolute neutrophil count <1500 $\times$ 10^9/L) followed by thrombocytopenia and anemia.
      - Dose-related.
      - Nadir of white blood cell count occurs 7–14 days after intravenous administration (lymphocyte nadir day 7, granulocyte nadir day 14) with bone marrow recovery at 21 days.
   b. Risk of infections especially with concomitant use of GCs:
      - Bacterial and fungal infections.
      - Pneumocystis jirovecii.
      - Herpes zoster.
      - Reactivation of human papillomavirus.
   c. Alopecia: Diffuse thinning with onset 3–6 weeks after starting CYC.
   d. Gastrointestinal: Nausea, vomiting, abdominal pain, diarrhea, stomatitis, mucositis.
   e. Gonadal toxicity:
      - Related to cumulative total CYC dose.
      - Females: Infertility and premature ovarian failure, especially in those treated over the age of 30 years.
      - Males:
        - Oligospermia, especially with cumulative doses of >200 mg/kg.
        - Recovery of normal spermatogenesis more likely in men who received a cumulative dose <7.5 g/m^2.
        - Risk for genetic anomalies within sperm highest within 1–2 weeks of CYC dosing.
   f. Teratogenicity (CYC embryopathy):
      - Growth restriction, ear and facial abnormalities, absence of digits, and hypoplastic limbs.

g. Malignancy:
   - Greatest risk in those treated for more than 2–3 years.
   - Increased risk of myelodysplastic syndrome, lymphoma, myeloproliferative disease, and skin cancer.

h. Bladder toxicity:
   - Related to exposure to acrolein.
   - Hemorrhagic cystitis.
   - Bladder cancer.

i. Electrolyte abnormalities:
   - Hyponatremia due to syndrome of inappropriate antidiuretic hormone (SIADH).
   - Hypomagnesemia.

j. Cardiac toxicity: May occur if there is decreased myocardial contractility at baseline.

k. Pulmonary fibrosis (rare): Related to prolonged treatment in those using relatively low doses.

5. Pretreatment evaluation:

a. Assess for possible contraindications:
   - Non-immune mediated neutropenia.
   - Pregnancy and lactation.

b. Check for potential drugs that may interact with CYC.

c. Infection screen:

i. Check for active infection.
   - For IV CYC infusion, ensure that there were no active infections in the last 2 weeks.

ii. Screen for varicella-zoster virus (VZV) infection.
   - Check history for VZV infection or immunization.
   - Confirm if patient is immune to varicella-zoster (VZV-IgG titers).
   - Check if patient has been recently exposed (within 3 weeks of contact) to VZV.
     - If in doubt, check VZV-IgM titers.

iii. Hepatitis B surface antigen (HBsAg) and antibody (anti-HBs), and anti-hepatitis B core antibody (anti-HBc).

iv. Hepatitis C serology.

v. Tuberculosis (TB)
   - Check family history for TB.
   - Consider a chest X-Ray to exclude latent TB.
   - TB screen if positive contact history or is living in a high endemic area:
     - Tuberculin skin test in patients aged <2 years.
     - Interferon-gamma release assay in patients aged ≥2 years:
       - ✓ TB T-spot test (preferred in immunocompromised patients).
       - ✓ TB Quantiferon (less sensitive in immunocompromised patients).

vi. SARS-CoV-2 DNA nucleic acid amplification if clinically indicated.

d. Counsel for gonadal toxicity:

i. In post-pubertal adolescent boys, consider a referral for cryopreservation of ejaculated semen either before or at least 6–12 months after completing CYC course.

ii. Post-pubertal adolescent girls can be offered:
   - Gonadotrophin-releasing hormone (GnRH) agonists for ovarian suppression.
   - Long-acting reversible contraceptives if sexually active.

e. Screening for cervical cancer in sexually active adolescent girls.
   - Papanicolaou (Pap) test (cytology)
   - Cervical testing for human papillomavirus (HPV) testing for oncogenic strains (high-risk HPV).

6. Pneumocystis jirovecii pneumonia prophylaxis:

a. Co-trimoxazole oral 3 mg/kg/dose alternate days.

b. In glucose-6-phosphate dehydrogenase (G6PD)-deficient patients, use aerosolized pentamidine 300 mg monthly (via Respigard nebulizer).

c. In patients who are allergic to co-trimoxazole, alternative drugs include:
   - Dapsone 2 mg/kg daily (maximum 100 mg).
   - Atavaquone 30 mg/kg daily (maximum 1500 mg).

C. Azathioprine (AZA)

1. Mechanism of action:
   a. AZA is the 1-methyl-4-nitro-5-imidazolyl derivative of thioguanine, a purine-mimic antimetabolite.
      i. Principle active metabolite is 6-mercaptopurine (6-MP), formed by the action of glutathione in red blood cells.
      ii. Metabolic pathways:
         - Xanthine oxidase-dependent catabolic oxidation of 6-MP to 6-thiouric acid, an inactive metabolite, in the intestine and liver.
         - Thiopurine S-methyltransferase (TPMT) and hypoxanthine-guanine phosphoribosyl transferase (HGPRT)-dependent anabolic pathway where 6-MP is metabolized to several metabolites, including 6-methylmercaptopurine (6-MMP), 6-methyl-thioinosine 5′-monophosphate, and 6-thioguanine (6-TG).
         - Nucleoside triphosphate diphosphatase or nucleoside diphosphate-linked moiety X-type motif 15 (NUDT15) metabolizes the active thiopurine metabolite thioguanosine triphosphate (TGTP) to inactive thioguanosine monophosphate (TGMP).
   b. 6-MP and its metabolites result in decreased numbers of circulating B and T lymphocytes, reduced immunoglobulin synthesis, and diminished interleukin (IL)-2 secretion through the following mechanisms:
      i. Inhibiting intracellular purine synthesis:
         - Thioinosinic and thioguanylic acid produced by intracellular metabolism of 6-MP by HGPRT suppress inosinic acid synthesis, thereby interfering with adenine and guanine ribonucleotide production.
      ii. Inducing T-cell apoptosis:
         - Thioguanine inhibits costimulatory binding by CD28 on the surface of CD4+ T cells to CD80 and CD86 (B7-1 and B7-2) molecules on antigen-presenting cells.
2. Drug dosing:
   a. 25–75 mg/m^2 or 1–3 mg/kg.

b. Correction for abnormal kidney function:
   - Creatinine clearance 10–50 ml/min/1.73m^2: 75% of the dose.
   - Creatinine clearance <10 ml/min/1.73m^2: 50% of the dose.
   - Hemodialysis: Administer 50% of the dose with a supplement 0.25 mg/kg (approximately 45% removed in 8 hours).
   - Continuous kidney replacement therapy: Administer 75% of the dose.

3. Pharmacogenetics and dose adjustment:
   a. AZA toxicity:
      i. Hematologic toxicity due to AZA and 6-MP is predominantly related to the activity of TPMT and/or NUDT15 genetic variants in the population.
         - Deficiency of TPMT causes 6-MP to be preferentially metabolized to 6-TG nucleotides, accounting for hematologic toxicity, and is the primary genetic cause of thiopurine intolerance in European and African ancestry.
         - Variants of *NUDT15*, particularly, NUDT15 c.415C>T, have been associated with hematologic toxicity, especially in East Asian populations (2% of studied populations have poor metabolizer phenotype) and Hispanics.
         - AZA-related adverse effects are also associated with polymorphisms of glutathione-S-transferase.
      ii. Hepatotoxicity has been associated with the inactive metabolite 6-MMP
   b. Consider genotyping TPMT and NUDT15 first before starting AZA:
      i. TPMT/NUDT15 poor metabolizers are at a very high risk of life-threatening myelosuppression on conventional AZA doses, while intermediate metabolizers tolerate 30–60% of conventional doses of AZA.
      ii. Patients can be assigned a TPMT and NUDT15 phenotype (poor/intermediate/possible intermediate/normal) based on genotypes on both alleles for each gene.
         - An updated reference of genotype-phenotype correlations can be found on the Clinical Pharmacogenetics Implementation Consortium (CPIC) website (https://cpicpgx.org).

- Overall AZA metabolism is described by the poorer of TPMT and NUDT15 metabolism, e.g., if the patient is a TPMT normal metabolizer and NUDT15 poor metabolizer, he/she is considered overall a poor metabolizer.

iii. Dosing recommendations based on a metabolizer status:

Metabolizer Status	Dosing Recommendations
Normal	• Start with normal starting dose. • Allow 2 weeks to reach steady-state after each dose adjustment.
Intermediate/ possible intermediate	• Start with 30–80% of normal starting dose. • Allow 2 to 4 weeks to reach steady-state after each dose adjustment.
Poor	• Consider alternative immunosuppression. • If unavailable, start with 10% of normal starting dose. • For TPMT poor metabolizers, reduce the dosing frequency to 3 times per week. • Allow 4 to 6 weeks to reach steady-state after each dose adjustment.

4. Drug monitoring:
   a. FBC 2 weekly for the first month, then monthly for at least a year, then 3 monthly.
      - Omit if absolute neutrophil count is $<1.5 \times 10^9$/L.
   b. Liver function should be tested monthly for the first year, then 3 monthly.
5. Drug interactions:
   a. Xanthine oxidase inhibitors:
      - Slow the elimination of 6-MP.
      - Avoid concomitant usage of allopurinol and febuxostat.
   b. Angiotensin-converting enzyme inhibitors (ACEi):
      - May enhance myelosuppressive effects of AZA.
   c. Anti-tumor necrosis factor (TNF) agents:
      - Increased risk of non-Hodgkin's T-cell lymphoma including hepatosplenic T-cell lymphoma.

d. Ribavirin (oral inhalation and systemic):
   - Increase the serum concentration of potentially myelotoxic methylated metabolites.
e. Trimethoprim and sulfamethoxazole:
   - Enhance the myelosuppressive effect of AZA.
f. Warfarin:
   - Decreases the effect of vitamin K.
g. 5-aminosalicylic acid derivatives such as sulfasalazine:
   - Enhance the myelosuppressive effect of AZA due to exposure to active 6-TG.
h. Cyclophosphamide:
   - AZA enhances the hepatotoxic effect of cyclophosphamide.

6. Adverse effects:
   a. Hematologic toxicity: Leukopenia, thrombocytopenia, macrocytic anemia and/or pancytopenia.
   b. Hepatotoxicity: Increased alkaline phosphatase, transaminases and bilirubin.
      - Rarely hepatic sinusoidal obstruction syndrome.
   c. Gastric: diarrhea and vomiting.
   d. Fever, myalgia and rarely arthralgia.
   e. Infections including reactivation of latent infections.
   f. Malignancy risk in particular post-transplant lymphoproliferative disease and hepatosplenic T-cell lymphoma.
   g. Progressive multifocal leukoencephalopathy.

D. Mycophenolic Acid (MPA)

1. Mechanism of action:
   a. Reversibly inhibits inosine monophosphate (IMP) dehydrogenase, which catalyzes the conversion of IMP to guanosine monophosphate (GMP), the rate-limiting step in purine nucleotide synthesis specifically in lymphocytes.
   b. Specifically binds type II isoform of IMP dehydrogenase expressed by activated lymphocytes.
   c. These properties result in:
      - Decreased B- and T cell proliferation and antibody production.
      - Induction of apoptosis of activated T lymphocytes.

d. Inhibition of adhesion molecule expression and lymphocyte recruitment.

2. Formulations:
   a. Mycophenolate mofetil (MMF): Prodrug (morpholinoethyl ester) of MPA.
      - Cellcept®.
   b. Enteric-coated mycophenolate sodium (ECMS) (Myfortic®): Reduces incidence of gastrointestinal side effects, primarily diarrhea, through the delayed release of MPA into the small intestine.
   c. Dose equivalence:
      Myfortic® 180 mg = 250 mg Cellcept®.
      Myfortic® 360 mg = 500 mg Cellcept®.
3. Drug dosing:
   a. MMF: 600 mg/m²/dose 12 hourly (15–23 mg/kg/dose 12 hourly).
      - Maximum adult dose: 1–1.5 g 12 hourly.
   b. ECMS: 400 mg/m²/dose 12 hourly.
      - Maximum adult dose: 720 mg 12 hourly.
   c. May require a reduced dosage in kidney failure (avoid doses >1 g 12 hourly).
4. Drug monitoring:
   a. Monitor FBC monthly to 3 monthly.
      - Omit if absolute neutrophil count $<1.5 \times 10^9$/L.
   b. Consider monitoring serum mycophenolate levels if necessary (target 2–4 mg/L).
   c. Estimation of MPA area under the time–concentration curve (AUC):

AUC Formula (mg L^{-1} hour)	Assay#	Reference
$0.98*[C_1] + 2.38*[C_2] + 4.86*[C_6] + 10.75$	EMIT	(Filler and Mai, 2000)
$18.6 + 4.3*[C0] + 0.54*[C0.5] + 2.15*[C2]$	EMIT	(Weber *et al.*, 2006))
$7.75 + 6.49*[C_0] + 0.76*[C_{0.5}] + 2.43*[C_2]$	CEDIA	(Pawinski *et al.*, 2009)
Bayesian estimator	HPLC	(Woillard *et al.*, 2014)

#EMIT: Enzyme multiplied immunoassay test
CEDIA: Cloned enzyme donor immunoassay
HPLC: High-performance liquid chromatography

- Target MPA AUC 30–60 mg*h/L.

d. Food and drug interactions:
   i. Decrease in absorption:
      - High fat meal.
      - Antacids.
      - Minerals: Magnesium, calcium, iron.
      - Sevelamer.
      - Bile acid sequestrants: Cholestyramine.
      - Proton pump inhibitors, e.g., pantoprazole and lansoprazole.
   ii. Decreased serum concentration of MPA:
      - Rifampicin.
   iii. Increased serum concentration of MPA:
      - Acyclovir, valacyclovir.
      - Probencid.
e. Adverse effects:
   i. Bone marrow suppression: Neutropenia (especially at 1–6 months of therapy), anemia, and thrombocytopenia (rare).
   ii. Gastrointestinal: Gastritis, peptic ulceration, abdominal colic, diarrhea, gastrointestinal hemorrhage, and perforation.
      - Histopathologic changes suggestive of inflammatory bowel disease (or colitis) have been described.
   iii. Viral infections such as cytomegalovirus and herpes zoster.
   iv. Progressive multifocal leukoencephalopathy (rare).
   v. Malignancy including lymphomas.
   vi. Pregnancy:
      - First-trimester pregnancy loss.
      - Congenital malformations including cleft lip and palate, anomalies of the distal limbs, heart, esophagus, and kidneys.
f. Start famotidine prophylactically at 0.5–1 mg/kg/day once nightly or divided dose 12 hourly (maximum 40 mg), or rabeprazole 0.5–1.0 mg/kg once nightly or divided dose 12 hourly (maximum 40 mg).
g. Avoid MPA in:
   - Pregnancy: Stop the drug for at least 3 months prior to attempting conception.
   - Breastfeeding as MPA is excreted into breast milk.

E. Calcineurin Inhibitors (CNI)

1. Mechanism of action:
   a. Cyclosporine (CsA) and tacrolimus (Tac) selectively inhibit calcineurin, a calcium- and calmodulin-dependent phosphatase, by binding to cyclophilin and FK-binding protein respectively.
   b. This process leads to the inhibition of transcription of IL-2 and other cytokine genes, namely, tumor necrosis factor (TNF)-α, IL-3, IL-4, CD40L, granulocyte-macrophage colony-stimulating factor, and interferon-γ, resulting in the reduction of T lymphocyte proliferation.
   c. CNIs act primarily on T helper cells, with some effect on the T suppressor and T cytotoxic cells.
   d. CsA also increases the expression of transforming growth factor (TGF)-β, which is pro-fibrotic and may therefore be associated with renal fibrosis.
2. Formulations:

CNI	Formulation	Strength	Switching Formulation	Notes
CsA[b] (non-modified)	Oral capsules *(Sandimmune/ Generics)*	25 mg 50 mg 100 mg	▪ 1:1 conversion with modified formulation ▪ 40:1 conversion from CsA to Tac	▪ Depends on bile for absorption, therefore, absorption is erratic ▪ Solution should be mixed with milk, chocolate milk or orange juice at room temperature
	Oral solution[a]	100 mg/ ml (50 ml bottles)		
	Parenteral	50 mg/ ml in 5 ml ampules	▪ Dose is 1/3 the oral dose	▪ Use polyvinyl chloride (PVC)-free IV containers and tubings ▪ Infuse over 2–6 hours BD

(*Continued*)

CNI	Formulation	Strength	Switching Formulation	Notes
CsA[b] (modified) Micro-emulsion	Oral capsules *(Neoral/ Generics)*	10 mg 25 mg 100 mg	▪ 1:1 conversion with non-modified formulation ▪ 40:1 conversion from CsA to Tac	▪ Does not depend upon bile salts for absorption ▪ Increased bioavailability and more consistent absorption ▪ Solution should be mixed with water, orange juice or apple juice
	Oral solution[a]	100 mg/ ml (50 ml bottles)		
Tac[a,d]	Immediate release capsules *(Prograf)*[b]	0.5 mg 1 mg 5 mg	▪ 1:1 conversion with extended release capsules ▪ 5:4 conversion with extended release tablets ▪ 40:1 conversion from CsA to Tac	▪ Sublingual Tac is 50% the oral Tac dose

(*Continued*)

(*Continued*)

CNI	Formulation	Strength	Switching Formulation	Notes
	Extended release capsules[c] (*Astagraf XL/ Advagraf*)	0.5 mg 1 mg 5 mg	▪ 1:1 conversion with immediate release capsules ▪ 5:4 conversion with extended release tablets ▪ 40:1 conversion from CsA to Tac	▪ Should not be crushed or chewed
Tac[a,d]	Extended-release tablets[c] (*Envarsus XR*)	0.75 mg 1 mg 4 mg	▪ 80% of total daily dose of immediate-release tacrolimus	▪ Should not be crushed or chewed
	Parenteral	5 mg/ml in 1ml ampules	▪ Dose is 1/3 to 1/5 the daily oral dose	▪ Given as continuous 24-hour infusion

[a]Avoid plastic cups and utensils as CNI solutions and granules may adhere to plastic.
[b]Missed dose should be taken as soon as possible within 4 hours, without doubling the next dose.
[c]Missed dose of extended-release Tac should be taken as soon as possible within 14–15 hours after missing the dose, and if not possible, to wait until the usual scheduled time to take the next daily dose without doubling it.
[c]Consumption of alcohol may increase the release rate of extended-release Tac, adversely affecting the effectiveness and safety.
[d]Sodium bicarbonate, magnesium hydroxide and aluminum hydroxide should be given at least 2 hours apart from Tac because this may affect bioavailability by causing pH-mediated degradation, i.e., lowering the Tac levels.

3. Drug dosing:
   a. CsA: Starting dose: 4–10 mg/kg/day given 12 hourly.
   b. Tac (immediate release): Starting dose: 0.1–0.2 mg/kg/day given 12 hourly.
4. Drug monitoring:
   a. CsA:
      i. 12-hour trough (C_0).
      ii. 2-hour post-dose (C_2).
      iii. CsA pharmacokinetics study:
         - AUC = 2.4*[C_2] + 7.7*[C_6] + 195.8 (Amante and Kahan, 1996)
         - AUC = 335.9 + 1.1*[C_1] + 1.1*[C_2] + 5.4*[C_4] (Kelles *et al.*, 1999)
         - $\text{Average concentration } (C_{AV}) = \dfrac{\text{AUC}}{\text{Dosing Interval}}$
   b. Tac:
      i. 12-hour or 24-hour trough (C_0).
      ii. Tac pharmacokinetics study:
         - AUC = 16.2 + 2.4*[C2] + 5.9*[C4] (Wong *et al.*, 2000)
   c. Target concentrations depend on the disease being treated.
   d. Dose adjustments:
      i. Steady-state concentrations reached after 4–6 doses.
      ii. Hold dose if the drug concentration is supratherapeutic until drug concentrations return to therapeutic range:
         - CsA: C_0 >400 ng/ml.
         - Tac: C_0 >20 ng/ml.
      iii. If creatinine increases by 25% and CNI nephrotoxicity is suspected, reduce CNI dose by 20% to determine if this is the cause.
5. Food interactions:
   a. Avoid grapefruit or grapefruit juice, which contains furanocoumarins, potent inhibitors of cytochrome P-450 3A4 enzyme, resulting in an increase in systemic exposure to CNI.
   b. High-fat meal affects absorption, decreasing maximum concentration (C_{max}) and area under the curve (AUC).
      - Tac absorption is more affected than CsA.

6. Drug interactions:
   a. Mechanism of action:
      i. CNIs are substrates for cytochrome P-450 3A4/5 (CYP3A4/5) enzymes, and therefore any drug that is metabolized by these enzymes or affects metabolism by these enzymes can potentially interact with CNIs.
      ii. CsA and not Tac, is an inhibitor of P-gp, which may lead to nephrotoxicity due to the increased kidney exposure when interacting with drugs that inhibit P-gp-mediated efflux of CsA from tubular epithelial cells.
      iii. Absorption of CNI is influenced by drugs that affect gastrointestinal motility or emptying.
      iv. Divalent cations influence absorption of tacrolimus.
   b. Decrease CNI levels:
      i. Inducers of CYP3A4/5:
         - Anti-epileptic agents: Phenytoin, carbamazepine, phenobarbitone, primidone, eslicarbazepine.
         - Anti-tuberculous agents: Isoniazid, rifampin.
         - Anticoagulants: Heparin, warfarin.
         - Antibiotics: Co-trimoxazole.
         - Estrogens: Estradiol, norethindrone.
         - Prednisolone, dexamethasone.
         - Endothelin receptor antagonist: Bosentan.
         - Cystic fibrosis treatment: Lumacaftor, lumacaftor-ivacaftor.
         - St. John's wort.
      ii. Decrease in bioavailability:
         - Laxatives (decrease intestinal transit time).
         - Sodium bicarbonate.
   c. Increase in CNI levels:
      i. Inhibitors of CYP3A4/5:
         - Macrolide antibiotics: Erythromycin, clarithromycin, azithromycin
         - Azole antifungals: Ketoconazole, variconazole, fluconazole, itraconazole, posaconazole.
         - Non-dihydropyridine calcium channel blockers: Diltiazem, verapamil.
         - Anti-arrhythmic agents: Amiodarone, dronedarone.

- Antiviral agents:
  - Hepatitis C: Ombitasvir, paritaprevir, ritonavir, dasabuvir.
  - Human immunodeficiency virus (HIV): Indinavir, lopinavir, nelfinavir, saquinavir, fosamprenavir.
  - Cytomegalovirus: Letermovir.
- Methylprednisolone (high dose).
- Cimetidine (weak inhibitor, associated with about 15% increase in serum creatinine due to the inhibition of proximal tubular secretion of creatinine).
- Androgens: Methyltestosterone.
- Schisandra.

ii. Inhibitor of P-gp:
- Carvedilol (increases CsA levels).

iii. Increase in bioavailability:
- Prokinetic agents (hasten gastric emptying into small intestines): Erythromycin, metoclopramide.
- Narcotics (prolong intestinal transit time).
- Divalent cations: Aluminum hydroxide, magnesium hydroxide (may increase Tac AUC).

d. Potentiate acute nephrotoxicity:
   i. Antimicrobial agents: Aminoglycosides, amphotericin B, acyclovir, sulfonamides including co-trimoxazole, rifampicin.
   ii. Non-steroidal anti-inflammatory drugs (NSAIDs).
   iii. Phenobarbitone.
   iv. Renin-angiotensin system blockers (RASB).
   v. Diuretics: Furosemide.
   vi. Colchicine.

e. Other interactions:
   i. Imipenem: Central nervous system disturbance including seizures.
   ii. Digoxin: Increase in serum digoxin levels.
   iii. 3-hydroxy-3-methylglutaryl coenzyme A (HMG CoA) reductase inhibitors: Rhabdomyolysis, myalgia and muscle weakness.

7. Adverse effects:
   a. Acute reversible kidney injury.

b. Hypertension due to renal vasoconstriction and sodium retention.
   - Calcium channel blockers useful to reverse acute renal vasoconstriction.

c. Thrombotic microangiopathy.

d. Acid-base and electrolyte abnormalities:
   i. Hyperkalemia.
      - Aggravated by the concurrent use of renin-angiotensin system blockers (RASBs), aldosterone antagonists, amiloride, triamterene, trimethoprim, and co-trimoxazole.
      - Concurrent use of beta-blockers with CsA may also result in the transient elevation of plasma potassium concentration due to the movement of potassium out of the cells into the extracellular fluid.

   ii. Hypomagnesemia due to renal magnesium wasting.
   iii. Renal tubular acidosis type 4.
   iv. Hypophosphatemia.
   v. Hypercalciuria.

e. Neurotoxicity (more common with Tac than CsA):
   i. Tremors.
   ii. Reversible posterior leukoencephalopathy syndrome (PRES):
      - Severe headache, visual abnormalities, seizures.
      - Brain imaging: Posterior leukoencephalopathy.

   iii. Akinetic mutism, encephalopathy, seizures, focal neurologic abnormalities, coma:
      - Reported with Tac.

   iv. CNI pain syndrome:
      - Symmetrical pain in lower limbs, in particular, bones of feet, ankles, knees.
      - MRI: Marrow edema.
      - Symptoms improve with the use of calcium channel blockers.

f. Metabolic abnormalities:
   i. Glucose intolerance and diabetes mellitus:
      - Tac causes worse toxicity to islet cells in the pancreas.

   ii. Hyperlipidemia:
      - Dose-dependent association of CsA with hypercholesterolemia.

iii. Hyperuricemia and gout:
   - Worse with CsA due to reduced uric acid secretion by renal tubules.

g. Increased risk of infections.
h. Risk of malignancy:
   i. Benign or malignant lymphoproliferative disorders.
   ii. Squamous cell skin cancer.
i. Gastrointestinal side effects:
   i. Anorexia, nausea, vomiting diarrhea, abdominal discomfort:
      - More frequent with Tac.
   ii. Elevated transaminases with mild hyperbilirubinemia:
      - Reversible with dose reduction or discontinuation of CNI.
j. Cosmetic:
   i. Gingival hyperplasia and fibromatosis:
      - Associated with CsA.
      - Advise on good dental hygiene to prevent gingival hyperplasia.
      - Treatment of mild or early hyperplasia: Azithromycin for 3 consecutive days or Metronidazole for 2 weeks.
   ii. Hirsutism:
      - Associated with CsA.
   iii. Alopecia:
      - Associated with Tac.

F. Mammalian (Mechanistic) Target of Rapamycin Inhibitor (mTORi)

1. Mechanism of action:
   a. Sirolimus (SRL) and everolimus (EVL) exert their antiproliferative effects by binding to the FK binding protein and modulating the activity of mTOR.
      - mTOR inhibits IL-2-mediated signal transduction, resulting in cell-cycle arrest in the G1-S phase.
   b. SRL and EVL block the response of T and B cell activation by cytokines, which prevent cell-cycle progression and proliferation.
   c. SRL inhibits proliferation of smooth muscle cells.

   d. EVL inhibits the expression of vascular endothelial growth factor (VEGF) and hypoxia-inducible factor (HIF-1) causing antiangiogenic effects.

2. Formulations:
   a. SRL
      - Available in 0.5 mg, 1 mg and 2 mg tablets and a 1 mg/ml oral solution.
      - Oral solution should be taken with water and orange juice.
   b. EVL [40-O-(2 hydroxyethyl) derivative of sirolimus]
      - Certican®: 0.25 mg and 0.75 mg tablets
      - Afinitor®: 2.5 mg, 5 mg and 10 mg tablets
3. Drug dosing:
   a. SRL:
      i. Children:
         - Loading dose on Day 1: 3–5 mg/m²/day divided every 12 hours.
         - Maintenance dose: 3 mg/m²/day divided every 12 hours.
      ii. Adolescents (weight <40 kg):
         - Loading dose on Day 1: 3 mg/m²/day divided every 12 hours.
         - Maintenance dose: 1 mg/m²/day divided every 12 hours.
      iii. Adolescents (weight >40 kg):
         - Loading dose on Day 1: 6 mg daily.
         - Maintenance dose: 2 mg daily.
      iv. Dose adjustment:
         - Dosages should be adjusted to maintain trough whole blood concentrations within the desired range.
         - Dosage should be adjusted at 7–14 days intervals due to the long half-life.
         - Patients on twice-daily doses should have their levels checked earlier than 7 days due to pharmacokinetic differences.
         - New sirolimus dose = current dose × (target concentration/current concentration)
         - If a large dose increase is required, consider a loading dose: Loading dose = 3 × (new maintenance dose − current maintenance dose)
            - If the required dose >40 mg/day, divide over 2 days as the maximum adult daily dose is 40 mg.

b. EVL:
   - Starting dose: 0.8 mg/m^2 12 hourly.
   - Adult dose: 0.75 mg 12 hourly (Maximum 1.5 mg 12 hourly).

c. mTORi should only be started 1 month after kidney transplantation due to the increased risk of graft arterial and venous thrombosis and poor wound healing.

4. Drug monitoring:
   a. Trough whole blood levels of SRL and EVL correlate well with AUC.
   b. Whole blood concentrations of SRL are measured by chromatographic and immunoassay methods.
   c. Steady-state concentrations:
      - SRL: 5–7 days after the initiation of therapy or change in dose.
      - EVL: 4–5 days.
5. Dosing of mTORi in hepatic impairment:
   a. No dose adjustment is needed for patients with mild hepatic impairment (Child-Pugh Class A).
   b. In patients with moderate hepatic impairment (Child-Pugh Class B), the daily dose needs to be reduced by one-half the recommended initial daily dose, and blood concentrations should be monitored to make further adjustments as necessary.
   c. There is no information on the effects of severe hepatic impairment (Child-Pugh Class C) on everolimus pharmacokinetics.
6. Food interactions:
   a. Avoid grapefruit or grapefruit juice as it may increase plasma concentrations.
   b. High-fat meals affect absorption, decrease the maximum concentration (C_{max}), and increase the AUC and the time to C_{max}.
7. Drug interactions:
   a. SRL and EVL are substrates for cytochrome P450 3A4 and P-gp, resulting in high pharmacokinetic variability.
   b. SRL is counter-transported in the gut lumen by P-gp, accounting for low bioavailability.
   c. Increase plasma concentration of MTOR inhibitors:
      i. Inhibitors of CYP3A and/or P-gp:
         - Macrolide antibiotics: Erythromycin, clarithromycin, azithromycin.

- Azole antifungals: Voriconazole, fluconazole, posaconazole, ketaconazole.
- Non-dihydropyridine calcium channel blockers: Diltiazem, verapamil.
- Anti-arrhythmic agents: Amiodarone.
- Antiviral agents: Ritonavir.
- CNIs: CsA, Tac.

ii. Inhibitors of P-gp:
- Carvedilol.
- CNIs: CsA, Tac.

d. Decrease plasma concentration of MTOR inhibitors by the inducers of CYP3A:

i. Anti-epileptic agents:
- Phenytoin, carbamazepine, primidone, phenobarbitone.

ii. Anti-tuberculous agents:
- Rifampin, rifabutin, rifapentine.

iii. Dexamethasone.

iv. St. John's wort.

e. Higher mean AUC for MPA when used in combination with SRL.
- Dose reduction of MMF required to avoid potential toxicity.

f. Increased risk of angioedema when MTORi is taken with angiotensin-converting enzyme inhibitors (ACEi).

g. Increased risk of rhabdomyolysis in transplant patients when EVL is taken with HMG-CoA reductase inhibitors: Simvastatin, lovastatin.

8. Adverse effects:

a. Kidney:

i. Acute kidney injury.

ii. Proteinuria:
- Due to reduced tubular protein reabsorption and podocyte dysregulation.
- May develop collapsing focal segmental glomerulosclerosis (FSGS) with sirolimus.
- Consider for use only in patients with mild proteinuria and an eGFR >40 ml/min/1.73m^2.
- Treatment: Mild proteinuria may be treated with RASBs, and heavy proteinuria may require drug discontinuation.

iii. Hemolytic uremic syndrome/thrombotic microangiopathy.
   - Reported with a combination of SRL and CsA.

iv. Renal arterial and venous thrombosis associated with EVL.

v. Delayed allograft function:
   - Seen mainly with SRL.

vi. Cast nephropathy (rare):
   - Associated with delayed allograft function and extensive tubular damage when Tac is administered together with SRL.

vii. Myoglobinuria associated with SRL.

b. Cardiovascular:

i. Pericardial effusion associated with SRL.

ii. Pleural effusion.

iii. Hypertension.

c. Dermatology:

i. Acne-like eruption.

ii. Scalp folliculitis.

iii. Hidradenitis suppurativa.

iv. Peripheral edema and angioedema (especially with the use of ACEi).

v. Leukocytoclastic vasculitis.

vi. Poor wound healing.

d. Hematological:

i. Anemia:
   - Combination of MPA and SRL associated with an increased incidence of anemia.

ii. Thrombocytopenia.
   - Dose-related.
   - Occurs 9–10 days after initiation of treatment.
   - Normalization within 2 weeks of discontinuation.

iii. Leukopenia.
   - Occurs within 2 weeks of initiation of therapy and reversible on discontinuation.

e. Gastrointestinal system:

i. Constipation or diarrhea.

ii. Dyspepsia, nausea and vomiting.

iii. Painful mouth ulcers.

iv. Delayed healing of gastric or duodenal ulcers.

f. Metabolic effects:
   i. Hyperlipidemia:
      - Hypercholesterolemia due to the inhibition of lipoprotein lipase.
      - Hypertriglyceridemia.
   ii. Hyperglycemia and new-onset diabetes mellitus associated with SRL.

g. Respiratory system: Interstitial pneumonitis associated with SRL and abnormal kidney function.
   - Complete recovery within 6 months of SRL withdrawal.

h. Arthralgia:
   i. Pain may be disabling and is caused by changes in bone circulation.
   ii. Worse with concomitant use of CsA due to intraosseous vasoconstriction.
   iii. Usually resolves with dose reduction.

i. Malignancy:
   i. Post-transplant lymphoproliferative disease.
   ii. Skin malignancies.

j. Teratogenicity and fertility:
   i. Absolute contraindication in pregnancy.
   ii. Associated with impaired spermatogenesis.

Recommended Reading

1. Amante AJ, Kahan BD. (1996) Abbreviated area-under-the-curve strategy for monitoring cyclosporine microemulsion therapy in immediate posttransplant period. *Clin Chem* **42**:1294–1296.
2. Kelles A, Herman J, Tjandra-Maga TB, Van Damme-Lombaerts R. (1999) Sandimmune to Neoral conversion and value of abbreviated AUC monitoring in stable pediatric kidney transplant recipients. *Pediatr Transplant* **3**:282–287.
3. Wong KM, Shek CC, Chau KF, Li CS. (2000) Abbreviated tacrolimus area-under-the-curve monitoring for renal transplant recipients. *Am J Kidney Dis* **35**:660–666.
4. Filler G, Mai I. (2000) Limited sampling strategy for mycophenolic acid area under the curve. *Ther Drug Monit* **22**:169–173.
5. Weber LT, Hoecker B, Armstrong VW, Oellerich M, Tönshoff B. (2006) Validation of an abbreviated pharmacokinetic profile for the estimation of mycophenolic acid exposure in pediatric renal transplant recipients. *Ther Drug Monit* **28**:623–631.

6. Pawinski T, Kunicki PK, Sobieszczanska-Malek M, Gralak B, Szlaska I. (2009) A limited sampling strategy for estimating mycophenolic acid area under the curve in adult heart transplant patients treated with concomitant cyclosporine. *J Clin Pharm Ther* **34**:89–101.
7. Liu D, Ahmet A, Ward L, Krishnamoorthy P, Mandelcorn ED, Leigh R, Brown JP, Cohen A, Kim H. (2013) A practical guide to the monitoring and management of the complications of systemic corticosteroid therapy. *Allergy Asthma Clin Immunol* **9**:30. doi: 10.1186/1710-1492-9-30.
8. Woillard JB, Bader-Meunier B, Salomon R, Ranchin B, Decramer S, Fischbach M, Berard E, Guigonis V, Harambat J, Dunand O, Tenenbaum J, Marquet P, Saint-Marcoux F. (2014) Pharmacokinetics of mycophenolate mofetil in children with lupus and clinical findings in favour of therapeutic drug monitoring. *Br J Clin Pharmacol* **78**:867–876.
9. Relling MV, Schwab M, Whirl-Carrillo M, Suarez-Kurtz G, Pui CH, Stein CM, Moyer AM, Evans WE, Klein TE, Antillon-Klussmann FG, Caudle KE, Kato M, Yeoh AEJ, Schmiegelow K, Yang JJ. (2019) Clinical pharmacogenetics implementation consortium guideline for thiopurine dosing based on TPMT and NUDT15 genotypes: 2018 update. *Clin Pharmacol Ther* **105**:1095–1105.
10. Clouse MB, McCune JW. (2020, updated) General toxicity of cyclophosphamide in rheumatic diseases. Edited by Frust DE, Curtis MR. *UpToDate ONLINE.* http://www.uptodate.com.
11. Hardinger K, Brennan DC. (2020, updated) Pharmacology of mammalian (mechanistic) target of rapamycin (mTOR) inhibitors. Edited by Legendre C, Vella J. *UpToDate ONLINE.* http://www.uptodate.com.
12. Seo P. (2020, updated) Mycophenolate: Overview of use and adverse effects in the treatment of rheumatic diseases. Edited by Furst DE, Curtis MR. *UpToDate ONLINE.* http://www.uptodate.com.
13. McCune JW, Clowse MB. (2020, updated) General principles of the use of cyclophosphamide in rheumatic diseases. Edited by Frust DE, Curtis MR. *UpToDate ONLINE.* http://www.uptodate.com.
14. Hardinger K, Magee CC. (2021, updated) Pharmacology cyclosporine and tacrolimus. Edited by Furst DE, Brennan DC, Lam AQ. *UpToDate ONLINE.* http://www.uptodate.com.
15. Nieman LK. (2021, updated) Pharmacologic use of glucocorticoids. Edited by Lacroix A, Martin KA. *UpToDate ONLINE.* http://www.uptodate.com.
16. Belmont HM. (2021, updated) Pharmacology and side effects of azathioprine when used in rheumatic diseases. Edited by Furst DE, Romain PL. *UpToDate ONLINE.* http://www.uptodate.com.

13 Methylprednisolone Pulse Therapy

Yap KH, Teo S and Resontoc LP

A. Indications

1. Treatment of various immune disorders.
2. Anti-rejection therapy for allograft rejection.

B. Pre-Infusion Monitoring

1. Infection screening:
   a. Varicella-zoster virus (VZV) infection
      i. Check past history of VZV infection or VZV immunization.
      ii. Confirm if patient is immune to varicella-zoster (VZV-IgG titers).
      iii. Check if patient has recently been exposed (within 3 weeks of contact) to VZV. If in doubt, check VZV-IgM titers.
   b. Hepatitis B surface antigen (HBsAg) and antibody (anti-HBs), and anti-hepatitis B core antibody (anti-HBc).
   c. Tuberculosis (TB)
      i. Check family history for TB.
      ii. Consider a chest X-Ray to exclude latent TB.
      iii. TB screen if positive contact history or is living in a high endemic area:
         - Tuberculin skin test in patients aged <2 years.
         - Interferon-gamma release assay in patients aged ≥2 years:
           - TB T-spot test (preferred in immunocompromised patients).
           - TB Quantiferon (less sensitive in immunocompromised patients).

d. SARS-CoV-2 nucleic acid amplification if clinically indicated.
e. Ensure patient has no active infections within the last 2 weeks.

2. Ensure blood pressure is within the normal range prior to starting the methylprednisolone infusion.
3. Check blood glucose level prior to the first dose.

C. Treatment Protocol

1. Stop oral prednisolone.
2. Dose of IV methylprednisolone: 10–30 mg/kg/day or alternate day according to protocol (maximum single dose 1 g/day).
3. Give IV furosemide 0.5–2 mg/kg (depending on kidney function), prior to a methylprednisolone infusion.
4. Dilute the calculated dose of methylprednisolone in 20 ml of 5% dextrose, 5% dextrose in 0.45% saline or normal saline.
   - In patients with no volume restriction, the dose can be diluted in 50–100 ml if there is infusion pain.
5. Infuse over 30–60 mins.
6. Doses less than 250 mg may be given as a slow bolus.
7. Monitor vitals including pulse, respiration, and blood pressure every 15 minutes during infusion, then hourly for the first 4 hours (post-infusion).
   - Consider monitoring for 24 hours if patient is hypertensive.

D. Adverse Effects

1. Adverse effects requiring no intervention:
   a. Facial flushing.
   b. Metallic taste in the mouth.
   c. Hyperactivity
   d. Bradycardia.
   e. Mood changes.
2. Adverse effects that may require intervention:
   a. Stinging during infusion.
      - Slow the rate.
      - Give in a more dilute solution.

b. Hypertension.
  - Slow down infusion rate and repeat blood pressure reading in 30 minutes.
  - If blood pressure is persistently elevated, consider nifedipine.

c. Hypotension.
  - Stop the infusion and observe.
  - Consider restarting at a lower infusion rate when blood pressure has normalized.

d. Severe tachycardia.
  - Stop the infusion and observe.
  - Consider restarting at a lower infusion rate when heart rate has decreased.

3. Extremely rare adverse effects requires that infusion be discontinued:
   a. Altered conscious state.
   b. Seizures.
   c. Psychosis.
   d. Cardiac arrhythmias.
   e. Circulatory collapse and cardiac arrest due to large bolus doses (that contain benzyl alcohol).

14 Intermittent Intravenous Cyclophosphamide Therapy for Glomerulonephritis

Teo S, Resontoc LP and Yap HK

A. Indications

1. Anti-neutrophil cytoplasmic antibodies (ANCA)-associated vasculitis with necrotizing glomerulonephritis or crescentic glomerulonephritis.
2. Lupus nephritis.
3. Anti-glomerular basement membrane disease.
4. Primary membranous nephropathy.
5. Immunoglobulin A (IgA) nephropathy.
6. IgA vasculitis nephritis.

B. Pre-infusion Monitoring

1. Check weight and height and calculate body surface area (BSA) on admission.
2. Infection screen:
   a. Varicella-zoster virus (VZV) infection
      i. Check past history of VZV infection or immunization.
      ii. Confirm if patient is immune to varicella-zoster (VZV-IgG titers).
      iii. Check if patient has been recently exposed (within 3 weeks of contact) to VZV. If in doubt, check VZV-IgM titers.
   b. Hepatitis B surface antigen (HBsAg) and antibody (anti-HBs), and anti-hepatitis B core antibody (anti-HBc).
   c. Hepatitis C serology.

d. Tuberculosis (TB)
  i. Check family history for TB.
  ii. Consider a chest X-Ray to exclude latent TB.
  iii. TB screen if positive contact history or living in a high endemic area:
    - Tuberculin skin test in patients aged <2 years.
    - Interferon-gamma release assay in patients aged ≥2 years:
      - TB T-spot test (preferred in immunocompromised patients).
      - TB Quantiferon (less sensitive in immunocompromised patients).

e. SARS-CoV-2 nucleic acid amplification if clinically indicated.
f. Ensure the patient has no active infections within the last 2 weeks before infusion.

3. Laboratory tests:
   a. Full blood count.
   b. Blood urea, creatinine, sodium, potassium, chloride, bicarbonate, calcium, phosphate, and uric acid.
   c. Serum magnesium.
   d. Liver function test.
   e. Urine microscopy.
   f. Urine protein:creatinine ratio.
4. Administer dose only if:
   a. Total white blood cell count $>4.0 \times 10^9$/L OR
   b. Absolute neutrophil count $>1.5 \times 10^9$/L.
5. Nadir of white blood cell count occurs 7–14 days after administration (lymphocyte nadir day 7, granulocyte nadir day 14) with bone marrow recovery at 21 days:
   a. Repeat full blood count at 7, 10 and 14 days.
   b. If the nadir of the absolute neutrophil count $<1.0 \times 10^9$/L, decrease the next dose by 20%.
   c. If the nadir white cell count is stable and does not fall significantly, the dose may be increased by 250 mg/m^2 (maximum 1000 mg/m^2).

C. Protocol

1. Cyclophosphamide (CYC) dosing:
   a. Dose = 500 mg/m², 750 mg/m², 1000 mg/m²
      - Select the lower dose range and increase monthly until the suitable dose is reached.
   b. Dose adjustment in patients with abnormal kidney function:
      i. Estimated glomerular filtration rate (eGFR) <15 ml/min/1.73m²: 75% of the usual dose.
      ii. Hemodialysis: 50% of the usual dose to be given after dialysis.
         - Approximately 20–50% of the dose is dialyzable.
      iii. Peritoneal dialysis: 75% of the usual dose.
      iv. Continuous kidney replacement therapy: 100% of the usual dose.
2. Ensure adequate hydration to prevent hemorrhagic cystitis:
   a. Intravenous fluid requirements: 5% Dextrose + 0.45% saline, especially in patients with edema, at 3 L/m²/day.
   b. Give intravenous furosemide 1–2 mg/kg if the patient is oliguric.
   c. Consider IV albumin 20% 1g/kg over 4–6 hours for patients with nephrotic syndrome.
      - Start IV mesna and CYC midway during the albumin infusion (i.e., at 2–3 hours).
      - Give IV furosemide midway and at the end of albumin infusion.
3. For patients with eGFR >60 ml/min/1.73m² and urine output >0.5 ml/kg/hour:

Time (T)	Procedure
T = −1 to −2 hour	Start 125 ml/m²/hour of IV 5% Dextrose + 0.45% saline.
T = −30 minutes	PO Diphenhydramine 1–2 mg/kg/dose (maximum 100 mg). IV Ondansetron 0.15 mg/kg (maximum 8 mg).
T = −15 minutes	IV Mesna (as 20 mg/ml in 5% Dextrose) given over 15 minutes. Dose (mg) = 0.2 × CYC dose.

(Continued)

(*Continued*)

Time (T)	Procedure
T = 0 minutes	IV CYC infusion. ▪ Infuse in 100–150 ml 5% Dextrose or 0.9% saline over 1 hour. IV Furosemide 1 mg/kg if urine output <1.5 ml/kg/hour.
T = 60 minutes	Resume pre-CYC IV fluid administration.
T = 3.5 hour	IV Mesna [Dose (mg) = 0.2 × CYC dose].
T = 6 to 9 hour	PO Mesna (400 mg tablet) [Dose (mg) = 0.3 × CYC dose] at 6 and 9 hours post CYC. Can stop IV hydration and discharge the patient if: ▪ Urine output is adequate (>1.5 ml/kg/hour). ▪ Tolerating oral fluids. ▪ No macroscopic hematuria.
Next 24 hours	Drink at least 3 L/m^2 of water over the next 24 hours.

4. **For patients with eGFR <60 ml/min/1.73m^2 or urine output <0.5 ml/kg/hour:**

Time (T)	Procedure
T = –1 to –2 hour	Start 125 ml/m^2/hour of IV 5% Dextrose + 0.45% saline.
T = –30 minutes	PO Diphenhydramine 1–2 mg/kg/dose (maximum 100 mg). IV Ondansetron 0.15 mg/kg (maximum 8 mg).
T = –15 minutes	IV Mesna (as 20 mg/ml in 5% Dextrose) given over 15 minutes. Dose (mg) = 0.2 × CYC dose.
T = 0 minutes	IV CYC infusion. ▪ Infuse in 100–150 ml 5% Dextrose or 0.9% saline over 1 hour.
T = 60 minutes	Resume pre-CYC IV fluid administration.
T = 90 minutes	IV furosemide 1–2 mg/kg over 15 minutes.
T = 3.5 hour	IV Mesna [Dose (mg) = 0.4 × CYC dose].
T = 6.5 hour	IV Mesna [Dose (mg) = 0.4 × CYC dose]. IV fluid can decrease to maintenance rate of 1500 ml/m^2/day.
T = 12–24 hour	Discontinue hydration and discharge the patient if well.

5. For patients with nephrotic syndrome in full relapse and urine output <0.5 ml/kg/hour:

Time (T)	Procedure
T = –2 hour	Start 1 g/kg 20% albumin (given over 4 hours).
T = –30 minutes	PO Diphenhydramine 1–2 mg/kg/dose (maximum 100 mg). IV Ondansetron 0.15 mg/kg (maximum 8 mg).
T = –15 minutes	IV Mesna (as 20 mg/ml in 5% Dextrose) given over 15 minutes. Dose (mg) = 0.2 × CYC dose.
T = 0 minutes	IV CYC infusion. ▪ Infuse in 100–150 ml 5% Dextrose or 0.9% saline over 1 hour. IV furosemide 1–2 mg/kg over 15 minutes.
T = 60 minutes	Resume IV 20% albumin infusion to completion
T = 3 hour	End of 20% albumin infusion. IV furosemide 1–2 mg/kg over 15 minutes. IV Mesna [Dose (mg) = 0.4 × CYC dose]. Start 5% Dextrose + 0.45% saline at maintenance rate of 1500 ml/m^2/day.
T = 6.5 hour	IV Mesna [Dose (mg) = 0.4 × CYC dose].
T = 12–24 hour	Discontinue hydration and discharge the patient if well.

6. Monitoring:
   a. Hourly temperature, pulse rate, respiratory rate, and 4-hourly blood pressure.
   b. Strict intake/output chart.
   c. Ensure the child is able to void every 2 hours while awake and every 3 hours while asleep to prevent hemorrhagic cystitis.
   d. Dipstick all urine:
      - Inform if urine microscopic hematuria increases by 2 grades.
      - Consider increasing hydration or administering extra doses of Mesna.

D. Acute Side Effects

1. Gastrointestinal irritation: Nausea, vomiting and abdominal pain.
2. Electrolyte abnormalities: Hyponatremia due to syndrome of inappropriate antidiuretic hormone secretion (SIADH) and hypomagnesemia.
3. Hemorrhagic cystitis.

Note: See chapter "Immunosuppressive Medications" for a full list of adverse effects and pre-treatment evaluation.

E. Pneumocystis Jirovecii Pneumonia Prophylaxis

1. Check glucose-6-phosphate dehydrogenase (G6PD) status.
2. Prophylactic agents:
   a. Co-trimoxazole oral 3 mg/kg/dose alternate days.
   b. In G6PD-deficient patients, use aerosolized pentamidine 300 mg monthly (via a Respigard nebulizer).
   c. In patients who are allergic to co-trimoxazole, alternative drugs include:
      - Dapsone 2 mg/kg daily (maximum 100 mg).
      - Atovaquone 30 mg/kg/daily (maximum 1500 mg).

Recommended Reading

1. Lehman TJ, Sherry DD, Wagner-Weiner L, McCurdy DK, Emery HM, Magilavy DB, Kovalesky A. (1989) Intermittent intravenous cyclophosphamide therapy for lupus nephritis. *J Pediatr* **114**:1055–60.
2. Bosch X, Guilabert A, Espinosa G, Mirapeix E. (2007) Treatment of antineutrophil cytoplasmic antibody-associated vasculitis. *JAMA* **298**:655–669.
3. Basiaga M, Engberg R, Ford R, Hrachovec J, Kroon L, Mark D, Okamura D, Ohare P, Stanford S, Vilavicencio C; Seattle Children's Hospital (2018) Cyclophosphamide recurring infusion pathway. http://www.seattlechildrens.org/pdf/cyclophosphamide-pathway.pdf.
4. McCune JW, Clowse MB. (2020, updated) General principles of the use of cyclophosphamide in rheumatic diseases. Edited by Frust DE, Curtis MR. *UpToDate ONLINE*. http://www.uptodate.com.

15 Anti-CD20 Monoclonal Antibody Therapy for Nephrotic Syndrome

Teo S, Leow EH, Ng KH and Yap HK

A. Indications

I. Rituximab:

1. Idiopathic childhood nephrotic syndrome including:
   - Minimal change disease.
   - Focal segmental glomerulosclerosis.
   - Focal global glomerulosclerosis.
   - Focal mesangial proliferative glomerulonephritis.
   - Diffuse mesangial proliferative glomerulonephritis (excluding IgA nephropathy).
   - IgM nephropathy
   - C1q nephropathy.
2. Primary membranous nephropathy.

II. Obinutuzumab:

1. Nephrotic syndrome resistant to Rituximab therapy.
2. Anaphylactic reactions to Rituximab.
3. Anti-chimeric (Rituximab) antibodies as evidenced by:
   - High antibody titer.
   - Time to B-cell repopulation shortening after each Rituximab cycle.

B. Pathophysiologic Considerations

I. Rituximab:

1. Chimeric type I anti-CD20 monoclonal antibody.
2. Depletion of peripheral, circulating CD19+/CD20+ B cells are usually achieved by a single infusion of Rituximab, and this can modulate T-B cell interactions leading to response in diseases predominantly mediated by T-cells.
3. Rituximab preserves sphingomyelin phosphodiesterase acid-like 3b (SMPDL-3b) activity, which seems to be important in the preservation of podocyte function and prevention of proteinuria.

II. Obinutuzumab:

1. Fully humanized type II anti-CD20 monoclonal antibody that may be more potent as a B-cell depleting agent when compared to Rituximab.
2. Binds to an overlapping epitope of CD20 in a different orientation when compared to Rituximab, preventing the internalization of the CD20/antibody complex.
3. Obinutuzumab is glycol-engineered, which results in an enhanced affinity of the drug for FcgammaRIIIa on the B-cells which causes increased ability to bind and recruit effector cells and therefore higher antibody dependent cytotoxicity and less dependence on complement-mediated activity.
4. Induces a direct cell death mediated by lysosomes and has less dependence on high levels of B-cell activating factor (BAFF), which contributes to a greater depletion of memory B-cells that classically are more resistant to the effect of Rituximab.

C. Pre-infusion Monitoring

1. Infection screen:
   a. Varicella-zoster virus (VZV) infection:
      i. Check past history for VZV infection or immunization.
      ii. Confirm if patient is immune to varicella-zoster (VZV-IgG titers).

iii. Check if patient has been recently exposed (within 3 weeks of contact) to VZV. If in doubt, check VZV-IgM titers.

b. Hepatitis B surface antigen (HBsAg) and antibody (anti-HBs), and anti-hepatitis B core antibody (anti-HBc).
c. Tuberculosis (TB)
   i. Check family history for TB.
   ii. Consider a chest X-Ray to exclude latent TB.
   iii. TB screen if positive contact history or living in a high endemic area:
      - Tuberculin skin test in patients age <2 years.
      - Interferon-gamma release assay in patients age ≥2 years:
         - TB T-spot test (preferred in immunocompromised patients).
         - TB Quantiferon (less sensitive in immunocompromised patients).
d. SARS-CoV-2 Nucleic acid amplification if clinically indicated.
e. Spinal fluid examination for JC polyomavirus if suggestive neurological symptoms, including rapidly progressive focal neurologic deficits without signs of increased intracranial pressure, are present.
f. Ensure patient has no active infections within the last 2 weeks before infusion.

2. Baseline investigations at first course:
   a. Full blood count (FBC).
   b. Liver function test.
   c. Urea, creatinine, sodium, potassium, chloride, bicarbonate, calcium, phosphate, and uric acid.
   d. Serum immunoglobulin G (IgG).
   e. Fasting glucose, triglycerides, total cholesterol, low-density lipoprotein (LDL)-cholesterol, and high-density lipoprotein (HDL)-cholesterol.
   f. 24-hour urinary protein.
   g. Creatinine clearance.
   h. Urine microscopy.
   i. Serum complements C3 and C4.
   j. Glucose-6-phosphate dehydrogenase (G6PD) (if not checked previously).
   k. CD19 count.

3. Mandatory investigations at subsequent courses:
   a. FBC.
   b. Liver function test.
   c. Urea, creatinine, sodium, potassium, chloride, bicarbonate, calcium, phosphate, and uric acid.
   d. Serum IgG.
   e. Urine protein:creatinine ratio.
   f. Urine microscopy.

D. Treatment Protocol

I. Rituximab:

1. Dosing:

Steroid-dependent	IV Rituximab 375 mg/m^2 (maximum dose 1 g) once
Steroid-resistant and/or calcineurin inhibitor-resistant	IV Rituximab 375 mg/m^2 (maximum dose 1 g) 2-weekly x 2 doses

   - Rituximab should preferably be started during remission of nephrotic syndrome.
   - Consider repeating the Rituximab course if there is a relapse of proteinuria, especially if CD19 counts have recovered.
2. Premedication 30 minutes prior to infusion:
   a. Paracetamol 10–15 mg/kg (maximum 1 g).
   b. IV Hydrocortisone 4–10 mg/kg (maximum 500 mg).
   c. IV Diphenhydramine 1 mg/kg (maximum 50 mg).
3. IV Rituximab infusion:
   a. Dilute Rituximab to 1 mg/ml.
   b. Start at 5 ml/hour and increase by 5 ml every ½ hour as tolerated by blood pressure (BP) and heart rate (HR).
   c. Maximum infusion rate 50 ml/hour unless the patient had a previous reaction, then the maximum infusion rate should be capped at 25 ml/hour.
   d. Monitor HR, respiratory rate (RR), BP, temperature, oxygen saturation (SpO_2) every 15 minutes for the first hour. Then hourly if there are no problems.

e. If BP falls <100/60 mm Hg, HR >120/minute, SpO_2 <95% on room air, stop the infusion and recheck. Inform the Pediatric Nephrologist on-call immediately.
f. When the parameters stabilize, restart the infusion at the previously tolerated rate.

II. Obinutuzumab:

1. Dosing for each course:
   a. First Dose: IV Obinutuzumab 1000 mg/1.73 m^2 (maximum 1000 mg) on day 1.
   b. Second Dose: IV Obinutuzumab 1000 mg/1.73 m^2 (maximum 1000 mg) on day 8 or day 15.
2. Premedication 30 minutes prior to infusion:
   a. Paracetamol 10–15 mg/kg (maximum 1 g).
   b. IV Hydrocortisone 4–10 mg/kg (maximum 500 mg).
   c. IV Diphenhydramine 1 mg/kg (maximum 50 mg).
3. IV Obinutuzumab infusion:
   a. Comes in 1000 mg/40 ml (25 mg/ml) single dose vial.
   b. Dilute dose in 250 ml of 0.9% sodium chloride (not compatible with 5% dextrose).
   c. Administer at a final concentration of 0.4–4 mg/ml.
   d. Start at a rate of 25 mg/hour and observe for at least 4 hours.
      - Rate of infusion subsequently can be escalated in 50 mg/hour increments every 30 minutes to a maximum of 400 mg/hour.
      - For the second dose onwards, if there are no infusion reactions, the starting rate can be 100 mg/hour and increased by 100 mg/hour every 30 minutes (maximum 400 mg/hour).
   e. Monitor HR, RR, BP, temperature, and SpO_2:
      - Every 15 minutes for the first hour.
      - Hourly for the rest of the infusion.
      - If BP <100/60 mmHg, HR >120/minute, SpO_2 <95% on room air, stop the infusion and recheck. Inform the Pediatric Nephrologist on-call immediately.
      - When the parameters stabilize, restart the infusion at the previously tolerated rate.

III. Maintenance immunosuppressive agents post anti-CD20 antibody therapy:

1. For patients on a combination of mycophenolate, calcineurin inhibitor, and prednisolone:
   a. Discontinue mycophenolate, restarting at 1-month post anti-CD20 antibody therapy if absolute neutrophil count is normal.
   b. Begin tapering prednisolone if the patient is in remission, followed by calcineurin inhibitor once prednisolone is discontinued.
2. For patients on a calcineurin inhibitor and/or prednisolone:
   a. Begin tapering prednisolone if the patient is in remission, followed by a calcineurin inhibitor once prednisolone is discontinued.
   b. Start mycophenolate after one month.
3. For patients on prednisolone and mycophenolate:
   a. Begin tapering prednisolone once patient is in remission.
   b. Do not discontinue mycophenolate.

E. Post-therapy Monitoring

1. CD19 monthly starting 3 months post-infusion until CD19 recovery.
2. Daily urine protein dipstick monitoring.
3. Urine protein:creatinine ratio and FBC monthly.
4. Urea, creatinine, sodium, potassium, chloride, bicarbonate, calcium, phosphate, uric acid, and liver function test 3-monthly for 1 year.
5. Creatinine clearance and a 24-hour urine protein excretion 6-monthly for 1 year.
6. Serum IgG at 1 month and subsequently monthly if low until recovery.

F. Complications

I. Acute:

1. Infusion reactions:
   a. Most develop within 24 hours of the first infusion and is dose-dependent.

b. Include low-grade fever, chills, hypotension, hypertension, rigors, flushing, rash, headaches, dizziness, throat irritation, rhinitis, nausea, vomiting, diarrhea, dyspnea, and chest discomfort.
c. Hypotension may occur as part of the infusion reaction.
    - Consider withholding antihypertensive treatment for 12 hours prior to and the first hour after adminstration until BP is stable.
d. Systemic inflammatory response syndrome (SIRS)-like reactions or cytokine release syndrome is a severe infusion reaction characterized by severe dyspnea, often accompanied by bronchospasm and hypoxia.
    - Usually manifests itself within 1–2 hours of starting the first infusion.
    - Do a chest X-Ray to look for pulmonary infiltrates.
e. Management:
    i. Slow the infusion rate by half or stop infusion temporarily, especially if there is a severe reaction.
    ii. If required, give diphenhydramine, paracetamol, oxygen, intravenous 0.9% saline, bronchodilators, or corticosteroids.
    iii. Upon resolution of symptoms and chest X-Ray is clear in patient with SIRS-like syndrome, consider restarting the infusion at no more than half the previous rate.
    iv. If there is no further reaction, the infusion rate escalation may resume.
    v. If the same severe adverse reactions occur a second time, stop treatment immediately.

2. Hypersensitivity reactions:
    a. Immediate-onset hypersensitivity: Dyspnea, bronchospasm, hypotension, urticaria, angioedema, and tachycardia.
        - Send blood for tryptase within 1–2 hours of reaction to confirm anaphylaxis.
    b. Late-onset hypersensitivity or serum sickness: Chest pain, diffuse arthralgia and fever.
    c. Very rarely occurs with the first infusion.
    d. Infusion must be stopped and treatment permanently discontinued.

II. Chronic:

1. Neutropenia:
   a. Can occur during treatment or late-onset (occurring more than 28 days after completion of treatment) and/or prolonged (lasting longer than 28 days).
   b. Consider administration of granulocyte colony-stimulating factors (GCSF) if the absolute neutrophil count <1 × 10^9/L.
2. Thrombocytopenia.
3. Hypogammaglobulinemia:
   - Consider monthly intravenous immunoglobulin 0.5 g/kg in cases with persistently low serum IgG and recurrent/severe infections.
4. Hepatitis B virus reactivation:
   a. Defined as an abrupt increase in hepatitis B virus (HBV) replication manifesting as a rapid increase in serum HBV DNA level or detection of HBsAg in a person who was previously HBsAg negative and anti-HBc positive.
   b. Monitor patients with evidence of current or prior HBV infection for clinical and laboratory signs of hepatitis or HBV reactivation monthly for 3 months following treatment.
5. Interstitial lung disease:
   a. Diagnosis should be considered in patients who present with fever, cough and breathlessness, with no clear evidence of infection.
   b. Prompt diagnosis and early institution of corticosteroid therapy are essential.
6. Erythema nodosum.
7. Progressive multifocal leukoencephalopathy:
   a. Caused by reactivation of the polyomavirus JC virus.
   b. Suspected in patients who present with subacute neurologic deficits that do not conform to vascular territories, and focal or multifocal white matter lesions on brain magnetic resonance imaging (MRI) without mass effect.

G. Pneumocystis Jirovecii Prophylaxis

1. Co-trimoxazole oral 3 mg/kg/dose alternate days for 3 months.
2. In G6PD-deficient patients, use aerolized pentamidine 300 mg monthly (via Respigard nebulizer).

3. In patients who are allergic to co-trimoxazole, use dapsone 2 mg/kg daily (maximum 100 mg).

Recommended Reading

1. Iijima K, Sako M, Nozu K, Mori R, Tuchida N, Kamei K, Miura K, Aya K, Nakanishi K, Ohtomo Y, Takahashi S, Tanaka R, Kaito H, Nakamura, Kenji Ishikura H, Ito S, Ohashi Y, on behalf of the Rituximab for Childhood-onset Refractory Nephrotic Syndrome (RCRNS) Study Group. (2014) Rituximab for childhood-onset, complicated, frequently relapsing nephrotic syndrome or steroid-dependent nephrotic syndrome: A multicentre, double-blind, randomised, placebo-controlled trial. *Lancet* **384**:1273–1281.
2. Sinha A, Bhatia D, Gulati A, Rawat M, Dinda AK, Hari P, Bagga A. (2015) Efficacy and safety of rituximab in children with difficult-to-treat nephrotic syndrome. *Nephrol Dial Transplant* **30**:96–106.
3. Gagez AL, Cartron G. (2014) Obinutuzumab: A new class of anti-CD20 monoclonal antibody. *Curr Opin Oncol* **26**:484–491.
4. Freeman CL, Sehn LH. (2018) A tale of two antibodies: Obinutuzumab versus Rituximab. *Br J Haematol* **182**:29–45.
5. Klomjit N, Fervenza FC, Zand L. (2020) Successful treatment of patients with refractory PLA2R-associated membranous nephropathy with obinutuzumab: A Report of 3 Cases. *Am J Kidney Dis* **76**:883–888.
6. Majeranowski A, Okrój M. (2021) Regarding. A global anti-B cell strategy combining obinutuzumab and daratumumab in severe pediatric nephrotic syndrome. *Pediatr Nephrol* **36**:1175–1182.

16 Eculizumab (Anti-C5 Monoclonal Antibody) Therapy for Complement-Mediated Injury

Teo S, Dela Cruz RC, Resontoc LP, Lau PYW and Yap HK

A. Mechanism of Action

1. Eculizumab is a recombinant, humanized, monoclonal immunoglobulin G antibody that targets complement component C5.
2. Eculizumab blocks the cleavage of C5 to C5a and C5b, ultimately preventing the generation of the proinflammatory peptide C5b and the cytotoxic membrane attack complex C5b-9.

B. Indications

1. Atypical hemolytic uremic syndrome (aHUS).
2. Paroxysmal nocturnal hemoglobinuria (PNH).
3. Antibody-mediated rejection with thrombotic microangiopathy.
4. Severe antibody-mediated rejection with a poor response to conventional therapy.
5. Refractory generalized myasthenia gravis with anti-acetylcholine receptor antibody.
6. Neuromyelitis optica spectrum disorder (NMOSD) with anti-aquaporin-4 antibody.

C. Contraindications

1. Hypersensitivity to eculizumab.
2. Unresolved *Neisseria meningitides* infection.
3. In patients who are not currently vaccinated against *Neisseria meningitides* or have not received prophylactic treatment with appropriate antibiotics until 2 weeks after vaccination.

D. Pre-infusion Preparation

1. Patients must be vaccinated at least 2 weeks prior to the first dose of Eculizumab with meningococcal vaccine (tetravalent, conjugated, vaccine against serotypes A, C, Y and W 135 is recommended).
   - A booster dose should be given 8 weeks after starting Eculizumab.
   - If available, meningococcal vaccine against serotype B (Bexcero) should also be given.
2. Patients <18 years of age must be vaccinated against *Haemophilus influenza* and pneumococcal infections, and strictly adhere to the national vaccination recommendations for each age group.

E. Pre-infusion Monitoring

1. Full blood count.
2. Sodium, potassium, chloride, bicarbonate, urea, creatinine, calcium, phosphate, and uric acid.
3. Serum lactate dehydrogenase.
4. Urine microscopy.
5. Urine protein:creatinine ratio.
6. Serum complements C3, C4 and CH50.

F. Treatment Protocol

Patient Body Weight	Initial Phase	Maintenance Phase
≥40 kg	900 mg weekly × 4	1,200 mg at week 5; then 1,200 mg every 2 weeks
30 to <40 kg	600 mg weekly × 2	900 mg at week 3; then 900 mg every 2 weeks
20 to <30 kg	600 mg weekly × 2	600 mg at week 3; then 600 mg every 2 weeks
10 to <20 kg	600 mg weekly × 1	300 mg at week 2; then 300 mg every 2 weeks
5 to <10 kg	300 mg weekly × 1	300 mg at week 2; then 300 mg every 3 weeks

1. *Dosage form:*

a. Eculizumab 10 mg/mL solution (Soliris®), 30 mL vial.
b. Withdraw:
   - 30 ml for 300 mg
   - 60 ml for 600 mg
   - 90 ml for 900 mg
   - 120 ml for 1200 mg

   Note: Preferable to use a needle and syringe to withdraw the drug.
c. Dilute in equal volumes of 0.9% saline, 0.45% saline, 5% dextrose-water, or Ringer's lactate to a final volume of:
   - 60 ml for 300 mg
   - 120 ml for 600 mg
   - 180 ml for 900 mg
   - 240 ml for 1200 mg
d. After dilution, the final concentration of the solution to be infused is 5 mg/ml.
e. Diluted Eculizumab is stable for 24 hours refrigerated (2° or 8°C) or at room temperature.
f. Can be given through a peripheral vein.

2. *IV Eculizumab infusion:*

a. Allow to reach room temperature.
b. Infuse over 60 minutes.
c. Monitor heart rate (HR), respiratory rate (RR), blood pressure (BP), temperature, and oxygen saturation (SpO_2) every 15 minutes.
   - If BP falls <100/60 mm Hg, HR >120/minute, SpO_2 <95% on room air, stop infusion and recheck.
   - Inform the Pediatric Nephrologist on-call immediately.
d. When the parameters stabilize, restart infusion at a lower infusion rate.
   - Do not exceed 2 hours in adults and adolescents and 4 hours in children <12 years.

3. *Supplemental dosing:*

Required in the setting of concomitant plasmapheresis or plasma exchange, or fresh frozen plasma infusion:

Type of Plasma Intervention	Most Recent Eculizumab Dose	Supplemental Dose with each Plasma Intervention	Timing of Supplemental Dose
Plasmapharesis or plasma exchange	300 mg	300 mg each plasmapheresis or plasma exchange session	Within 60 minutes after each plasmapheresis or plasma exchange
	≥600 mg	600 mg each plasmapheresis or plasma exchange session	
Fresh frozen plasma infusion	≥300 mg	300 mg per unit of fresh frozen plasma	60 minutes prior to each unit of fresh frozen plasma infusion

G. Post-Eculizumab Monitoring (Prior to Each Dose)

1. Full blood count.
2. Sodium, potassium, chloride, bicarbonate, urea, creatinine, calcium, phosphate, and uric acid.
3. Serum lactate dehydrogenase.
4. Serum complement C3.
5. Urine microscopy.
6. Urine protein:creatinine ratio.
7. Monitor the patient for early signs and symptoms of meningococcal infections and evaluate immediately if an infection is suspected.

Note: Patients who discontinue treatment with Eculizumab should be monitored closely for at least 12 weeks for signs and symptoms of severe thrombotic microangiopathy complications.

H. Antibiotic Prophylaxis

1. Indicated in patients who have not been immunized with meningococcal vaccine, and have been given the vaccine one day before the start of Eculizumab.
2. Antibiotics at therapeutic doses should be given for 2 weeks during the course of the Eculizumab to prevent infection with encapsulated bacteria.
3. Choice of antibiotic:
   a. Methylpenicillin (Penicillin V):
      - 2 months to 12 years: 250 mg OM.
      - >12 years: 250 mg BD.
   b. Azithromycin (if allergic to penicillin):
      - 10 mg/kg single dose (maximum 500 mg) and repeated a week later.

I. Clinically Significant Adverse Drug Reactions

1. Very common (≥1/10)
   a. Leukopenia.
   b. Headache.

2. Common (≥1/100 to <1/10)
    a. Infections.
    b. Anaphylactic reaction.
    c. Thrombocytopenia, hemolysis.
    d. Dizziness, dysgeusia, paresthesia.
    e. Accelerated hypertension.
    f. Upper respiratory tract infection.
    g. Abdominal pain, constipation, diarrhea, dyspepsia, nausea, vomiting.
    h. Alopecia, dry skin, pruritus, rash
    i. Arthralgia, back pain, myalgia.
    j. Dysuria.
    k. Chest discomfort, chills, fatigue, asthenia, edema, pyrexia.

Recommended Reading

1. Loirat C, Fremeaux-Bacchi V. (2011) Atypical haemolytic uremic syndrome. *Orphanet J Rare Dis* **6**:60.
2. Loirat C, Fakhouri F, Ariceta G, Besbas N, Bitzan M, Bjerre A, Coppo R, Emma F, Johnson S, Karpman D, Landau D, Langman CB, Lapeyraque AL, Licht C, Nester C, Pecoraro C, Riedl M, van de Kar NC, Van de Walle J, Vivarelli M, Frémeaux-Bacchi V; HUS International. (2016) An international consensus approach to the management of atypical hemolytic uremic syndrome in children. *Pediatr Nephrol* **31**(1):15–39.
3. Soliris. (2020) Soliris Official FDA information, side effects and uses.

17 Adjunctive Therapy in Glomerular Disease

Resontoc LP, Teo S, Liu ID, Ng KH and Yap HK

A. Adjunctive Agents to Decrease Proteinuria and Progression of Chronic Kidney Disease

I. Renin-angiotensin system blockers (RASBs):

1. Angiotensin-converting enzyme inhibitors (ACEi) and angiotensin receptor blockers (ARB) should be used for control of blood pressure (BP) and proteinuria.
2. In children, expert opinion suggests a favorable outcome when time-averaged proteinuria is reduced to <0.5 g/day/1.73m^2 or urine protein:creatinine ratio (UPCR) <0.05 g/mmol.
3. ACEi dose:
   a. Captopril:
      - Infants: 0.05 mg/kg/dose 4 times a day (maximum 6 mg/kg/day).
      - Children: 0.5 mg/kg/dose 3 times a day (maximum 6 mg/kg/day).

   b. Enalapril 0.08 mg/kg/day 12–24 hourly (maximum 1.0 mg/kg/day 12–24 hourly or 40 mg daily).
   c. Ramipril 0.05 mg/kg/day daily (maximum 0.2 mg/kg/day daily or 10 mg daily).
   d. Lisinopril 0.1 mg/kg/day daily (maximum 1 mg/kg/day daily or 20 mg daily).
4. ARB dose:
   a. Losartan 0.5–0.7 mg/kg/dose daily (maximum 1.4 mg/kg/dose daily or 100 mg daily).
   b. Valsartan 0.8–3.0 mg/kg/dose daily (maximum 160 mg daily).
   c. Telmisartan 1–2 mg/kg/day once daily (maximum 80 mg).

5. Side effects:
   a. Hypotension.
   b. Hyperkalemia.
   c. Rising serum creatinine:
      - ACEi and ARBs lower the glomerular filtration rate, resulting in a 10–20% increase in serum creatinine; therefore, this should not prompt a withdrawal of the medications unless the serum creatinine continues to rise.
      - Increased risk of acute kidney injury, especially if the patient is hypovolemic.
   d. Chronic cough associated with ACEi use:
      - Related to increased local concentrations of kinins, substance P, prostaglandins, or thromboxane.
      - Cough resolves in 4–7 days after discontinuation of ACEi use.
      - Can switch to ARB, which has a lower rate of cough.
   e. Anemia:
      - ACEi and ARBs can suppress erythropoietin production in patients with chronic kidney disease (CKD).
      - Related to the accumulation of N-acetyl-seryl-aspartyl-lysyl-proline, which inhibits stem cell multiplication.
6. Monitor serum potassium and creatinine 3 days after commencing ACEi or ARB or increasing the dose, and at least 3–6 monthly thereafter.
7. Consider using ACEi and ARB in combination in patients with persistent proteinuria, but should be approached with caution in view of the potential adverse effects.
8. Post-pubertal girls should be informed of the teratogenic risks of ACEi and ARB:
   - ACEi and ARB should be discontinued at least 6 weeks before pregnancy is planned.
   - Contraception should be offered to sexually active females on these drugs.

II. Aldosterone antagonists:

1. Aldosterone antagonists may have an additive effect in reducing proteinuria when used in combination with ACEi or ARB.

2. Aldosterone antagonists also have an anti-fibrosis or anti-proliferation effect in animal studies.
3. Spironolactone dose:
   - Body weight:
     - 0–10 kg: 6.25 mg 12 hourly.
     - 11–20 kg: 12.5 mg 12 hourly.
     - 21–40 kg: 25 mg 12 hourly.
     - >40 kg: 25 mg 8 hourly.
4. Eplerenone dose:
   - 0.5–1 mg/kg (adult dose: 25–50 mg) 12–24 hourly.
5. Side effects:
   a. Risk of hyperkalemia, especially in patients already on ACEi or ARB.
   b. Gynecomastia occurs in about 10% of adult patients with spironolactone, but not with eplerenone.

III. Sodium-glucose co-transporter 2 (SGLT-2) inhibitors:

1. SGLT-2 inhibitors slow the rate of progression of CKD by promoting natriuresis and reducing intraglomerular pressure and glomerular hyperfiltration.
2. Beneficial effects attributed to:
   a. Glycosuria leading to osmotic diuresis and increased urine output.
   b. Decreasing glucose levels and glycated hemoglobin (HbA1c).
   c. Lowering systolic blood pressure.
   d. Weight loss.
   e. Less estimated glomerular filtration rate (eGFR) decline.
   f. Reduction in albuminuria.
3. Adjunctive therapy in emerging adults ≥18 years of age.
   a. Not studied in children and patients with eGFR <25 ml/min/1.73m^2.
   b. Contraindicated when eGFR <30 ml/min/1.73m^2.
4. Dosing:
   a. Dapagliflozin 5–10 mg once daily.
   b. Empagliflozin 10–25 mg once daily.
   c. Canagliflozin 100–300 mg once daily.

   Note:
   - Correct volume depletion before initiation of therapy.
   - Assess kidney function prior to initiation of therapy.

5. Adverse effects:
   a. Reversible decline in eGFR when SGLT2 inhibitors are first initiated.
      - Secondary to hemodynamic effect and changes in kidney blood flow.
      - Occurs over 6 weeks with eGFR dip of up to 6 ml/min/1.73m^2.
   b. Polyuria.
   c. Nasopharyngitis.
   d. Urinary tract infection.
   e. Nausea.
   f. Dyslipidemia.
   g. Constipation.
   h. Pain in the extremities.
   i. Hypersensitivity in <1%.
   j. Rash.
   k. Ketoacidosis.
   l. Female genital mycotic infection.
   m. Necrotizing fasciitis of the perineum.

B. BP Control

1. Good BP control is essential to delay the progression of CKD.
2. Target for BP control:
   a. Age <18 years:
      - <90th percentile (clinic BP)
      - <50th percentile if there is proteinuria >1 g/day/1.73m^2.
   b. Age ≥18 years:
      - <130/80 mmHg (clinic BP)
      - <120/80 mmHg if there is proteinuria >1 g/day/1.73m^2.
3. Choice of antihypertensive drugs.
   a. ACEi and ARB should be used preferentially to other agents for BP control, in the absence of other contraindications.
   b. Non-dihydropyridine calcium channel blockers are useful for control of proteinuria but dihydropyridine calcium channel blockers may be required for BP control.
   c. Beta-blockers can also be used.

C. Control of Hyperlipidemia

1. Treatment of hyperlipidemia in patients with glomerular disease should follow the guidelines for those at high risk of cardiovascular disease.
2. Statins: 3-hydroxy-3-methylglutaryl coenzyme A (HMG CoA) reductase inhibitors are more effective in correcting the lipid profile than the use of dietary restriction of fats and cholesterol in patients with glomerular disease, in particular, nephrotic syndrome.
3. Statins may also have some effect on delaying the progression of CKD.
4. Statin therapy should be introduced in patients with low-density lipoprotein (LDL)-cholesterol >3.36 mmol/L.
5. Choice of statins:
   a. Avoid simvastatin due to the increased risk of rhabdomyolysis, especially with the concomitant use of calcineurin inhibitors (CNIs).
   b. Rosuvastatin in combination with CNI has the lowest risk of rhabdomyolysis.
   c. Rosuvastatin 5–20 mg nightly.
      - For children on CNI, the dose should not exceed 5 mg.
   d. Lovastatin 0.4–0.8 mg/kg nightly.
      - Dose can be increased monthly, up to 12-hourly dosing (maximum 40 mg 12 hourly).
   e. Atorvastatin 0.2–1.6 mg/kg nightly.
      - Dose can be increased monthly (maximum 80 mg nightly).
6. Monitoring:
   a. Monitor liver panel and serum creatine kinase monthly for the first 3 months, then 3-monthly.
   b. Cholesterol profile should be repeated every 6 months after the initiation of statin therapy.

D. Salt and Water Regulation

1. Fluid and salt intake should be restricted if there is evidence of fluid overload.
2. Diuretics may be used to regulate salt and water homeostasis.

3. Prolonged severe hypokalemia should be avoided as this may exacerbate tubular damage and fibrosis.
4. Combination of loop diuretics with aldosterone antagonists may be useful in preventing hypokalemia, as well as an additive effect on reducing proteinuria.

E. Avoidance of Further Insults

1. Avoid agents that can cause tubulointerstitial injury:
   a. Non-steroidal anti-inflammatory agents.
   b. Penicillin antibiotics.
   c. Certain traditional medicines.
2. Avoid smoking.
3. Control each component of the metabolic syndrome.
4. Consider the use of allopurinol or febuxostat to alleviate the pro-inflammatory effect of uric acid on vascular cells in patients with hyperuricemia.

Recommended Reading

1. Floege J, Eitner F. (2011) Current therapy for IgA nephropathy. *J Am Soc Nephrol* **22**:1785–1794.
2. Navaneethan SD, Nigwekar SU, Sehgal AR, Strippoli GF. (2009) Aldosterone antagonists for preventing the progression of chronic kidney disease: a systematic review and meta-analysis. *Clin J Am Soc Nephrol* **4**:542–551.
3. Kelly MS, Lewis J, Huntsberry AM, Dea L, Portillo I. (2019) Efficacy and renal outcomes of SGLT2 inhibitors in patients with type 2 diabetes and chronic kidney disease. *Postgrad Med* **131**:31–42.
4. Stotter BR, Ferguson MA. (2019) Should ACE inhibitors and ARBs be used in combination in children? *Pediatr Nephrol* **34**:1521–1532.
5. Heerspink HJL, Stefánsson BV, Correa-Rotter R, Chertow GM, Greene T, Hou FF, Mann JFE, McMurray JJV, Lindberg M, Rossing P, Sjöström CD, Toto RD, Langkilde AM, Wheeler DC; DAPA-CKD Trial Committees and Investigators. (2020) Dapagliflozin in Patients with Chronic Kidney Disease. *N Engl J Med* **383**:1436–1446.
6. Cattran DC, Appel GB, Hunder GG. (2021, updated) Treatment and prognosis of IgA nephropathy. Edited by Glassock RJ, Fervenza FC, Forman JP. *UpToDate ONLINE*. http://www.uptodate.com.

1 Chronic Kidney Disease Staging

Yap HK, Liu ID, Qader MA, Resontoc LP and Ng KH

A. Definition of Chronic Kidney Disease (CKD)

1. CKD is defined as abnormalities of kidney structure or function, presenting for greater than 3 months with health implications.
2. Criteria for CKD staging: Either of the following presents for more than 3 months.

Markers of kidney damage (one or more)	Albuminuria* (AER ≥30 mg/24 hours/1.73m^2; ACR ≥3 mg/mmol or ≥30 mg/g). Urine sediment abnormalities. Electrolytes and other abnormalities due to tubular disorders. Abnormalities detected by histology Structural abnormalities detected by imaging. History of kidney transplantation.
Decreased GFR	GFR# ≤60 ml/min/1.73m^2 (GFR categories G3a–G5).

*AER = albumin excretion rate; ACR = albumin:creatinine ratio
#GFR = glomerular filtration rate

B. Classification of CKD

1. CKD is classified based on CGA criteria:
   - Cause.
   - Glomerular filtration rate (GFR) category.
   - Albuminuria category.

2. GFR category:

CKD Stage	Description	eGFR (ml/min/1.73m²)
G1	Normal or high	≥90
G2	Mildly decreased	60–89
G3a	Mildly to moderately decreased	45–59
G3b	Moderately to severely decreased	30–44
G4	Severely decreased	15–29
G5	Kidney failure	<15

- **A GFR-estimating equation may be used for initial assessment.**
- **In the absence of evidence of kidney damage, neither GFR categories G1 nor G2 fulfil the criteria for CKD.**

3. **Criteria for persistent albuminuria/proteinuria:**

Measure	Categories		
	A1	A2	A3
	Normal to Mildly Increased	Moderately Increased	Severely Increased*
Albumin excretion rate ($mg/1.73m^2/24$ hours)	<30	30–300	>300
Protein excretion rate ($mg/1.73m^2/24$ hours)	<150	150–500	>500
Albumin:creatinine ratio (ACR) (g/mmol) (mg/mmol) (mg/g)	<0.003 <3 <30	0.003–0.03 3–30 30–300	>0.03 >30 >300
Protein:creatinine ratio (PCR) (g/mmol) (mg/mmol) (mg/g)	<0.015 <15 <150	0.015–0.05 15–50 150–500	>0.05 >50 >500

(*Continued*)

Measure	Categories		
	A1	A2	A3
	Normal to Mildly Increased	Moderately Increased	Severely Increased*
Protein reagent strip#	Negative to trace	Trace to +	+ or greater

* Includes nephrotic syndrome.
\# Protein reagent strip is not recommended if quantitative measurements are available.

- The relationship between albumin excretion rate and albumin:creatinine ratio, and between protein excretion rate and protein:creatinine ratio are based on the assumption that the average creatinine excretion rate is approximately 1 g/day or 10 mmol/day.
- An early morning urine sample is preferred for ACR or PCR.
- There are no normal standards for ACR or AER in children <24 months old.

4. Children <2 years of age do not fit this classification system.
   a. Normative GFR values increase in a non-linear fashion over the first 2 years of life.
   b. GFR is generally lower in this age group even after correcting for body surface area.
   c. Should be categorized according to age-adjusted GFR as:
      - Normal.
      - Moderately reduced: Below mean by >1 but ≤2 SD (standard deviation).
      - Severely reduced: >2 SD below mean.

   Normal GFR for age <2 years:

Age	Mean GFR ± SD (ml/min/1.73m²)
1 week	41 ± 15
2 to 8 weeks	66 ± 25
>8 weeks to <2 years	96 ± 22

5. Example of nomenclature and comments in CGA staging of CKD: A 15-year-old boy had an acute kidney injury in infancy following an episode of vomiting and severe dehydration, secondary to duodenal stenosis. On his latest follow-up, his weight and height were 25 kg and 154 cm, respectively, his serum creatinine was 104 μmol/L, and his urine protein:creatinine ratio was 51.3 mg/mmol.

Cause	Ischemic Nephropathy
GFR category	G3a (eGFR = 54 ml/min/1.73m^2)
Albuminuria/proteinuria category	A3 (urine PCR 51.3 mg/mmol)
Criteria for CKD	Imaging abnormality and low eGFR
Comment	Expected outcome of an acute kidney injury in infancy

Recommended Reading

1. Hogg RJ, Furth S, Lemley KV, Portman R, Schwartz GJ, Coresh J, Balk E, Lau J, Levin A, Kausz AT, Eknoyan G, Levey AS; National Kidney Foundation's Kidney Disease Outcomes Quality Initiative. (2003) National Kidney Foundation's Kidney Disease Outcomes Quality Initiative clinical practice guidelines for chronic kidney disease in children and adolescents: Evaluation, classification, and stratification. *Pediatrics* **111**:1416–1121.
2. KDIGO. (2012) Clinical practice guideline for the evaluation and management of chronic kidney disease.
3. Inker LA, Astor BC, Fox CH, Isakova T, Lash JP, Peralta CA, Tamura MK, Feldman HI. (2014) KDOQI US commentary on the 2012 KDIGO clinical practice guideline for the evaluation and management of CKD. *Am J Kidney Dis* **63**:713–735.
4. Wong CS, Warady BA. (2020, updated) Chronic kidney disease in children: Definition, epidemiology, etiology, and course. Edited by: Mattoo TK, Kim MS. *UpToDate ONLINE.* http://www.uptodate_online.com.

2 Estimation of Glomerular Filtration Rate

Ng KH, Teo S and Yap HK

	Recommended	eGFR Equation
Pre-term infants (0–12 months)	Revised Schwartz (Adjusted)	$22.1 \times L/Cr$
Full-term infants (0–12 months)	Revised Schwartz (Adjusted)	$30.1 \times L/Cr$
Child (1–12 years)	Revised Schwartz	$36.5 \times L/Cr$
Adolescents (12–17 years)	Revised Schwartz	$36.5 \times L/Cr$
Adult (≥18 years#)	CKD-EPI	$141 \times \min [\{Cr/(k*88.4)\},1]^{\alpha} \times \max [\{Cr/(k*88.4)\},1]^{-1.209} \times 0.993^{age} \times 1.018^{(if\ female)}$
Patients with abnormal muscle mass or body habitus	Cystatin C levels	
Acute kidney injury	Cystatin C levels	

eGFR : In ml/min/1.73m^2
L : Length or height in cm
Cr : Serum creatinine in μmol/L
k : Constant (0.7 for females and 0.9 for males)
α : Constant (–0.329 for females and –0.411 for males)
min : Minimum
max : Maximum
\# : Consider the average of Revised Schwartz + CKD-EPI equations for 18–26 years

A. General Considerations in Estimating Glomerular Filtration Rate (GFR)

I. Principles

1. Kidney function may be inferred using absolute serum creatinine or cystatin C levels, or using GFR-estimation equations (eGFR), which are most often based on serum creatinine and/or cystatin C.
2. The accuracy of GFR estimations is often based on measured GFR by standard means such as ^{99Tm}Tc-DTPA, iohexol, iothalamate, ^{51}Cr-EDTA, or inulin clearances.
3. eGFR in children is standardized to a body surface area (BSA) of 1.73 m^2.

II. Limitations of GFR estimation

GFR estimation may not be accurate in the following circumstances:

1. Patient factors:
   a. Healthy individuals.
      - Most equations are derived from patients with decreased GFR.

   b. Patients whose muscle mass deviate from the mean of persons of his/her age, sex and ethnic origin in the population.
   c. Patients who are not in a steady state such as in the presence of an acute kidney injury.
   d. Patients with extremes of GFR (normal or very low).
2. Laboratory factors:
   a. Assay methodology for creatinine and cystatin C may differ from the assay used in derivation studies.
   b. Calibration of the assay should be done using standard reference materials.

III. Serum creatinine

1. Serum creatinine should be measured using an assay with calibration traceable to the international standard reference materials and

with minimal bias, compared to isotope-dilution mass spectrometry (IDMS) reference methodology.

2. Creatinine-based estimating GFR equations include anthropometric data such as age, sex and ethnicity, which compensate for the influence of muscle mass, as serum creatinine depends on muscle mass.
3. Provide GFR estimates from 20–60 ml/min/1.73m^2 with good accuracy but poor bias and precision.

IV. Serum Cystatin C

1. Cystatin C:
   a. Important inhibitor of cysteine proteinase, produced by all nucleated cells.
   b. Freely filtered in glomerulus, reabsorbed and catabolized in the proximal tubule.
   c. Not secreted by the tubules.
   d. Minimal extra-renal elimination.
   e. Depends almost entirely on GFR and is not substantially affected by diet, nutritional status, inflammatory or malignant disease.
2. Advantages:
   a. Not affected by gender, body weight and muscle mass.
   b. Constant production rate.
   c. Lower variability of measurements compared to serum creatinine.
   d. Sensitive for detecting mild GFR reduction between 60 and 90 ml/min/1.73m^2.
   e. Shorter half-life and lower distribution volume: Potentially better marker in an acute kidney injury, as it increases earlier compared to serum creatinine.
   f. Does not pass through the placenta, therefore cystatin C levels reflect the neonate's GFR.
3. Disadvantages:
   a. Limited reference standards.
   b. No extensive validation studies, especially in Asia.

c. Affected by:
   - Thyroid status: Hyperthyroidism elevates cystatin C while hypothyroidism reduces cystatin C.
   - High glucocorticoid doses following transplantation increase cystatin C.
   - High cardiovascular morbidity increases cystatin C, possibly due to atherosclerosis.
   - Inflammation.

4. Reference ranges:
   a. Levels highest in the first few days of life with a rapid decrease in the first 4 months:

Age	Cystatin C (mg/L)	
	Median	Range
24–28 weeks gestational age	1.48	0.65–3.37
29–36 weeks gestational age	1.65	0.62–4.42
0–3 months	1.37	0.81–2.32
4–11 months	0.98	0.65–1.49
1–17 years	0.80	0.50–1.27

Note: Data from 244 patient samples (Finnery *et al.*, 2000).

   b. In healthy children, cystatin C concentrations stabilize from the second year of life and the reference range is identical to adults (0.51–0.98 mg/L).

B. GFR-Estimation Equations in Children (<18 Years Old)

I. Revised Schwartz Formula (Simplified CKiD bedside equation, $CKiD_{SCr}$):

1. Simplified version of the CKiD equation.

$$eGFR = 36.5 \times L/Cr$$

2. eGFR is expressed in ml/min per 1.73 m^2 BSA, L represents the body length in cm, Cr represents serum creatinine concentration in μmol/L.
3. Recommended for use in children >1 year old.
4. For infants aged 0–12 months, the revised Schwartz Formula can be adjusted with a proportionality constant to account for the change in creatinine assay (not validated):

$$eGFR = K \times L/Cr$$

	K
Preterm infants, 0–12 months	22.1
Full-term infants, 0–12 months	30.1

II. CKiD Equation based on serum cystatin C and creatinine ($CKiD_{SCr\text{-}Cys}$):

$$eGFR = 39.8[(height \times 88.4)/Cr]^{0.456} \times [1.8/cystatin\ C]^{0.418} \times [10.71/serum\ urea]^{0.079} \times [1.076]^{male} \times [height/1.4]^{0.179}$$

1. eGFR is expressed in ml/min per 1.73 m^2 BSA, height is measured in meters, Cr represents serum creatinine concentration in μmol/L, serum cystatin C is measured by immunonephelometric assay in mg/L, serum urea is measured in mmol/L, and male=1 and female=0.
2. Equation is most robust:
   - At GFR 15–75 ml/min/1.73m^2, though probably accurate up to 90 ml/min/1.73m^2.
   - For children 6–14 years old, as it tends to underestimate the GFR in adolescents 14–17 years old and in healthy subjects with normal GFR.
3. For eGFR outside of 15–75 ml/min/1.73m^2, it is best to report it as <15 or >75 ml/min/1.73m^2 rather than absolute values.

C. GFR-Estimation Equations in Adults (≥18 Years Old)

I. Chronic Kidney Disease Epidemiology (CKD-EPI)$_{SCr}$ equation:

$$eGFR = 141 \times \min[(Cr/k), 1]^{\alpha} \times \max[(Cr/k), 1]^{-1.209} \times 0.993^{age} \times 1.018^{(\text{if female})}$$

1. eGFR is expressed in ml/min per 1.73 m^2 BSA, age is expressed in years, Cr is standardized creatinine in mg/dL and k is a constant (0.7 for females and 0.9 for males) and α is a constant (–0.329 for females and –0.411 for males), min indicates the minimum while max indicates the maximum.
   [Cr in μmol/L / 88.4 = Cr in mg/dL]
2. Does not perform as well in Asians compared to Americans or Europeans.

II. Average of CKiD$_{SCr}$ and CKD-EPI$_{SCr}$ equations:

1. In emerging adults 18–26 years, the adult eGFR equation overestimated while the pediatric equation underestimated the measured GFR.
2. The CKD-EPI$_{SCr}$ equation is approximately 14 ml/min/1.73m^2 higher than the CKiD$_{SCr}$ equation.
3. Accuracy of GFR estimation is improved in emerging adults with CKD by taking the simple average of CKiD$_{SCr}$ and CKD-EPI$_{SCr}$ equations.

$$eGFR = (CKiD_{SCr} + CKD\text{-}EPI_{SCr})/2$$

D. Choice of GFR-Estimation Equations Using Serum Creatinine

Patient	Expected GFR (ml/min/1.73m²)	CKiD or Revised Schwartz£	CKD-EPI
Child (1–12 years)	>75	↓**¥	
	15–75	↔*	
	<15	↑**	
Adolescent (12–17) years	>60	↓↓**	
	<60	↓**	
Adult (≥18 years)	>60	↓↓	↑*#
	20–60	↓↓	↑*#
	<20	↓↓	**#

↑ Overestimate
↓ Underestimate
↔ Accurate
* Recommended
** Recommended but use with caution
£ Most robust for 6–14-year-olds
¥ Probably accurate up to 90 ml/min/1.73m²
\# Average of $CKiD_{SCr}$ and CKD-EPI_{SCr} equations recommended for 18–26 years

Recommended Reading

1. Schwartz GJ, Brion LP, Spitzer A. (1987) The use of plasma creatinine concentration for estimating glomerular filtration rate in infants, children, and adolescents. *Pediatr Clin North Am* **34**:571–590.
2. Finney H, Newman DJ, Thakkar H, Fell JM, Price CP. (2000) Reference ranges for plasma cystatin C and creatinine measurements in premature infants, neonates, and older children. *Arch Dis Child* **82**:71–75.
3. Herget-Rosenthal S, Bokenkamp A, Hofmann W. (2007) How to estimate GFR-serum creatinine, serum cystatin C or equations? *Clin Biochem* **40**:153–161.
4. Levey AS, Stevens LA, Schmid CH, Zhang YL, Castro AF, 3rd, Feldman HI, Kusek JW, Eggers P, Van Lente F, Greene T, Coresh J. (2009) A new equation to estimate glomerular filtration rate. *Ann Intern Med* **150**:604–612.
5. Schwartz GJ, Munoz A, Schneider MF, Mak RH, Kaskel F, Warady BA, Furth SL. (2009) New equations to estimate GFR in children with CKD. *J Am Soc Nephrol* **20**:629–637.

6. Lemley KV. (2009) Pediatric nephrology: Estimating GFR in children: Schwartz redux. *Nat Rev Nephrol* **5**:310–311.
7. Stevens LA, Claybon MA, Schmid CH, Chen J, Horio M, Imai E, Nelson RG, Van Deventer M, Wang HY, Zuo L, Zhang YL, Levey AS. (2011) Evaluation of the Chronic Kidney Disease Epidemiology Collaboration equation for estimating the glomerular filtration rate in multiple ethnicities. *Kidney Int* **79**:555–562.
8. Schwartz GJ, Schneider MF, Maier PS, Moxey-Mims M, Dharnidharka VR, Warady BA, Furth SL, Muñoz A. (2012) Improved equations estimating GFR in children with chronic kidney disease using an immunonephelometric determination of cystatin C. *Kidney Int* **82**:445–453.
9. Earley A, Miskulin D, Lamb EJ, Levey AS, Uhlig K. (2012) Estimating equations for glomerular filtration rate in the era of creatinine standardization: A systematic review. *Ann Intern Med* **156**:785–795.
10. Mian AN, Schwartz GJ. (2017) Measurement and estimation of glomerular filtration rate in children. *Adv Chronic Kidney Dis* **24**:348–356.
11. Ng DK, Schwartz GJ, Schneider MF, Furth SL, Warady BA. (2018) Combination of pediatric and adult formulas yield valid glomerular filtration rate estimates in young adults with a history of pediatric chronic kidney disease. *Kidney Int* **94**:170–177.

3 Anemia of Chronic Kidney Disease

KWY Kyaw, Yap HK, Teo S, Qader MA, Resontoc LP and Ng KH

A. Contributory Factors

1. Factors contributing to anemia of chronic kidney disease (CKD) include:
   - Iron and folate deficiency.
   - Shortened red cell survival.
   - Mineral bone disease with hyperparathyroidism.
   - Aluminum toxicity.
   - Elevated hepcidin levels.
   - Inhibition of erythropoiesis.
2. Erythropoietin (EPO) deficiency is the most important contributory cause of anemia of CKD as kidney function declines.
3. Mechanisms underlying anemia of CKD:

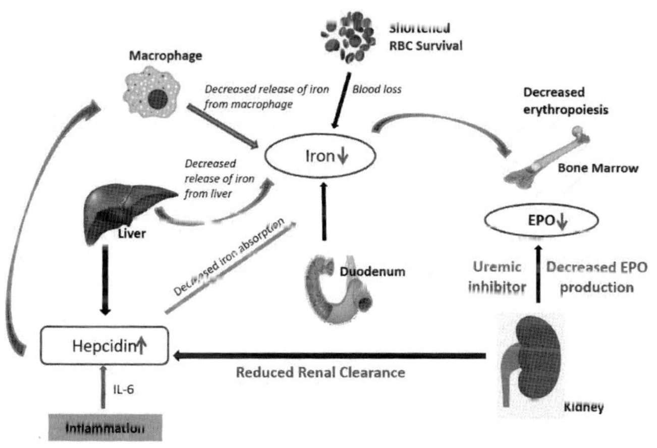

B. Diagnosis of Anemia

1. In otherwise healthy children with anemia, studies have shown a diminution of exercise capacity, suggesting that normative age-appropriate hemoglobin (Hb) levels for children should be used.
2. Evaluation of anemia should be undertaken when Hb falls to <5th centile (2 standard deviations) of age-sex adjusted norms:

Age	Mean Hb (g/dL)	5th Centile Hb (g/dL)
Term (cord blood)	16.5	13.5
1–3 days	18.5	14.5
1 week	17.5	13.5
2 weeks	16.5	12.5
1 months	14.0	10.0
2 months	11.5	9.0
3–6 months	11.5	9.5
6–24 months	12.0	10.5

Age	5th Centile Hb (g/dL)	
	Males	Females
1–2 years	10.7	10.8
3–5 years	11.2	11.1
6–8 years	11.5	11.5
9–11 years	12.0	11.9
12–14 years	12.4	11.7
15–19 years	13.5	11.5
Adult	13.5	12.0

3. Hb concentrations for the diagnosis of anemia of CKD (KDIGO, 2012):

Age	Hb (g/dL)
6 months to 5 years	<11.0
5–12 years	<11.5
12–15 years	<12.0
>15 years and adults:	
Males	<13.0
Females	<12.0

4. Frequency of testing for anemia:
   a. For CKD patients without anemia, measure Hb concentration when clinically indicated and:
      i. At least annually in patients with CKD G3.
      ii. At least twice per year in patients with CKD G4–5.
      iii. At least every 3 months in patients with CKD G5D.
   b. For CKD patients with anemia not being treated with an erythropoietin stimulating agent (ESA), measure Hb concentration when clinically indicated and:
      i. At least every 3 months in patients with CKD G3–5 and CKD G5D on peritoneal dialysis (PD).
      ii. At least monthly in patients with CKD 5D on hemodialysis (HD).

C. Evaluation of Anemia

1. Initial assessment:
   a. Full blood count (FBC) including red blood cell indices:
      - Mean corpuscular hemoglobin (MCH).
      - Mean corpuscular volume (MCV).
      - Mean corpuscular hemoglobin concentration (MCHC).
   b. Mentzer index = MCV(fl)/RBC count (10^9/L)
      - >13 suggestive of iron deficiency.
      - <13 suggestive of thalassemia.
   c. Reticulocyte profile:

i. Absolute reticulocyte count.
ii. Percent hypochromic red cells (HRC):
- Must be processed within 6 hours of blood collection.
- Cannot be used in the presence of hemoglobinopathies.

iii. Reticulocyte Hb concentration (CHr) or reticulocyte Hb equivalent (Ret-He):
- Cannot be used in the presence of hemoglobinopathies.

d. Iron panel:
- Serum ferritin to assess iron stores.
- Iron.
- Transferrin.
- Total iron binding capacity (TIBC) = 0.26 × Transferrin.
- Transferrin saturation (TSAT) = iron/TIBC × 100 (%).

e. Serum vitamin B12 and folate levels.

2. Diagnosis of iron deficiency:

a. Estimation of Hb content of red blood cells to diagnose iron deficiency (both absolute and functional):
- Percent HRC >6%.
- CHr or Ret-He <29 pg.

b. Absolute iron deficiency defined as a marked reduction or absent storage iron in bone marrow, liver and spleen:

i. TSAT ≤20%.
ii. Serum ferritin levels:
- ≤100 ng/ml (non-dialysis and PD).
- ≤200 ng/ml (HD).

c. Functional iron deficiency is characterized by the presence of adequate iron stores but insufficient iron availability for incorporation into erythroid precursors:

i. Distinguished from absolute iron deficiency by TSAT ≤20% and high serum ferritin levels >200–500 ng/ml.
ii. Related to ESA therapy:
- Adequate iron stores defined by stainable iron in bone marrow.
- Release of iron from stores not rapid enough to support increased erythropoietic rate driven by ESA.
- Responds to intravenous iron in association with a concomitant increase in ESA dose, with a decrease in ferritin levels.

iii. Anemia of chronic disease:
- Related to underlying inflammatory state.
- Mediated in part by upregulation of hepcidin by inflammatory cytokines.
- Administration of intravenous iron fails to increase erythropoiesis despite increasing ESA dose, but increases ferritin levels.

D. Iron Therapy

1. Goal of iron therapy is to correct absolute iron deficiency in order to increase Hb level to the desired level.
2. Consider iron supplementation in CKD patients:
   a. Children: TSAT ≤20% and serum ferritin ≤100 ng/ml.
   b. Adults: TSAT ≤30% and serum ferritin ≤500 ng/ml.
   Note: Consider stopping iron if TSAT >30% or serum ferritin >500 ng/ml since such patients are unlikely to respond to iron.
3. Monitor Hb and iron status (TSAT and ferritin):
   a. At least every 3 months during ESA therapy.
   b. More frequently when:
      i. Initiating or increasing ESA dose.
      ii. Blood loss is present.
      iii. Monitoring response to iron supplementation.
4. Target iron status as follows:
   a. CKD G3–5 and 5D on PD: Serum ferritin ≥100 ng/ml and TSAT ≥20%.
   b. CKD G5 on HD: Serum ferritin ≥200 ng/ml and TSAT ≥20%.
   c. If iron status is normal but the child is still anemic, check Ret-He, targeting levels ≥29 pg.
5. Oral iron supplementation:
   a. Dose:
      i. Recommended dose of elemental iron: 3–4 mg/kg/day up to 6 mg/kg/day (maximum 150–300 mg/day in 2–3 divided doses).
      ii. Take 2 hours before or 1 hour after all calcium-containing binders and food.

b. Iron preparations:

Oral Iron Preparation	Elemental Iron (%)
Ferrous fumarate, 200 mg tablet	66 mg (33%)
Ferrous gluconate, 300 mg tablet	36 mg (12%)
Iron polymaltose, 50 mg/ml drops (Maltofer®)	50 mg/ml (100%)
Iron polymaltose, 100 mg tablet (Maltofer®)	100 mg (100%)
Ferric citrate, 1000 mg tablet*	210 mg (21%)

*Used in adults for the treatment of iron deficiency in non-dialysis-dependent CKD patients and hyperphosphatemia in dialysis patients.

c. Causes of failure of oral iron therapy:
   i. Non-compliance.
   ii. Poor absorption in uremia.
   iii. Decreased dietary absorption due to inhibition by phosphate binders or functional achlorhydria with the use of H_2-blockers or proton-pump blockers.
   iv. Functional iron deficiency related to ESA therapy.
   v. Functional iron deficiency due to chronic inflammation.

6. Parenteral ferric carboxymaltose (Ferinject®):
   a. Preparation: Each 10 ml ampoule contains 50 mg/ml iron corresponding to 500 mg of iron per ampoule.
   b. Indications:
      i. Iron deficiency not responding to oral iron therapy.
      ii. Non-adherence to oral iron therapy.
      iii. Intolerance to oral iron preparation.
      iv. Functional iron deficiency, not responding to ESA.
      v. Severe anemia (Hb <7 g/dL) in asymptomatic patients to minimize the need for blood transfusions.

      Note: Preferred therapy for HD patients.
   c. Dosage:
      i. The dose and dosage schedule must be individually estimated for each child based on the calculation of total iron deficit.

Iron deficit [mg] = Weight [kg] × (Target Hb – Actual Hb) [g/dL] × 2.4 + Depot Iron [mg]

- <35 kg (BW): Target Hb = 11.0 g/dL and depot iron = 15 mg/kg (maximum 500 mg).
- ≥35 kg (BW): Target Hb = 11.5 g/dL and depot iron = 500 mg.

ii. Calculation of total iron deficit (mg):

Body Weight (kg)	Hb (g/dL)								
	6.0	6.5	7.0	7.5	8.0	8.5	9.0	9.5	10
10	270	258	246	234	222	210	198	186	174
15	405	387	369	351	333	315	297	279	261
20	540	516	492	468	444	420	396	372	348
25	675	645	615	585	555	525	495	465	435
30	810	774	738	702	666	630	594	558	522
35	962	920	878	836	795	752	710	668	626
40	1028	980	932	884	836	788	740	692	644
45	1094	1040	986	932	878	824	770	716	662
50	1160	1100	1040	980	920	860	800	740	680
55	1226	1160	1095	1028	962	896	830	764	698
60	1292	1220	1148	1076	1004	932	860	788	716
65	1358	1280	1290	1124	1046	968	890	812	734
70	1424	1340	1256	1172	1088	1004	920	836	752

iii. Ferinject® dosage:

- Calculated based on iron deficit.
- Start at 15 mg/kg (maximum 750 mg), which can be repeated after at least 7 days to the maximum allowable cumulative dose.
- Maximum allowable cumulative dose for body weight should not be exceeded:

Hb (g/dL)	Maximum Ferrinject® Dosage For Body Weight:		
	<35 kg	35–70 kg	≥70 kg
<10	500 mg	1500 mg	2000 mg
≥10	500 mg	1000 mg	1500 mg

d. Contraindications:
   i. Hypersensitivity to ferric carboxymaltose complex.
   ii. Anemia not attributed to iron deficiency.
   iii. Evidence of iron overload or disturbances in the utilization of iron.
   iv. Presence of active infection.

e. Administration:
   i. Intravenous injection:
      - May be administered undiluted up to 15 mg/kg iron (maximum 1000 mg iron).
      - For iron dosage ≤500 mg, administer at a rate of 100 mg/min.
      - For iron dosage 501–1000 mg, administer over 15 minutes.
   ii. Intravenous infusion:
      - Dilute in 0.9% saline only.
      - 100–200 mg iron: Dilute in 50 ml 0.9% saline, infuse over 15 minutes.
      - 201–500 mg iron: Dilute in 100 ml 0.9% saline, infuse over 15 minutes.
      - 501–1000 mg iron: Dilute in 250 ml 0.9% saline, infuse over 30 minutes.
   iii. Injection into hemodialyzer:
      - A single maximum daily dose of 200 mg iron should not be exceeded.
   iv. Ferinject® must not be administered by subcutaneous or intramuscular route.

f. Monitoring during therapy:
   i. Facilities for cardiopulmonary resuscitation must be available as there is a risk of hypersensitivity reactions.
   ii. Vital signs monitoring (pulse rate, respiratory rate, blood pressure [BP], oxygen saturation):
      - Baseline weight, temperature, pulse rate, respiratory rate, BP, and oxygen saturation.
      - Pulse rate and BP every 15 minutes during infusion.
      - Pulse rate and BP every 30 minutes for 1 hour after infusion.
   iii. Inform pediatric nephrologist **immediately** if:
      - Tachycardia (pulse rate >120/min).
      - Hypotension (diastolic BP <60 mmHg, systolic BP <80 mmHg).

Note: Lowest systolic BP = 70 + [2 × age (in years)] mmHg.
- Urticarial rash.

g. Management of adverse reactions:
   i. Anaphylaxis:
      - Stop Ferinject® infusion immediately.
      - Cardiopulmonary resuscitation.
      - IV adrenaline (1:10000) 0.05–0.1 ml/kg.
      - IV hydrocortisone 5 mg/kg.
   ii. Mild allergic reaction:
      - Stop Ferinject® infusion.
      - Consider intravenous drip infusion (slower rate of infusion) if intravenous injection (slow small bolus regime) was given.
      - Chlorpheniramine PO 0.1 mg/kg (maximum 4 mg) OR IV diphenhydramine 0.5–1.0 mg/kg (maximum 50 mg) OR IV hydrocortisone 5 mg/kg depending on severity.

h. Follow-up and monitoring following intravenous iron therapy:
   i. FBC and absolute reticulocyte count weekly, then monthly, if there is a good response.
   ii. Monitoring iron status:
      - TSAT and ferritin monthly, then 3 monthly when target Hb is achieved.
   iii. Patients are unlikely to respond with further increase of Hb if TSAT ≥50% and/or serum ferritin ≥800 ng/ml.

E. Treatment with Erythropoietin-Stimulating Agents (ESAs)

1. Initiation of ESA therapy:
   a. Before starting patients on ESAs, the following factors must be addressed:
      i. Adequate nutrition.
      ii. Give hematinics such as iron, folate and vitamin B12.
      iii. Correction of severe hyperparathyroidism.
      iv. Avoidance of aluminum toxicity.
      v. Treat chronic infection or inflammation.
   b. Use ESA with caution in CKD patients with active or previous malignancy.

c. Consider starting treatment with ESAs:
   i. Children: When Hb ≤10 g/dL.
   ii. Adults: When Hb ≤9–10 g/dL.
   iii. If the patient is symptomatic and Hb >10 g/dL and may benefit from improvement in quality of life.
d. Consider intravenous or subcutaneous administration of ESA for those on HD, and subcutaneous administration for non-dialysis patients and those on PD.

2. Dose adjustments:
   a. Based on patient's Hb concentration, rate of change of Hb, current ESA dose, and clinical circumstances.
   b. Target rate of increase of Hb ≈ 0.25 g/dL per week.
      i. Do not exceed an increase of Hb >0.5 g/dL per week.
      ii. If Hb is higher than desired, decreasing ESA dose is preferable to withholding it.
3. Monitoring:
   a. If adjustments are made in ESA dose, 1–2 weekly FBC with absolute reticulocyte count may be required until the target is reached.
   b. Once target Hb is reached and the patient is on a stable dose of ESA, monitor monthly FBC and iron panel.
4. Recommended Hb targets while on ESA therapy:
   a. For pediatric patients, aim for a Hb target of 11–12 g/dL.
   b. For adults, suggested Hb target is ≤10–11.5 g/dL.
      - Target Hb should not be ≥13 g/dL, as studies have shown a greater risk for death, serious cardiovascular events, and strokes.
      - Hb targets for maintenance ESA therapy should generally not be >11.5 g/dL, but can be individualized with risks and benefits informed, as some patients may have improvements in their quality of life.

F. Types of ESAs

I. Intravenous rhEPO-alfa (Eprex®)

1. Recommended for patients on HD.
2. Dosing:
   a. Starting dose: 50–75 IU/kg three times a week, checking Hb 1–2 weekly until target Hb is reached.

   b. Increase to a maximum of 240 IU/kg/dose 3 times a week if target Hb is not attained.
   c. Maintenance dose: 100–300 IU/kg/week.
3. Monitor blood pressure to watch for worsening of hypertension, which must be treated urgently.
4. It is strongly recommended that rhEPO-alfa (Eprex®) should not be administered subcutaneously because of the risk of pure red cell aplasia.

II. rhEPO-beta (Recormon®)

1. Recommended for pre-dialysis patients and those on PD.
2. Use rhEPO-beta for subcutaneous route of administration, as rhEPO-alpha has been associated with the complication of pure red cell aplasia.
3. Dosing:
   a. Correction phase: 75–150 IU/kg/week.
      i. Increase the dose by 25–50 IU/kg/week monthly to a maximum of 240 IU/kg/week.
      ii. Target Hb should be reached within 3 months.
   b. Maintenance phase:
      i. Once target Hb has been achieved in the correction phase, the dose should be reduced by 25–50% in order to maintain Hb at that level.
      ii. If required, a further dose reduction may be instituted to ensure that Hb level does not exceed 13 g/dL.
   c. If the rise in Hb is >2 g/dL in 4 weeks, the dose should be reduced by 25–50%.
4. The half-life is shorter for intravenous administration, compared to subcutaneous. Consider shorter dosing intervals for intravenous route.
   a. Half-life for intravenous route: 4–12 hours.
   b. Half-life for subcutaneous route: 13–28 hours.
5. Patients who are stable on a once-weekly subcutaneous dosing regimen may be switched to a once every two weeks administration. A dose increase may be necessary.

III. Darbepoietin-alfa

1. Analogue of rhEPO with 2 extra oligosaccharide chains, resulting in a more prolonged effect, hence requiring less frequent dosing than rhEPO.
2. Pharmacokinetics in children 7–16 years:
   a. Terminal half-life for intravenous (IV) administration is 21 hours (range 12–25 hours).
   b. Terminal half-life for subcutaneous (SC) administration is 33 hours (range 16–44 hours).
   c. SC bioavailability is 52% (range 32–70%).
3. Starting dose: SC or IV 0.45 mcg/kg given weekly (estimated equivalent to rhEPO 100 IU/kg/week).
4. Substitution of rhEPO with darbepoetin-alfa:
   a. Substitution of rhEPO with darbepoetin-alfa for rhEPO should be based on the patient's rhEPO dose at the time of substitution, and the same route of administration should be used.
   b. Patients previously receiving rhEPO <100 IU/kg/week should receive a 25–50% reduced dose of darbepoietin-alfa by weight.
5. FDA-approved ESA conversion table for darbepoietin-alfa:

Weekly rhEPO-alfa Dose (IU/week)	Darbepoetin-alfa Conversion Dose (Adult)	Darbepoetin-alfa Conversion Dose (Pediatrics)
<1500	6.25	*
1500 to 2499	6.25	6.25
2500 to 4999	12.5	10
5000 to 10999	25	20
11000 to 17999	40	40
18000 to 33999	60	60
34000 to 89999	100	100
≥90000	200	200

*For pediatric patients receiving a weekly rhEPO-alfa dose of <1500 IU/week, the available data is insufficient to determine darbepoietin-alfa conversion dose.

6. Dose interval for darbepoietin-alfa:
   a. Administer darbepoietin once weekly in patients who were receiving rhEPO-alfa 2–3 times weekly.
   b. Administer darbepoietin-alfa once every 2 weeks in patients who were receiving rhEPO-alfa once weekly.
   c. The dose conversions in the FDA-approved conversion table do not accurately estimate the once-monthly dose of darbepoietin-alfa in patients with CKD not on dialysis.
7. Subsequent dose titration of darbepoetin-alfa:
   a. Check FBC 2–4 weekly.
   b. If Hb does not increase by at least 1 g/dL within 4 weeks and iron stores are adequate:
      - Increase darbepoetin-alfa by 25%.
      - Further increases may be made at 4-week intervals until the desired response is attained.
   c. If Hb increases by more than 2.5 g/dL within 4 weeks, the dose of darbepoetin-alfa should be decreased by 25–50%, depending on the rate of increase.
   d. If Hb >13 g/dL:
      - Discontinue darbepoetin-alfa until Hb decreases to <12 g/dL.
      - Then restart darbepoetin-alfa at a dose approximately 25% below the previous dose.
   e. Dose changes in the maintenance phase of treatment should not be made more frequently than every 2 weeks.
   f. The maximum amount of darbepoetin-alfa that can be safely administered in single or multiple doses has not been determined.
      - Doses >3 mcg/kg/week for up to 28 weeks have been administered to patients with CKD without any direct toxic effects of darbepoetin-alfa itself
   g. Changing route of administration: The same dose should be used and Hb monitored so that appropriate darbepoetin-alfa dose adjustments can be made to keep Hb at the desired concentration.

h. Table for calculation of darbepoetin-alfa dose and adjustments:

Weight (kg)	Dose (mcg):	Interval (days)	Low Hb <10.0 g/dL, Increase Dose 25–50%	High Hb >12.5 g/dL, Decrease Dose 25–50%
56–75	40	Q 10	40 mcg Q 7	40 mcg Q 14
46–55	40	Q 14	40 mcg Q 10	40 mcg Q 21
38–45	20	Q 7	40 mcg Q 14	20 mcg Q 10
26–37	20	Q 10	20 mcg Q 7	20 mcg Q 14
23–25	20	Q 14	20 mcg Q 10	20 mcg Q 21
20–22	20	Q 18	20 mcg Q 10	20 mcg Q 21
14–19	20	Q 21	20 mcg Q 14	20 mcg Q 28
10–13	10	Q 14	10 mcg Q 10	10 mcg Q 21
8–9	10	Q 21	10 mcg Q 14	10 mcg Q 28

IV. *Methoxy polyethylene glycol-epoetin beta (Mircera®)*

1. **C**ontinuous **e**rythropoietin **r**eceptor **a**ctivator (CERA) is the generic term for the class of third-generation ESAs.
2. Mircera®, one of the CERAs available in the market, is structurally similar to previous synthetic EPOs except that it is connected to polyethylene glycol (PEG), which confers its longer half-life (6 times longer than darbepoetin-alfa and 20 times longer than rhEPO-alfa).
3. Pharmacokinetics:
   a. Following IV administration to CKD patients, the half-life for Mircera® was 134 hours (or 5.6 days) and the total systemic clearance was 0.494 ml/hour/kg.
   b. Following SC administration, the observed terminal elimination half-life was 139 hours (or 5.8 days) in patients.
4. Starting dose adjustment:
   a. Starting dose is 0.6 mcg/kg body weight, administered once every 2 weeks via IV or SC in order to increase Hb ≥11 g/dL.
   b. If Hb level ≥11 g/dL is reached, Mircera® may be continued once monthly, using a dose that is twice the previous one.
   c. If the rate of rise in the Hb is <1.0 g/dL over a month, the dose may be increased by ~25% of the previous dose.

   d. Further increases of ~25% may be made at monthly intervals until the individual target Hb level is obtained.

5. Subsequent dose titration:
   a. Monitor FBC once monthly.
   b. If the rate of Hb rise is >2 g/dL in 1 month or if Hb level is increasing and approaching 12 g/dL, the dose should be reduced by ~25%.
   c. If Hb level continues to increase, therapy should be interrupted until Hb level begins to decrease, at which point therapy should be restarted at a dose ~25% below the previously administered dose.
   d. After dose interruption, Hb decrease of ~0.35 g/dL per week is expected.
   e. Dose adjustments should not be made more frequently than once a month.
   f. The following table outlines the conversion of weekly rhEPO-alfa and darbepoietin-alfa to Mircera® once monthly:

Previous Weekly rhEPO-alfa IV or SC Dose		Darbepoietin-alfa IV or SC Weekly Dose		Monthly Mircera® Starting Dose IV or SC Dose	
IU/week	<8000	mcg/week	<40	mcg/monthly	120
	8000–16000		40–80		200
	>16000		>00		360
IU/kg/week	120	mcg/kg/week	0.54	mcg/kg/monthly	3.2

G. Problems Associated with ESA Therapy

1. Side effects:
   a. Hypertension.
   b. Seizures.
   c. Hyperkalemia.
   d. Thrombosis of arteriovenous fistula or graft.
   e. Decreased dialyzer clearances.
   f. Hyperphosphatemia due to increased appetite and decreased clearances.

2. Contraindications:
   a. Uncontrolled hypertension.
   b. Known hypersensitivity to erythropoietin or any of the excipients.
   c. Known sensitivity to products derived from mammalian cells when using recombinant human EPOs.
3. ESA hyporesponsiveness:
   a. Definition: Continued need for higher than 300 IU/kg/week doses of EPO or a 1.5 mg/kg/week dose of darbepoetin-alfa.
      i. Initial hyporesponsiveness: No increase in Hb from baseline after the first month of ESA treatment on appropriate weight-based dosing.
      ii. Acquired hyporesponsiveness: Increases in ESA doses up to 50% above their stable dose.
   b. Avoid repeated escalations in ESA dose beyond double the initial weight-based dose.
   c. Possible causes:
      i. Blood loss:
         - Mean daily gastrointestinal blood loss in children is 6 ml/m^2 compared to 11 ml/m^2 in pediatric HD patients.
         - HD patients have a potential for blood loss in the bloodlines and dialyzer, and this can be up to 8 ml/m^2 per treatment.
      ii. Hemolysis.
      iii. Absolute or functional iron deficiency.
      iv. Vitamin B12 or folate deficiency.
      v. Malnutrition.
      vi. Underdialysis.
      vii. Hypothyroidism.
      viii. Hyperparathyroidism.
      ix. Use of angiotensin-converting enzyme inhibitors or angiotensin receptor blockers.
      x. Infection or inflammation.
      xi. Malignancy.
      xii. Pure red cell aplasia due to anti-EPO antibodies.
      xiii. Bone marrow disorders.
4. Antibody-mediated pure red cell aplasia:
   a. Suspected when a patient who had received ESA for more than 8 weeks develops:
      - Sudden rapid decrease in Hb at a rate of 0.5–1.0 g/dL per week, OR

- Requirement for transfusions at a rate of 1–2 per week, AND
- Normal platelet and white cell counts, AND
- Absolute reticulocyte count <10000/µl.

b. Exclude parvovirus infection.

c. Definitive diagnosis: Presence of neutralizing antibodies against EPO.

d. Bone marrow biopsy characteristically shows reduced numbers or the absence of erythroblasts.

e. Treatment:

   i. Stop all ESAs.

   ii. Transfuse if severe symptomatic anemia.

   iii. Consider immunosuppressive drugs.

H. Algorithm for the Management of Anemia of CKD in Children

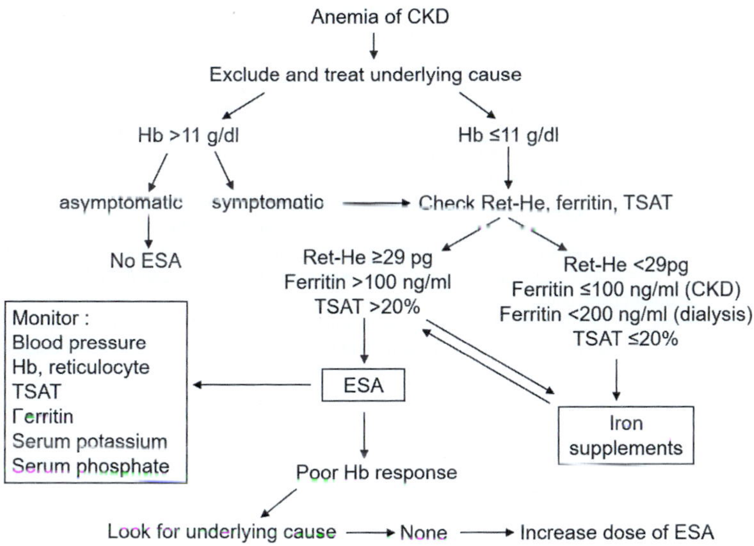

Recommended Reading

1. Amgen Inc. (2019) Conversion dosing guide for epoetin alfa to Aranesp® in patients with anemia due to CKD on dialysis. https://www.anemiahub.com/~/media/amgen/full/www-anemiahub-com/files/brochures/_aranesp-dosing-conversion-guide.ashx.
2. Vifor (International) Inc. (n.d.) Prescribing Information: Ferinject®.
3. Lexicomp® (n.d.) Ferric carboxymaltose: Drug information Lexicomp®.
4. Hoffmann-La Roche Ltd. (n.d.) Brief prescribing information: MIRCERA® -F.
5. Hoffmann-La Roche Ltd. (n.d.) Prescribing information: Recormon®.
6. Geary DF, Keating LE, Vigneux A, Stephens D, Hebert D, Harvey EA. (2005) Darbepoetin alfa (Aranesp) in children with chronic renal failure. *Kidney Int* **68**:1759–1765.
7. Yap HK. (2005) Anemia, renal osteodystrophy, growth failure in chronic renal failure. In: *Practical Paediatric Nephrology. An Update of Current Practices*, edited by: Chiu MC, Yap HK. Medcom Limited, Hong Kong. pp 253–261.
8. Cano F, Alarcon C, Azocar M, Lizama C, Lillo AM, Delucchi A, Gonzalez M, Arellano P, Delgado I, Droguett MT. (2001) Continuous EPO receptor activator therapy of anemia in children under peritoneal dialysis. *Pediatr Nephrol* **26**:1303–10.
9. KDIGO. (2012) KDIGO clinical practice guideline for anemia in chronic kidney disease. *Kidney Int* **2**(Suppl):279–335.
10. Kliger AS, Foley RN, Goldfarb DS, Goldstein SL, Johansen K, Singh A, Szczech L. (2013) KDOQI US commentary on the 2012 KDIGO clinical practice guideline for anemia in CKD. *Am J Kidney Dis* **62**:849–859.
11. Locatelli F, Bárány P, Covic A, De Francisco A, Del Vecchio L, Goldsmith D, Hörl W, London G, Vanholder R, Van Biesen W; ERA-EDTA ERBP Advisory Board. (2013) Kidney Disease: Improving Global Outcomes guidelines on anaemia management in chronic kidney disease: A European Renal Best Practice position statement. *Nephrol Dial Transplant* **28**:1346–1359.
12. Berns JS. (2020, updated) Treatment of iron deficiency in hemodialysis patients. Edited by: Golper TA, Motwani S. *UpToDate ONLINE*. http://www.uptodateonline.com.
13. Srivastava T, Warady BA. (2021, updated) Chronic kidney disease in children: Overview of management. Edited by: Mattoo TK, Kim MS. *UpToDate ONLINE*. http://www.uptodateonline.com.
14. Berns JS. (2020, updated) Diagnosis of iron deficiency in chronic kidney disease. Edited by: Golper TA, Motwani S. *UpToDate ONLINE*. http://www.uptodateonline.com.

4 Chronic Kidney Disease — Mineral and Bone Disorder

Pinapala A, Yap HK, Liu ID, Ng KH and Qader MA

A. Definition: Chronic Kidney Disease — Mineral and Bone Disorder (CKD-MBD)

1. Kidney Disease Improving Global Outcome (KDIGO):
   A systemic disorder of mineral and bone metabolism due to CKD manifested by either one or a combination of the following (syndrome of biochemical, bone and extra-skeletal calcification):
   - Abnormalities of calcium, phosphorous, parathyroid hormone (PTH), or vitamin D metabolism.
   - Abnormalities in bone turnover, mineralization, volume, linear growth, or strength.
   - Vascular or other soft tissue calcification.
2. Kidney Disease Outcomes Quality Initiative (K/DOQI) (children):
   - The effects of abnormal bone and mineral metabolism on endochondral ossification during growth, resulting in complications in the epiphyseal region that are unique to children with CKD.
   - An early and universal feature of CKD that may develop prior to any clinical manifestations of kidney failure.

B. Renal Osteodystrophy (ROD)

1. Definition of ROD:
   - Alteration of bone morphology in patients with CKD.
   - One measure of the skeletal component of the systemic disorder of CKD-MBD that is quantifiable by histomorphometry of bone biopsy.

2. Classification of ROD:
   a. TMV system
      i. Bone turnover:
         - Reflects rate of skeletal remodeling: Bone resorption and formation.
         - Assessed histomorphometrically by dynamic measurements of double tetracycline labeling to measure osteoblast function.
      ii. Mineralization:
         - Reflects how well bone collagen becomes calcified during the formation phase of skeletal remodeling.
         - Assessed histomorphometrically by:
           ▪ Static measurements of osteoid volume and thickness.
           ▪ Dynamic measurements of tetracycline-based measurement of mineralization lag time and osteoid maturation time.
      iii. Volume:
         - Indicates the amount of bone per unit volume of tissue.
         - Assessed histomorphometrically by static measurements of bone volume in cancellous bone.

Turnover	Mineralization	Volume
Low	Normal	Low
Normal	Abnormal	Normal
High		High

   b. Histologic classification:

Type	Etiology	Description
High-turnover bone disease (Osteitis fibrosa)	• Hyperparathyroidism.	• Increased bone formation, resorption and osteoid deposition. • Disorganized collagen (woven bone), marrow fibrosis.

(*Continued*)

Type	Etiology	Description
Low-turnover: (I) Adynamic bone	• Relatively low PTH. • Calcium load, vitamin D metabolites. • Uremic toxins. • Altered cytokines or growth factors.	• Low bone formation and resorption rate. • Decreased osteoid deposition.
(II) Osteomalacia	• Aluminium. • Unknown factors.	• Accumulation of osteoid. • Inhibition of the mineralization process.
Mixed disease	• Hyperparathyroidism. • Aluminium. • Unknown factors.	• Increased remodeling, resorption and osteoid. • Areas of low bone formation.

3. Expected biochemical changes in children with abnormal bone turnover and/or mineralization:

		Markers		
		PTH	ALP	Calcium
High turnover	Abnormal mineralization	↑↑↑	↑↑	↓, variable
	Normal mineralization	↑↑	↑	Normal-variable
Normal turnover	Abnormal mineralization	↑↑	↑, variable	↓, variable
	Normal mineralization	Normal-variable	Normal-variable	Normal-variable
Low turnover	Abnormal mineralization	↑, variable	Variable	↓, variable
	Normal mineralization	↓, variable	↓, variable	↑, variable

C. Clinical Evaluation of CKD-MBD

I. Clinical manifestations:

1. Bone involvement:
   - Linear growth failure with delayed skeletal maturation and epiphyseal closure.

- Slipped epiphyses.
- Skeletal deformities resembling Vitamin D deficient rickets genu valgum and genu varum of the knees, valgus deformity of the ankles.
- Avascular necrosis and spontaneous tendon rupture.
- Meniscal tears.
- Bone pains.
- Fractures.

2. Proximal myopathy:
   - Progressive muscle weakness.
   - Waddling gait.
3. Hormonal abnormalities:
   - Altered Vitamin D metabolism.
   - Secondary hyperparathyroidism.
4. Metabolic abnormalities:
   - Hypocalcemia.
   - Hyperphosphatemia.
5. Ocular disease:
   - Conjunctival calcification presenting as "red eyes".
   - Band keratopathy.
   - Corneal calcification.
6. Dermatological disease:
   - Pruritus.
   - Skin ulceration and soft tissue necrosis.
7. Gastrointestinal complications:
   - Constipation.
   - Peptic ulcer.
   - Pancreatitis.
8. Extraskeletal calcification:
   - Soft tissue calcification of blood vessels, lung, kidney, myocardium, coronary arteries, and cardiac valves.
9. Radiographic abnormalities:
   - Subperiosteal resorption.
   - Osteosclerosis.

II. Frequency of clinical assessment:

1. All children with CKD should be examined for CKD-MBD-related bone disease.

2. The frequency of assessment should be based on the underlying cause and stage of CKD, the patient's age, symptoms, presence of comorbidities, and extent of abnormalities in previous CKD-MBD measures.
3. More frequent assessment during periods of rapid growth in infancy and adolescence is required.
4. Frequency of clinical evaluation including history, length/height and physical examination:

CKD Stage	Frequency of Monitoring (Months)			
	Age 0–1 years	Age 1–3 years	Age >3 years	Puberty
G2	1–3	3–6	3–6	3–6
G3	0.5–2	1–3	3–6	1–3
G4	0.5–2	1–2	1–3	1–3
G5 G5D	0.5–1	1–2	1–3	1–3

D. Evaluation of Calcium and Phosphorus Metabolism

I. Frequency of monitoring

1. Serum levels of calcium (albumin-corrected calcium), phosphorus, alkaline phosphatase (ALP), bicarbonate, and intact PTH (iPTH) should be measured in all patients with CKD G2 to G5D to determine the need for treatment.
   - Ionized calcium should be used if feasible.
2. Serum calcidiol or 25-hydroxyvitamin D_3 [25(OH)D_3] should be measured in all patients with CKD G2 to G5D, especially if serum PTH levels are above the target range for the stage of CKD.

CKD Stage	Serum Calcium, Bicarbonate, Phosphate	Serum ALP, iPTH	Serum 25(OH)D_3
G2	At least every 6 months	Annually	Annually
G3	At least every 6 months	At least every 6 months	At least every 6 months

(Continued)

(*Continued*)

CKD Stage	Serum Calcium, Bicarbonate, Phosphate	Serum ALP, iPTH	Serum 25(OH)D_3
G4	At least every 3 months	At least every 3 months	At least every 3 months to 6 monthly
G5 G5D	At least every month	At least every month to 3 monthly	At least every 3 months to 6 monthly

II. Target levels:

1. Representative normal values for serum phosphorus, albumin-corrected total calcium, and blood ionized calcium levels:

Age	Phosphorus (mmol/L)	Corrected Total Calcium* (mmol/L)	Ionized Calcium (mmol/L)
0–5 months 6–12 months	1.68–2.71 1.61–2.52	2.18–2.83 2.18–2.75	1.22–1.40 1.20–1.40
1–5 years	1.45–2.10	2.35–2.70	1.22–1.32
6–12 years	1.16–1.87	2.35–2.58	1.15–1.32
≥13 years	0.74–1.45	2.2–2.55	1.12–1.30

*Corrected calcium (CaC) = Ca + 0.02 × (40-ALB) where ALB is serum albumin in g/L.

2. Representative normal values for ALP levels:

Age and Sex	ALP (U/L)
0–15 days	90–273
15–30 days	134–518
1 to <10 years	150–369
10 to <13 years	141–460
13 to <15 years, females 13 to <15 years, males	62–280 127–517

(*Continued*)

Age and Sex	ALP (U/L)
15 to <17 years, females 15 to <17 years, males	54–128 89–365
17 to <19 years, females 17 to <19 years, males	48–95 59–164

3. In CKD G1 to G4, the serum corrected total calcium and phosphorus levels should be maintained between age-appropriate lower and upper limits.
4. Target levels for serum phosphorus and calcium for CKD G5 and G5D are as shown:

CKD Stage	Age (Years)	Corrected Total Calcium (mmol/L)	Phosphorus (mmol/L)
G5 and G5D	1–12	2.3–2.6	1.29–1.93
	>12	2.2–2.5	1.13–1.78

5. Target iPTH range in children with CKD G2–G5D are shown in the table below:

CKD Stage	GFR (ml/min/1.73m^2)	Target iPTH Range pmol/L* (pg/ml)
G2	60–89	3.7–7.4 (35–70)
G3	30–59	3.7–7.4 (35–70)
G4	15–29	7.4–11.7 (70–110)
G5 G5D	<15 Dialysis	21.2–31.8 (200–300)

*pmol/L = (pg/ml) × 0.106

6. Serum bicarbonate should be monitored regularly and maintained within the normal range.

III. Other studies:

1. Bone radiographs:
   a. Done when results are expected to impact treatment decisions.
   b. Indicated in patients with:
      - Clinical manifestations of avascular necrosis.
      - Symptomatic slipped capital femoral epiphysis (SCFE).
      - Rickets.
      - Assessment of bone pain.
      - Suspected atraumatic fractures.
      - Genetic diseases with specific bone involvement.
      - Assessment of skeletal maturation (X-Ray left wrist).
2. Bone mineral density (Dual-energy X-Ray absorptiometry):
   a. Should not be used routinely in children with CKD-MBD.
   b. Can be considered for assessment of fracture risk in patients with CKD G3a to G5D with evidence of CKD-MBD and/or risk factors of osteoporosis, if results will impact treatment decisions.
3. Bone biopsy:
   a. Most accurate diagnostic test for determining the type of bone disease associated with CKD.
   b. Done on the iliac crest.
   c. Involves double tetracycline labeling and bone histomorphometric analysis.
   d. Should be considered if knowledge of the type of ROD will impact treatment decisions in patients with the following:
      - Severe bone pain or deformity.
      - Fractures with minimal or no trauma (pathological fractures).
      - Suspected aluminium bone disease based on clinical symptoms or history of aluminium exposure.
      - Persistent hypercalcemia (serum corrected total calcium >2.54 mmol/L) with iPTH levels between 42.4 and 63.6 pmol/L despite optimizing treatment.
      - Unexplained hypophosphatemia despite optimizing treatment.
      - Prior to initiating bisphosphonate therapy.
4. Vascular imaging:
   a. Chest (PA) and lateral abdominal X-Rays to screen for vascular and soft-tissue calcifications.
   b. 2-D echocardiogram for valvular calcifications.

E. Management

I. Control of serum phosphate levels:

1. Guiding principles:
   a. Since hyperphosphatemia is an independent risk factor for secondary hyperparathyroidism, ROD and vascular calcifications, optimal control of serum phosphate levels is the crucial element of preventive management.
   b. Assessment of dietary intake of phosphate with due consideration to phosphate additives and dietary counseling should begin as early as CKD G2.
   c. Treatment for hyperphosphatemia should be initiated based on the trend of serial results rather than a single result.
   d. Elevated phosphate levels should be lowered toward the normal range.
2. Hypophosphatemia should be avoided as it may induce hypophosphatemic osteomalacia.
3. Diet control:
   a. Dietary phosphorus should be decreased to:
      i. Suggested Dietary Intake (SDI) for age when:
         - Serum PTH is above the target range for the stage of CKD.
         - Serum phosphorus is within the target range.
      ii. Lower limit of the SDI for age when:
         - Serum PTH is above the target range for the stage of CKD.
         - Serum phosphorus is above the target range.
      iii. SDI of phosphorus in children:*

Age	SDI (mg/day)
0–4 months	120
4–12 months	275–420
1–3 years	250–500
4–10 years	440–800
11–17 years	640–1250

*Avoid processed food as the bioavailability of inorganic phosphate is 100%.

b. Dietary intake of phosphate should be increased in those with persistent hypophosphatemia.
   - Phosphorus supplements may be necessary with intensified dialysis or renal phosphate wasting.

c. In CKD G5D, adequate protein intake must be maintained while reducing the phosphate intake to as low as possible:
   - 1 g protein = 10–12 mg phosphate.

4. Phosphate binders:

   a. If serum phosphate levels cannot be controlled within the target range for age and stage of CKD despite dietary phosphorus restriction, phosphate binders should be prescribed.

   b. Phosphate binders should be taken immediately before, during or immediately after meals to maximize efficacy, and the amount prescribed should be proportionate to the amount of phosphorus-containing foods.

   c. The decision to use a calcium-based or non-calcium-based phosphate binder depends on the serum calcium levels.

   d. Calcium-based phosphate binders should be used as the initial binder therapy in infants and young children <6 years of age, while non-calcium-based phosphate binders can be used as primary therapy in older children and adolescents.

   e. Calcium-based phosphate binders:

      i. The total dose of elemental calcium provided by calcium-based phosphate binders and dietary calcium should not exceed up to 2x SDI for calcium based on age, or 2600 mg/day.

      ii. The dosage of calcium-based phosphate binders should be lowered in dialysis patients with:
         - Hypercalcemia and corrected serum calcium ≥2.54 mmol/L.
         - Serum iPTH levels <16.6 pmol/L on 2 consecutive measurements due to low-turnover bone disease.

   f. Sevelamer:

      i. Non-absorbable cationic polymer that binds phosphate through ion exchange.

      ii. Sevelamer hydrochloride is associated with metabolic acidosis.

      iii. Acts as a cholesterol-binding resin, and binds fat-soluble vitamins.

iv. Pre-treatment of oral or enteral nutrition:
- 800 mg added in up to 400 ml of breast milk or 100 ml of infant formula and tube feeding and cow's milk.
- After sitting for 10 minutes, decant the liquid from the precipitate at the bottom.
- Reduces phosphate by >85% in breast milk, 42% in cow's milk, 48% in tube feeding, and 68% in infant formula.

g. Lanthanum carbonate:
   i. Gastrointestinal side effects common.
   ii. Accumulates in bone, but long-term effects on growing bone are unknown.

h. Sucroferric oxyhydroxide:
   i. Gastrointestinal side effects: Diarrhea, nausea.
   ii. Contraindications:
   - Hemochromatosis.
   - Other iron accumulation disorders.
   - History of peritonitis in the last 2 months, or ≥3 episodes in the last 12 months.
   - Significant gastric or hepatic disorders (alanine aminotransferase or aspartate aminotransferase >3 times the upper limit of normal).
   - Major gastrointestinal surgery.

Compound	Formulation	Calcium Content (%)	Calcium Absorbed When Taken With Food (%)	Phosphate Bound/g Compound (Phosphate Bound/ Calcium Absorbed)	Comment (Maximum/ day)
Calcium carbonate	625 mg	40	20–30	30 mg/g (1 mg/8 mg)	Chew, needs acidic pH in stomach[#] (10 tablets)

(*Continued*)

(*Continued*)

Compound	Formulation	Calcium Content (%)	Calcium Absorbed When Taken With Food (%)	Phosphate Bound/g Compound (Phosphate Bound/ Calcium Absorbed)	Comment (Maximum/ day)
	1250 mg	40	20–30	39 mg/g (1 mg/8 mg)	Chew, needs acidic pH in stomach[#] (5 tablets)
Calcium acetate	667 mg	25	22 (between meals, 40)	45 mg/g (1 mg/3 mg)	Swallow (15 tablets)
Sevelamer* (Polyallyl-amine)	Renagel® Sevelamer hydrochloride 400 mg	0	0	80 mg/g	Swallow, decreases cholesterol (12 tablets)
	Renvela® Sevelamer carbonate 800 mg	0	0	80 mg/g	Swallow, decreases cholesterol (6 tablets)
Lanthanum carbonate	500 mg, 750 mg, 1000 mg	0	0	90 mg/g	Chew. Should be taken during or after meals (4500 mg)
Sucroferric oxy-hydroxide	2.5 g	Iron content 500 mg		52 mg/g	Chew 6 tablets

*Additional supplements of 400 to 800 mg can be taken with snacks when needed.
*Caution is needed when crushing the tablets as this may make it more difficult to swallow and can cause choking.
[#]Avoid concomitant use of proton-pump inhibitors or H2 antagonists.

a. Avoid using the following phosphate binders:
   i. Aluminium hydroxide due to problems of aluminium bone disease, neurocognitive defects, and hematological complications.
      - Recommended for use only as "rescue therapy" in severe hyperphosphatemia in adolescents.
      - For short-term therapy only, up to 4–6 weeks.
   ii. Magnesium-containing antacids due to the risk of hypermagnesemia and diarrhea.
   iii. Calcium citrate due to increased absorption of dietary aluminium.

5. In dialysis patients who remain hyperphosphatemic despite the use of phosphate binders, the dialysis prescription can be modified to improve hyperphosphatemia.
   a. Peritoneal dialysis (PD):
      i. In high transporters, increase the total therapy volume and number of cycles.
      ii. In high-average, low-average and low transporters, consider longer dwells and increasing PD duration.
      iii. For patients on nightly automated PD, consider addition of a day dwell, a mid-day exchange, or conversion to CAPD.
      iv. Increase convective clearance by increasing ultrafiltration.
      v. Consider measuring the ratio of dialysate phosphate to plasma phosphate levels (D/P phosphate).
         - Optimal dwell time for phosphate clearance is the time when D/P phosphate is at least 0.6.
   b. Hemodialysis (HD):
      i. Optimize vascular access and blood flow rate.
      ii. Check for recirculation.
      iii. Consider use of high-flux dialyzers, increasing the frequency of sessions or changing to hemodiafiltration.

II. Control of serum calcium levels:

1. Guiding principles:
   a. In children with CKD G3 to G5D, serum calcium should be maintained within the age-appropriate normal range, as growing bones need calcium.

b. To prevent the development of hypercalcemia:
   i. In patients receiving calcium-based phosphate binders, low calcium-containing dialysate should be used:
      - Peritoneal dialysis: 1.3 mmol/L.
      - Hemodialysis: 1.25 mmol/L.
   ii. In patients not receiving calcium-based phosphate binders, dialysate calcium should be targeted to 1.25–1.5 mmol/L based on serum calcium levels and need for active vitamin D_3.

2. SDI of calcium:

Age (years)	SDI (mg/day)
0–0.5	220
0.5–1.0	330–540
1–3	450–700
4–8	700–1000
9–18	1300
>18	900–1300

Note: Gastrointestinal calcium absorption:
- 19% of dietary calcium absorbed without active vitamin D.
- 25% of dietary calcium absorbed with active vitamin D.

3. Management of hypocalcemia (serum total corrected calcium <2.20 mmol/L):
   a. Increase calcium intake above 200% SDI for short periods under close medical supervision.
   b. Treatment with calcium salts:

Calcium Preparation	Elemental Calcium (%)
Calcium gluconate	9
Calcium lactate	13
Calcium acetate	25
Calcium carbonate	40
Calcium lactogluconate (765 mg/5 ml)	7.7 (100 mg/5 ml)

- Elemental calcium 125 mg = 3.1 mmol.
- Avoid calcium chloride in uremic patients as this may cause metabolic acidosis.

c. Oral active vitamin D sterols should be initiated as a single daily morning dose or twice-daily dose.

d. Change low calcium to normal calcium dialysate.
   - Peritoneal dialysis: 1.8 mmol/L.
   - Hemodialysis: 1.5 mmol/L.

4. Management of hypercalcemia (serum total corrected calcium >2.54 mmol/L):
   a. Stop all calcium supplements.
   b. Discontinue all calcium-based phosphate binders and use non-calcium-based phosphate binders.
   c. Discontinue native or active vitamin D sterols until serum calcium returns to the target range, and then restart at a lower dose.
   d. Consider using lower dialysate calcium for 3–4 weeks.
   e. Consider a transient reduction of dietary calcium without compromising adequate nutrition.

III. Vitamin D therapy:

1. Guiding principles:
   a. Cholecalciferol (vitamin D_3) or ergocalciferol (vitamin D_2) supplementation is necessary for patients with CKD G2 to G5D, and patients with $25(OH)D_3$ deficiency, as activation via peripheral 1α-hydroxylation is required for normal cellular function in certain cells such as immune cells.
   b. Active vitamin D therapy should be started when serum PTH is above the target range for the stage of CKD.
   c. Active vitamin D therapy and vitamin D analogs may be considered to maintain serum calcium levels in the age-appropriate normal range.
   d. Close monitoring is important when therapy with vitamin D sterols is initiated due to the risk of arterial and soft tissue calcification:
      i. Serum calcium and phosphorus levels:
         - Monthly in CKD G2 to G4 for 3 months, and then at least 3-monthly thereafter.

- 2-weekly in CKD G5 and G5D for 1 month then monthly thereafter.

ii. Serum iPTH levels:
- At least 3-monthly in CKD G2 to G4.
- Monthly in CKD G5 and 5D for 6 months, then at least 3-monthly when target levels are stably achieved.

2. Cholecalciferol (vitamin D_3) or Ergocalciferol (vitamin D_2) supplementation:
   a. Supplementation with cholecalciferol (preferred because of longer half-life) or ergocalciferol should be initiated when serum 25(OH)D_3 is <30 ng/ml OR serum iPTH is high OR serum calcium is low.
   b. Recommended supplementation for vitamin D deficiency/insufficiency in patients with CKD G2 to G5D:

Serum 25(OH)D_3 (ng/ml)	Definition	Vitamin D Dose (Intensive Replacement Phase)
<5	Severe vitamin D deficiency	• 8000 IU/day orally for 4 weeks, then 4000 IU/day for 2 months OR • 50000 IU/week for 4 weeks, then 50000 IU/2 weeks for 2 months.
5–15	Vitamin D deficiency	• 4000 IU/day orally for 12 weeks OR • 50000 IU every other week for 12 weeks
16–30	Vitamin D insufficiency	• 2000 IU/day orally for 12 weeks OR • 50000 IU every month for 12 weeks

Note: 40 IU ergocalciferol (D_2) or cholecalciferol (D_3) = 1 μg D_3

   c. Mega-dose vitamin D therapy such as the stoss regimen is not recommended in children with CKD because:
   - It can cause fractures especially in the first 3 months of therapy.
   - Associated hypercalcemia can cause an acute decline in kidney function.
   - Increase in fibroblast growth factor-23 (FGF23) levels is associated with adverse cardiac effects.

d. Monitor serum 25(OH)D_3 levels after 3 months of supplementation.
   - If levels are normal, continue maintenance dose of vitamin D supplementation and measure the levels every 6 months.
   - If low levels persist, consider one repeat course of "intensive" replacement treatment and repeat levels in 3 months.

e. Once patients are replete with vitamin D, continue supplementation with a vitamin D-containing multivitamin preparation at maintenance dose:
   - 0–12 months: 400 IU/day.
   - >1 year: 400–1000 IU/day.

f. To avoid hypercalcemia, patients with CKD G5 and G5D and high serum iPTH levels should either:
   - Continue with vitamin D supplementation together with calcimimetics or selective vitamin D receptor analogs
     OR
   - Discontinue vitamin D supplementation when starting active vitamin D_3 unless serum 25(OH)D_3 levels decrease below the normal range.

g. Vitamin D supplementation should be stopped when serum 25(OH)D_3 level is 48 ng/ml.
   - Symptomatic toxicity from vitamin D is defined as serum 25(OH)D_3 level ≥100 ng/ml.

3. Active vitamin D_3 sterol:

   a. Available as calcitriol (1,25-dihydroxycholecalciferol) or alfacalcidol (1-α-hydroxycholecalciferol).
   b. Efficacy of calcitriol appears to be better (1.5–2x) than alfacalcidol for the treatment of CKD-MBD.
   c. Active vitamin D_3 will suppress the hyperactive parathyroid gland through its action on PTH synthesis via the vitamin D receptor, as well as on PTH secretion through the calcium-sensing receptor.
   d. Intermittent administration of active vitamin D_3 by intravenous or oral routes is as effective as daily oral dosing in lowering serum iPTH levels.
   e. In patients with CKD G2 to G4, therapy with active oral vitamin D sterol should be initiated only when serum levels of PTH are persistently above the target range for the CKD stage and:
      - Serum 25(OH)D_3 >30 ng/ml.
      - Serum calcium level is <2.37 mmol/L.

- Serum phosphorus is less than the age-appropriate upper limits for the stage of CKD.

f. In patients with CKD G5 and 5D, treatment with active vitamin D_3 is recommended as follows:
- Start if the serum iPTH levels are >31.8 pmol/L.
- Reduce the serum iPTH levels to the target range of 21.2–31.8 pmol/L.
- Do not reduce the serum iPTH levels <10.6 pmol/L to avoid adynamic bone disease.

g. Initial active vitamin D_3 dosing recommendations for children with CKD:

CKD Stage	Serum iPTH (pmol/ml)	Serum Calcium (mmol/L)	Serum Phosphorus (mmol/L)	Initial Dose of Oral Active Vitamin D_3
G2 to G3	>7.4	<2.37	≤age-appropriate levels	<10 kg: 0.05 µg EOD 10–20 kg: 0.1–0.15 µg/day >20 kg: 0.25 µg/day
G4	>11.7	<2.37	≤age-appropriate levels	<10 kg: 0.05 µg EOD 10–20 kg: 0.1–0.15 µg/day >20 kg: 0.25 µg/day
G5D	31.8–53.0	<2.37	<1.93 (C)* <1.78 (A)#	0.0075 µg/kg/dose 3x/week (maximum 0.25 µg/dose 3x/week)
G5D	53.0–106.0	<2.37	<1.93 (C)* <1.78 (A)#	0.015 µg/kg/dose 3x/week (maximum 0.5 µg/dose 3x/week OR 0.25 µg daily)
G5D	>106.0	<2.50	<1.93 (C)* <1.78 (A)#	0.025 µg/kg/dose 3x/week (maximum 1 µg/dose 3x/week OR 0.25 µg daily)

*(C) denotes infants and children of 1–12 years of age.
#(A) denotes adolescents of >12 years of age.

h. Active vitamin D_3 should be given at night to minimize the absorption of calcium from food.

i. Dosage of active vitamin D_3 sterols should be adjusted upward by 50% if the serum iPTH levels fail to decrease by at least 30%

after the initial 3 months of therapy, and the serum calcium and phosphorus levels are within the target ranges based on CKD stage.

j. Maximum daily dose of active vitamin D_3 should not exceed 1.5 μg.
k. Treatment should be based on the trend of serial iPTH results rather than a single result.
l. If serum levels of iPTH decrease to values below the target range for the CKD stage:
   - Active vitamin D_3 should be held off until serum levels of iPTH increase to above the target range.
   - Treatment should then be resumed at half the previous dose of active vitamin D_3, or alternate day dosing can be used.
m. Intravenous calcitriol can be considered in children on HD who are poorly adherent to oral active vitamin D3:
   - Calcijex® (Abbott) 1 μg/ml.
   - Dose: 0.01–0.05 μg/kg 3x/week.
n. Pulse calcitriol therapy:
   i. Can be initiated if the serum iPTH levels remain at ≥106 pmol/L after 6 months of active vitamin D_3 therapy, and the serum corrected total calcium <2.50 mmol/L, and serum phosphorus <1.98 mmol/L (age 1 to 12 years) or <1.78 mmol/L (age >12 years).
   ii. Duration of treatment should be at least 6 months.
   iii. Effective in improving osteitis fibrosa but may have an adverse effect of linear growth due to adynamic bone disease.
   iv. Oral pulse calcitriol:
      - ≥30 kg: 4 μg 3x/week.
      - <30 kg: 3 μg 3x/week.

IV. Calcimimetic agents:

1. Guiding principles
   a. Class of compounds that bind to the parathyroid calcium-sensing receptor, increasing its sensitivity to ionized calcium and dose dependently decreasing plasma PTH levels by up to 80%.
   b. Used as a form of "medical parathyroidectomy".

2. Cinacalcet:
   a. Type II calcimimetic agent (positive allosteric modulator) with a serum half-life of 30–40 hours.
   b. Indications:
      - Children >3 years of age with CKD G5D and persistent, severe hyperparathyroidism in the presence of high or high-normal calcium levels, despite optimized conventional management.
   c. Contraindications for starting cinacalcet:
      - Albumin-corrected serum calcium levels <2.37 mmol/L (ionized calcium <1.11 mmol/L).
      - Prolonged QT interval.
   d. Caution should be exercised in children with the following:
      - History of seizures.
      - Arrhythmias.
      - Significant liver disease.
      - Poor medication adherence.
      - Drugs that may prolong QT interval or affect cinacalcet metabolism:

Mechanism	Drugs Contraindicated
Potential to increase QTc	Ondansetron Salbutamol
Inhibitors of CYP3A4	Grapefruit juice Erythromycin Clarithromycin Ketoconazole Itraconazole
Inhibitors of CYP2D6	Flecanide Propafenone Metoprolol Desipramine Nortriptyline Clomipramine

   e. Side effects:
      - Nausea and vomiting.
      - Headache.
      - Hypocalcemia.
      - Reduces testosterone levels by 30%.

f. Recommended dosage:
   i. Start with ≤0.2 mg/kg/day based on the dry weight.
   ii. Take with meals or immediately following; do not crush, chew or cut tablets.
   iii. Dosage adjustments should not be made more frequently than 4 weeks.
   iv. Titrate dose accordingly:

Criteria	Dose Titration
iPTH >31.8 pmol/L Total corrected calcium >2.2 mmol/L	• Titrate dose upward slowly (not more frequent than 4-week intervals) by 0.2 mg/kg/day increments to a target iPTH of 21.2–31.8 pmol/L. • Maximum dose: 2.5 mg/kg/day (not exceeding 180 mg/day).
iPTH >21.2 and <31.8 pmol/L Total corrected calcium >2.2 mmol/L	• Continue with current dose.
iPTH between 10.6–15.9 pmol/L OR Declining too rapidly	• Decrease dose.
iPTH <10.6 pmol/L on 2 consecutive measurements	• Discontinue cinacalcet.
Corrected total serum calcium <2.2 mmol/L or ionized calcium <1.1 mmol/L	• Withhold cinacalcet and restart when calcium levels increase to the higher end of normal range.
Symptomatic hypocalcaemia: Paresthesia, myalgia, cramps, tetany, convulsions, long QT interval, or severe side effects.	• Withdraw cinacalcet.

   v. Monitor serum calcium within 1 week of starting cinacalcet, then weekly during titration phase, and then monthly during maintenance phase, as hypocalcemia occurs commonly.
   vi. iPTH levels should be checked monthly.
   vii. Restart active vitamin D3 at 0.25 μg 3x/week once serum calcium levels have decreased to the target range.

F. Parathyroidectomy

1. Guiding principles:
   - Effective surgical therapy of severe hyperparathyroidism can be accomplished by subtotal parathyroidectomy or total parathyroidectomy with parathyroid tissue autotransplantation.
2. Indications:
   a. Severe hyperparathyroidism with persistent serum levels of iPTH >110 pmol/L and disabling bone deformities associated with hypercalcemia, and/or hyperphosphatemia that is refractory to medical therapy.
   b. Calciphylaxis (calcific uremic arteriopathy) with serum iPTH levels >55.0 pmol/L.
      - Syndrome characterized by the development of progressive ischemic skin ulcerations involving the fingers, toes, thighs, legs, and ankles.
      - Almost always accompanied by vascular calcification involving the media of the arteries.
      - Usually exhibit X-Ray evidence of subperiosteal bone resorption.
      - Serum calcium is usually normal and occasionally elevated, and a period of hyperphosphatemia will have been present for some time before the appearance of this syndrome.
      - Lesions may be preceded or accompanied by severe pain.
      - Before the appearance of ulcerations or tissue necrosis, tender, slightly erythematous, subcutaneous nodules may develop, or there may be blotchy, bluish discoloration of the skin.
      - Raynaud's phenomenon may also precede lesions of the fingers or toes.
      - The ulcers may develop slowly over several months, or may appear and progress rapidly over a few weeks.
      - Infection may supervene, leading to sepsis and death.
3. Imaging
   a. Parathyroid imaging is not usually required pre-operatively.
   b. Parathyroid imaging with ^{99m}Tc-sestamibi scan, ultrasound, CT scan or MRI should be done prior to re-exploration parathyroid surgery.

4. Pre- and post-operative management:
   a. Active vitamin D_3 should be given 72 hours prior to parathyroidectomy to reduce post-operative hypocalcemia.
   b. Blood level of ionized calcium should be measured every 4 to 6 hours for the first 24 hours after surgery, then 8 to 12 hourly until stable.
   c. Consider placing a central line for intravenous calcium infusion post-operatively.
   d. If the level of ionized calcium <1 mmol/L, corresponding to corrected total calcium of 1.8 mmol/L, intravenous calcium gluconate infusion should be initiated at a rate of 0.025 to 0.05 mmol/kg/hour or 1 to 2 mg/kg/hour of elemental calcium, and adjusted to maintain ionized calcium in the normal range (1.15 to 1.36 mmol/L).
      Note: 10 ml of 10% calcium gluconate contains 90 mg (2.32 mmol) of elemental calcium.
   e. When oral intake is possible, the patient should receive:
      - Elemental calcium 1 to 2 g three times a day.
      - Active vitamin D_3 1 to 2 μg/day.
   f. If patients are hypocalcemic, normal calcium dialysate is recommended.
      i. Calcium content of peritoneal dialysate:
         - Dianeal Normal Calcium: 1.8 mmol/L.
         - Dianeal Low Calcium: 1.3 mmol/L.
      ii. Calculation to prepare a 5 L Normal Calcium Dianeal from a Low Calcium Dianeal:
         Amount of calcium to be added to 1 L: (1.8–1.3) mmol = 0.5 mmol/L.
         For every 5-L-bag amount of calcium to be added: (0.5 × 5) mmol = 2.5 mmol.
         10 ml of 10% calcium chloride ($CaCl_2$) contains 7 mmol calcium (Ca^{2+}) and 14 mmol chloride (Cl^-).
         Total amount of 10% calcium chloride to be added: (2.5 × 10) ÷ 7 ml = 3.6 ml.

G. Bone Disease in Kidney Transplantation

1. Guiding principles:
   a. Successful kidney transplantation corrects many of the underlying abnormalities contributing to bone disease in children with CKD.
   b. Hyperphosphatemia, pre-existing hyperparathyroidism, and glucocorticoid therapy may impair healing of renal bone disease and lead to bone loss.
2. Monitoring:
   a. Frequency of measurement of calcium, phosphate, magnesium, bicarbonate, iPTH, and $25(OH)D_3$ after kidney transplantation:

<table>
<tr><th rowspan="2">Screening Test or Evaluation</th><th colspan="5">Screening Intervals By Time After Transplantation</th></tr>
<tr><th>Month 1</th><th>Month 2–3</th><th>Month 4–6</th><th>Month 7–12</th><th>>Month 12</th></tr>
<tr><td>Calcium and phosphate</td><td>Weekly</td><td colspan="3">Monthly</td><td>Monthly to 2-monthly</td></tr>
<tr><td>Magnesium</td><td>Weekly</td><td colspan="3">Monthly</td><td>Monthly to 2-monthly</td></tr>
<tr><td>Bicarbonate</td><td>Weekly</td><td colspan="3">Monthly</td><td>Monthly to 2-monthly</td></tr>
<tr><td>iPTH</td><td>Once</td><td colspan="4">3 monthly if abnormal after transplant or eGFR <60 ml/min/1.73m²</td></tr>
<tr><td>$25(OH)D_3$</td><td></td><td colspan="4">3 monthly</td></tr>
<tr><td>Urine calcium: creatinine ratio</td><td>Once</td><td colspan="4">6 monthly if on vitamin D therapy</td></tr>
</table>

   b. 6 months after transplantation, the frequency of measurements should follow the recommendations mentioned earlier for CKD G2 to G5, depending on the stage of CKD.
3. Treatment:
   a. Kidney transplant recipients who develop persistent hypophosphatemia (below the age-appropriate lower limits) should be treated with phosphate supplementation.

b. The care of CKD-MBD in kidney transplant patients reaching CKD G2 to G4 should follow the guidelines established for native CKD.

H. Algorithms for the Management of CKD-MBD

1. Management of hyperphosphatemia:

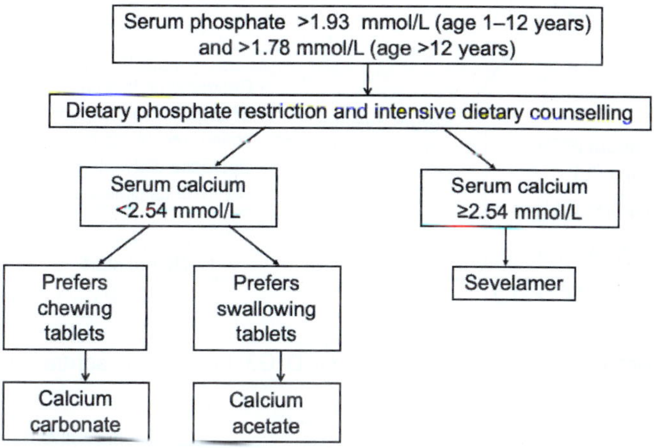

2. Vitamin D_3 or D_2 supplementation based on serum 25(OH)D_3 levels:

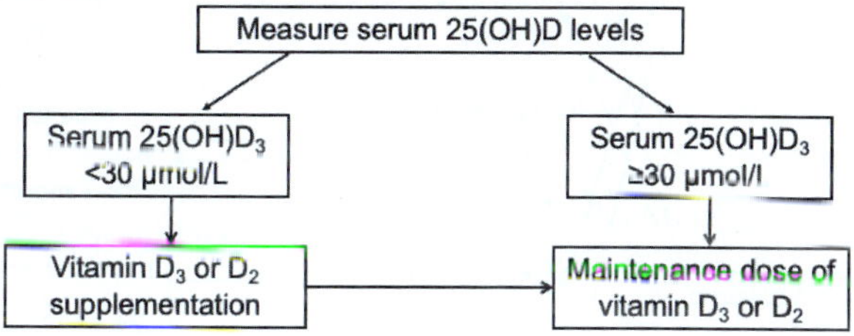

3. Initiate active vitamin D_3 therapy based on serum calcium and iPTH levels:

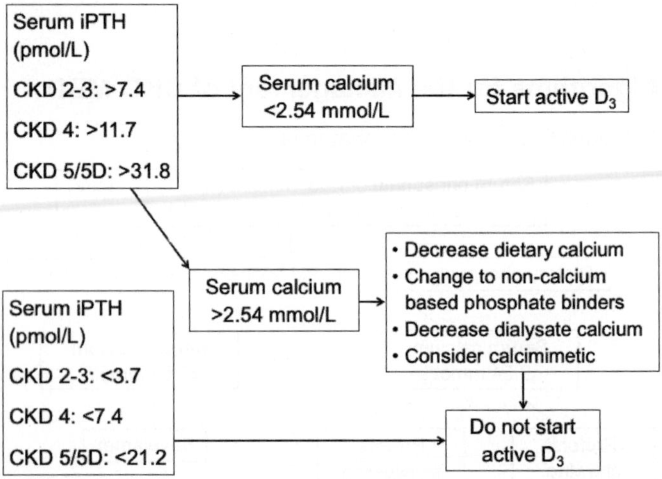

4. Active vitamin D_3 therapy in CKD G3 to G5 with serum calcium ≤2.54 mmol/L:

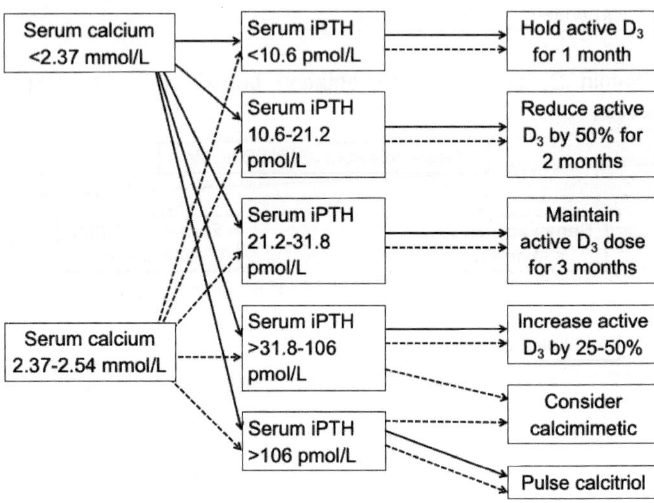

5. Active vitamin D_3 therapy in CKD G3 to G5 with serum calcium >2.54 mmol/L:

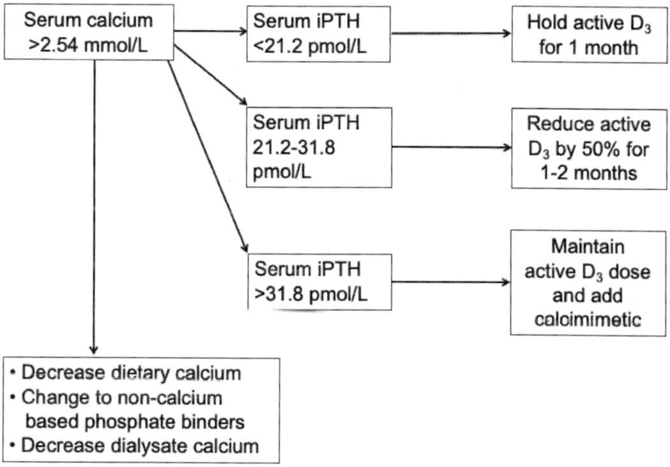

Recommended Reading

1. K/DOQI. (2005) K/DOQI clinical practice guidelines for bone metabolism and disease in children with chronic kidney disease. *Am J Kidney Dis* **46**:S1–S102.
2. Katherine W, Sevcan B, Salusky I. (2008) Chronic kidney disease mineral and bone disorder in children. *Pediatr Nephrol* **23**:195–207.
3. Kidney Disease: Improving Global Outcomes (KDIGO) CKD–MBD Work Group. (2009) KDIGO clinical practice guideline for the diagnosis, evaluation, prevention, and treatment of chronic kidney disease–mineral and bone disorder (CKD–MBD). *Kidney Int* **76**(Suppl 113):S1–S130.
4. Kidney Disease: Improving Global Outcomes (KDIGO) CKD-MBD Update Work Group. (2017) KDIGO 2017 clinical practice guideline update for the diagnosis, evaluation, prevention, and treatment of chronic kidney disease–mineral and bone disorder (CKD-MBD). *Kidney Int* **7**:1–59.
5. Shroff R, Wan M, Nagler EV, Bakkaloglu S, Cozzolino M, Bacchetta J, Edefonti A, Stefanidis CJ, Vande Walle J, Ariceta G, Klaus G, Haffner D, Schmitt CP; European Society for Paediatric Nephrology Chronic Kidney Disease Mineral and Bone Disorders and Dialysis Working Groups. (2017) Clinical practice recommendations for treatment with active vitamin D analogues in children with chronic kidney disease stages 2–5 and on dialysis. *Nephrol Dial Transplant* **32**:1114–1127.

6. Srivastava T, Warady BA. (2018, updated) Pediatric chronic kidney disease-mineral and bone disorder (CKD-MBD). Edited by: Mattoo TK, Kim MS. UpToDate ONLINE. http://www.uptodateonline.com.
7. Bacchetta J, Schmitt CP, Ariceta G, Bakkaloglu SA, Groothoff J, Wan M, Vervloet M, Shroff R, Haffner D; European Society for Paediatric Nephrology and the Chronic Kidney Disease-Mineral and Bone Disorders and Dialysis Working Group of the ERA-EDTA. (2020) Cinacalcet use in paediatric dialysis: A position statement from the European society for paediatric nephrology and the chronic kidney disease-mineral and bone disorders working group of the ERA-EDTA. *Nephrol Dial Transplant* **35**:47–64.
8. McAlister L, Pugh P, Greenbaum L, Haffner D, Rees L, Anderson C, Desloovere A, Nelms C, Oosterveld M, Paglialonga F, Polderman N, Qizalbash L, Renken-Terhaerdt J, Tuokkola J, Warady B, Walle JV, Shaw V, Shroff R. (2020) The dietary management of calcium and phosphate in children with CKD stages 2–5 and on dialysis-clinical practice recommendation from the Pediatric Renal Nutrition Taskforce. *Pediatr Nephrol* **35**:501–518.
9. Bakkaloglu SA, Bacchetta J, Lalayiannis AD, Leifheit-Nestler M, Stabouli S, Haarhaus M, Reusz G, Groothoff J, Schmitt CP, Evenepoel P, Shroff R, Haffner D; European Society for Paediatric Nephrology (ESPN) Chronic Kidney Disease Mineral and Bone Disorder (CKD-MBD) and Dialysis working groups and CKD-MBD working group of the European Renal Association–European Dialysis and Transplant Association (ERA-EDTA). (2021) Bone evaluation in paediatric chronic kidney disease: Clinical practice points from the European Society for Paediatric Nephrology CKD-MBD and Dialysis working groups and CKD-MBD working group of the ERA-EDTA. *Nephrol Dial Transplant* **36**:413–425.

5 Calciphylaxis

Teo S, Yap HK and Ng KH

A. Definition of Calciphylaxis

1. Calciphylaxis or calcific uremic arteriolopathy (CUA) is a potentially life-threatening vasculopathy of the skin and subcutaneous tissues.
2. Calciphylaxis is characterized by systemic medial calcification of the arterioles that leads to ischemia and subcutaneous necrosis.
3. Histologic inspection may reveal small vessel mural calcification with or without endovascular fibrosis, extravascular calcification (amorphous luminal calcium), and thrombotic vaso-occlusion (leading to ischemic skin necrosis).

B. Epidemiology

1. The incidence of CUA is ~4% in patients on dialysis and <1% in patients with chronic kidney disease (CKD).
2. CUA has a high mortality rate, with a 1-year survival rate of 45% and a 5-year survival rate of 35%.

C. Risk Factors for CUA

1. Caucasian race.
2. Female gender.
3. Comorbid conditions:
   - CKD.
   - Obesity.

- Diabetes mellitus.
- Liver disease.
- Malignancy.
- Hypercoagulable states, such as protein C and S deficiency and antiphospholipid syndrome.

4. Biochemical abnormalities:
   - Hypercalcemia.
   - Hyperphosphatemia.
   - Elevated calcium-phosphate product.
5. Medications:
   - Vitamin D analogs.
   - Calcium containing phosphate binders.
   - Corticosteroids.
   - Vitamin K antagonists.
   - Iron.
6. Specific risk factors for dialysis patients:
   - Long periods on dialysis.

D. Pathophysiology

1. Disturbances of calcium-phosphate homeostasis are thought to be the main pathogenic event.
2. Imbalance between factors favoring and resisting precipitation of calcium phosphate in tissues and leading to pathologic calcification.
3. Low levels of calcification inhibitors such as fetuin A and carboxylated matrix Gla protein (MGP) have been reported.
4. MGP requires vitamin K to carry out its biological functions, hence treatment with a vitamin K antagonist, warfarin, is a risk factor for CUA.
5. Vascular thrombosis, which is an important feature of CUA, is likely secondary to arterial narrowing and endothelial injury.

E. Clinical Features

1. CUA has an insidious onset.
2. Livedo-reticularis-like skin lesions in areas with increased subcutaneous fat tissue (abdomen, buttocks and thighs).

3. Lesions transform into painful, subcutaneous, purpuric plaques and nodules and subsequently necrotic ulcers covered by eschars (dry scabs or sloughs formed on the skin) over a period of days to weeks.
4. The areas of ischemic, necrotic skin, and subcutaneous fat can extend into deeper tissues, including muscle and can become infected.
5. CUA can less commonly affect distal extremities such as the hands or lower legs.
6. Systemic involvement with ischemic infarction of the bowel, myocardium, brain, optic nerve, or muscles (painful proximal myopathy) has also been reported rarely.
7. Presence of peripheral pulses distinguishes CUA from atherosclerosis.
8. Death is predominantly the result of infectious complications.

F. Diagnosis

1. Diagnosis is usually clinical.
2. Laboratory studies:
   a. Elevation of serum calcium and phosphate are not specific as both values may be normal or low; however, a review of laboratory values may reveal a trend for increasing the calcium-phosphate (Ca x P) product and parathyroid hormone (PTH) levels.
   b. Serum lipase and amylase to detect pancreatic involvement.
   c. Do an erythrocyte sedimentation rate, and C-reactive protein, anti-nuclear antibodies, rheumatoid factor, anti-neutrophil cytoplasmic antibodies, anti-hepatitis C antibody, and cryoglobulin to exclude vasculitis.
   d. Exclude hypercoagulable states: Prothrombin time, activated partial thromboplastin time, anti-thrombin III, protein C, protein S, anti-phospholipid antibodies, homocysteine, and factor V Leiden level.
3. Imaging studies:
   a. Plain X-Ray of the affected extremity to look for arborization or a net-like pattern of vascular calcification within the dermis and subcutaneous tissues or the affected part to look for calcification.

b. Three-phase technetium 99m methylene diphosphate scan can also be used to assess soft tissue calcification.
c. High resolution CT or mammogram to distinguish calcium from surrounding non-calcium containing radiolucent tissues.

4. Skin biopsy:
   a. Incisional skin biopsy is diagnostic.
   b. Not generally recommended as this can lead to non-healing ulcerations, which increases the mortality rate by two-fold.
5. Differential diagnosis:
   a. Benign nodular calcification (common in CKD patients).
   b. Systemic vasculitis.
   c. Erythema nodosum.
   d. Cryoglobulinemia.
   e. Pyoderma gangrenosum.
   f. Nephrogenic systemic fibrosis.
   g. Oxalosis.
   h. Warfarin induced skin necrosis.
   i. Atherosclerotic peripheral vascular disease.
   j. Cholesterol embolization.

G. Treatment

I. Reduce serum levels of procalcifying factors:

1. Increase frequency of hemodialysis (HD).
2. Switch from peritoneal dialysis (PD) to HD to increase phosphate clearance.
3. Use low calcium dialysate.
4. Avoid vitamin D and calcium supplements.
5. Administer calcium-free phosphate binders.
6. Manage hyperparathyroidism with cinacalcet or parathyroidectomy.

II. Increase serum levels of calcification inhibitors:

1. Halt administration of vitamin K antagonists (warfarin).
2. Treat infections or other proinflammatory stimuli aggressively to increase fetuin-A levels.

III. Sodium thiosulfate for prevention or reversal of calcium-phosphate deposition:

1. Mechanism of action:
   a. Sodium thiosulfate ($Na_2S_2O_3$) is a reducing agent that forms water-soluble complexes with many metals.
   b. Sodium thiosulfate has a dual therapeutic action in CUA:
      - Formation of highly soluble calcium thiosulfate complexes.
      - Antioxidant activity.
2. Pharmacokinetics:
   a. Intestinal absorption of sodium thiosulfate is poor.
   b. Approximately 20–50% of the thiosulfate dose is rapidly excreted unchanged in the urine; the rest is eliminated by metabolic oxidation to sulfite and subsequently, sulfate.
   c. Serum half-life of 15 minutes in individuals with normal kidney function.
   d. When administered as a slow infusion during HD, about 50% of the dose is estimated to be eliminated by dialysis.
3. Dose:
   a. 12 g/1.73m^2.
   b. Maximum dose of 25 g (100 ml of 25% solution).
4. Mode of infusion:
   a. In HD patients, give sodium thiosulfate intravenously over 30–60 minutes during the last hour of HD 3×/week (maximum infusion rate 5 ml/min).
   b. In PD patients, give sodium thiosulfate 3×/week over 60 minutes.
      - If patients have significant residual kidney function, the frequency can be increased to 4×/week as tolerated.
      - Can also be given intraperitoneally: 12.5 g in 2 L of long dwell dialysate 3×/week, but there is a risk of chemical peritonitis.
   c. In patients not on dialysis:
      - Estimated glomerular filtration rate (eGFR) <60 ml/min/1.73m^2: Administer sodium thiosulfate 2×/week initially, then gradually increase to 4×/week if there is no metabolic acidosis.
      - eGFR >60 ml/min/1.73m^2: Administer sodium thiosulfate 2×/week initially, then gradually increase to 5x/week if there is no metabolic acidosis.
   d. Duration of infusion can be increased by an additional 30–60 minutes if patients experience gastrointestinal side effects.

5. Duration of treatment:
   a. Can range from weeks to months.
   b. Pain relief occurs within a few days to up to 2 weeks, possibly as a result of the effect of thiosulfate on the vasa nervorum of peripheral nerves.
   c. Complete healing of the ulcers takes several months.
6. Monitoring:
   a. Monitor heart rate, respiratory rate, and blood pressure:
      - Every 15 minutes during the infusion and the first hour after completion of the infusion.
      - Every 30 minutes for the next hour.
      - Then hourly for 4 hours.
   b. Continuous oxygen saturation monitoring for the above period.
   c. For those with cardiac involvement, continuous cardiac monitoring should be done during infusion.
7. Adverse effects:
   a. Frequently reported:
      - Nausea and vomiting.
      - Headache.
      - Decreased serum bicarbonate level.
      - Increased serum anion gap.
      - Increased serum sodium levels.
   b. Rarely reported:
      - Rhinorrhea.
      - Sinus congestion.
      - Neurological effects (bad taste, periorbital tingling, decreased hearing).
      - Hypocalcemia with increased corrected QT interval.
      - Hunger.
      - Weakness.

IV. Adjunctive care

1. Wound care:
   a. Avoid local tissue trauma by implementing atraumatic wound care with a gentle debridement of necrotic tissue and avoiding subcutaneous injections.
   b. Improve the oxygen supply by use of hyperbaric oxygen therapy.

2. Implement pain management measures.
3. Consider intravenous heparin infusion in patients with documented conditions of hypercoagulability.

Recommended Reading

1. Araya CE, Fennel RS, Neiberger RE, Dharnidharka VR. (2006) Sodium thiosulfate treatment for calcific uremic arteriolopathy in children and young adults. *Clin J Am Soc Nephrol* **1**:1161–1166.
2. Schlieper G, Brandenburg V, Ketteler M, Floege J. (2009) Sodium thiosulfate therapy for calcific uremic arteriolopathy. *Nat Rev* **5**:539–543.
3. Nigwekar SU, Thadhani R, Brandenburg VM. (2018) Calciphylaxis. *N Eng J Med.* **378**(18):1704–1714.
4. Nigwekar SU, Thadhani RI. (2021, updated) Calciphylaxis (calcific uremic arteriolopathy). Edited by: Goldfarb S, Motwani S. *UpToDate ONLINE*. http://www.uptodate online.com.

6 Immunization Guidelines for Children and Adolescents with Chronic Kidney Disease

Koh CT, Dela Cruz RC, Teo S, Ng KH, Lau PYW and Yap HK

A. Principles

1. Immunization should be updated as early as possible in the course of kidney disease and should be as complete as possible prior to transplant because vaccines, noted to be safe for administration after transplantation, may not be sufficiently immunogenic after transplantation.
2. A vaccine series does not need to be restarted, regardless of the time that has elapsed between doses.
3. Always use this guideline in conjunction with the national infant and adolescent immunization schedules.
4. All live vaccines must be given either on the same day or separated by at least 1 month.
5. Immunize at least 4–8 weeks before potent immunosuppression.
6. Wait 3 months after treatment with intravenous immunoglobulin (IVIG) and cytomegalovirus (CMV) hyperimmune immunoglobulin before giving vaccines.
7. Response to live vaccines is most effective when given after 1 year of age once passive maternal antibodies have waned.
   - Some live vaccines can be safely administered as early as 6–9 months if needed.
8. Transplantation should not be done within 1 month of receiving a live vaccine.
9. Live vaccine is contraindicated post-transplant.
10. Timing of resumption of non-live vaccination series post-transplant is usually 6 months post-transplant and following acute rejection, with the exception of inactivated influenza vaccine, which can be given as early as 1-month post-transplant.

11. Immunocompromised patients should not handle diapers of infants who were given rotavirus vaccines for at least 1 month.
12. Family members should be immunized against influenza.

B. Singapore Immunization Schedule for Infants and Adolescents

1. Available vaccines in Singapore:

	Vaccines		Brand Name
Live Attenuated Vaccines	BCG		
	Measles, Mumps, Rubella		MMR-II
	Varicella		Varivax
	MMRV		Proquad
Inactivated Vaccines	Hepatitis B		Engerix
	Diphtheria, Tetanus, Pertussis	DTaP	—
		TdaP	Boostrix
	Diphtheria, Tetanus	Td	Tetadif
	Inactivated polio	IPV	Imovax
	Haemophilus influenzae type B	Hib	Hiberix
	Pneumococcal	PCV13	Prevnar 13
		PPSVS23	Pneumovax 23
	Meningococcal (ACWY)	MCV4-D (conjugated)	Menactra
		MCV4-TT (conjugated)	Nimenrix
	Hepatitis A		Vaqta
	Influenza		VaxigripTetra
	Human papilloma virus	HPV9	Gardasil-9
		HPV4	Gardasil
		HPV2	Cervarix
Combination Vaccines	DTaP + IPV + Hib	5-in-1	Pentaxim
	DTaP + IPV + Hib + Hep B	6-in-1	Hexaxim
	MMR + Varicella	MMRV	Proquad

2. Singapore Immunization Schedule for infants and adolescents (November 2020):

		Months							Years		
Vaccine	Birth	2	3	4	6	12	15	18	6–7	10–11	≥12
Routine											
BCG	D1										
Hepatitis B	D1	D2			D3						
DTaP/TdaP		DTaP D1		DTaP D2	DTaP D3			DTaP B1		TdaP B2	
IPV		IPV D1		IPV D2	IPV D3			IPV B1		IPV B2	
Hib		D1		D2	D3			B1			
MMR						D1	D2				
Pneumococcal (Prevenar 13)				D1	D2	B1					
Recommended											
Rotavirus		D1 6 weeks	D2								
Varicella						2 doses given 6–10 weeks apart					
Hepatitis A						2 doses 6 months apart					
Influenza					From 6 months: 2 doses 1 month apart for 1st-time vaccination (<9 years), then 1 dose every 6 months to a year						
HPV (HPV4)*									9–14 years: 2 doses at least 5 months apart; ≥15 years: 3 doses at 0, 2 and 6 months.		

*Patients with CKD (9–26 years): 3 doses at 0, 2 and 6 months.

C. Deferment of Immunization Following Augmentation of Immunosuppression

<table>
<tr><th colspan="2">Immunosuppression</th><th colspan="2">No vaccination within:</th></tr>
<tr><td colspan="2">Steroid pulse
Thymoglobulin
Rituximab</td><td colspan="2">3 months
1 year
1 year (at least 6 months if expedited vaccination needed)</td></tr>
<tr><td colspan="2"></td><td>Live vaccines</td><td>Non-live vaccines</td></tr>
<tr><td colspan="2">Mycophenolate/Tacrolimus/ Cyclosporin/Cyclophosphamide/ Azathioprine</td><td>3 months after cessation</td><td></td></tr>
<tr><td colspan="2">High dose corticosteroid given as a daily dose or on alternate days for $>$14 days:
• $>$2 mg/kg if body weight $<$10 kg
• ≥20 mg if body weight ≥10 kg</td><td>1 month after cessation</td><td></td></tr>
<tr><td rowspan="2">Blood products</td><td>Packed cells</td><td>5 months</td><td rowspan="2"></td></tr>
<tr><td>Platelets
Plasma</td><td>7 months</td></tr>
<tr><td rowspan="2">IVIG</td><td>High dose (≥1600 mg/kg)</td><td>11 months</td><td rowspan="2">Can be given, but response is unknown</td></tr>
<tr><td>Low dose (400 mg/kg)</td><td>8 months</td></tr>
</table>

D. Catch-up Immunization Schedules

The following tables provide catch-up schedules and minimum intervals between doses for children whose vaccinations have been delayed.

1. Children aged 4 months through 6 years:

<table>
<tr><th rowspan="2"></th><th rowspan="2">Minimum Age For Dose 1</th><th colspan="4">Minimum Interval Between Doses</th></tr>
<tr><th>Dose 1 to 2</th><th>Dose 2 to 3</th><th>Dose 3 to 4</th><th>Dose 4 to 5</th></tr>
<tr><td>BCG</td><td>Birth</td><td></td><td></td><td></td><td></td></tr>
<tr><td></td><td colspan="5">• Tuberculin skin testing/T-Spot (age ≥2 years)/Interferon-γ Release Assay (IGRA) (age ≥5 years) prior to BCG vaccination in the following circumstances:
a. Children aged 3 months to <6 years in at-risk environment, including those:
▪ Who are contacts of a pulmonary tuberculosis case.
▪ From an area of high endemicity.
▪ Whose parents are from an area of high endemicity.
▪ Who have household contacts belonging to an at-risk group for tuberculosis.
b. Infants and children <6 years of age with a history of residence or prolonged stay (>3 months) in a country of high endemicity, that is, countries with a tuberculosis incidence rate of ≥20 per 100000 population.
c. Close contact with a person with known tuberculosis.
d. History of tuberculosis in a household contact in the last 5 years.
• If positive testing without active disease, give isoniazid for 1 year (no need to delay transplant); treatment should continue post-transplant with increased surveillance for active disease.
• Should be avoided in patients receiving:
a. Immunosuppressive drugs.
b. Corticosteroids with dose:
>2 mg/kg body weight (<10 kg)
≥20 mg total daily dose or on alternate days for >14 days.
• Once corticosteroids are discontinued, vaccination should be delayed for at least 1 month.
• Contraindicated in the post-kidney transplant patient.</td></tr>
</table>

(*Continued*)

	Minimum Age For Dose 1	Minimum Interval Between Doses			
		Dose 1 to 2	Dose 2 to 3	Dose 3 to 4	Dose 4 to 5
Hepatitis B	Birth	4 weeks	8 weeks and at least 16 weeks after the 1st dose.		
	• Post-vaccination testing (anti-HBs antibody) is recommended 1–2 months after the primary series is completed, with up to 3 additional doses if protective antibody levels (>10 mIU/ml) are not achieved. • Give special double dose formulation for dialysis patients according to age. • Annual testing of anti-HBs antibody is required in immunocompromised patients and transplant recipients. • Booster dose in transplant recipient if anti-HBs antibody titer <10 mIU/ml.				

	Minimum Age For Dose 1	Minimum Interval Between Doses			
		Dose 1 to 2	Dose 2 to 3	Dose 3 to 4	Dose 4 to 5
Diphtheria Tetanus Pertussis (DTaP)	6 weeks	4 weeks	4 weeks	6 months (minimum age of 4 years for the final dose).	6 months
	• A 4th dose is not necessary if the 3rd dose was administered at age of 4 years or older and at least 6 months after the previous dose. • The 5th dose is not necessary if the 4th dose was administered at age 4 years or older.				

	Minimum Age For Dose 1	Minimum Interval Between Doses			
		Dose 1 to 2	Dose 2 to 3	Dose 3 to 4	Dose 4 to 5
Inactivated poliovirus (IPV)	6 weeks	4 weeks	4 weeks	6 months (minimum age of 4 years for final dose).	
	• 4th dose is not necessary if the 3rd dose was administered at age ≥4 years and at least 6 months after the previous dose. • Booster should be given every 10 years for transplant recipients with ongoing travel to polio endemic areas.				

	Minimum Age For Dose 1	Minimum Interval Between Doses			
		Dose 1 to 2	Dose 2 to 3	Dose 3 to 4	Dose 4 to 5
Haemophilus influenzae type b	6 weeks	If 1st dose is given at age <1 year: 4 weeks. If 1st dose is given at age 12–14 months: 8 weeks (final dose). If 1st dose is given at age ≥15 months: No further doses needed.	If current age is <1 year and 1st dose is given at age <7 months: 4 weeks. If current age is <1 year with 1st dose is given at age 7–11 months and 2nd dose is given at least 4 weeks later: At least 8 weeks at age 12–15 months (as final dose).	This dose is only necessary for children age 1 to <5 years who received 3 doses before age 1 year: 8 weeks (final dose).	

(*Continued*)

	Minimum Age For Dose 1	Minimum Interval Between Doses			
		Dose 1 to 2	Dose 2 to 3	Dose 3 to 4	Dose 4 to 5
			If current age is ≥1 year with 1st dose given at age <1 year and 2nd dose given at age <15 months: 8 weeks (as final dose). If previous dose is given at age ≥15 months: No further doses needed.		
	• Booster every 5 years if patient is on the deceased donor waiting list.				

	Minimum Age For Dose 1	Minimum Interval Between Doses			
		Dose 1 to 2	Dose 2 to 3	Dose 3 to 4	Dose 4 to 5
MMR	12 months	4 weeks			
	• Should be avoided in patients receiving: a. Immunosuppressive drugs. b. Corticosteroids with dose: >2 mg/kg body weight (<10 kg). ≥20 mg total daily dose or on alternate days for >14 days. • Once corticosteroids are discontinued, vaccination should be delayed for at least 1 month. • Contraindicated in the post-kidney transplant patient. • Could be administered as early as 6 months of age for infants preparing for transplant. If transplantation still has not occurred by the time the infant is 1 year of age, the dose should be repeated.				

	Minimum Age For Dose 1	Minimum Interval Between Doses			
		Dose 1 to 2	Dose 2 to 3	Dose 3 to 4	Dose 4 to 5
Pneumococcal	6 weeks (PCV13)	If 1st dose is given at age of <1 year: 4 weeks. If 1st dose is given at age ≥1 year or current age is 2 to <6 years: 8 weeks.	If current age is <1 year: 4 weeks. If the current age is ≥1 year: 8 weeks.	8 weeks (final dose).	PPSV23 to be given at least 8 weeks after PCV13.
	• Children age 2 to <6 years who received at least 3 doses of either PCV7 or PCV13 before age 2 years: Single dose of PCV13 is recommended at least 8 weeks after the most recent dose, then PPSV23 at least 8 weeks after PCV13 dose.				

(*Continued*)

	Minimum Age For Dose 1	Minimum Interval Between Doses			
		Dose 1 to 2	Dose 2 to 3	Dose 3 to 4	Dose 4 to 5
	• Children age 2 to <6 years previously unvaccinated or with <3 doses of either PCV7 or PCV13: 2 dose series of PCV13, then PPSV23 at least 8 weeks after the final dose of PCV13. • Booster dose of PPSV23: 5 years from the last dose. • Booster dose of PPSV23 after transplantation, if not completed before.				

	Minimum Age For Dose 1	Minimum Interval Between Doses			
		Dose 1 to 2	Dose 2 to 3	Dose 3 to 4	Dose 4 to 5
Varicella	12 months	3 months			
	• Should be avoided in patients receiving immunosuppressive drugs, including corticosteroids. • Once corticosteroids are discontinued, vaccination should be delayed for at least 1 month. • Contraindicated in the post-kidney transplant patient. • Could be administered as early as age 9 months for infants preparing for transplant. The 2nd dose can be administered as early as 3 months later.				

	Minimum Age For Dose 1	Minimum Interval Between Doses			
		Dose 1 to 2	Dose 2 to 3	Dose 3 to 4	Dose 4 to 5
Influenza	6 months	1 month			
	• Should be given yearly. • Patients on dialysis and those post-kidney transplant should only receive the inactivated vaccine, not the intranasal influenza vaccine. • Inactivated influenza vaccination can be given as early as 1 month post-transplantation.				

	Minimum Age for Dose 1	Minimum Interval Between Doses			
		Dose 1 to 2	Dose 2 to 3	Dose 3 to 4	Dose 4 to 5
Meningococcal	6 weeks if MCV4-TT (Nimenrix) 2 months if MCV4-CRM (Menveo) 9 months if MCV4-D (Menactra).	8 weeks			
	• Tetravalent conjugated vaccine preferred (A/C/Y/W-135 conjugate vaccine). • Menactra must be administered at least 4 weeks after completion of PCV13 series. • Booster every 5 years if patient is on the deceased donor waiting list and in transplant recipient who is at high risk of invasive meningococcal infection.				

	Minimum Age For Dose 1	Minimum Interval Between Doses			
		Dose 1 to 2	Dose 2 to 3	Dose 3 to 4	Dose 4 to 5
Hepatitis A	12 months	6 months			

2. Children and adolescents aged 7 through 18 years:

	Minimum Age For Dose 1	Minimum Interval Between Doses		
		Dose 1 to 2	Dose 2 to 3	Dose 3 to 4
Hepatitis B	Birth	4 weeks	8 weeks and at least 16 weeks after 1st dose.	

(Continued)

	Minimum Age For Dose 1	Minimum Interval Between Doses		
		Dose 1 to 2	Dose 2 to 3	Dose 3 to 4
	• Post-vaccination testing (anti-HBs antibody) is recommended 1–2 months after the primary series is completed, with up to 3 additional doses if protective antibody levels (>10 mIU/ml) are not achieved. • Give special double dose formulation for dialysis patients: Children age 7–10 years: 20 mcg. Children age >10–19 years: 40 mcg. • Annual testing of anti-HBs antibody is required in immuno-compromised patients. • Booster dose in transplant recipient if anti-HBs antibody titer <10 mIU/ml.			

	Minimum Age For Dose 1	Minimum Interval Between Doses		
		Dose 1 to 2	Dose 2 to 3	Dose 3 to 4
Tetanus, diphtheria (Td) Tetanus, diphtheria, pertussis (TdaP)	7 years	4 weeks	If 1st dose (DTaP) is given at age <1 year: 4 weeks. If 1st dose (DTaP or TdaP) is given at age ≥1 year: 6 months (final dose).	If 1st dose (DTaP) is given at age <1 year: 6 months.
	• TdaP vaccine should be substituted for a single dose of Td in the catch-up series; if additional doses are needed, use Td vaccine every 5 years as booster dose. • An inadvertent dose of DTaP vaccine administered to children age 7–10 years can count as part of the catch-up series. This dose can count as the adolescent TdaP dose, or the child can later receive a TdaP booster dose at 11–12 years. • TdaP can be given between age 7–10 years if they are not fully vaccinated with DTaP. • Adolescents should get at least one vaccination of TdaP, then subsequent boosters with Td or TdaP (every 10 years).			

	Minimum Age For Dose 1	Minimum Interval Between Doses		
		Dose 1 to 2	Dose 2 to 3	Dose 3 to 4
Inactivated polio (IPV)	6 weeks	4 weeks	4 weeks	6 months
	• 4th dose is not necessary if the 3rd dose was administered at age ≥4 years and at least 6 months after the previous dose. • Booster should be given every 10 years for transplant recipients with ongoing travel to polio-endemic areas.			

	Minimum Age For Dose 1	Minimum Interval Between Doses		
		Dose 1 to 2	Dose 2 to 3	Dose 3 to 4
Haemophilus influenza type b	6 weeks			
	• Booster every 5 years if patient is on the deceased donor waiting list.			

	Minimum Age For Dose 1	Minimum Interval Between Doses		
		Dose 1 to 2	Dose 2 to 3	Dose 3 to 4
MMR	1 year	4 weeks		
	• Should be avoided in patients receiving: a. Immunosuppressive drugs. b. Corticosteroids with dose: ≥20 mg total daily dose or on alternate days for >14 days. • Once corticosteroids are discontinued, vaccination should be delayed for at least 1 month. • Contraindicated in the post-kidney transplant patient.			

	Minimum Age For Dose 1	Minimum Interval Between Doses		
		Dose 1 to 2	Dose 2 to 3	Dose 3 to 4
Pneumococcal	PCV13: 6 weeks. PPSV23: 2 years.			

(*Continued*)

	Minimum Age For Dose 1	Minimum Interval Between Doses		
		Dose 1 to 2	Dose 2 to 3	Dose 3 to 4
	• Single dose of PCV13 should be given regardless of previous history of PCV7 or PPSV23. • Patients unvaccinated with PPSV23: PPSV23 at least 8 weeks after PCV13. • Booster dose of PPSV23: 5 years from the last dose. • Booster dose of PPSV23 after transplantation, if not completed before.			

	Minimum Age For Dose 1	Minimum Interval Between Doses		
		Dose 1 to 2	Dose 2 to 3	Dose 3 to 4
Varicella	1 year	If the current age is <13 years: 3 months. If the current age is ≥13 years: 4 weeks.		
	• Should be avoided in patients receiving immunosuppressive drugs, including corticosteroids. • Once corticosteroids are discontinued, vaccination should be delayed for at least 1 month. • Contraindicated in the post-kidney transplant patient.			

	Minimum Age For Dose 1	Minimum Interval Between Doses		
		Dose 1 to 2	Dose 2 to 3	Dose 3 to 4
Influenza	6 months	If the age is <9 years: 1 month.		
	• Should be given yearly. • Patients on dialysis and kidney transplant recipients should only receive the inactivated vaccine, not the intranasal influenza vaccine. • Inactivated influenza vaccination can be given as early as 1 month, post-transplantation.			

	Minimum Age For Dose 1	Minimum Interval Between Doses		
		Dose 1 to 2	Dose 2 to 3	Dose 3 to 4
Hepatitis A	1 year	6 months		

	Minimum Age For Dose 1	Minimum Interval Between Doses		
		Dose 1 to 2	Dose 2 to 3	Dose 3 to 4
Meningococcal	6 weeks if MCV4-TT (Nimenrix) 2 months if MCV4-CRM (Menveo) 9 months if MCV4-D (Menactra)	8 weeks		
	• Tetravalent conjugated vaccine preferred (A/C/Y/W-135 conjugate vaccine). • Menactra must be administered at least 4 weeks after completion of PCV13 series. • Booster every 5 years if patient is on the deceased donor waiting list and in a transplant recipient who is at high risk of invasive meningococcal infection. • Meningococcal B vaccine (Bexcero) is recommended for children age ≥10 years who are at increased risk for serogroup B meningococcal disease (e.g., patients on eculizumab therapy or patients living in areas with serogroup B meningococcal disease outbreak).			

(*Continued*)

	Minimum Age For Dose 1	Minimum Interval Between Doses		
		Dose 1 to 2	Dose 2 to 3	Dose 3 to 4
Human papillomavirus	9 years	1 month	3 months and at least 5 months from dose 1 (repeat dose if administered too soon).	
	• HPV 9 vaccine recommended. • Routine recommended age for the 1st dose: 11–12 years for boys and girls. • Transplant recipients should receive a 3-dose series (healthy population only requires 2 doses if they receive dose 1 at age <15 years). • Not recommended in individuals with known immediate hypersensitivity to yeast.			

E. Travel Vaccines for the Immunocompromised Patient

1. Recommended vaccines for travel to endemic areas:
   a. DTaP/TdaP.
   b. IPV.
   c. IM typhoid.
   d. Pneumococcal vaccine.
   e. Rabies.
   f. Meningococcal (conjugated).
   g. Hib.
   h. Influenza.
   i. Oral cholera (killed whole-cell oral cholera vaccine, Dukoral)
      - 2 doses, 1–6 weeks apart for children aged >6 years.
      - 3 doses, 1–6 weeks apart for children aged 2–6 years.
   j. Japanese B encephalitis.

	Minimum Age For Dose 1	Minimum Interval Between Doses
		Dose 1 to 2
Japanese B encephalitis	2 months	1 month
	• Series should be completed at least 1 week prior to potential exposure. • Booster dose can be given in adolescents ≥17 years, prior to potential re-exposure if the primary series is completed >1 year previously.	

2. Contraindicated (live attenuated vaccines):
   - OPV.
   - Intranasal influenza.
   - MMR.
   - Varicella.
   - Oral typhoid.
   - Yellow fever.

F. COVID-19 Vaccines for the Immunocompromised Patient

1. Everyone should receive COVID-19 vaccines, irrespective of past COVID-19 infection or prior evidence of humoral immunity.
2. Currently, there is limited data on vaccine safety profile and effectiveness in the immunocompromised population, as well as the potential for reduced immunogenicity.
3. Recommended that all transplant candidates and their household members receive COVID-19 vaccination.
4. Recommendations for the transplant recipient:
   a. Vaccination should be completed >2 weeks prior to transplantation.
   b. Vaccination can be given 3 months post-transplant in the stable patient.

Company	Type of Vaccine	Minimum Age For Dose 1	Minimum Interval Between Doses
			Dose 1 to 2
Pfizer-BioNTech	mRNA	12 years	3 weeks
Moderna	mRNA	18 years	4 weeks
Astra-Zeneca	Viral vector	18 years	4 weeks
Sinovac (CoronaVac)	Inactivated virus	18 years	2 weeks (Emergency) 4 weeks (Routine)
Sinopharm	Inactivated virus	18 years	3–4 weeks
Sputnik V	Viral vector	18 years	3 weeks
Johnson & Johnson/Janssen	Viral vector	18 years (Single dose)	
Novavax	Protein-based	18 years	3 weeks

- These vaccines are not interchangeable.
- Absolute contraindication:
    a. Severe allergic reaction after a previous dose of an mRNA COVID-19 vaccine or any of its components.
    b. Immediate allergic reaction of any severity to a previous dose of an mRNA COVID-19 vaccine or any of its components (including polyethylene glycol).
    c. Immediate allergic reaction of any severity to polysorbate (due to potential cross-reactive hypersensitivity with the vaccine ingredient such as polyethylene glycol).

Recommended Reading

1. Centers for Disease Control and Prevention. (2010) Prevention of pneumococcal disease among infants and children — Use of 13-valent pneumococcal conjugate vaccine and 23-valent pneumococcal polysaccharide vaccine. Recommendations of the Advisory Committee on Immunization Practices (ACIP). *Morb Mortal Wkly Rep* **59**:1–18.
2. American Academy of Pediatrics. Committee on Infectious Diseases. (2012) HPV vaccine recommendation. *Pediatrics* **129**:602–605.
3. World Health Organization. (2018) Immunization, vaccines and biologicals: Cholera. http://www.who.int/immunization/diseases/cholera/en/.
4. Lexicomp, Inc. (n.d.) Japanese encephalitis virus vaccine (inactivated). Pediatric drug information Lexicomp®. *UpToDate ONLINE*. http://www.uptodateonline.com.

5. Danzinger-Isakov L, Kumar D; AST Infectious Diseases Community of Practice. (2019) Vaccination in solid organ transplant candidates and recipients: Guidelines from the American society of transplantation infectious diseases community of practice. *Clin Transplant* e13563.
6. Fox TG, Nailescu C. (2019) Vaccinations in pediatric kidney transplant recipients. *Pediatr Nephrol* **34**:579–591.
7. Centers for Disease Control and Prevention. (2020) Recommendations of the Advisory Committee on Immunization Practices (ACIP): Recommended immunization schedules for persons aged 0 through 18 years. www.cdc.gov/vaccines/hcp/acip-recs/index.
8. Centers for Disease Control and Prevention. (2021) Different COVID-19 vaccines.

7 Recommended Dietary Intake in Children with Chronic Kidney Disease

Pinapala A, Teo S, Ng KH and Yap HK

A. Acceptable Macronutrient Distribution Ranges

Macronutrient	Age		
	<1 year	1–3 years	4–18 years
Carbohydrate	36–56%	45–65%	45–65%
Fat	40–54%	30–40%	25–35%
Protein	7–12%	5–20%	10–30%

B. Suggested Dietary Intake (SDI) for Energy

1. The lower and upper limits of the SDI for energy fall within the average amount given in the published values, that is, the daily amount of energy considered sufficient to meet the needs of half the population.
2. The initial prescription for energy intake in children with chronic kidney disease stages 2-5D (CKD2-5D) should approximate that of healthy children of the same chronological age.
3. To promote optimal linear growth in those with suboptimal weight gain, energy intake should be adjusted towards the higher end of the SDI.
4. In overweight or obese children, energy intake should be adjusted to achieve appropriate weight gain, without compromising nutrition.

5. SDI for energy:
   a. Age ≤1 year:

Months	SDI (kcal/kg/day)
0	93–107
1	93–120
2	93–120
3	82–98
4	82–98
5	72–82
6–9	72–82
10–11	72–82
12	72–120

   b. Age 2–17 years:

Years	SDI Males (kcal/kg/day)	SDI Females (kcal/kg/day)
2	81–95	79–92
3	80–82	76–77
4–6	67–93	64–90
7–8	60–77	56–75
9–10	55–69	49–63
11–12	48–63	43–57
13–14	44–63	39–50
15–17	40–55	36–46

6. SDI for energy has been adjusted to account for Physical Activity Level (PAL):
   - 1–3 years PAL: 1.4 times
   - 4–9 years PAL: 1.6 times
   - 10–17 years PAL: 1.8 times

C. SDI for Protein

1. In children with CKD2-5D:
   a. Target protein intake should be at the upper end of the SDI to promote optimal growth.

   b. The protein intake should not be reduced below the lower end of the SDI.
2. Children on dialysis may need higher protein intake compared to non-dialysis patients to account for dialysate protein losses:
   a. Peritoneal dialysis (PD): 0.28 g/kg/day in infants to 0.1 g/kg/day in adolescents.
   b. Hemodialysis (HD): 0.1 g/kg/day.
3. In children with persistently high blood urea levels, protein intake should be adjusted towards the lower end of the SDI, after excluding other causes of high blood urea levels.
4. SDI for protein:
   a. Age ≤1 year:

Months	SDI Protein (g/kg/day)
0	1.52–2.5
1	1.52–1.8
2	1.4–1.52
3	1.4–1.52
4	1.3–1.52
5	1.3–1.52
6–9	1.1–1.3
10–11	1.1–1.3
12	0.9–1.14

   b. Age 2–17 years:

Years	SDI Protein (g/kg/day)
2	0.9–1.05
3	0.9–1.05
4–6	0.85–0.95
7–8	0.9–0.95
9–10	0.9–0.95
11–12	0.9–0.95
13–14	0.8–0.9
15–17	0.8–0.9

D. Nutrition in Infants with CKD

1. Breastfeeding is the preferred method for feeding an infant with CKD.
2. Whey-dominant infant formulas should be used if needed.
3. Breastmilk and infant formulas can be fortified when there is a prescribed fluid restriction or when more energy or nutrient-dense feed is required.
4. Suggested addition of energy modules to formulas:

Energy Module	Age	Amount of Carbohydrate/ Fat (g) Added to 100 ml Formula*	Final Concentration of Carbohydrate or Fat (g/100ml)
Glucose polymer	<6 months	3–5	10–12
	6 months to 1 year	5–8	12–15
	>1 year	8–18	20–30
Fat emulsion (50% fat content)	<1 year	1.5–2.5 (3–5 ml)	5–6
	>1 year	4.5 (9 ml)	9

*Infant formula typically contains 7 g of carbohydrates and 3.5 g of fat per 100 ml. Pediatric formula typically contains 12 g of carbohydrates and 4.5 g of fat per 100 ml.

E. Dietary Recommendation for Fats

1. Recommended fat requirements:
   a. Neonates: 2–3 g/kg/day (up to 4 g/kg/day).
   b. Infants and preschool children: 1–3 g/kg/day.
   c. Adults and school-age children: 1–2 g/kg/day.

2. Recommendations on specific types of fats and carbohydrates:

Macronutrient	Recommendation
Dietary cholesterol	As low as possible while consuming a nutritionally adequate diet.
Trans-fatty acids	As low as possible while consuming a nutritionally adequate diet.
Saturated fatty acids	As low as possible while consuming a nutritionally adequate diet.
Added sugars	Limit to a maximal intake <25% of the total energy.

3. Dietary recommendations for children with CKD5D with dyslipidemia:

Macronutrient	Serum LDL-cholesterol >2.60 mmol/L	Serum Triglyceride >1.70 mmol/L
Energy		If associated with excess weight, then energy balance and activity recommendations as for weight loss.
Dietary fat	<30% of calories	Low
Dietary cholesterol	<200 mg/day	
Trans-fatty acids	Avoid	
Saturated fatty acids	<7% of calories	
Carbohydrates		Low simple carbohydrates.

F. Vitamin and Trace Element Requirements

1. Children on dialysis should receive a water-soluble vitamin supplement.
2. Dietary intake consisting of at least 100% of the dietary recommended intake (DRI) for thiamine (B_1), riboflavin (B_2), niacin (B_3), pantothenic acid (B_5), pyridoxine (B_6), biotin (B_8), cobalamin (B_{12}), ascorbic acid (C), retinol (A), α-tocopherol (E), vitamin K, folic acid, copper, and zinc should be provided.
3. Recommended dietary allowances for normal individuals:

Age	Vit A (mcg)	Vit D (mcg)	Vit B1 (mg)	Vit B2 (mg)	Vit B3 (mg)	Vit B6 (mg)	Vit B12 (mcg)	Folic Acid (mcg)	Folic Acid in CKD§ (mcg)
3–<6 mos	300	10.0	0.28	0.42	4.6	0.1	0.4	65	250/kg*
6–<9 mos	300	10.0	0.32	0.49	5.3	0.3	0.5	80	250/kg*
9–<12 mos	300	10.0	0.38	0.57	6.3	0.3	0.5	80	250/kg*
1–<2 years	250	10.0	0.46	0.69	7.6	0.5	0.9	150	2500
2–<3 years	250	10.0	0.54	0.81	8.9	0.6	1.1	200	2500
3–<5 years	300	10.0	0.62	0.93	10.2	0.6	1.1	200	2500
Males									
5–<7 years	300	10.0	0.74	1.11	12.2	0.6	1.1	200	5000
7–<10 years	400	2.5	0.84	1.26	13.9	1.0	1.8	300	5000
10–<12 years	575	2.5	0.88	1.32	14.5	1.0	1.8	300	5000
12–<14 years	725	2.5	0.96	1.44	15.8	1.4	2.4	350	5000
14–<16 years	725	2.5	1.06	1.59	17.5	1.4	2.4	350	5000
16–<18 years	750	2.5	1.14	1.71	18.8	1.4	2.4	350	5000
18–<30 years	750	2.5	1.18	1.77	19.5	1.3	2.4	400	5000
Females									
5–<7 years	300	10.5	0.70	1.05	11.6	0.6	1.1	200	5000
7–<10 years	400	2.5	0.72	1.08	11.9	1.0	1.8	300	5000
10–<12 years	575	2.5	0.78	1.17	12.9	1.0	1.8	300	5000
12–<14 years	725	2.5	0.84	1.26	13.9	1.2	2.2	350	5000

Age	Vit A (mcg)	Vit D (mcg)	Vit B1 (mg)	Vit B2 (mg)	Vit B3 (mg)	Vit B6 (mg)	Vit B12 (mcg)	Folic Acid (mcg)	Folic Acid in CKD§ (mcg)
14–<16 years	725	2.5	0.86	1.29	14.2	1.2	2.2	350	5000
16–<18 years	750	2.5	0.86	1.29	14.2	1.2	2.2	350	5000
18–<30 years	750	2.5	0.84	1.26	13.9	1.3	2.4	400	5000
Preparations									
Renalmin (per tablet)	—	—	1.5	1.7	20.0	10.0	6.0	1000	1000
Polyvitamin (per mL)	450 (1500 IU)	10 (400 IU)	0.5	0.6	8.0	0.4	2.0	—	—

§Amount of folate to lower homocysteine levels in CKD.

*Max of 2500 mcg daily.

Recommended Reading

1. KDOQI. (2009) KDOQI clinical practice guidelines for nutrition in children with chronic kidney disease: 2008 update. *Am J Kidney Dis* **53**(Suppl 2):S35–S47.
2. Shaw V, Polderman N, Renken-Terhaerdt J, Paglialonga F, Oosterveld M, Tuokkola J, Anderson C, Desloovere A, Greenbaum L, Haffner D, Nelms C, Qizalbash L, Vande Walle J, Warady B, Shroff R, Rees L. (2020) Energy and protein requirements for children with CKD stages 2–5 and on dialysis-clinical practice recommendations from the Pediatric Renal Nutrition Taskforce. *Pediatr Nephrol* **35**:519–531.

8 Contrasted Magnetic Resonance Imaging in Kidney Failure

Teo S, Yap HK and Liu ID

A. Nephrogenic Systemic Fibrosis (NSF)

1. Linked to gadolinium-based contrast agents (GBCAs).
2. Related to the dissociation of unexcreted gadolinium from the chelate in patients with poor kidney function.
3. Excess gadolinium infiltrates multiple organs inciting an inflammatory response that causes thickening of collagen bundles with an increased number of fibrocytes.
4. Typically bilateral and symmetrical, most commonly affecting the skin of the distal extremities, with involvement of the lower limbs more than the upper limbs.
5. Skeletal muscles, pleura, diaphragm, pericardium, and myocardium can also be affected.
6. Fibrocyte and mucin infiltration result in muscle weakness, contractures and arthralgias.
7. Symptoms appear 2–11 weeks after gadolinium exposure in up to 5% of patients at risk.

B. Agents Associated With NSF

Group I: Agents associated with the greatest number of NSF cases.	Gadodiamide Gadopentetate dimeglumine Gadoversetamide
Group II: Agents associated with few, if any, unconfounded cases of NSF.	Gadobenate dimeglumine Gadobutrol Gadoterate acid Gadoteridol

(Continued)

(*Continued*)

Group III: Agents for which data remains limited regarding NSF risk, but for which few, if any unconfounded cases of NSF have been reported.	Gadoxetate disodium

1. Patients with chronic kidney disease (CKD) stage G5 (estimated glomerular filtration rate [eGFR] <15 ml/min/1.73m^2) have a 1–7% chance of developing NSF after one or more exposures to group I GBCAs.
2. NSF occurs most commonly in patients who have received high doses of GBCA (0.3 mmol/kg), either as a single administration or cumulatively, in multiple administrations over months to years.
3. Risk of NSF among patients exposed to standard or lower dose of Group II GBCAs is low or possibly nonexistent.

C. Preventive Measures

1. Patients with the following conditions should be considered at risk of developing NSF after receiving Group I and III GBCAs:
   a. Dialysis-dependent.
   b. CKD stage 4 or 5 with eGFR <30 ml/min/1.73m^2 without dialysis.
   c. Acute kidney injury.
2. Group II agents may be used in patients at risk of NSF.
3. Guidelines for hemodialysis (HD) patients:
   a. Dialysis should be performed within 2–3 hours of administration of intravenous GBCA.
      - To facilitate GBCA clearance, dialysis times and flow rates can be increased.
   b. Second HD should be performed within 24 hours after gadolinium-based contrast administration.
4. Guidelines for peritoneal dialysis (PD) patients:
   a. Temporary intensive automated PD regimen aimed at maximizing clearance of the GBCA immediately after exposure may be an effective alternative when the institution of HD is problematic.

- One study showed that 90% of the gadolinium was removed from the circulation in 2 days, with a regimen of 10–15 exchanges per day of PD.

b. Perform automated PD within 2–3 hours of gadolinium administration: 15–20 full volume hourly exchanges for 2 days.

Recommended Reading

1. Kanal E, Barkovich AJ, Beli C, Borgstede JP, Bradley WG Jr, Froelich JW, Gilk T, Gimbel JR, Gosbee J, Kuhni-Kaminski E, Lester JW Jr, Nyenhuis J, Parag Y, Schaefer DJ, Sebek-Scoumis EA, Weinreb J, Zaremba LA, Wilcox P, Lucey L, Sass N; ACR Blue Ribbon Panel on MR Safety. (2007) ACR guidance document for safe MR practices: 2007. *Am J Roentgenol* **188**:1447–1474.
2. Murashima M, Drott HR, Carlow D, Shaw LM, Milone M, Bachman M, Tsai DE, Yang SL, Bloom RD. (2008) Removal of gadolinium by peritoneal dialysis. *Clin Nephrol* **69**:368–372.
3. Agarwal R, Brunelli SM, Williams K, Mitchell MD, Feldman HI, Umscheid CA. (2009) Gadolinium-based contrast agents and nephrogenic systemic fibrosis: A systematic review and meta-analysis. *Nephrol Dial Transplant* **24**:856–863.
4. American College of Radiology (ACR) Committee on Drugs and Contrast Media. (2021) Nephrogenic systemic fibrosis (NSF). In: *ACR Manual on Contrast Media*, version 2021, pp 83–91.

9 Initiation of Kidney Replacement Therapy

Koh LJ, Teo S, Ng KH and Yap HK

A. Preparation

1. Patients and their family should receive education about kidney failure and options for its treatment when chronic kidney disease (CKD) stage 4 is reached.
   - Options for treatment include kidney transplantation, peritoneal dialysis, hemodialysis, and conservative treatment.
2. Ensure immunizations are up to date.

B. Timing for Initiation

1. Kidney replacement therapy should be considered when patients reach CKD stage G5, with a glomerular filtration rate (GFR) of 9–14 ml/min/1.73m².
2. Kidney replacement therapy is recommended if GFR ≤8 ml/min/1.73m².
3. Consider early kidney replacement therapy in the presence of:
   a. Intractable fluid overload.
   b. Intractable hyperkalemia.
   c. Refractory hypertension due to fluid overload.
   d. Growth failure.
   e. Malnutrition.
   f. Uremic neurological dysfunction.
   g. Uremic serositis.
   h. Refractory hyperphosphataemia.
   i. Refractory metabolic acidosis.

4. Kidney replacement therapy may be delayed after reaching CKD stage G5 if the patient is:
   a. Asymptomatic.
   b. Awaiting imminent kidney transplant.
   c. Has chosen conservative therapy.

C. Modality Selection

1. Modality selection should take into account patient/family choice, patient's size, medical comorbidities, and family support.
2. Types of kidney replacement therapy include:
   a. Automated peritoneal dialysis.
   b. Chronic ambulatory peritoneal dialysis.
   c. Hemodialysis.
   d. Pre-emptive kidney transplantation.
3. Peritoneal dialysis is the preferred initial long-term dialysis for pediatric patients with CKD stage G5, especially in the small child where maintenance of functional and complication-free vascular access can be problematic.
4. Contraindications to hemodialysis include:
   a. Contraindications to the use of anticoagulation.
   b. Cardiovascular instability.
5. Contraindications to peritoneal dialysis in children include:
   a. Absolute
      - Omphalocele.
      - Gastroschisis.
      - Bladder exstrophy.
      - Diaphragmatic hernia.
      - Obliterated peritoneal cavity.
      - Peritoneal membrane failure.
   b. Relative
      - Fresh intra-abdominal foreign bodies including gastrostomy.
      - Recent ventricular-peritoneal shunt.
      - Peritoneal leaks.
      - Body size limitations including morbid obesity.

- Intolerance to peritoneal dialysis volumes necessary to achieve adequate peritoneal dialysis dose.
- Advanced lung disease.
- Recurrent hydrothorax.
- Inflammatory or ischemic bowel disease.
- Abdominal wall or skin infection.

Recommended Reading

1. European Best Practice Guidelines for Peritoneal Dialysis. (2005) Adequacy of peritoneal dialysis. *Nephrol Dial Transplant* **20**(Suppl 9):ix1–ix35.
2. National Kidney Foundation. (2015) KDOQI clinical practice guidelines for hemodialysis adequacy: 2015 update. *Am J Kidney Dis* **66**(5):884–930.
3. Nehus E, Mitsnefes MM. (2019) When to initiate dialysis in children and adolescents: Is waiting worthwhile? *Am J Kidney Dis* **73**:762–764.

1 Hemodialysis Orders

Ng KH, Teo S, Resontoc LP, Sathe KP and Yap HK

A. Types of Hemodialysis (HD)

1. Modality:
   a. Hemodialysis: Removes solutes with molecular weights (MW) <500 Da.
   b. Hemodiafiltration (HDF): Better clearance of middle molecules (<300–500 Da) and larger molecules (>15–60 kDa) (Reference molecule: β2-microglobulin).
      - Solute clearance is dictated by UF volume and sieving coefficient.
      - HDF is effective in removing solutes with larger MW <40 kDa.
2. Regimes:
   a. Conventional HD: Standard frequency: ≥4 hours, 3 times per week.
   b. Intensified HD
      - Short daily HD: 2–3 hours/day for 5–7 days a week.
      - Nocturnal HD: 6–8 hours/night for 4–7 days a week.

B. Vascular Access

1. Subcutaneously tunneled central venous catheters:
   a. Type of catheter:
      i. Use tunneled catheters if the expected time for use is more than 2 weeks.
      ii. Recommendation is to change non tunneled internal jugular catheters after 3 weeks and femoral catheters after 5 days.

b. Position of HD catheter:
   i. Most commonly placed in the internal jugular vein and tunneled superficially to exit on the upper anterior chest.
   ii. Catheter tip should be located at the junction of the superior vena cava (SVC) and right atrium or in the right atrium to provide adequate dialysis.
   iii. Catheters located in the SVC may have inadequate blood flow, as they tend to abut the vessel wall, sealing off the entry and exit sites.
   iv. Femoral vein catheters:
      - Tip of femoral hemodialysis catheters should be placed in the distal inferior vena cava (IVC) to minimize recirculation.
      - Should only be used as temporary access as damage to the IVC may compromise future kidney transplantation.
   v. Avoid the subclavian vein if possible as there is a high risk of stenosis, which will compromise successful fistula formation in the future.
c. Size of catheters:
   - Select the largest diameter catheter with the shortest length where possible

Body Weight	Double Lumen
<4 kg	6.5–7 F
4–10 kg	8 F
10–20 kg	9–10 F
20–40 kg	10–12.5 F
40–50 kg >50 kg	12–12.5 F 12–14.5 F

d. Perioperative care of catheter placement.
   i. Refer to chapter "Hemodialysis Catheter Infections" (Section: "Prevention of Catheter Infections").
   ii. Desmopressin (DDAVP) should be given on-call to the Diagnostic Imaging department at a dose of 0.3 mcg/kg (maximum 10 mcg) as a 30-minute intravenous infusion.

2. Native arteriovenous fistulas (AVF):
   a. Preferred modality as this has the longest lifespan with the least complications.
   b. Anastomosis: End-to-side, vein-to-artery.
      i. Radiocephalic or wrist fistula: Radial artery and cephalic vein.

ii. Brachiocephalic or upper arm fistula: Brachial artery and cephalic vein. The former can be difficult in small children due to vessel size.
iii. Transposed brachiobasilic fistula:
- 2-stage basilic vein transposition may be preferred in small patients.
- Arterialized vein is moved to a more superficial position about two months after the anastomosis has been created.

c. Time to cannulation:
i. Cannulation before 2 weeks should be avoided.
ii. Cannulation after 4 weeks if the fistula is clinically mature.

3. Synthetic arteriovenous grafts (AVG):
a. Synthetic conduit, usually expanded polytetrafluoroethylene (ePTFE), between an artery and a vein.
b. Conduit can be straight or looped and ranges between 4 to 8 mm in diameter.
c. Common graft locations:
i. Straight forearm: Radial artery to cephalic vein.
ii. Looped forearm: Brachial artery to cephalic vein.
iii. Straight upper arm: Brachial artery to axillary vein.
iv. Looped upper arm: Axillary artery to axillary vein.
v. Others: Leg grafts, looped chest grafts, axillary-axillary (necklace), and axillary-atrial grafts.
d. Time to cannulation.
i. Grafts can be cannulated for HD earlier than AVF.
ii. Cannulation can be performed within 24 to 72 hours of placement with newer synthetic grafts.

C. Dialyzers and Lines

1. Types of dialyzers:
a. Low or high-flux.
b. High-flux dialyzers have large pores that allow for enhanced permeability of larger molecules, which can enhance removal of toxins and improve outcome.
c. If the water system is of high quality, high-flux dialyzers are preferable.
2. Dialyzer surface area should be as big as possible and comparable to the child's surface area.

3. Characteristics of dialyzers:

Dialyzer	Membrane	Sterilization	KoA (ml/min)	Kuf (ml/hour × mmHg)	Surface Area (m^2)	Fill Volume (ml)	Blood Flow (ml/min)
High-flux							
FX paed	Helixone®	Steam	170	7	0.2	18	30–100
FX CorDiax 40	Helixone® plus	Steam	547	21	0.6	32	50–200
Polyflux 6H	PAES/PVP/PA	Steam	465	33	0.6	52	50–300
FX CorDiax 50	Helixone® plus	Steam	886	33	1.0	53	100–300
FX CorDiax 60	Helixone® plus	Steam	1164	47	1.4	74	150–400
Revaclear 300	PAES/PVP*	Steam	1186	48	1.4	74	200–500
FX 80	Helixone®	Steam	1292	59	1.8	95	200–500
Polyflux 170H	PAES/PVP/PA*	Steam	1153	70	1.7	115	250-500
Low-flux							
F4 HPS	Polysulfone	Steam	495	8	0.8	51	50–200
F5 HPS		Steam	606	10	1.0	63	100–300
F6 HPS		Steam	746	13	1.3	78	150–400
F7 HPS		Steam	789	16	1.6	96	200–500
F8 HPS		Steam	848	18	1.8	113	250–600

Kuf = UF coefficient; PA = polyamide; PAES = polyarylethersulfone; PVP = polyvinylpyrrolidone; *bisphenol A (BPA)-free

4. Fill volumes of dialysis lines:

Lines	Fill Volume (ml)
Neonatal	34 (14 ml arterial + 20 ml venous)
Pediatric	74
Adult	149

D. Dialysate Solutions

1. Potassium: 2 mmol/L
2. Bicarbonate: 35 mmol/L
3. Calcium:
    - Normal calcium (1.75 mmol/L): Hypocalcemic patients, young age <12 months, or patients at risk of seizures.
    - Low calcium (1.25 mmol/L): Most patients on chronic HD (to decrease calcium load).
4. Glucose: 0.2% (2 g in 1 L)
    - For young, diabetic or malnourished patients.
5. Sodium: 132–140 mmol/L, or within 4–5 mmol/L of pre-dialysis serum sodium.

E. Blood Flow Rate

1. Depends on the size of access.
2. Ideally, maximum blood flow should be up to the extracorporeal volume (ECV).
    - For example, blood flow is up to 80 ml/min if the ECV (dialyzer + lines) is 80 ml.
3. Suggested flow rate:

	Blood Flow Rate (ml/kg/min)	Typical Ranges (ml/min)
Neonates and small infants	10–12	30–80
Infants	10–12	50–100
Children	4–6	100–150
Adolescents	2–4	150–250
Adults	—	150–250

4. Adults: 150–250 ml/min.
   Children: 150–200 ml/m²/min or 5–7 ml/kg/min (minimum 3–5 ml/kg/min).
   BW <10 kg: Blood flow ≤100 ml/min (where BW = body weight).
   BW 10–40 kg: Blood flow (ml/min) = 2.5 × BW (kg) + 100 ml/min.
   BW >40 kg: Blood flow up to 250 ml/min.

F. Dialysate Flow Rate

1. Typically, 300 ml/min for a smaller child and 500 ml/min for a larger child.
2. For maximum dialysate saturation, the dialysate flow is 2x of the blood flow.

G. Ultrafiltration (UF)

1. UF volumes = desired net negative volume + rinsing volume + volume of infusions during HD (e.g., packed red cells, intradialytic nutrition).
2. Starting net negative fluid removal rate can be 5–10 ml/kg/hour, maximum 13 ml/kg/hour, or 1–2% of body weight per hour.
3. UF rates that are too high can result in:
   i. Cramps and hypotension during HD.
   ii. Loss of residual kidney function and cardiovascular morbidities.
4. Aim to achieve optimal dry weight, which results in normal blood pressure at the end of each HD session without the need for antihypertensive medications.
5. Machine accuracy in measuring volume of removed fluid:
   i. Gambro AK 96: ± 30 ml or ± 1% of reading, whichever is larger.
   ii. Gambro AK 98: ± 50 ml or ± 50 ml/hour x passed treatment time (h) or 2.5% of total UF removed, whichever is larger.
   iii. Fresenius 4008: ± 0.5%.
   iv. Fresenius 5008: ±1%.

H. Priming Solutions

1. Calculation of patient's blood volume:
   i. <10 kg child: 80 ml/kg.
   ii. >10 kg child: 70 ml/kg.
   iii. Adolescent or adult: 60 ml/kg.

2. Calculate ECV / patient's blood volume to determine the priming solution:
   i. ECV ≤10% of patient's blood volume: 0.9% saline.
   ii. ECV 10–15% of patient's blood volume:
      • Normal Hb: 5% albumin.
      • Low Hb (<7 g/dL): Packed red cells.
   iii. ECV >15% of patient's blood volume: Packed red cells.
3. Consider diluting packed red cells with 0.9% saline to decrease load of potassium and acids from the transfusion.

I. Anticoagulation

I. Types of anticoagulation

1. Unfractionated heparin:
   a. Dosing: Start with low-dose heparin dosing.

Unfractionated Heparin	Loading Bolus (U/kg)	Maintenance Infusion (U/kg/hour)	Monitoring
Low dose	>15 kg: 10–20 ≤15 kg: 5–10 (Adult: 1000 U)	5–10 (Adult: 500 U/hour)	Keep ACT 150–200 sec
Regular dose	50 (Adult: max 2000 U)	10–50 (Adult: 750 U/hour)	Keep ACT 200–250 sec

Note: Maintenance dose without loading bolus in patients at risk of bleeding.

   b. Stopping of heparin:
      i. Catheter: 30 minutes before circuit termination.
      ii. AVF/AVG: 60 minutes before circuit termination.
         • If clotting develops, stop 30 minutes before termination.
   c. Adjustments:
      i. Prolonged bleeding from needle sites post-dialysis: Lengthen the time between heparin cessation and circuit termination.
      ii. High clotting tendency:
         • If there are clots in the first half of the session, increase bolus dose in the next session.

- If there are clots in the second half of the session, increase infusion rate in the next session.
- If there is recurrent/refractory circuit clotting, evaluate for access inflow or outflow stenosis.

2. Low molecular weight heparin (LMWH):
   a. Considerations:
      i. More prolonged half-life and more unpredictable pharmacokinetics than unfractionated heparin.
      ii. No evidence it increases filter lifespan more than unfractionated heparin.
   b. Enoxaparin dose: (0.01 ml = 1 mg = 100 IU).
      i. Initial bolus: 50–100 IU/kg = 0.5–1 mg/kg per HD session.
         - If fibrin rings are found, a further dose of 0.5–1.0 mg/kg may be given.
      ii. For patients at risk of thrombosis or if HD >4 hours:
         - Can increase initial bolus to 0.8–1 mg/kg OR
         - Give lower initial bolus of 0.4 mg/kg, followed by second bolus at 3 hours of 0.4 mg/kg, OR
         - Give a second dose at half the initial dose.
      iii. For patients at risk of hemorrhage:
         - Keep initial bolus at 0.5 mg/kg.
      iv. Higher dose may be needed in high flux dialyzers.
   c. Administration:
      i. High flux dialyzer: Preferably administered into the venous limb of the circuit because up to 80% is cleared if injected into the arterial port.
      ii. Low flux dialyzer: No difference between arterial and venous administration.
   d. Dose adjustment:
      i. Routine monitoring of anti-Xa activity is not required as dose adjustment can be made by clinical monitoring.
      ii. Increase dose if there is evidence of clotting tendency:
         - Extremely dark blood in the venous bubble trap.
         - Shadows or black streaks in the dialyzer.
         - Foaming with clot formation in drip chambers and venous trap.

- Clots at the arterial side header.
- Increased transmembrane and venous pressure.

iii. Decrease dose if there is evidence of increased bleeding tendency:

- Prolonged bleeding upon removal of the needle.

e. Target anti-Xa levels:

i. During dialysis (2 hours after administration): 0.2–0.4 IU/ml.

ii. For patients at risk of recurrent thrombosis: 0.4–0.6 IU/ml.

iii. Patients on HD >3x/week and/or <3 hours per session may be at risk of drug accumulation:

- Maintain the pre-dialysis trough level <0.1 IU/ml.

3. No anti-coagulation:

a. 0.9% saline flush every 30–60 minutes: Flushing volume is half of the ECV volume.

- Flushing volumes should be added to the UF volume.

b. Minimize clotting by:

- Pre-treating circuit with heparinized saline (5000 U/L) and flushing out the heparinized saline prior to connecting to the patient.
- Using vascular access of the largest possible diameter and higher blood flow.
- Adding higher prefilter replacement flow rates.

II. Reversal of anticoagulant effect

1. Management of anticoagulant-associated bleeding:

a. Hold further doses of anticoagulant.

b. Consider antidote.

c. Supportive treatment:

- Volume resuscitation and inotropes as needed.
- Transfusion (red cells, platelets, fresh frozen plasma) as indicated.

d. Local or surgical hemostatic measures including topical agents:

- Epsilon-aminocaproic acid (EACA).
- Tranexamic acid.
- Adrenaline.

2. Reversal of anticoagulant effect with protamine:
   a. Use depends on location and severity of bleeding.
   b. Dose:

Anticoagulant	Dosage of Protamine Sulfate	Monitoring for Reversal
Heparin	1 mg/100 U heparin. Based on administered heparin dose and elapsed time from the last heparin dose (heparin half-life is short at ~30–60 minutes).	Activated partial thromboplastin time (aPTT)
Enoxaparin given <8 hours	1 mg/100 units or 1 mg enoxaparin.	Anti-Xa activity
Enoxaparin given >8 hours	0.5 mg/100 units or 1 mg enoxaparin.	Anti-Xa activity

   c. Administration:
      - Slow intravenous infusion not >20 mg/min.
      - Infusion should not exceed 50 mg in any 10-minute period.
   d. Protamine is derived from fish sperm and has a small but potential risk of anaphylaxis in individuals who have previously been exposed:
      - Diabetic patients who have received protamine-containing insulin.
      - Patients with fish allergy.
3. Minimum duration of cessation of anticoagulant prior to surgery in HD patients:
   a. Heparin: At least 4–6 hours.
   b. Enoxaparin: At least 24–36 hours.

J. Investigations

1. Pre-dialysis:
   - Hemoglobin, hematocrit.
   - Urea, creatinine, sodium, potassium, bicarbonate, calcium, phosphate.
2. Post-dialysis (ideally should be done 30 minutes after stopping dialysis):
   - Hemoglobin, hematocrit.
   - Urea, creatinine.
   - Potassium (if high pre-dialysis).
3. Glucose monitoring in at-risk patients (young age, malnourished, diabetic): Pre-and post-HD, and during HD (1–2 hourly).

K. HD Duration Based on Urea Clearance

1. One-Compartment Model:

$$\frac{Kt}{V} = -\ln \frac{C_1}{C_0},$$

   where K = Dialyzer urea clearance at specific blood flow (ml/min)
   t = Time (min)
   V = Total body water (ml)
   C_1 = Post-dialysis urea levels
   C_0 = Pre-dialysis urea levels
2. Dialyzer urea clearance (K):
   a. The mass transfer area coefficient KoA is the theoretical maximum urea clearance at infinite blood and dialysate flow.
   Estimated dialyzer urea clearances (ml/min) at specific blood flow rates are shown, calculated based on manufacturers' KoA reduced by 25%, UF of 0 L/hour and dialysate flow of 500 ml/min, except for FX paed, which is 300 ml/min:

Dialyzer	KoA (urea) (ml/min)	Blood Flow (ml/min)								
		50	75	100	125	150	200	250	300	400
FX paed	170	40	52	**76**/60	—	—	—	—	—	—
FX CorDiax 40	547	45	67	88	107	124	**175**/151	170	—	—
Polyflux 6H	465	**50**/45	67	**97**/87	105	**136**/120	**167**/144	160	171	—
FX CorDiax 50	886	—	—	89	111	132	**191**/169	195	**255**/215	—
FX CorDiax 60	1164	—	—	—	—	133	**196**/174	205	**271**/229	**319**/263
Revaclear 300	1186	—	—	—	—	—	**196**/174	196/205	**272**/230	**323**/265
FX80	1292	—	—	—	—	—	**197**/175	208	**276**/234	270
Polyflux 170 H	1153	—	—	—	—	—	—	205	**270**/229	**321**/263
F4HPS	495	45	66	86	102	117	**170**/138	—	—	
F5HPS	606	—	67	88	106	122	**179**/148	165	**227**/177	—
F6HPS	746	—	—	—	109	127	**186**/157	177	**243**/192	213
F7HPS	789	—	—	—	—	128	**188**/159	180	**247**/196	218
F8HPS	848	—	—	—	—	—	**190**/162	184	**252**/201	**290**/224

Numerals in bold are urea clearances obtained in the manufacturer's *in vitro* testing.

3. Calculation of total body water (V):
   a. Watson formula (age >23 years):
      Male: V (L) = 2.447 – (0.09156*age) + (0.1074*Ht) + (0.3362*Wt)
      Female: V (L) = –2.097 + (0.1069*Ht) + (0.2466*Wt)
      Note: Wt = kg, Ht = cm
   b. Morgenstern equation (age ≤23 years):
      Boys: $V (L) = 0.10 \times (Ht*Wt)^{0.68} - 0.37 \times Wt$
      $V (L) = 20.88 \times BSA - 4.29$
      Girls: $V (L) = 0.14 \times (Ht*Wt)^{0.64} - 0.35 \times Wt$
      $V (L) = 16.92 \times BSA - 1.81$
      Note: BSA = body surface area in m^2
   c. Bioimpedance spectroscopy measures total body water composition (L) of various tissue compartments.
   d. Nomograms for estimation of V based on heavy water dilution method using the Morgenstern equation in Appendix 3.
4. Determination of desired urea reduction ratio:
   a. Aim to increase the urea reduction ratio gradually over 3–4 sessions (see the steps on how to prevent dialysis disequilibrium in chapter "Acute Complications in Hemodialysis").
   b. Calculation of $\ln(C_1/C_0)$:

Urea Reduction Ratio (%)	C_1/C_0	$\ln(C_1/C_0)$
90	0.1	–2.302
80	0.2	–1.609
70	0.3	–1.204
60	0.4	–0.916
50	0.5	–0.693
40	0.6	–0.511
30	0.7	–0.357
20	0.8	–0.223
10	0.9	–0.105

5. Calculation of HD duration:
   - Duration of HD (t) can be calculated using this equation.

$$\frac{Kt}{V} = -\ln \frac{C_1}{C_0}$$

   - Worked example:
     A 12 kg boy is scheduled for acute HD using an FX CorDiax 40. The blood flow is 50 ml/min and this is his first session. The target urea reduction ratio is 30%. The estimated time of HD required for his first dialysis is as follow:
     Weight = 12 kg, Height = 90.5 cm
     Total body water V = 7100 ml
     Dialyzer urea clearance K = 45 (for BF 50 ml/min)
     Kt/V = $-\ln C_1/C_0 = -\ln 0.7 = -0.357$
     t = 7100 – (–0.357) / 45 = 56 mins ~ **1 hour**
6. For the first few HD sessions, the pre- and post-dialysis urea levels should be measured to calculate the actual urea reduction ratio obtained.

Recommended Reading

1. Preka E, Shroff R. (2018) Hemodialysis. In: *Critical Care Nephrology and Renal Replacement Therapy in Children*. Edited by: Deep A, Goldstein SL. Springer. pp. 271–289.
2. Rees L. (2020, updated) Hemodialysis for children with chronic kidney disease. Edited by: Mattoo TK, Kim MS. *UpToDate ONLINE*. http://www.uptodateonline.com.
3. Kovalik EC. (2020) Anticoagulation for the hemodialysis procedure. Edited by: Schwab SJ, Motwani S. *UpToDate ONLINE*. http://www.uptodateonline.com.
4. Mailloux LU. (2020, updated) Dialysis disequilibrium syndrome. Edited by: Berns JS, Motwani S. *UpToDate ONLINE*. http://www.uptodateonline.com.

2 Hemodialysis Adequacy

Ng KH, Teo S, Liu ID, Todi VK and Yap HK

A. Criteria for Adequate Hemodialysis (HD)

1. Good control of fluid status, blood pressure, and cardiovascular health.
2. Good electrolyte and acid-base balance.
3. Good control of mineral bone disease.
4. Adequate growth and nutrition.
5. Good quality of life and achieved patient-centered outcomes.

B. Measures of HD Adequacy

1. Weekly Kt/V_{urea}:
   - Reflects small molecule clearance.
   - Kt/V_{urea} = Urea clearance × time normalized by total body water.
2. Urea reduction ratio (URR):
   - Fractional excretion of urea caused by dialysis.
3. Fluid status and dry weight.
4. Normalized protein catabolic rate (nPCR):
   - Takes into account both protein catabolic rate and protein losses.
   - Used to estimate dietary protein intake (DPI) in steady-state.

C. Urea Kinetic Modeling

1. Urea distribution and movement (concept of urea rebound):
   a. Urea is evenly distributed across a patient's total body water, in both intracellular and extracellular compartments

b. Urea is removed from the intravascular space during HD, with almost instantaneous equilibration between extravascular and intravascular components of the extracellular space.
c. Urea movement from intracellular to extracellular space is limited by cellular transport characteristics and occurs more slowly, lasting up to 1 hour after the end of HD.
d. This constitutes the phenomenon of serum urea rebound.

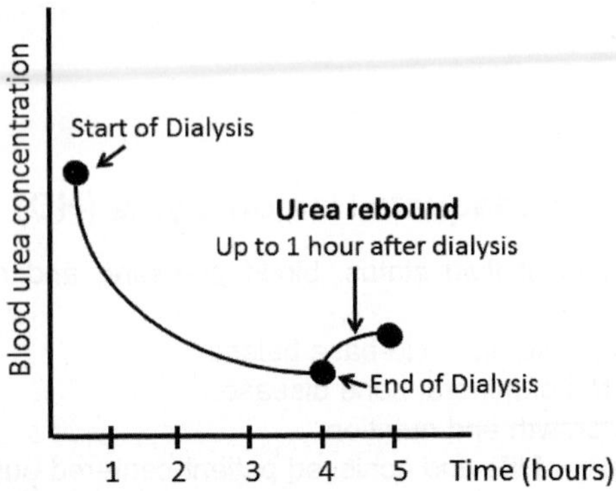

2. Urea generation:
   a. Urea steadily increases after HD due to protein intake.
   b. The amount of urea generated between dialysis treatments can be used to calculate the nPCR.

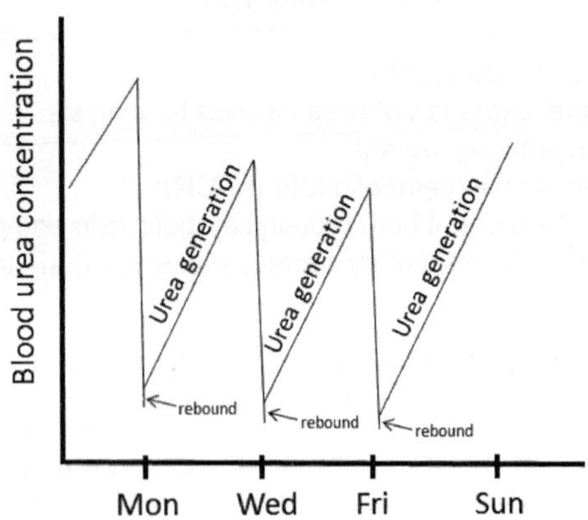

D. Measurement of HD Adequacy

I. Small solute clearance

1. Urea Reduction Ratio:
   a. $\text{URR}(\%) = \dfrac{(C_2 - C_1) \times 100}{C_2}$,

      where C_1 = Post-dialysis blood urea nitrogen (BUN) (mg/dL) or urea (mmol/L)
      C_2 = Pre-dialysis BUN (mg/dL) or urea (mmol/L)
   b. Does not take into account urea generation during dialysis, urea removed by convection, and contraction of total body water during dialysis.
2. Dialysis Kt/V_{urea}:
   a. Measures the fractional urea clearance.
      i. K_{urea} is the effective (delivered) dialyzer urea clearance in ml/min integrated over the entire dialysis duration.
      ii. t is the time in minutes measured from the beginning to the end of dialysis.
      iii. V_{urea} is the patient's volume of urea distribution in ml.
   b. Obtained by urea kinetic modeling and takes into account intradialytic urea generation, decrease in urea concentration during dialysis, and contraction of total body water during dialysis.
   c. Single pool Kt/V (spKt/V) based on single compartment kinetics (Daugirdas II formula):
      i. $\text{spKt/V} = -\ln\left(\dfrac{C_1}{C_2} - 0.008t\right) + \left[\left(4 - 3.5\dfrac{C_1}{C_2}\right)\left(\dfrac{UF}{W}\right)\right]$,

         where C_1 = Post-dialysis BUN (mg/dL) or urea (mmol/L)
         C_2 = Pre-dialysis BUN (mg/dL) or urea (mmol/L)
         t = Duration of dialysis session (hours)
         UF = Ultrafiltration volume (L)
         W = Post-dialysis weight (kg).
      ii. spKt/V does not take into account the urea rebound and hence tends to overestimate the true urea mass removed.
      iii. spKt/V should be measured during the mid-week dialysis session.

iv. Post-dialysis urea can be obtained immediately after dialysis by the following methods:
- Slow-Blood-Flow method:
  - Dialysate flow is turned off, and UF rate decreased to 50 ml/hour or off.
  - Decrease the blood flow to 100 ml/min for 15 seconds (longer if the blood line volume to the sampling port is >15 ml), to reduce the entry of dialyzed blood into the access in order to avoid cardiopulmonary and access recirculation.
  - The venous pressure limits may need to be adjusted downwards to prevent pump shut-off.
  - Either stop the blood pump or leave the blood flow at 100 ml/min while the sample is being drawn.
- Stop-Dialysate-Flow method (not validated in pediatrics):
  - Dialysate flow is turned off, and UF rate decreased to 50 ml/hour or off.
  - Wait 3 minutes without reducing blood flow rate.
  - Stop blood pump just prior to blood sampling.

d. Double-pool or equilibrated Kt/V (eKt/V) based on double compartment kinetics:

i. Ideally, calculate using Daugirdas II spKt/V formula using BUN obtained by a blood sample drawn at 1 hour after the end of the dialysis (BUN_{60min}).

ii. Alternative methods of calculation:
- Obtain blood samples immediately after dialysis for post-dialysis blood urea, calculate spKt/V as per Daugirdas II formula, and estimate eKt/v based on the following equation:

$$\text{Estimated epKt/V} = \text{spKt/V}\left(1-\frac{0.6}{t}\right)+0.03,$$

where t = duration of dialysis session (hours).

- Obtain blood samples at 15 minutes and 30 seconds, respectively, after termination of HD (BUN_{15min} and BUN_{30s}), and calculate the estimated BUN (estBUN):
  - $$estBUN = \left[\frac{(BUN_{15min} - BUN_{30s})}{0.69}\right] + BUN_{30S}.$$
  - estBUN is entered into the Daugirdas II equation to obtain eKt/V as shown below:

    $$eKt/V = -\ln\left(\frac{C_1}{C_2} - 0.008t\right) + \left[\left(4 - 3.5\frac{C_1}{C_2}\right)\left(\frac{UF}{W}\right)\right],$$

    where C_1 = estBUN (mg/dL)
    C_2 = Pre-dialysis serum BUN (mg/dL)
    t – Duration of dialysis session (hours)
    UF = Ultrafiltration volume (L)
    W = Post-dialysis weight (kg).

    Note: To convert blood urea (mmol/L) to BUN (mg/dL), multiple by 2.808.

e. Weekly standard Kt/Vurea (stdKt/V):
   i. Hypothetical continuous urea clearance that would achieve a constant blood urea concentration identical to the mean pre-dialysis urea concentration for a given HD session.
   ii. Normalizes and expresses the dose of HD independent of frequency, duration or modality of HD.
   iii. stdKt/V can be derived using the Leypoldt equation:

$$spKt/V = \frac{168\dfrac{1-e^{-e^{-eKt/V}}}{t}}{\dfrac{1-e^{-eKt/V}}{eKt/V} + \dfrac{168}{Nt} - 1},$$

where t = Dialysis duration in hours
N = The number of sessions per week
eKt/V is derived from Daugirdas II (estBUN as C1).

iv. stdKt/V in children can be estimated using the following table for a given spKt/V and dialysis frequency:

spKt/V	Frequency of Dialysis (Sessions per Week)					
	2x	3x	4x	5x	6x	7x
0.9	1.15	1.74	2.34	2.95	3.56	4.19
1.0	1.15	1.66	2.23	2.81	3.41	4.01
1.1	1.23	1.86	2.51	3.16	3.83	4.51
1.2	1.31	1.99	2.68	3.38	4.09	4.82
1.3	1.36	2.06	2.77	3.50	4.24	5.00
1.4	1.42	2.15	2.89	3.65	4.43	5.22
1.5	1.47	2.23	3.00	3.79	4.60	5.42
1.6	1.50	2.28	3.07	3.88	4.71	5.56
1.7	1.55	2.35	3.17	4.01	4.87	5.75
1.8	1.57	2.38	3.21	4.06	4.93	5.83
1.9	1.64	2.49	3.36	4.25	5.16	6.10
2.0	1.63	2.48	3.35	4.24	5.15	6.08

3. Correcting for residual kidney function:
   a. Patients with residual kidney function will require less HD compared to those with no residual kidney function.
   b. Residual kidney urea clearance (KRU):
      i. KRU is best measured with mid-week interdialytic urine collected from the end of one dialysis session to the beginning of the next dialysis session.
      ii. $$\text{KRU(ml/min)} = \frac{(U_{urea} * U_{vol})}{t[(P_{urea1} * 0.25) + (P_{urea2} * 0.75)]}$$
      where U_{urea} = Urine urea concentration (mmol/L)
      U_{vol} = Urine volume (ml)
      t = Duration of the interdialytic urine collection (min)
      P_{urea1} = Blood urea at beginning of urine collection (mmol/L)
      P_{urea2} = Blood urea at end of urine collection (mmol/L).
   c. Kr = KRU standardized to body surface area of $1.73m^2$.
      i. Patients with Kr ≥2 ml/min/$1.73m^2$ are considered to have significant residual kidney function.

ii. Dialysis Kt/V targets are lower in patients with significant residual kidney function.

II. Normalized protein catabolic rate (nPCR)

1. A measure of the amount of protein catabolized to yield the interdialytic urea generation rate.
2. Varies directly with Kt/V and used in conjunction with Kt/V to assess the adequacy of dialysis and dietary protein intake.
3. Reflects nutritional status more accurately than serum albumin at steady state, in the absence of protein catabolism or protein losses such as burns or urinary losses.
4. Patients with high catabolic rates due to infection, inflammation or malnutrition will have rapidly rising nPCR or nPCR >1.4 g/kg/day.
   - Consider this especially in the setting of weight loss and/or decline in serum albumin.
5. Calculation of the nPCR from the modified Borah equation:

$$\text{nPCR(g/kg/day)} = \left(5.43\frac{\text{estG}}{V_1}\right) + 0.17,$$

$$\text{estG} = \frac{(C_2 * V_2) - (C_1 * V_1)}{t},$$

where estG = urea generation rate (mg/min)

C_1 = Post-dialysis BUN (mg/dL)
C_2 = Pre-dialysis BUN (mg/dL)
V_1 = Post-dialysis TBW (dL) = 5.8*post-dialysis weight (kg)
V_2 = Pre-dialysis TBW (dL) = 5.8*post-dialysis weight (kg)
t = Time from end of dialysis to the beginning of next dialysis (min).
Note: To convert blood urea (mmol/L) to BUN (mg/dL), multiple by 2.808.

III. Optimization of fluid status

1. Dry weight:
   a. Definition: Post-dialysis weight at which the patient is euvolemic, below which there will be hypotension.
   b. Needs regular assessment in a growing child.

2. Methods to estimate dry weight are:
   a. Clinical and laboratory assessment:
      i. Jugular venous pressure (most accurate marker in absence of cardiac failure) and edema.
      ii. Trends in interdialytic weight gain, post-dialysis weight, and blood pressure.
      iii. Laboratory parameters such as hematocrit, albumin and sodium.
   b. Ultrasound-guided measurement of the supine inferior vena cava (IVC) diameter and their decrease upon deep inspiration:
      i. Collapse index (CI) = [(end-expiratory IVC diameter – end-inspiratory IVC diameter)/end-expiratory IVC diameter]*100
      ii. Shown to correlate with right atrial pressure and circulating blood volume.
      iii. Hypervolemia:
         - Mean right atrial pressure >7 mmHg.
         - IVC diameter >11.5 mm/m^2.
         - CI >0.75 (decrease in IVC diameter during inspiration <25% of the baseline diameter during expiration).
      iv. Hypovolemia:
         - Mean right atrial pressure <3 mmHg.
         - IVC diameter <8 mm/m^2.
         - CI <0.4 (decrease in IVC diameter during inspiration >60% of the baseline diameter during expiration).
      v. Problems:
         - Wide interpatient variability.
         - No pediatric normal standards.
         - Results are influenced by the timing of the measurement after dialysis and are difficult to interpret in patients with heart failure or tricuspid regurgitation.
   c. Bioelectric impedance:
      i. Allows accurate assessment of the patient's fluid status by measuring extracellular water (ECW), intracellular water (ICW), and total body water (TBW).
         - TBW = ECW + ICW
      ii. The difference between "normal" ECW and measured ECW is the overhydration volume.
         - Overhydration fluid is almost 100% extracellular.

iii. Parameters used to assess fluid status:

Parameter	Normal Reference Range
ECW/ICW	Dependent on age and gender
ECW/TBW (%)	Boys: 40.02 + 0.0714*age (years) Girls: 43.28 + 0.0470*age (years)
Absolute overhydration (L)	>10 years old: ± 1.1L <10 years old: Dependent on age and gender
Relative overhydration (%) $= \frac{\text{overhydration(L)}}{\text{ECW (L)}} \times 100\%$	± 7% (up to +15% before a dialysis session)

iv. Standard values are derived from the normal population rather than dialysis patients.
   - There is limited data on normal ranges in children.

d. Intradialytic non-invasive blood volume (hematocrit) monitoring (see chapter "Acute Complications in Hemodialysis").
e. Trends in N-terminal pro b-type natriuretic peptide (NT-pro BNP).

E. Timing of Assessment

1. Kt/V and nPCR should be assessed monthly in patients undergoing HD at least 3 times a week and 3 hours per session.
2. Kr should be assessed at least 3 monthly if:
   a. Kr is at least 2 ml/min/1.73m^2.
   b. HD dose is decreased because of residual kidney function.
   c. There is an acute change in urine output.
3. Dry weight assessment should be performed monthly, or if there are changes in the patient's clinical status:
   a. Hypotension or hypertension during dialysis.
   b. Symptomatic hypovolemia such as cramps.
   c. Recent acute illness.
   d. Malnutrition or poor dietary intake.

F. Adjustment of HD Prescription

1. Improving solute clearance (Kt/V):
   a. Optimize blood flow:
      i. Increasing effective blood flow rates has the biggest effect in increasing clearance.
      ii. Ensure appropriate catheter, needle sizes, and location.
      iii. Treat catheter dysfunction.
      iv. Decrease access recirculation.
   b. Dialyzer:
      i. Use a dialyzer with appropriate surface area.
      ii. Consider high flux dialyzers, which have higher urea clearances.
   c. Increase the dialysate flow rate.
   d. Optimize anticoagulation to decrease dialyzer clotting.
   e. Increase frequency and/or duration of each dialysis session.
   f. Evaluate dry weight as the patient may have gained weight.
   g. Evaluate post-dialysis blood sampling methods for blood urea testing.
      - Technical errors leading to a falsely low pre-dialysis blood urea or high post-dialysis blood urea may result in decreased Kt/V.
2. Optimize fluid control while avoiding intradialytic symptoms:
   a. Increase frequency of dialysis and/or duration of dialysis.
   b. Isolated UF and UF profiling with or without combined sodium profiling.
   c. Sodium profiling while avoiding high time-averaged dialysate sodium concentration.
   d. Non-invasive blood volume monitoring to allow maximal removal of fluid.
   e. Avoid excessive interdialytic weight gain with salt and water restriction.
   f. Loop diuretics can preserve urine output and improve fluid control.
   g. Judicious use of anti-hypertensive medications as this may result in intradialytic hypotension and inability to remove fluid.

3. Efforts should be made to minimize missed or shortened dialysis sessions.
4. Improving nutrition, including dietary protein intake (nPCR):
   a. Nutritional counseling.
   b. Adjust dialysis prescription to increase Kt/V.
   c. Consider intradialytic parenteral nutrition.
5. Improving cardiovascular outcomes (extrapolated from adult studies)
   a. Use of high flux dialyzers (instead of low flux).
   b. Optimal fluid status.
   c. Optimal phosphate control.

   Note: Increasing Kt/V urea *per se* above the target does not improve cardiovascular outcomes.

G. Targets for Adequate Dialysis

1. Children should receive at least the recommended dialysis dose for the adult population.
2. Younger children may require higher dialysis doses.
3. Recommendation for stdKt/V in children:
   a. Minimally adequate dose is 2.0.
   b. Target dose is 2.2.
4. For patients with Kr <2 ml/min/1.73m^2:
   a. Minimally adequate dose for thrice-weekly HD:
      - spKt/V >1.2 and eKt/V >1.03 per dialysis session.
      - Minimum URR for HD of <5 hours should be 65%.
   b. Target dose for thrice-weekly HD:
      - spKt/V in children and adolescents >1.4 and eKt/V >1.2 per dialysis session.
      - spKt/V in infants should be >2.
      - Target URR for HD of <5 hours should be 70%.
   c. Minimum HD duration for thrice-weekly HD should be at least 3 hours.
   d. Minimum dialysis spKt/V needed to achieve stdKt/V of 2.0 per week based on HD frequency and duration (assuming dialysis duration is constant, UF is 7 L/week, symmetric schedule) is shown in the table:

Kr <2 ml/min/1.73m²			
Sessions per Week	Dialysis Duration (hours)		
	2.0	3.5	8.0
2	—	—	3.00
3	—	1.22	1.06
4	0.87	0.77	0.68
5	0.64	0.57	0.51
6	0.51	0.45	0.40
7	0.42	0.38	0.34

Note: Target spKt/v should be at least 15% greater than the minimum dose.

e. High Kt/V may reflect adequate clearance or a low total body water volume related to malnutrition.

5. For patients with Kr ≥2 ml/min/1.73m²:
   a. Minimally adequate dose of dialysis can be reduced, but this may limit other potential benefits of HD, including salt and water control.
   b. Reduction of dialysis dose can be done using the following table.
      - The minimum dialysis spKt/V needed to achieve stdKt/V of 2.0 per week (assuming the dialysis duration is constant, UF is 7 L/week, symmetric schedule) is as shown:

Kr ≥2 ml/min/1.73m²			
Sessions per Week	Dialysis Duration (hours)		
	2.0	3.5	8.0
2	—	1.93	1.68
3	0.94	0.85	0.77
4	0.62	0.56	0.52
5	0.46	0.42	0.39
6	0.37	0.34	0.31
7	0.31	0.28	0.26

Note: Target spKt/V should be at least 15% greater than the minimum dose.

6. nPCR
   a. nPCR fluctuates rapidly in response to daily protein intake.
   b. The trend of nPCR over several months is more informative than single values.
      - Monthly nPCR allows for monitoring of trends in a particular patient.
   c. Adolescents and adults:
      - Target >1.4 g/kg/day.
      - Minimum >1.2 g/kg/day.
   d. In children, nPCR minimum targets follow the age-specific protein intake recommendations for HD patients.

Age	Protein Intake (g/kg/day)
0–6 months	1.60
7–12 months	1.40
1–3 years	1.15
4–13 years	1.05
>13 years	1.20

   e. nPCR should be interpreted together with Kt/V, especially in patients with low predialysis serum urea, to determine whether this is due to inadequate dialysis or poor protein intake.

H. Other Issues

1. Cardiovascular risk status:
   a. Regular monitoring of blood pressure with strict blood pressure control at the 50th centile for gender, height and age.
   b. Consider the use of high flux membranes to remove middle molecules.
   c. Avoid interdialytic weight gain of >5%.
   d. Dietary sodium intake per day should not be more than 5 g of sodium chloride.
   e. Echocardiograms yearly.
   f. Lipid monitoring yearly and consider statins or ezetimibe in lowering cholesterol levels.
   g. Monitoring of fasting glucose 6 monthly.

2. Special considerations:
   a. Patients with weight or body mass index <3rd centile or poor weight gain should have an increase in the minimally adequate dialysis dose and/or a change to a more frequent dialysis schedule.
   b. Patients with hyperphosphatemia or chronic fluid overload may benefit from more frequent dialysis schedule.
3. Quality of life issues:
   a. Cognitive development, school attendance, and performance are key issues to be monitored and may influence the choice of dialysis modality.
   b. Changing to a more frequent dialysis schedule in children may improve quality of life, quality of sleep, growth, sensitivity to erythropoietin, and decrease the need for phosphate binders.

Recommended Reading

1. National Kidney Foundation. (2006) KDOQI clinical practice guidelines and clinical practice recommendations for 2006 updates: Hemodialysis adequacy, peritoneal dialysis adequacy and vascular access. *Am J Kidney Dis* **48**(Suppl 1):S1–S322.
2. Cherry M, Stuart LG, Ruth M, Colin TW. (2010) Standard Kt/V thresholds to accurately predict single-pool Kt/V targets for children receiving thrice-weekly maintenance haemodialysis. *Nephrol Dial Transplant* **25**:3044–3050.
3. Benz MR, Schaefer F. (2012) Technical aspects of hemodialysis in children. In: *Pediatric Dialysis* 2nd edition. Edited by: Warady BA, Schaefer F, Alexander SR. pp. 287–311.
4. Preka E, Shroff R. (2018) Hemodialysis. In: *Critical Care Nephrology and Renal Replacement Therapy in Children*. Edited by: Deep A, Goldstein SL. Springer. pp. 271–289.
5. Qunibi WY. (2020, updated) Prescribing and assessing adequate hemodialysis. Edited by: Schwab SJ, Motwani S. *UpToDate ONLINE*. http://www.uptodateonline.com
6. Rees L. (2020, updated) Hemodialysis for children with chronic kidney disease. Edited by: Mattoo TK, Kim MS. *UpToDate ONLINE*. http://www.uptodateonline.com

3 Intra-Dialytic Parenteral Nutrition

Ng KH, Qader MA, Teo S and Yap HK

A. Indications for IDPN

1. Malnourished children on hemodialysis (HD) with body mass index (BMI)-for-height-age <5th percentile.
2. Unable to meet nutritional requirements through oral and tube feeding.
3. Three-month average serum albumin <34 g/L or normalized protein catabolic rate (nPCR) below age-specific limits.

Age	nPCR (g/kg/day)
0–6 months	1.60
7–12 months	1.40
1–3 years	1.15
4–13 years	1.05
>13 years	1.20

B. Contraindications

1. Hemodynamically unstable.
2. Excessive chronic fluid overload and heart failure.
3. Allergy to eggs, corn, sulfites, soy, and legumes because Intralipid 20% is derived from these ingredients.

C. Composition and Administration

1. Principles:
   a. The ideal weight of the patient should be used for calculations.

- The ideal weight is defined as the weight at the same percentile as the child's height percentile for the same age and gender.

b. Parenteral nutrition should be infused into the venous limb of the dialysis circuit to prevent clearance of amino acids and trace elements.

c. The volume of IDPN fluid should be added to the total ultrafiltration volume.

d. If the combination of enteral intake and IDPN is below the caloric and protein requirements, consider a daily total or partial parenteral nutrition.

2. Carbohydrate:
   a. Glucose infusion rate 5–9 mg/kg/min.
   b. **Aim to keep serum glucose 6–11 mmol/L.**
   c. Available dextrose preparations:

Preparation	Content	Infusion Rate
Dextrose 20%	20 g glucose/100 ml	1.5–2.7 ml/kg/hour
Dextrose 50%	50 g glucose/100 ml	0.6–1.08 ml/kg/hour

   d. Trace elements may be added to the dextrose solution.

3. Protein:
   a. Aim for recommended daily allowance of protein for age.
   b. Do not exceed 0.5–1.5 g/kg/session.
   c. Infuse over 3–4-hour dialysis period.
   d. Available amino acid preparations:

	Aminoplasmal 10% E		Vaminolact
Osmolarity (mOsm/L)	1030		510
Total amino acid (g/L)	100		65.3
Total nitrogen (g/L)	15.8		9.3
Caloric value (kcal/L)	400		240
Electrolytes (mmol/L)	Sodium	50	None
	Acetate	46	
	Potassium	25	
	Chloride	57	
	Magnesium	2.6	
	H_2PO_4	9.0	

4. Fat:
   a. Recommended lipid infusion rate ≤0.2–0.3 g/kg/hour.
   b. **Lipid infusion rate should not exceed 12.5 g/hour (62.5 ml/hour of Intralipid 20%).**
      Note: For total parenteral nutrition, daily lipid infusion should be administered over a minimum of 16 hours.
   c. Available preparation: 20% Intralipid infusion.
      - Intralipid volume should not be more than 25% of the combined volume of dextrose and amino acids.
      - Keep lipid infusion in a separate bottle from the dextrose and amino acid solutions.
      - For the first session of IDPN, start lipid infusion at 0.5 ml/kg/hour for 30 minutes. Observe and stop if adverse reactions occur.
      - If there are no reactions, infusion rate can be increased to 1.0 ml/kg/hour.
      - Too rapid infusion can lead to fluid and/or fat overload: Electrolyte abnormalities, overhydration, congested states, pulmonary edema, impaired pulmonary diffusion capacity, hyperketonemia, and/or metabolic acidosis.
      - Acute reactions: Dyspnea, nausea, vomiting, cyanosis, allergic reactions, hyperlipemia, hypercoagulability, headache, flushing, hyperthermia, sweating, chills, sleepiness, chest and back pain.
      - Delayed reactions: Hepatomegaly, cholestatic jaundice, splenomegaly, thrombocytopenia, leukopenia, transient transaminitis, and fat overload syndrome.

D. Monitoring

1. IDPN monitoring:

	Pre-treatment	Pre-HD after IDPN	Weekly
FBC	X		X
Urea, creatinine, sodium, potassium, chloride, bicarbonate, calcium, phosphate, magnesium	X	X	X
Liver panel	X		X
Triglycerides/cholesterol	X	X	X

2. Serum glucose monitoring:

During IDPN					
Time to measure serum glucose	0 minute	30 minutes	1.5 hours	2.5 hours	3.5 hours
After IDPN					
Time to measure serum glucose	15–30 minutes	1–2 hours if there are problems during IDPN			

E. Management of Complications

Complications	Parameter/Possible Cause	Management
Hyperglycemia	• If serum glucose >16 mmol/L.	• Decrease dextrose infusion rate by 2 mg/kg/min. • If serum glucose is still >16 mmol/L, start insulin and monitor serum glucose every 30 minutes. • Insulin starting dose: 5 units insulin (Actrapid) per 125 g dextrose or 4 units insulin (Actrapid) per 500 ml 20% dextrose. • Titrate dose with incremental doses of 2 units as needed.
Hypoglycemia	• If serum glucose <6 mmol/L 30 minutes before the end of HD.	• Give a snack of 15–30 g carbohydrate (1–2 slices of white bread or 2–4 biscuits or 120–240 ml of milo) near the end of the HD run. • Consider ending IDPN at the same time as HD. • Consider using glucose-containing dialysate in subsequent HD sessions.

(*Continued*)

Complications	Parameter/Possible Cause	Management
Electrolytes abnormalities associated with refeeding syndrome	• Hypophosphatemia. • Hypomagnesemia. • Hypokalemia.	• Routine monitoring of potassium, magnesium and phosphate. • Withold phosphate binders if hypophosphatemia persists. • Give supplements if needed.
Electrolyte abnormalities associated with ineffective HD	• Post-HD hyperkalemia due to IDPN with higher glucose driving potassium into the cells leading to ineffective potassium extraction.	• Monitor serum potassium on non-HD days and consider treatment of hyperkalemia if serum potassium ≥6 mmol/L.
Abnormal liver and lipid function	• Hepatic steatosis. • Hypertriglyceridemia. • Lipid intolerance is indicated by a 50% rise of serum triglyceride levels above baseline between 2 treatments.	• Avoid excessive lipid or carbohydrate intake. • Mandatory testing of liver and lipid function. • Control serum glucose. • Prescribe appropriate amount and infusion rates of macronutrients. • Discontinue lipid administration.
Respiratory distress	• Excessive carbohydrate load resulting in increased CO_2 production. • Too rapid infusion of IDPN. • Most likely to occur when glucose is the sole non-protein energy source (e.g., no lipid).	• Observation and evaluation of pulmonary status. • Provide dextrose and lipid in a 50:50 energy ratio. • Ensure patient's dry weight is achieved by the end of HD.
Painful arm cramps	• High osmolality IDPN solution • Too rapid infusion of IDPN	• Lengthen HD session. • Give infusion slowly. • Check osmolality of IDPN solution.

F. Criteria for Discontinuation

1. Improving nutrition:
   a. Adequate dry weight gain.
   b. Increase in oral intake to meet caloric and protein requirements.
2. No improvement in nutritional status after 4–6 months of IDPN.
3. Refractory complications or intolerance to IDPN.

G. Sample Calculation

Case example:
16-year-old boy: Patient dry weight (BW) 30 kg.

Carbohydrate calculations:
Rate (8 mg/kg/min) × BW (30 kg) × HD run time in minutes (180 min) = 43.2 g of carbohydrate = 216 ml Dextrose 20%

Protein calculations:
1.0 g protein/kg/day × BW (30 kg) = 30 g protein = 300 ml of Aminoplasmal 10%

Lipid calculations:
Rate (0.2 g/kg/hour) × BW (30 kg) × HD run time in hours (3 hr) = 18 g lipid = 90 ml Intralipid 20%
Combined carbohydrate and protein volume = 216 ml + 300 ml = 516 ml
Therefore, total lipid volume = 90/516 × 100% = 17.4% **(<25%)**
Lipid infusion rate should not exceed 62.5ml/hour

Final IDPN prescription:
IV Dextrose 20%: 216 ml (172.8 kcal)
IV Aminoplasmal 10%: 300 ml (120 kcal)
IV Intralipid 20%: 90 ml (162 kcal)
Total calories: 454.8 kcal per session.

Recommended Reading

1. IDPN Working Group. (2008) BC provincial guidelines. Intradialytic Parenteral Nutrition (IDPN).

2. KDOQI. (2009) KDOQI clinical practice guidelines for nutrition in children with chronic kidney disease: 2008 update. *Am J Kidney Dis* **53**(Suppl 2):S35–S47.
3. Rocco MV, Ikizler TA. (2015) Nutrition. In: *Handbook of Dialysis*, 5th edition. Edited by: Dauguirdas JT, Blake PG, Ing TS. Wolters Kluwer. pp. 535-554.
4. Shaw V, Polderman N, Renken-Terhaerdt J, Paglialonga F, Oosterveld M, Tuokkola J, Anderson C, Desloovere A, Greenbaum L, Haffner D, Nelms C, Qizalbash L, Vande Walle J, Warady B, Shroff R, Rees L. (2020) Energy and protein requirements for children with CKD stages 2–5 and on dialysis-clinical practice recommendations from the Pediatric Renal Nutrition Taskforce. *Pediatr Nephrol* **35**:519–531.

4 Acute Complications in Hemodialysis

Ng KH, Koh LJ, KT Ya, Liu ID and Yap HK

A. Intradialytic Hypotension

I. Pathophysiology:

1. Definition:
   a. Adults:
      - Decrease in systolic blood pressure (BP) ≥20 mmHg or a decrease in mean arterial pressure (MAP) by 10 mmHg, which is associated with clinical events and need for nursing interventions (National Kidney Foundation-Kidney Disease Outcomes Quality Initiative 2006).

   b. Children:
      - Symptomatic decrease in systolic BP according to the following table:

Age	Systolic BP (mmHg)
Term neonates: 0–28 days	<60
Infants: 1–12 months	<70
Children: 1–10 years	<70 + (age in years x 2)
Children: >10 years	<90

2. Implication:
   - Dialysis treatment is less effective when complicated by hypotension since treatments may be stopped early and the target weight may not be achieved.

3. Etiology:
   a. Dialysis-related factors:
      i. Patient:
         - Excessive interdialytic weight gain (>3% of body weight).
         - Incorrect dry weight calculation.
         - Antihypertensive or other medications that lower BP before dialysis.
         - Intradialytic food consumption.
      ii. Dialyzer and circuit:
         - Blood and dialyzer membrane reactions.
         - Too large extracorporeal volume (>10%).
         - Too rapid ultrafiltration (UF) rate (inadequate vascular refilling).
         - Too rapid blood flow rate.
         - Use of citrate anticoagulant.
      iii. Dialysate:
         - Acetate dialysate.
         - Low sodium dialysate.
         - High dialysate temperature.
   b. Cardiac dysfunction:
      i. Left ventricular hypertrophy.
      ii. Diastolic dysfunction.
      iii. Arrhythmia.
      iv. Pericardial tamponade.
      v. Myocardial infarction.
      vi. Air embolism.
   c. Sepsis.
   d. Severe hemorrhage:
      i. Gastrointestinal bleed.
      ii. Blood line disconnection.
   e. Electrolyte abnormalities, including acidosis.
   f. Autonomic neuropathy:
      - Downregulation of α-adrenergic receptors, which diminishes the hemodynamic response to endogenous catecholamines during UF.
   g. Anaphylaxis.

II. Clinical evaluation:

1. Presenting symptoms:
   a. Cramps.
   b. Dizziness and excessive fatigue.
   c. Nausea and vomiting.
   d. Dyspnea.
   e. Vagal symptoms, including yawning, sighing and hoarseness.
2. Exclude serious causes of intradialytic hypotension, including:
   a. Hemolysis: Port-wine appearance of blood in the venous line.
   b. Dialyzer reaction: Chest pain, back pain, and allergic symptoms such as urticaria, flushing, coughing and wheezing.
   c. Air embolus: Characteristic heart sounds.

III. Acute management:

1. Decrease or stop UF depending on the severity of hypotension.
2. Decrease the blood flow rate.
3. Place the patient in a Trendelenburg position.
4. Give the patient oxygen.
5. Give intravenous (IV) 0.9% saline or 5% albumin 10 ml/kg.
6. Consider dopamine infusion if dialysis is to be continued.
7. Stop dialysis if the patient is refractory to initial management.
8. Treat intradialytic hypocalcemia.
9. If recurrent, consider midodrine:
   - Dose: 0.06 mg/kg (adult: 2.5 mg).
   - May be repeated if BP does not increase in 30 minutes or systolic BP decreases to <75 mmHg.
   - Maximum cumulative dose 7.5 mg per 3-hour hemodialysis (HD) session.
   - Avoid in the last 30 minutes of dialysis.
10. Investigate for possible causes:
    a. Examine HD access for evidence of infection.
    b. Urgent ECG to exclude acute myocardial infarction and pulmonary embolism.

IV. *Prevention of recurrent episodes*

1. Step 1:
   a. Avoid antihypertensive medications before dialysis:
      - Take once daily medications at night.
      - Try to avoid antihypertensive drugs that require twice or more daily dosing.

   b. Avoid food during dialysis.
      - Ingestion of food results in a drop in peripheral vascular resistance 20–120 minutes later.

   c. Reassess target dry weight.

   d. Avoid excessive interdialytic weight gain by restricting salt and fluid intake:
      - High sodium intake results in thirst and larger fluid volume gain, which needs to be removed by UF during each dialysis session.
      - A rapid UF rate to attain target dry weight by the end of the HD session can result in intradialytic hypotension.

   e. Correct anemia.

   f. Consider use of compression stockings for lower limbs.

2. Step 2:
   a. Review dialysis prescription:
      i. Decrease UF rate.
         - High UF rates defined as UF volume per session >5% of post-dialysis weight or >13 ml/kg/hr have been associated with increased cardiovascular mortality risk in HD patients.

      ii. Isolated UF (iso-UF) or sequential UF-HD.
         - Iso-UF has been shown to preserve plasma volume by maintaining high plasma refilling rate, mediated by a rapid rise in oncotic pressure.
         - This mechanism contributes to the good tolerance of sequential ultrafiltration-HD (SUFH).

      iii. Additional dialysis sessions per week or a longer dialysis time.

      iv. Consider hemodiafiltration.

   b. Review dialysate composition:
      i. Use bicarbonate dialysate instead of acetate dialysate.

ii. Sudden decline in plasma potassium and calcium due to alkalosis can lead to intradialytic vascular and cardiac instability.
    - Use normal calcium (≥1.5 mmol/L) dialysate, especially in an acute setting in patients with cardiac disease.

c. Consider intradialytic non-invasive blood volume monitoring:
   i. Allows real-time monitoring of the patient's intravascular blood volume (x-axis: time; y-axis: percent blood volume change or hematocrit), facilitating interventions during the dialysis treatment.
   ii. UF rate is too slow:

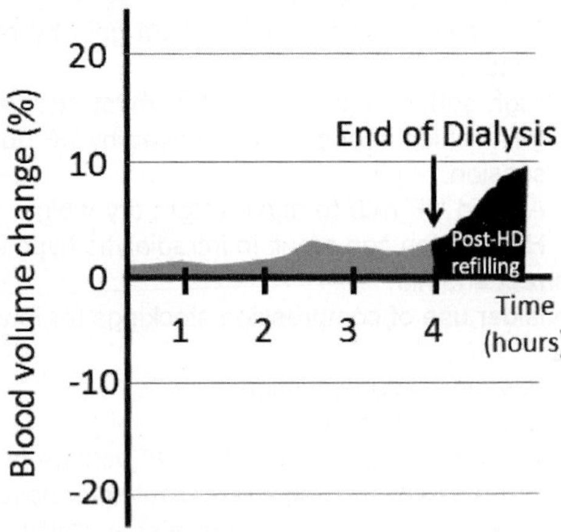

- Features suggesting that the patient's vascular refilling rate is occurring faster or at the same rate as the UF rate, implying that the current UF rate can be increased:
  - An increase in % of blood volume.
  - A decrease in hematocrit.
  - A flat slope.
  - Increase in hematocrit is <3% per hour.
- A steep slope of post-dialysis refilling (hematocrit decreases >0.5% or blood volume increases >1.5%) suggests the need to lower the post-dialysis weight.

iii. Optimal UF rate:

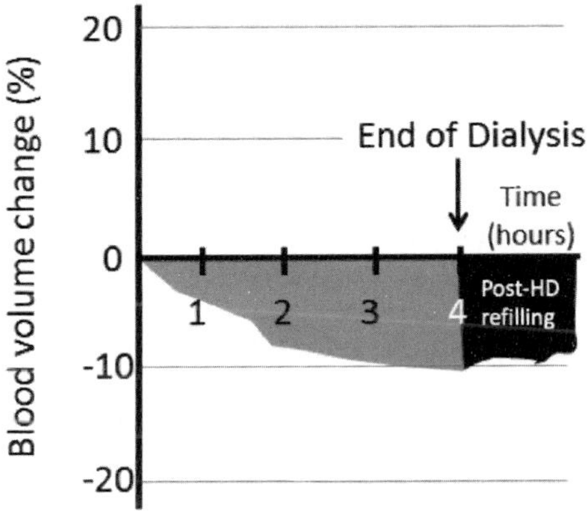

- A gradual decline in blood volume (3–8% per hour) or a gradual increase in hematocrit is ideal.
- Absence of or minimal post-dialysis refilling will imply that the patient is likely at dry weight.

iv. UF rate is too rapid:

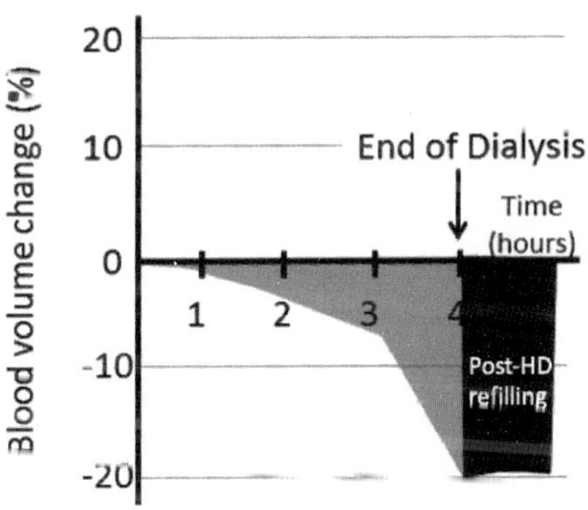

- Features suggesting a rapid decrease in blood volume and the patient is at risk for intradialytic symptoms, implying that the current UF rate should be decreased:
  - Rapid decrease in blood volume (>8% per hour).
  - Rapid increase in hematocrit despite a constant UF rate.
- "Crash" hematocrit: Hematocrit level at which blood volume change is >10% in 3 hours.
- The absence of post-dialysis refilling will also imply that the patient is likely below dry weight.

v. When setting up, set the hematocrit as 2 hematocrit units above the starting level.
- This limit may be increased 1 unit at a time with subsequent sessions if the patient is asymptomatic.

vi. Threshold for intradialytic symptoms varies between patients, depending on their cardiovascular status and other comorbidities but can be predictable within a patient.
- The relative blood volume threshold for each patient can be determined via trial and error over time.
- In general, blood volume percent change during dialysis should be ≤8% at the end of the first hour, and ≤4% per hour in subsequent hours, with a maximum overall change of 16% at the end of 4 hours.

vii. Hematocrit monitoring may be unreliable if the circuit is primed with blood or if there is intradialytic blood transfusion or active bleeding.

viii. Intradialytic noninvasive blood volume monitoring may guide UF profiling.

d. Consider sodium profiling in which dialysate sodium concentration is decreased in a step or linear manner:

i. For example, start with dialysate sodium 148 mmol/L and decrease in a linear or step manner to 138 mmol/L.
- Linear profiling: Steady decline of sodium throughout the session until the end.
- Step profiling: Initial sodium concentration is kept constant until 30 minutes before the end when sodium is decreased to final level.
- Step profiles are better in reducing intradialytic hypotension in children.

   ii. Use a sodium-neutral profile where time-averaged dialysate sodium concentration is kept at 138 mmol/L to reduce positive sodium balance and the consequence of increased thirst and interdialytic weight gain.
   iii. High dialysate sodium at the beginning causes diffusive sodium influx to counteract the initial decrease in plasma osmolarity, thus promoting vascular refilling.
   iv. Low dialysate sodium at the end allows the diffusive clearance of sodium load, decreasing the adverse effects of hypertonicity, namely hypertension and thirst.
 e. Consider different dry weight on different days:
   - Monday: Target 0.5 kg above dry weight.
   - Wednesday: Target dry weight.
   - Friday: Target 0.5 kg below dry weight.

3. Step 3:
 a. Assess for primary cardiac risk factors for intradialytic hypotension, including carnitine deficiency:
   - Consider IV L-carnitine 20 mg/kg into the dialysis venous port with each HD if there is carnitine deficiency.
 b. Decrease the dialysate temperature to increase hemodynamic stability:
   i. Empiric fixed reductions of dialysate temperature:
     - Reduce the dialysate temperature to 0.5–1.0°C below the patient's body temperature, lowering the temperature up to ~1°C.
     - Dialysate temperatures should not drop below 35°C.
     - Unacceptable side effects include chilling or cramping.
   ii. Isothermic dialysis using a biofeedback temperature-controlled device that cools the dialysate temperature, preventing a further increase in the patient's core temperature.
 c. Use of midodrine (selective α1-adrenergic agonist), especially if there is BP instability that is responsive to vasopressors:
   i. Consider in autonomic neuropathy or severe HD hypotension not responsive to the above.
   ii. Dose: Oral 0.06 mg/kg given 30 minutes predialysis.
     - The dose may be increased slowly in subsequent sessions to a maximum of 0.2 mg/kg (maximum 2.5 mg).
     - The dose may be repeated in the same session (maximum cumulative 7.5 mg per 3-hour HD session).

   iii. Contraindicated in patients with severe heart disease, uncontrolled hypertension, urinary retention, use of β-blockers, digoxin, and non-dihydropyridine calcium channel blockers.
   iv. Tachyphylaxis may occur.

d. Use of mannitol, especially if there is hypo-osmolality:
   - 1 g/kg in the first hour of the first dialysis session of the week, or 0.5 g/kg two times per week.

B. Cramps

I. Pathophysiology:

1. Definition:
   - Prolonged involuntary muscle contraction that occurs in a muscle that voluntarily contracts when it is already in its most shortened position.
2. Implication:
   - Often results in early termination of therapy with resultant underdialysis.
3. Etiology:
   a. Hypotension with blood volume contraction.
   b. Changes in plasma osmolarity.
   c. Hyponatremia.
   d. Tissue hypoxia.
   e. Hypomagnesemia.
   f. Hypocalcemia.
   g. Carnitine deficiency.
   h. Elevated serum leptin levels.

II. Clinical evaluation:

1. Commonly affecting the lower limbs.
2. Tend to occur most frequently towards the end of HD treatments:
   - Implying changes in plasma osmolarity and/or extracellular fluid volume as the underlying cause.
3. Check for intradialytic hypotension.

4. Check if UF is excessive:
   - UF >13 ml/kg/hr.
5. Check serum ionized calcium and magnesium levels.
6. Check sodium concentration of dialysate bath, in particular, low sodium concentrations.

III. Treatment of cramps during HD:

1. Treatment of patients with intradialytic hypotension:
   a. Decrease or stop the UF rate.
   b. Reduce blood flow rate.
   c. Place the patient in Trendelenburg position.
   d. IV 0.9% saline bolus 10 ml/kg.
   e. Address underlying cause of intradialytic hypotension.
2. Increase serum osmolarity by IV administration of:
   a. 50% dextrose 1 ml/kg (maximum 50 ml) (not recommended in diabetics) OR
   b. 20% mannitol 0.2–0.5 g/kg infusion (maximum 12.5–37.5 g) during the first 2 hours only, as it may accumulate if given near the end of dialysis.
3. Correct abnormalities in serum calcium, magnesium and phosphate.
4. Local therapy:
   a. Warm compress.
   b. Massaging the lower limbs.

IV. Prevention of recurrent cramps:

1. Minimize interdialytic weight gain:
   - Minimizes plasma volume contraction and hypoosmolarity that occurs with high rates of UF.
2. Prevention of dialysis-associated hypotension:
   a. Sequential UF-HD.
   b. Sodium profiling.
   c. Infusion of mannitol or dextrose to prevent hypotension during a dialysis session.

d. Oral salt supplementation:
    - May result in increased thirst and increase in interdialytic fluid gains.
3. Carnitine supplementation:
    a. IV infusion 20 mg/kg thrice weekly after HD.
    b. Oral carnitine should not be used for the following reasons:
        - Limited bioavailability requiring high oral doses.
        - Toxic metabolites, generated by intestinal metabolism accumulate between dialysis sessions.
4. Other prophylactic agents:
    a. Nifedipine: 0.25–0.5 mg/kg/dose (maximum 10 mg) per dialysis session.
    b. Vitamin E: 25–50 IU/kg nightly (maximum 400 IU).
    c. Gabapentin: 5–10 mg/kg every 48 hours on dialysis days, plus a top-up after HD (maximum 900 mg/day).
    d. Benzodiazepines.

    Note: The USA Food and Drug Administration's (FDA) warning against quinine sulfate for this indication is due to the risk of severe side effects, including cardiac arrhythmias, severe allergic reactions, and thrombotic thrombocytopenic purpura-hemolytic uremic syndrome (TTP-HUS).

C. Central Nervous System-Related Symptoms

I. Headache, nausea and vomiting:

1. HD-associated headaches defined by at least 3 acute headaches meeting at least 2 criteria of:
    a. Headache developing during HD.
    b. Headache relieved within 72 hours after HD.
    c. Headache episodes cease after transplantation and cessation of HD.
2. Etiology:
    a. Hypertension:
        - Intradialytic hypertension is defined as an increase in MAP of ≥15 mmHg during or after HD, or an increase in SBP of >10 mmHg from predialysis to post-dialysis.

   b. Hypotension.
   c. Metabolic disturbances:
      - Hypoglycemia.
      - Hypernatremia.
      - Hyponatremia.
      - Hypocalcemia.
   d. Dialysis disequilibrium syndrome.
   e. Uremic encephalopathy.
   f. Caffeine use.
   g. Medication-induced.
   h. Raised intraocular pressure.
3. Clinical evaluation:
   a. History of caffeine ingestion.
   b. Medication history, in particular, calcium channel blockers and erythropoietin (EPO) dose.
   c. Check BP profile during dialysis and its relation to UF rate:
      - Excessive UF rate can result in sympathetic overactivation leading to a rise in BP.
   d. Check blood glucose.
   e. Check electrolytes, in particular, sodium.
   f. Review dialysis prescription for risk of dialysis disequilibrium (see chapter "Hemodialysis Orders").
4 Acute treatment of headache:
   a. Symptomatic treatment of headaches with analgesics.
   b. Control of intradialytic hypertension:
      i. Oral nifedipine 0.25–0.5 mg/kg/dose (maximum 10 mg).
      ii. Consider serving antihypertensives if these have been withheld.
      iii. Angiotensin-converting enzyme (ACE) inhibitors (intradialytic hypertension can be due to inappropriate renin secretion).
      iv. More frequent HD: Restrict fluid removal to <4% of body weight per session.
5. Management of recurrent headaches:
   a. Correct underlying triggering factors.
   b. Modify dialysis prescription to be less intensive and more frequent.
   c. Prevention of intradialytic hypertension:

i. Restrict fluid and salt intake to avoid high interdialytic weight gain.
ii. Avoid antihypertensive drugs before dialysis as this may limit the rate of fluid removal.
iii. Avoid eating during dialysis.
iv. Correct anemia, slowly attaining target hemoglobin.
v. Reassess the patient's dry weight, blood flow rate, and UF rate.
vi. Consider the use of lower sodium dialysate (5 mmol/L below the predialysis serum sodium):
   - Avoid sodium profiling with high amounts of sodium dialysate.
vii. Consider increasing the dialysate temperature.
viii. Consider an additional dialysis session or a longer dialysis time.
ix. Optimize antihypertensive drug therapy if the dry weight is achieved and the patient is still hypertensive:
   - Carvedilol is useful for reflex sympathetic overactivation due to hypovolemia.
   - Calcium channel blockers and angiotensin receptor blockers are useful in left ventricular hypertrophy and diastolic dysfunction and are not dialyzable.
   - ACE inhibitors are removed by HD, but they are useful in renin-dependent intradialytic hypertension.

II. HD-associated seizures:

1. Definition:
   a. Seizures occurring during dialysis or within 12 to 24 hours of the dialysis procedure.
   b. Children have higher incidence of seizures than adults.
   c. Occurs more commonly in acute HD patients than those on chronic HD.
2. Etiology:
   a. Uremic encephalopathy.
   b. Dialysis disequilibrium syndrome:

- Reverse urea effect: Rapid urea clearance in HD creates an osmotic driving force that causes water to move into the brain.
- Idiogenic osmoles: Presence of other osmotically active substances in the brain.
- Paradoxical intracerebral acidosis: Rapid correction of metabolic acidosis causes secondary hypoventilation and rise in blood carbon dioxide, which diffuses into the cerebrospinal fluid more rapidly than serum bicarbonate, causing paradoxical acidemia in the brain and a cerebral edema and, subsequently, increase in brain water content.

c. Electrolyte and metabolic disorders:
  - Hyponatremia.
  - Hypernatremia.
  - Hypocalcemia.
  - Hypercalcemia.
  - Hypoglycemia.
  - Hyperglycemia.

d. Hypoxemia.

e. Hemodynamic instability: Rapid onset of hypotension or hypertensive encephalopathy.

f. Arterial air embolism through a patent foramen ovale or pulmonary circuit.

g. Rapid transfusion.

h. Drugs:
  - EPO due to a rapid rise in BP.
  - Imipenem.
  - Ertapenem.

i. Heparinization in the presence of intracranial bleeding.

j. Removal of anticonvulsant in patients with epilepsy:
  - Phenobarbitone (significant).
  - Gabapentin (significant).
  - Topiramate (significant).
  - Levetiracetam (significant).
  - Lamotrigine (partial).

k. Epileptogenic drugs requiring dose reduction:
  - Penicillin and cephalosporin.
  - Ciprofloxacin.
  - Meperidine (toxic metabolite normeperidine) — avoid entirely.

- Ethanol.
- Theophylline.
- Cyclosporin.
- Amantadine.
- Acyclovir.
- Aluminum-containing antacids.
- High doses of intravenous contrast agents.

l. Star-fruit ingestion.

3. Clinical evaluation:
   a. Obtain seizure history.
   b. Obtain drug history and use of epileptogenic drugs, as well as dialysable anticonvulsants.
   c. Check BP during dialysis.
   d. Check urea reduction ratio, serum sodium, calcium, magnesium, glucose, and acid-base status.
   e. Review dialysis prescription for the risk of dialysis disequilibrium (see chapter “Hemodialysis Orders”).
   f. Preemptive surveillance for seizures for 12–24 hours after HD in patients at increased risk.
   g. Consider the following investigations:
      - Diffusion-weighted MRI brain.
      - Electroencephalography.
4. Predialysis intervention to prevent seizures involves recognition and amelioration of the following risk factors:
   a. Uremic encephalopathy:
      - Initiate dialysis earlier.
      - Consider prophylactic anticonvulsants in high-risk patients, especially if blood urea ≥60 mmol/L with either phenobarbitone or phenytoin.
   b. Rapid acid-base and osmolarity changes with dialysis:
      - Treat severe predialysis hypocalcemia before correcting severe acidosis with dialysis.
   c. Hypoxia secondary to volume overload or underlying cardiac or pulmonary disease:
      - Ensure oxygen saturation is satisfactory.
      - Treat arrhythmias and stabilize patients with cardiac disease.

d. Hypotension and hemodynamic instability:
   - Consider peritoneal dialysis or continuous venovenous hemodiafiltration in high-risk patients with hemodynamic instability.

e. Anticoagulation in the presence of intracranial bleeding:
   - Reduce heparin or consider heparin-free dialysis.

f. Removal of anticonvulsant medications during dialysis:
   - Adjust doses post-dialysis and monitor therapeutic levels.

g. Hypertensive crisis, which may be induced by EPO therapy:
   - Limit the initial dose of EPO to 150 U/kg/week.
   - Consider subcutaneous dosing as IV dose may stimulate the release of endothelin-1, a potent vasoconstrictor.
   - Withhold initiating EPO therapy in patients with severe uncontrolled hypertension.

5. Treatment of seizures:
   a. Reduce the blood flow rate and avoid rapid or severe reductions in BP.
   b. Resuscitative measures include:
      - Securing the airway.
      - Administering supplemental oxygen.
   c. Consider stopping the dialysis session.
   d. Seizure control with IV lorazepam 0.05–0.1 mg/kg/dose.

6. Treatment of dialysis disequilibrium:
   a. Mild symptoms:
      i. Initiate sodium modeling or increase sodium in dialysate (see chapter "Hemodialysis Orders").
      ii. Stop HD if there is no clinical response in 30 minutes.
   b. Moderate/severe symptoms or mild cases refractory to initial treatment, increase serum osmolarity by either:
      i. IV 20% mannitol 0.25–1 g/kg (= 1.25–5 ml/kg) (maximum 62 ml = 12.5 g) over 1–2 hours, or
      ii. IV 3% NaCl 3–5 ml/kg over 60 minutes, or
      iii. IV 50% dextrose 1 ml/kg (maximum 50 ml) slow bolus (not recommended in diabetics).
   c. If hypertonic saline or mannitol has been given, stop dialysis and plan for slow low-efficiency, daily dialysis sessions.

D. Chest Pain

I. Etiology:

1. Hypotension.
2. Dialysis disequilibrium syndrome.
3. Angina.
4. Musculoskeletal cause.
5. Pulmonary embolism:
   - May occur after manipulation of a catheter-related thrombus and/or occlusion of the dialysis access.
6. Dialyzer reaction.
7. Hemolysis:
   a. Access problems:
      - Use of subclavian catheter.
      - Mismatch in blood flow rate and access size.

   b. Hypotonicity:
      - Due to an insufficient concentrate:water ratio.

   c. Overheated dialysate:
      - Temperature >42°C.

   d. Contamination with oxidizing agents:
      - Formaldehyde.
      - Bleach.
      - Chloramine or nitrates from the water supply.
      - Copper from copper tubing or piping.

   e. Dialysis machine and tubing:
      - Malfunctioning blood pump.
      - Arterial line collapse.
      - Kinked or obstructed tubing.
      - Manufacturing defects in tubing.
      - Contamination of tubing.
8. Air embolism with air entering the system mainly from the pre-pump section where there is a negative pressure system:
   a. Accidental disconnection of the HD catheter.
   b. Dislodgement of the arterial needle in arteriovenous fistulae or grafts.
   c. Air entry during the connection or disconnection of the dialysis circuit.

d. Loose connectors.
e. Defects in the HD catheter or tubing (pre-pump arterial segment).
f. During infusions into the dialysis circuit.
g. Fluid level in the venous chamber becomes too low.

II. Clinical evaluation:

1. Evaluate the nature of chest pain:
   a. Localized tenderness suggesting a musculoskeletal cause.
   b. Pain upon deep breathing, which suggests pleurisy.
   c. Retrosternal chest pain radiating to the left arm and jaw, which suggests angina.
   d. Accompanying dyspnea may suggest more serious problems including:
      - Acute myocardial infarction.
      - Dialysis disequilibrium.
      - Pulmonary embolism.
      - Acute hemolysis.
      - Air embolism.
2. Review vital signs, including heart rate, blood pressure, respiratory rate, and oxygen saturation.
3. Cardiac assessment including:
   a. History of exercise-induced chest discomfort.
   b. Looking for predisposing causes for pulmonary embolism.
   c. Reviewing records for pre-existing cardiac disease, including previous echocardiogram.
   d. Cardiac examination looking for:
      - Cardiomegaly.
      - Arrhythmias.
      - Abnormal heart sounds.
      - Pericardial effusion.
      - Cardiac failure.
   e. Electrocardiogram.
   f. Cardiac enzymes:
      - Creatine kinase MB fraction (CKMB).
      - Troponin-I.

   g. Consider referral to a pediatric cardiologist for an echocardiogram and stress testing if symptoms persist, are recurrent, or associated with recurrent intradialytic hypotension preventing the attainment of dry weight.
4. Exclude hemolysis:
   a. Complaints of chest pain, dyspnea and/or back pain.
   b. Port-wine appearance of the blood in the venous line.
   c. Pink color in the plasma in centrifuged specimens.
   d. Check full blood count, potassium, haptoglobin, lactate dehydrogenase (LDH), and bilirubin:
      - Acute decrease in hemoglobin.
      - Elevated free plasma hemoglobin.
      - Elevated serum lactate dehydrogenase.
      - Low serum haptoglobin.
      - Increase in plasma bilirubin.
      - Hyperkalemia.
   e. Intradialytic blood volume monitoring may reveal an increase in blood volume due to the decrease in hematocrit and release of water from hemolyzed cells.
   f. Review drug history and check for glucose-6-phosphate dehydrogenase (G6PD) deficiency.
5. Exclude air embolism:
   a. Severity of presenting symptoms depends on:
      - Amount and rate of air introduced.
      - Position of the patient, affecting the final location of the air embolus.
   b. Chest pain and dyspnea.
   c. Cardiovascular collapse:
      - May have an initial brief increase in cardiac output and blood pressure due to tachycardia.
      - This is followed by a decrease in cardiac output, hypotension and tachypnea.
   d. Foam in venous blood line.
   e. Seated patients:
      - Infused air tends to migrate into the cerebral venous system.
      - Results in altered level of consciousness, seizures or neurological deficits.

f. Recumbent patients:
   - Large air embolism may enter the heart, generating foam in the right ventricle, leading to a mill wheel murmur (loud churning sound throughout the cardiac cycle) along the left sternal border or arrhythmias.
   - The blood-air interface may activate the clotting cascade and release vasoactive substances to cause bronchospasm, pulmonary vasoconstriction, and non-cardiogenic pulmonary edema.

III. Management of chest pain during dialysis:

1. The decision to continue or stop HD because of chest pain depends on the underlying etiology and hemodynamic stability. If dialysis is continued:
   a. Administer supplemental oxygen.
   b. Reduce UF and/or blood pump speed.
   c. Consider administration of glyceryl trinitrate (GTN) if angina is suspected:
      - Administer sublingual GTN 0.5 mg single dose.
      - Terminate dialysis if there is no relief of pain in 5–10 minutes and refer the patient to a pediatric cardiologist for an evaluation.
   d. Consider use of nitrates and/or beta-blockers prior to HD to prevent angina; however, this may result in reduced dialysis efficacy due to hypotension.
2. Air embolus:
   a. Clamp the venous blood line and stop the blood pump to prevent further air infusion into the circulation.
   b. Place the patient in Trendelenburg position with his left side down to force air into the right ventricular apex where it is less likely to embolize, allowing blood flow into the pulmonary circulation.
   c. Perform resuscitation as required and administer 100% oxygen.
   d. Consider aspirating the air if a dialysis catheter is used.
   e. If there is a large air embolus in the heart, consider aspiration of air from the atrium or ventricle with a percutaneous inserted cardiac needle or cardiac catheterization.

3. Hemolysis:
   a. Stop dialysis immediately and do not return the blood.
   b. Resuscitation if necessary.
   c. Treat hyperkalemia and severe anemia if necessary.
   d. Investigate for etiology:
      i. Review blood flow rates and dialysate temperature.
      ii. Do not discard dialyzer and tubing to aid in investigations for manufacturing defects and kinking of tubing.
      iii. Check composition of dialysate (e.g., hypotonic dialysate).
      iv. If hemolysis is present in other patients:
         - Check for contamination of the water supply by trace elements and other chemicals (such as copper, zinc, lead, sulfates, and nitrates, chlorine and chloramine).
         - Consider manufacturer defects in the dialyzers or tubing.
      v. Use a different HD machine and water treatment for the next session.

E. Arrhythmias

I. Pathophysiology:

1. Cardiac rhythm disturbances are common in dialysis:
   - Ventricular and atrial ectopy.
   - Conduction abnormalities including first-degree atrioventricular block and bundle branch block.
   - Supraventricular tachycardias.
2. Proarrhythmic nature of the HD process:
   - Large or rapid alterations in extracellular fluid volume and electrolyte composition.
   - Risk of hypoxemia and hypotension.
3. High burden of structural heart disease in the dialysis population:
   - Left ventricular hypertrophy.
   - Myocardial ischemia.
   - Myocardial dysfunction.
4. Underlying autonomic dysfunction predisposes to arrhythmias.

II. Clinical evaluation:

1. Identify the type of arrhythmia on ECG.
2. Check for hemodynamic stability.
3. Look for factors that may precipitate arrhythmias:
   a. Acute volume shifts:
      - Check that UF rate is not excessive.
   b. Hypercalcemic dialysate:
      - Check dialysate composition.
   c. Disturbance of atrioventricular conduction system:
      - Check position of HD catheter by chest X-Ray or echocardiogram.
   d. Digoxin toxicity:
      - Check digoxin dose and send digoxin levels at least 12–24 hours after dosing.
   e. Electrolyte abnormalities, in particular, hypokalemia and hypomagnesemia:
      - Check serum electrolytes, including sodium, potassium, ionized calcium, and magnesium.
   f. Myocardial ischemia:
      - Look for ECG evidence of ischemia and consider sending cardiac enzymes if indicated.

III. Management of acute, unstable or life-threatening arrhythmias:

1. Definition: Heart rhythms associated with chest pain or are evidence of circulatory insufficiencies such as a frank shock and impaired mentation.
2. HD should be stopped unless a clear metabolic precipitant correctable by dialysis is present, such as hyperkalcmia-induced heart block.
3. Manage as per current Advanced Cardiac Life Support (ACLS) and Pediatric Advanced Life Support (PALS) guidelines.

IV. Prevention:

1. Strict control of interdialytic fluid gain and potassium intake to decrease the need for aggressive UF and low potassium dialysate.
2. Substitution of normal instead of the usual elevated calcium bath.
3. Consider discontinuing arrhythmogenic drugs such as digoxin.
4. Chronic use of antiarrhythmic drugs (with the exception of beta-blockers and calcium channel blockers) is best avoided.

F. Dyspnea

I. Etiology:

1. Volume overload.
2. Cardiac conditions:
   - Angina.
   - Pericardial effusion, with or without tamponade.
3. Pulmonary embolism.
4. Respiratory conditions:
   - Asthma.
   - Pneumonia.
5. Bacteremia.
6. Dialyzer reaction.
7. Hemolysis.
8. Air embolism.
9. Medications administered during HD:
   a. IV iron:
      - Allergic reaction.

   b. Heparin:
      - Heparin-induced thrombocytopenia resulting in clotting in the dialyzer and lines with resultant hypoxia and capillary leak syndrome.

II. Clinical evaluation:

1. Timing of onset of dyspnea:
   a. Before initiation of HD:
      - Volume overload and cardiac failure.

    - Acute asthma attack.
    - Pneumonia.
  b. During HD:
    - At initiation of HD: Air embolism.
    - 5–30 minutes after initiation: Type A dialyzer reaction.
    - 30–60 minutes after initiation: Type B dialyzer reaction.
    - Dialysis-induced hypoxemia peaks at 30 minutes, and improves in the second hour.
    - Hemolysis tends to occur in the first hour.
    - Intradialytic hypotension is more common in the later stages of dialysis.
    - Dialysis disequilibrium occurs towards the end of dialysis and after the ending.
  c. After access declotting:
    - Pulmonary embolism.
2. Presence of other associated symptoms:
    - Fever and chills.
    - Cough.
    - Chest pain.
    - Back pain.
    - Pruritus and urticaria.
3. Medications administered during HD.
4. Recurrent episodes occurring on dialysis is suggestive of dialyzer reactions.
5. Clinical signs:
    - Hypotension or hypertension.
    - Signs of fluid overload.
    - Cardiac signs including cardiomegaly, abnormal heart sounds, and pericardial rub.
    - Signs of allergy, including wheezing, urticaria and angioneurotic edema.
    - Pulmonary signs suggestive of pneumonia.
6. Consider chest X-Ray if dyspnea is persistent after adequate UF.
7. Consider cardiac evaluation to exclude myocardial dysfunction if symptoms are persistent or recurrent.

III. Management of dialyzer reactions:

	Type A (Anaphylactic)	Type B (Non-specific)
Incidence	• 5/100000 dialyzers.	• 3–5/100 dialyzers.
Pathogenesis	• Hypersensitivity reaction to a component in the dialysis circuit accompanied by signs and symptoms of anaphylaxis.	• Complement activation by hydroxyl groups on bioincompatible membranes with pulmonary sequestration.
Etiology	• Leachable substances such as ethylene oxide (first use). • Bacterial peptides. • AN-69 membrane. • Heparin. • Formaldehyde.	• Synthetic membranes (most biocompatible). • Reused cellulose. • Cellulosynthetic (Hemophan). • Substituted cellulose (cellulose acetate). • Cellulose (cuprophane) (least biocompatible).
Onset	• Within 5 to 30 minutes of blood returning to the patient.	• Delayed, usually 30–60 minutes after starting dialysis.
Severity	• Moderate or severe.	• Usually mild.
Symptoms	• Itching, urticaria, cough, sneezing, coryza, watery eyes, flushing. • Abdominal cramps or diarrhea. • Headache. • Wheezing, shortness of breath. • Hypotension, hypoxia, cardiovascular collapse and death.	• Chest pain and back pain. • Dyspnea, nausea, vomiting or hypotension. • Neutropenia and increased band forms. • Thrombocytopenia.

(*Continued*)

	Type A (Anaphylactic)	Type B (Non-specific)
Treatment	• Stop dialysis immediately without blood return. • Diphenhydramine IV 2 mg/kg (maximum 100 mg). • Adrenaline IV 0.1 ml/kg 1:10000. • Hydrocortisone IV 4 mg/kg (maximum 100 mg).	• Continue dialysis.
Prevention	• Rinse well. • Change dialyzer membrane. • Choose dialyzers with alternative methods of sterilization such as steam, gamma irradiation, and electron beam.	• Reuse without bleach.

H. Blood Leak

1. Disruption of dialyzer hollow fiber integrity, allowing blood to flow into the dialysate compartment.
2. Etiology:
   a. Dialyzer damage during transport.
   b. Manufacturing defects.
   c. Excessive transmembrane pressure.
3. Clinical presentation:
   a. Blood leak detector alarm is activated.
   b. Bloodstained dialysate in the absence of hemolysis.
4. Management:
   a. When blood leak detector alarms:
      - Blood pump stops automatically.
      - Check dialysate effluent for gross bloodstaining.
      - If dialysate effluent is clear, check effluent with a dipstick for blood.

   b. Stop dialysis immediately if blood is detected in the dialysate effluent.
      - Do not return the blood

c. Consider restarting dialysis with a new circuit on a different machine if necessary.
d. Send blood culture and start empiric antibiotic treatment untill the culture results are back.

Recommended Reading

1. Preka E, Shroff R. (2018) Hemodialysis. In: *Critical Care Nephrology and Renal Replacement Therapy in Children*. Edited by: Deep A, Goldstein SL. Springer. pp. 271–289.
2. K/DOQI Workgroup. (2005) K/DOQI clinical practice guidelines for cardiovascular disease in dialysis patients. *Am J Kidney Dis* **45**(Suppl 3):S1–153.
3. Kooman J, Basci A, Pizzarelli F, Canaud B, Haage P, Fouque D, Konner K, Martin-Malo A, Pedrini L, Tattersall J, Tordoir J, Vennegoor M, Wanner C, ter Wee P, Vanholder R. (2007) EBPG guideline on haemodynamic instability. *Nephrol Dial Transplant* **22**(Suppl 2):ii22–44.
4. Tattersall J, Martin-Malo A, Pedrini L, Basci A, Canaud B, Fouque D, Haage P, Konner K, Kooman J, Pizzarelli F, Tordoir J, Vennegoor M, Wanner C, ter Wee P, Vanholder R. (2007) EBPG guideline on dialysis strategies. *Nephrol Dial Transplant* **22**(Suppl 2): ii5–21.
5. Sherman RA, Daugirdas JT, Ing TS. (2015) Complications during hemodialysis. In: *Handbook of Dialysis*, 5th edition. Edited by Daugirdas JT, Blake PG, Ing TS. Wolters Kluwer. pp. 215–236.
6. Raina R, Lam S, Raheja H, Krishnappa V, Hothi D, Davenport A, Chand D, Kapur G, Schaefer F, Sethi SK, McCulloch M, Bagga A, Bunchman T, Warady BA. (2019) Pediatric intradialytic hypotension: Recommendations from the Pediatric Continuous Renal Replacement Therapy (PCRRT) Workgroup. *Pediatr Nephrol* **34**:925–941.
7. Bellucci A. (2019, updated) Reactions to the hemodialysis membrane. Edited by: Schwab SJ, Motwani S. *UpToDate ONLINE*. http://www.uptodate online.com.
8. Davis KA, Ogu I, Golpher TA. (2020, updated) Seizures in patients undergoing hemodialysis. Edited by: Berns JS, Motwani S. *UpToDate ONLINE*. http://www.uptodate online.com.
9. Holley JL. (2020, updated) Acute complications during hemodialysis. Edited by: Berns JS, Motwani S. *UpToDate ONLINE*. http://www.uptodate online.com.
10. Henrich WL. (2020, updated) Intradialytic hypotension in an otherwise stable patient. Edited by: Schwab SJ, Motwani S. *UpToDate ONLINE*. http://www.uptodate online.com.

5 Hemodialysis Catheter Dysfunction

Ng KH, KLL Shein, Chaturvedi S, Liu ID, Taylor R and Yap HK

A. Definition

1. Inability to achieve a volumetric blood flow (Qb) greater than the recommended blood flow for that size catheter during the first 60 minutes of hemodialysis (HD), despite at least one attempt to improve flow in a catheter that was working well previously.
2. National Kidney Foundation–Kidney Disease Outcomes Quality Initiative (NKF KDOQI) 2006 definition in adult-size catheters:
   - Inability to achieve Qb >300 mL/min during the first 60 minutes of HD despite at least one attempt to improve flow in a catheter previously able to deliver >350 ml/min at a pre-pump pressure of –250 mmHg.

B. Causes of Catheter Dysfunction

1. Early catheter failure:
   a. Defined as a catheter not functioning adequately after placement.
   b. Usually due to problems during catheter placement or positioning, such as:
      - Catheter malposition.
      - Catheter retraction.
      - Kinked catheter (angulation in tunnel).
      - Misplaced sutures that constrict the catheter.
      - Loss of catheter integrity, such as cracks and holes.
      - Pre-existing fibrin sheath

2. Late catheter failure:
   a. Defined as the inability to attain and maintain Qb sufficient to perform HD without significantly lengthening the HD treatment in a catheter that was previously working adequately.
   b. Usually caused by thrombosis.
3. Types of thrombotic occlusions:

Type	Features	Symptoms
a. Extrinsic (within vein)		
Central vein thrombus	Total thrombosis of the vessel within which the catheter resides.	Asymptomatic or upper limb swelling with dilated chest wall veins and pain at the base of neck.
Mural thrombus 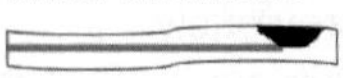	Fibrin from vessel wall injury binds to fibrin-covered catheter resulting in thrombus forming on the wall of the vein at its point of contact with the catheter tip, resulting in partial or complete venous occlusion.	Asymptomatic or leakage of infusate from the insertion site, swelling, pain, tenderness, and engorged vessels.
Atrial thrombus	Thrombus within the right atrium.	Asymptomatic.
b. Intrinsic (within catheter)		
Fibrin tail or flap 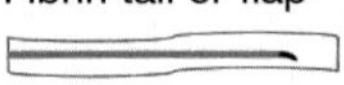	Fibrin extends from the end of the catheter causing partial occlusion (fibrin tail acts as a one-way valve-ball valve).	Ability to infuse but not withdraw blood.
Fibrin sheath (fibrin sleeve) 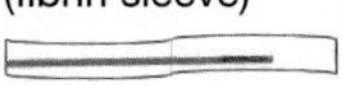	Fibrin adheres to the external surface encasing the catheter, possibly extending the length of the catheter; thrombi trapped between the sheath and catheter tip.	Inability to infuse and/or withdraw blood.
Intraluminal thrombus	Fibrin forms inside the catheter lumen, causing partial or complete occlusion.	Inability to infuse and/or withdraw blood.

C. Assessment for HD Catheter Dysfunction

1. Indicators of HD catheter dysfunction:
   a. Trend analysis of changes in access flow is the best predictor of access patency and risk for thrombosis.
      - Decline in Qb of >10% from baseline at the same negative pre-pump pressure, especially if progressive.
      - Qb <300 ml/min at a standardized arterial pressure of –250 mmHg for adult HD catheters.
      - Arterial pressure <–250 mmHg.
      - Venous pressure >+250 mmHg.
      - Conductance (the ratio of blood pump flow to the absolute value of pre-pump pressure) <1.2.
   b. Urea reduction rate progressively declines to <65%.
   c. Delivered Kt/V <1.2.
   d. Unable to aspirate blood freely (late manifestation).
   e. Frequent pressure alarms not responsive to patient repositioning or catheter flushing.
2. Bedside assessment:
   a. Position the patient in Trendelenburg position.
   b. Visually inspect the line for kinks and swelling beneath the exit site.
   c. Adjust dressing to prevent any inadvertent kinking of the catheter.
   d. Trial of manual 0.9% saline flush by using a 10–20 ml syringe, followed by an attempt to aspirate blood.
      - Repeat 3 times.
      - If blood can be aspirated, procedure should be repeated with a 10 ml syringe until free flow is achieved.
   e. If this fails, consider reversal of ports to continue the HD session.
3. Investigations:
   a. Chest X-Ray to look for catheter malposition or migration
   b. Duplex ultrasound to look for thrombus.
      - Noninvasive but low sensitivity.
   c. Venography has higher sensitivity and should be obtained if clinical suspicion of thrombosis remains high in the absence of sonography findings:
      - Needed for diagnosis of fibrin sheath.

- Consider renoprotective measures for preventing contrast-induced acute kidney injury in patients with significant residual kidney function.

d. 2D echocardiography (transthoracic and transesophageal) may be useful for diagnosis of atrial thrombi and embolism.

D. Initial Treatment of HD Catheter Thrombosis (Thrombolytic Therapy)

1. Urokinase protocol:
   a. Dilute 60000 U of urokinase (1 vial) in 12 ml of 0.9% saline to make a 5000 U/ml solution.
   b. Instill a volume equal to the stipulated priming volume of each affected port, then cap up.
   c. Dwell for 1 hour before trying to aspirate blood from the port.
   d. The process can be repeated to a total of 3 times in each setting.
2. Tissue plasminogen activator (t-PA) (Alteplase®):
   a. When t-PA is used for HD catheter thrombosis, the concentration in the circulation does not reach pharmacologic levels, and any t-PA released into the circulation is metabolized rapidly by the liver (plasma half-life <5 minutes), reducing the risk of systemic complications such as bleeding and intracranial hemorrhage.
   b. Use with caution in:
      i. Thrombocytopenia or coagulation defects.
      ii. Recent surgery <48 hours.
      iii. Recent puncture of non-compressible vessels.
      iv. An absolute contraindication is hypersensitivity to the drug or any component of its formulation, including t-PA, L-arginine, phosphoric acid, and polysorbate-80.
   c. t-PA instillation protocol:
      i. t-PA solution: 1 mg/ml.
         - Instill 110% of the internal volume of each lumen up to a maximum of 2 ml (2 mg).
      ii. Place a medication label on the catheter stating: "t-PA lock in progress, DO NOT USE".
      iii. Dwell for 60 or 120 minutes.

iv. This process can be repeated once.
v. Do not add heparin or antibiotics to t-PA.

d. Stopcock method (for completely occluded ports that can neither withdraw nor instill):
   i. Connect a three-way stopcock to the catheter using aseptic technique.
   ii. Connect a 10 ml Luer lock syringe (aspirating syringe) to one of the free ports and a smaller syringe containing the thrombolytic agent (t-PA syringe) to the remaining port.
   iii. With the stopcock set so that the t-PA syringe is off, withdraw the plunger of the aspirating syringe to the 3–5 ml mark.
   iv. Turn stopcock so that the aspirating syringe is off.
   v. Gently instill the thrombolytic agent into the catheter from the t-PA syringe.

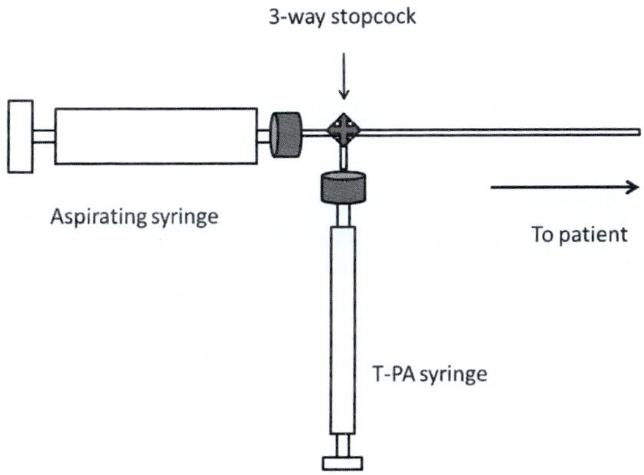

E. Second-Line Treatment of HD Catheter Thrombosis

1. Removal of fibrin sheath:
   a. Fibrin sheath stripping using a snare catheter.
      - The snare is introduced through the femoral vein and advanced up to the level of the dialysis catheter.
      - Reported success ranges from 75 to 98%.
   b. Fibrin sheath disruption with an angioplasty balloon.

2. Catheter exchange over a guidewire:
   a. Secondary treatment of choice for intrinsic catheter thrombosis.
   b. Important to obliterate a fibrin sheath that has been detected before performing a catheter exchange over a guidewire.
3. Indications for catheter removal:
   a. Symptomatic thrombosis with limb swelling/thromboembolism.
   b. Mural thrombus associated with catheter dysfunction.
   c. Atrial thrombus.
4. Systemic anticoagulation:
   a. Indications:
      i. When HD catheter is not removed.
      ii. Mural thrombi >1 cm.
      iii. Atrial thrombus >1.5 cm.
      iv. Patient with pro-thrombotic risk factors.
   b. Initial anticoagulation protocol with Enoxaparin:
      i. Starting dose: 1 mg/kg.
      ii. Therapeutic target for anti-Xa activity: 0.5–1.0 IU/ml.
      iii. Duration of initial treatment: 1 week.
      iv. Dosage adjustment:

Anti-Xa Level (IU/ml)	Dose Titration	Time to Repeat Anti-Xa Level
<0.35	Increase dose by 25%	4 hours after the next dose
0.35–0.49	Increase dose by 10%	4 hours after the next dose
0.5–1	Keep same dosage	Next day, then 1 week later, then monthly (4 hours after the dose)
1.1–1.5	Decrease dose by 20%	Before the next dose (trough)
1.6–2	Decrease dose by 30%	Before the next dose, then 4 hours after the next dose
>2	Hold all doses until anti-Xa is 0.5 IU/ml, then decrease dose by 40%	Before the next dose until anti-Xa <0.5 units/mL

c. Consider prophylactic anticoagulation for 3–12 months after catheter removal, especially in patients with a history of recurrent thrombosis:
   i. Enoxaparin:
      - Starting dose (subcutaneous): 0.5 mg/kg daily.
      - Therapeutic range for anti-Xa activity: 0.2–0.4 IU/ml.
      - Dosage adjustment:

Anti-Xa Level (IU/ml)	Dose Titration	Time to Repeat Anti-Xa Level
<0.1	Increase dose by 25%	4 hours after the next dose
0.1–0.19	Increase dose by 10%	4 hours after the next dose
0.2–0.4	Keep the same dosage	1 week later, then monthly (4 hours after the dose)
0.4–1.0	Decrease dose by 20%	4 hours after the next dose
>1.0	Hold all doses until anti-Xa is 0.2 IU/ml, then decrease the dose by 40%	Before the next dose (trough) until anti-Xa <0.2 units/mL

   ii. Warfarin: Aim for an international normalized ratio (INR) of 1.5–2.0.
   iii. Antiplatelet agents have not been proven efficacious.

F. Prevention of HD Catheter Thrombosis

1. Measures performed immediately post-HD to decrease risk of thrombosis:
   a. Proper flushing of HD catheter:
      i. Flush the catheter forcibly with 10 ml 0.9% saline to remove residual blood.
      ii. Clamp the catheter prior to removing syringe to prevent backflow of blood into the catheter.
      iii. Fill each limb of the HD catheter with the appropriate inscribed volume of locking solution.
   b. Locking solutions include:
      i. Heparin 5000 U/ml: Fill to the volume of each lumen.

ii. 4% sodium citrate: Fill to the volume of each lumen.
iii. t-PA 1 mg/ml (for recurrent blockages): Fill to the volume of each lumen + 0.1 ml.

G. Algorithm for Catheter Dysfunction

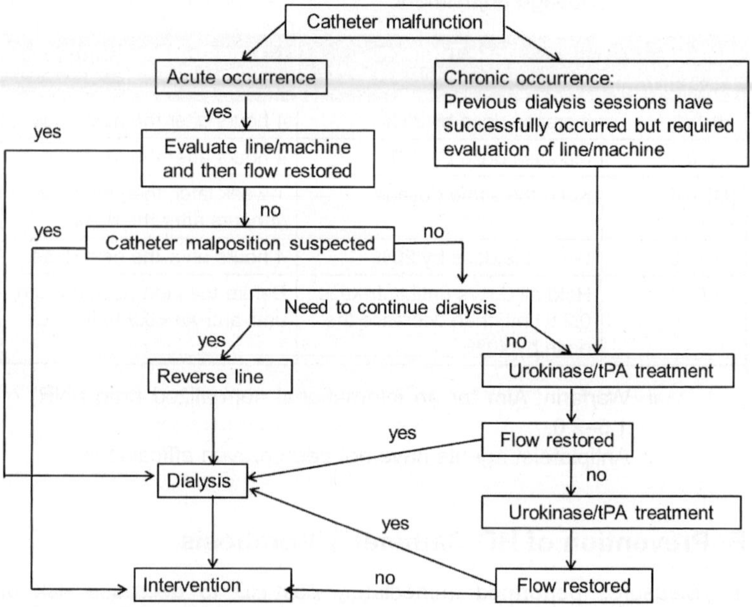

Recommended Reading

1. National Kidney Foundation. (2006) KDOQI clinical practice guidelines and clinical practice recommendations for 2006 updates: Hemodialysis adequacy, peritoneal dialysis adequacy and vascular access. *Am J Kidney Dis* **48**(Suppl 1):S1–S322.
2. Moran JE, Ash SR; Clinical Practice Committee. (2008) Locking solutions for hemodialysis catheters; heparin and citrate — A position paper by ASDIN. *Semin Dial* **21**(5):490–492.

3. Baskin JL, Pui CH, Reiss U, Wilimas JA, Metzger ML, Ribeiro RC, Howard SC. (2009) Management of occlusion and thrombosis associated with long-term indwelling central venous catheters. *Lancet* **374**:159–169.
4. Besarab A, Pandey R. (2011) Catheter management in hemodialysis patients: Delivering adequate flow. *Clin J Am Soc Nephrol* **6**:227–234.
5. Baskin JL, Ulrike R, Wilimas, JA, Metzger ML, Ribeiro RC, Pui CH, Scott CH. (2012) Thrombolytic therapy for central venous catheter occlusion. *Haematologica* **97**:641–650.
6. Beathard GA. (2020, updated) Malfunction of chronic hemodialysis catheters. Edited by: Dillavou ED, Berns JS, Schwab SJ, Collins KA, Motwani S. *UpToDate ONLINE*. http://www.uptodateonline.com.
7. Lexicomp Inc. (2020) Enoxaparin: Pediatric drug information. *UpToDate ONLINE*. http://www.uptodateonline.com.

6 Hemodialysis Catheter Infections

Ng KH, Isa MS, Teo S, Ambarsari CG, Liu ID and Yap HK

A. Definitions

Exit-site infection	Erythema, induration, and/or tenderness within 2 cm of the catheter exit site, not extending superiorly beyond the cuff if the catheter is tunneled: • May be associated with other signs and symptoms of infection, such as fever or purulent drainage emerging from the exit site. • Exudate culture positive, with or without concomitant bloodstream infection.
Tunnel infection	Tenderness, erythema, and/or induration >2 cm from the catheter exit site, along the subcutaneous tract of a tunneled catheter, with or without concomitant bloodstream infection.
Catheter-related blood stream infection (CRBSI)	A primary bloodstream infection in a patient who has a hemodialysis (HD) catheter.
a. Definite CRBSI	≥1 positive blood culture + Pathogenic organism* + Clinical signs/symptoms suggestive of infection#. + Absence of another source of infection. OR ≥2 positive blood cultures from ≥2 sites at the same time or within 14 days of each other + Same common skin organism@. + Clinical signs/symptoms suggestive of infection#. + Absence of another source of infection.

(*Continued*)

b. Probable CRBSI	1 catheter or circuit-drawn blood culture positive for skin organism[@^] + Clinical signs/symptoms suggestive of infection[#]. + Absence of another source of infection. +/– Concomitant negative peripheral-drawn blood cultures.
c. Possible CRBSI	Defervescence of symptoms after antibiotic treatment or after removal of catheter in the absence of positive blood culture in a patient with no other apparent source of infection.

*Pathogenic organisms: Non-skin, non-environmental microbes, e.g., *Staphylococcus aureus*, enterococci, gram-negative bacteria, *Candida*, non-tuberculous *Mycobacteria, Bacillus* species excluding *Bacillus anthracis*.

[@]Skin commensals: Microbes with skin colonization, e.g., coagulase-negative *Staphylococcus* (CoNS), *Corynebacterium* species excluding *Corynebacterium diphtheriae*, *Cutibacterium* species, viridans group streptococci, *diphtheroids*, *Micrococcus*.

[#]Clinical signs/symptoms suggestive of catheter-related infections include at least 1 of the following: Fever >38°C, hypotension, tachycardia, prolonged capillary refill time.

[^]A single catheter-drawn blood culture positive for skin organism, in the absence of clinical symptoms/signs and the presence of an alternative source of fever, may be due to catheter colonization. Consider repeat blood cultures.

B. Risk Factors

1. Risk of infection is approximately 10 times higher in patients with HD catheters than with arteriovenous fistula.
2. CRBSI is more frequent in non-tunneled versus tunneled catheters.
3. CRBSI arises from the following sources:
   a. Contamination of catheter connectors.
   b. Lumen contamination from infused solutions.
   c. Migration of the patient's skin flora through the puncture site and onto the catheter surface.
   d. Catheter colonization from remote sites during bacteremia.
   e. CoNS and *Staphylococcus aureus* account for up to 80% of infections.

C. Investigations

1. Septic workup:
   a. Full Blood Count (FBC).
   b. C-reactive protein (CRP) ± procalcitonin.
   c. Swab gram stain and culture of any discharge from the exit site or tunnel (catheter tip culture is not routinely used for diagnosis of CRBSI).
   d. Blood cultures before starting antibiotics for suspected infection:
      i. At least 10 ml should be obtained from each site.
      ii. Sites of blood cultures:
         - HD catheter.
         - HD circuit.
         - Peripheral vein.
      iii. Practical algorithm:
         - Ideally, 2 blood cultures, of which at least one from the peripheral vein.
         - Sampling from HD catheters can be from both lumens.

Onset of Symptoms	Blood Cultures
Within few hours prior to current HD session	• 1 sample from HD catheter and 1 sample from peripheral vein or HD circuit.
During HD session	• 2 samples from HD circuit, 15 minutes apart, or • 1 sample from HD circuit and 1 sample from peripheral vein.
Inter-dialytic period not shortly before HD session	• 1 sample from HD catheter and 1 sample from peripheral vein, or • 2 samples from HD catheter (both lumens), or • 2 samples from peripheral vein.

2. Exclude metastatic abscesses:
   a. In patients with:
      i. *Staphylococcus aureus* or fungal infection.
      ii. Persistent fever or bacteremia after 48–72 hours of adequate antibiotic therapy or following the removal of the catheter.

b. Consider the following investigations:
   i. Echocardiogram to exclude infective endocarditis.
   ii. Doppler ultrasound of the vessel to exclude suppurative thrombophlebitis.
   iii. Abdominal ultrasound to exclude hepatosplenic abscesses.
   iv. Ophthalmological examination to exclude endophthalmitis.
   v. Bone scan for osteomyelitis and septic arthritis.
   vi. Other imaging as indicated.

D. Antibiotic Therapy

I. Exit site infection

1. Topical antibiotics, namely, gentamicin is recommended if there are signs of exit-site infection with no fever, purulent discharge or CRBSI.
2. Change to topical mupirocin if exit site culture grows methicillin-resistant *Staphylococcus aureus* (MRSA).
3. Add oral cephalexin for 10 days if there is fever or purulent discharge.
4. If there is no improvement after 5 days, then IV antibiotics should be commenced based on culture result and sensitivities and continued for a total of 14 days.

II. Tunnel infection

1. Empiric treatment for tunnel infections without fever or CRBSI:
   a. IV cefazolin as first-line therapy.
   b. IV vancomycin if recent exit site culture (within 2 weeks) grew MRSA.
   c. Add IV ceftazidime if recent exit site culture (within 2 weeks) grew gram-negative organism.
2. Rationalize antibiotics according to exit site/tunnel swab culture results.
3. Duration of antibiotic treatment: 2 weeks.

III. CRBSI

1. Empiric antibiotic therapy:
   a. Initial selection of antibiotics should be based on:
      - Severity of symptoms.
      - Catheter infection history.
      - Patient's risk profile — history of infection and colonization pattern.
      - Local pattern of distribution of causative organisms and their antibiotic susceptibilities (antibiogram).

   b. Repeat blood cultures should be taken 48–72 hours after institution of treatment.
   c. Empiric treatment can stop if:
      - Both sets of initial blood cultures have negative results.
      - There is no other identified source of infection.
      - Signs and symptoms of bacteremia have resolved.
2. Choice of empiric antimicrobial agent:
   a. First-line empiric therapy in hemodynamically stable patients: IV cefazolin + ceftazidime to be administered via the catheter at the end of HD.
   b. IV vancomycin in place of cefazolin should be initiated if the patient is:
      - Hemodynamically unstable.
      - Allergic to beta-lactam.
      - Colonized with MRSA or resistant CoNS.

   c. If the patient is critically ill with septic shock, commence IV vancomycin + cefepime +/- amikacin.
   d. If known colonization with extended-spectrum beta-lactamases (ESBL) or a multi-drug resistant gram-negative organism, consider using cefepime or piperacillin-tazobactam or meropenem.
   e. Antibiotic dosing regime for patients on three times a week (high-flux) HD:

Antibiotic	Pediatric Patients	Adult Patients
Cefazolin*	25 mg/kg dose every 24 hours or post HD#	2 g post HD (Consider 3 g if next HD is 72 hours later)

(*Continued*)

Antibiotic	Pediatric Patients	Adult Patients
Ceftazidime	50 mg/kg* dose every 48 hours	1 g post HD (Consider 2 g if next HD is 72 hours later)
Cefepime	50 mg/kg post HD, or 50 mg/kg/dose* every 24 hours (if residual kidney function)	1.5≠–2 g post HD (Consider 2 g if next HD is 72 hours later)
Vancomycin^	10 mg/kg (dosing based on levels)	1 g post HD (up to 1500 mg/dose)
Amikacin	5–7.5 mg/kg dose post HD (dosing based on levels)	Up to 375 mg post HD

*Given after HD.

Extrapolated from adult studies as no pediatric studies are available.

Higher doses may be given if the drug was given in the last 1–2 hours during HD.

f. If yeast is grown, start empiric treatment with an echinocandin:
- IV anidulafungin 2–4 mg/kg/day loading dose then 1–2 mg/kg/day OR
- IV caspofungin 70 mg/m²/day loading dose (maximum dose 70 mg) then 50 mg/m² daily (maximum dose 50 mg) OR
- IV micafungin 2≠–4 mg/kg/day (maximum dose 100 mg).

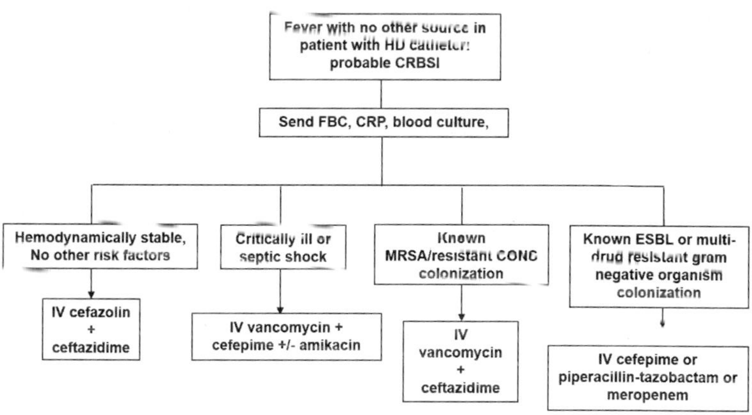

3. Tailored antibiotic therapy:
   a. Vancomycin:
      i. Dialyzability of vancomycin in high flux dialyzers (HD) is 25–50%.
      ii. Levels should be taken pre-HD because drug levels taken immediately post HD are unreliable due to drug rebound (up to 4 hours post-dialysis).
      iii. Trough levels of >15 μg/ml are associated with nephrotoxicity.
      iv. Target trough levels:
         - MRSA: 15–20 μg/ml.
         - CoNS: 10–15 μg/ml.
      v. Assuming 25–50% dialyzability (high flux HD, after drug rebound).

Target Trough Level (μg/ml)	Pre-dialysis Level (μg/ml)	Suggested Action
15–20	<15	Consider higher dose post-HD
	15–25	Dose post-HD
	>25	Withhold dose this HD session
10–15	<10	Consider higher dose post-HD
	10–20	Dose post-HD
	>20	Withhold dose this HD session

      vi. If dose is given over the last 1–2 hours of HD, a higher dose (up to 20 mg/kg) may be needed.
      vii. Check levels before every HD initially, then weekly if on stable dosing.
   b. For CRBSI due to *Enterococcus*:
      i. Ampicillin is the drug of choice for ampicillin-susceptible enterococci.
      ii. Vancomycin should be used if pathogen is resistant to ampicillin.
   c. For confirmed MRSA bacteremia with vancomycin minimum inhibitory concentration (MIC) >2 μg/ml, use daptomycin 6 mg/kg/day.

4. Duration of systemic antibiotic therapy in CRBSI:
   a. *Staphylococcus aureus*:
      - If HD catheter removed: 3 weeks.
      - If HD catheter retained: 4 weeks.
   b. Other gram-positive organisms including CoNS: 2 weeks.
   c. Gram-negative organisms: 2 weeks.
   d. Fungal organisms: 2 weeks.
   e. Presence of metastatic infection: 4–6 weeks.
5. Repeat blood cultures:
   a. Blood cultures from both lumens of the HD catheter should be drawn at every HD session until both lumen cultures are negative at 48 hours.
   b. If catheter is not removed or changed, duration of therapy is counted from first negative blood culture and resolution of fever.
      - Repeat blood cultures 7 days after completion of antibiotics.
      - If positive with the same organism, remove catheter and restart antibiotic treatment.
   c. If catheter is removed, duration of therapy is counted from first negative blood culture and resolution of fever, or date of catheter removal, whichever is later.

E. Management of HD Catheter

1. Indications for catheter removal:
   a. Tunnel infection if there is no improvement after 2 weeks of appropriate antibiotic therapy.
   b. Complicated CRBSI:
      - Sepsis with hemodynamic instability.
      - Suppurative thrombophlebitis.
      - Metastatic infection.

   Note: Patients who require emergency dialysis may be dialyzed once with the infected catheter before prompt removal after the HD.
   c. CRBSI due to *Staphylococcus aureus*, fungal elements, or multidrug resistant gram-negative bacteria.
      - Consider removal when causative organism comprise *Pseudomonas* sp., *Acinetobacter baumannii*, or *Stenotrophomonas maltophilia*.

d. Persistent bloodstream infection in spite of 48–72 hours of appropriate antibiotic therapy.

2. In rare cases where catheter removal is not feasible, long term systemic antibiotics with antibiotic lock and fungal prophylaxis may be considered.
3. Reinsertion of a new tunneled HD catheter should be performed only when the following criteria are met:
   a. Afebrile for 48–72 hours.
   b. At least 2 negative blood cultures.
   c. Normalization of CRP or procalcitonin.

   Note: If this interval needs to be extended, then a non-tunneled temporary catheter can be inserted as a short-term measure to provide dialysis.
4. Guidewire catheter exchange:
   a. Consider guidewire catheter exchange if the patient has complicated CRBSI and catheter removal is not feasible.
   b. The optimal time for guidewire exchange is after 48–72 hours of appropriate antibiotic therapy:
      - All the criteria for reinsertion of a new, tunneled HD catheter must be fulfilled.
      - There should be no evidence of tunnel tract involvement.
   c. Guidewire exchange increases the risk of venous wall stenosis and sclerosis.
5. Antibiotic lock solution is another option for salvage of tunneled catheters.
   a. Involves instilling a highly concentrated antibiotic solution into a catheter lumen and allowing the solution to dwell for a specified period.
   b. Consider in:
      i. Uncomplicated catheter-related infection in the absence of:
         - Persistent bacteremia.
         - Septic thrombosis.
         - Chorioretinitis.
         - Endocarditis.
         - Tunnel infection or abscess.
      ii. With infections caused by *Staphylococcus aureus* and CoNS.

c. Antibiotic solutions are stable in heparin for up to 72 hours without any significant precipitation.
d. Antibiotic locks should be instilled in both lumens of the HD catheter upon completion of each dialysis session, and withdrawn immediately prior to the next dialysis session.
e. Antibiotic locks should be continued as long as systemic antibiotic treatment is continued.
f. Antibiotic lock preparations should be instilled into the HD catheter in the appropriate luminal volume.
g. The type of antibiotics used is tailored according to the identified organisms.
h. Constituents of antibiotic lock preparations:

Antibiotic (Final Concentration)	Type of Lock Solution in 0.9% Saline (Final Volume 2 ml)				
	Vancomycin (Undiluted: 10 mg/ml)	Gentamicin (Undiluted: 8 mg/ml)	Cefazolin (Undiluted: 40 mg/ml)	Heparin* (Undiluted: 5000 U/ml)	0.9% saline
Vancomycin (2.5 mg/ml)	0.5 ml	—	—	1.0 ml	0.5 ml
Gentamicin (1 mg/ml)	—	0.25 ml	—	1.0 ml	0.75 ml
Vancomycin/ Gentamicin	0.5 ml	0.25 ml	—	1.0 ml	0.25 ml
Cefazolin (5 mg/ml)	—	—	0.25 ml	1.0 ml	0.75 ml
Cefazolin/ Gentamicin	—	0.25 ml	0.25 ml	1.0 ml	0.5 ml

*Final concentration of heparin = 2500 units/ml.

F. Prevention of Catheter Infections

1. For new patients planned for catheter insertion, the following measures should be instituted:
   a. Perform Hibiscrub® (4% chlorhexidine gluconate) body wash for at least 1 minute in the evening prior and the morning of catheter insertion.

  - For patients intolerant of chlorhexidine, Octenisan wash can be used.

b. Screen patient and caregivers for *Staphylococcus aureus* nasal carriage:
   i. If the first nasal swab culture is negative, repeat a second swab culture.
      - A person is deemed negative if both swabs are negative.
   ii. If nasal swab is positive, treat with 2% mupirocin nasal ointment for 5 days.
      - For patients, mupirocin 2% ointment should also be applied to the catheter exit site during each dressing change for a 2-week duration.

2. Antibiotic prophylaxis:
   a. There is insufficient data to recommend routine use of systemic antibiotics prior to HD catheter insertion.
   b. There is insufficient data to recommend routine use of antibiotic locks to prevent CRBSI.
   c. Routine application of topical antibiotics at the exit site reduces CRBSI; however, there is a risk of rapid emergence of antibiotic resistance as well as potential degrading effect of additives in the topical mupirocin on polyurethane catheters.
   d. In patients with exit site colonization or CRBSI due to MRSA:
      - Apply mupirocin 2% ointment to the catheter exit site during each dressing change for a 2-week duration.
      - Screen for MRSA carriage (nasal, axilla and groin).
      - Treat nasal carriage with 2% mupirocin nasal ointment for 5 days.

3. Handling catheter hubs:
   a. Catheters should be accessed by trained personnel under aseptic technique.
   b. Scrub the connection between the catheter cap and the catheter using aqueous iodine 10% for 1 minute, disconnect the catheter cap and scrub the catheter hub for another minute.
   c. When needleless connectors are used, scrub the connector using aqueous iodine 10% for 1 minute.

Recommended Reading

1. Mermel LA, Alon M, Bouza E, Craven DE, Flynn P, O'Grady NP, Raad II, Rijnders BJA, Sherertz RJ, Warren DK. (2009) Clinical practice guidelines for the diagnosis and management of intravascular catheter-related infection: 2009 Update by the Infectious Diseases Society of America. *Clin Infect Dis* **49**:1–45.
2. Vanholder R, Canaud B, Fluck R, Jadoul M, Labriola L, Marti-Monros A, Tordoir J, Biesen WV. (2010) Diagnosis, prevention and treatment of haemodialysis catheter-related blood stream infection (CRBSI): A position statement of European Renal Best Practice (ERBP). *Nephrol Dial Transplant Plus* **3**:234–246.
3. O'Grady NPO, Alexander M, Burns LA, Dellinger EP, Garland J, Heard SO, Lipsett PA, Masur H, Mermel LA, Pearson ML, Raad II, Randolph A, Rupp ME, Saint S, and the Healthcare Infection Control Practices Advisory Committee (HICPAC). (n.d.) 2011 Guidelines for the Prevention of Intravascular Catheter-Related Infections. https://www.cdc.gov/mmwr/preview/mmwrhtml/rr5110a1.htm.
4. Allon M, Sexton DJ. (2020, updated) Tunneled hemodialysis cathter-related bloodstream infection (CRBSI): Management and prevention. Edited by: Berns JS, Motwani S. *UpToDate ONLINE*. http://www.uptodateonline.com.
5. Cimino C, Burnett Y, Vyas N, Norris AH. (2021) Post-Dialysis Parenteral Antimicrobial Therapy in Patients Receiving Intermittent High-Flux Hemodialysis. *Drugs* **81**:555–574.
6. Chung E, Tjon JA, Nemec RM, Nalli N, Harvey EA, Licht C, Seto W. (2021) Pharmacokinetics of vancomycin in pediatric patients receiving intermittent hemodialysis or hemodiafiltration. *Kidney Int Rep* **6**:1003–1014.

7 Continuous Kidney Replacement Therapy

Ng KH, Teo S and Yap HK

A. Indications to Initiate Continuous Kidney Replacement Therapy

1. Acute kidney injury:
   a. Refractory metabolic acidosis, hyperkalemia or uremic organ involvement (pericarditis, encephalopathy, neuropathy, myopathy).
   b. Fluid overload: Consider continuous kidney replacement therapy (CKRT) when fluid overload is >10%, especially if >20%.
      - Equations for percent fluid overload (see chapter "Management of Acute Kidney Injury").
   c. Inability to provide adequate nutrition.
   d. Coagulopathy requiring large amounts of blood products.
2. Hyperammonemia or inborn errors of metabolism.
3. Intoxications (e.g., salicylates).
4. Decompensated liver failure.

B. Vascular Access

1. Location of catheters:
   a. Internal jugular catheters have longer circuit lifespans compared to femoral catheters.
   b. Left femoral catheter is preferred to the right, so as to preserve the right for future kidney transplant.
   c. Ideal position of the catheter tip:
      i. Femoral catheter: Inferior vena cava.
      ii. Internal jugular catheter: Right atrium or junction of superior vena cava and right atrium.

   d. If dialysis catheter tip is near to a central venous catheter for giving medications like inotropes and antibiotics, the medications may be siphoned to the dialysis machine due to the negative pressure applied to the dialysis catheter.

2. Size of catheters:

Body Weight	Double Lumen
<4 kg	6.5–7 F
4–10 kg	8 F
10–20 kg	9–10 F
20–40 kg	10–12.5 F
40–50 kg >50 kg	12–12.5 F (consider triple-lumen) 12–14.5 F (consider triple-lumen)

   - Select the largest diameter catheter with the shortest length where possible.

3. Tunneled versus non-tunneled catheters:
   - Tunneled catheters are preferred if the expected time for use is >2 weeks.

4. Catheter lock:
   a. Citrate lock:
      - 4% sodium citrate.
      - Fill to the volume of each lumen.
   b. Heparin lock:
      - 5000 U/ml.
      - Fill to the volume of each lumen.
      - Risk of spillage of heparin into circulation, resulting in clinically significant coagulopathy in at-risk patients (e.g., neonates, very septic patients).
   c. Tissue plasminogen activator (t-PA) lock:
      - 1 mg/ml.
      - Instill 110% of internal volume of each lumen up to a maximum of 2 ml (2 mg).

C. Modality

1. Modality choice should take solute clearance into consideration:
   a. Convection results in better clearance of middle and large molecules, including cytokines in cytokine storm, compared to diffusion.
      - Continuous venovenous hemofiltration (CVVHF): Primarily by convection.
      - Continuous venovenous hemodialysis (CVVHD): Primarily by diffusion.
      - Continuous venovenous hemodiafiltration (CVVHDF): By both convection and diffusion.
   b. CVVHDF provides the highest solute clearance and is generally preferred.
   c. CVVHD may be associated with longer circuit survival than CVVHF or CVVHDF.
      - Increased filtration fraction and transmembrane pressures seen with convective modalities are associated with increased risk of clotting.
2. CKRT circuit:

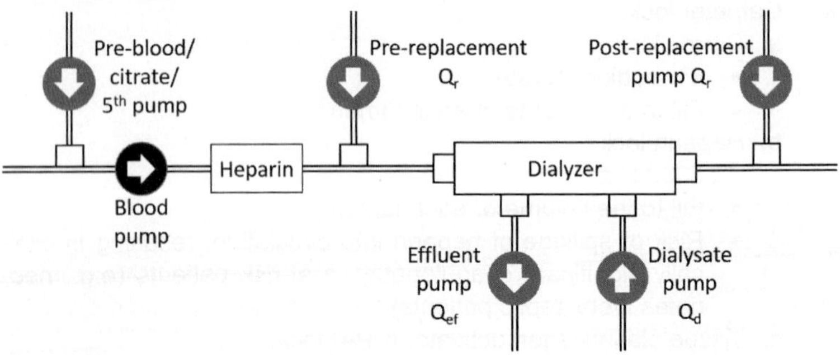

Note: Pre-blood pump *(PRISMAFLEX)*.
Citrate pump *(AQUARIUS)*.
5th pump *(INFOMED)*.

3. CKRT in an Extracorporeal Membrane Oxygenation (ECMO) circuit:

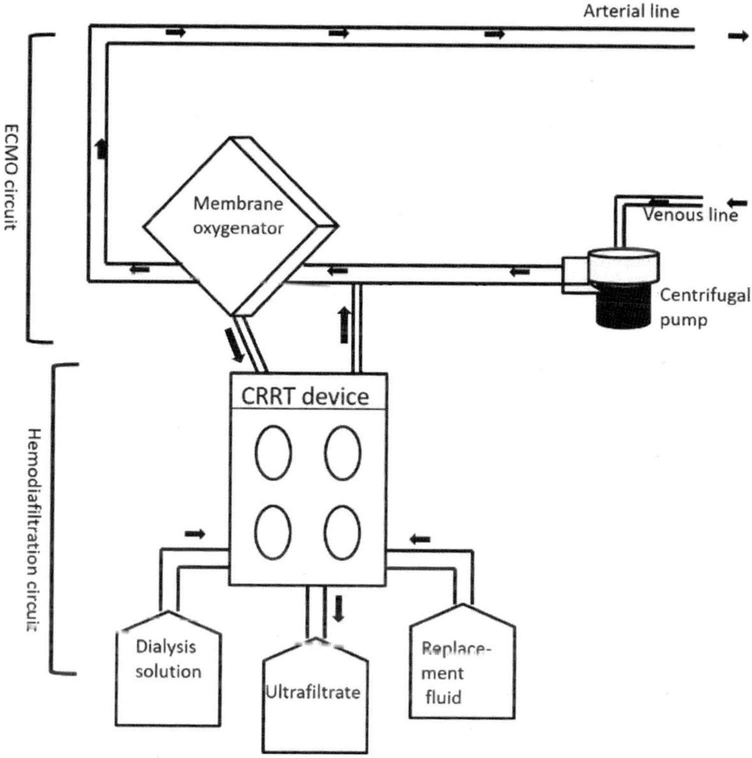

Note: Veno-arterial (VA) ECMO operates at much higher pressures than a venovenous (VV) ECMO.

4. Machine-specific considerations:
   a. *PRISMAFLEX*:
      i. CVVHF: Pre-replacement and post-replacement modes can be used simultaneously.
      ii. CVVHDF:
         - Set machine as CVVHDF (post-dilution) mode.
         - Pre-replacement flow rate is run via pre-blood pump and post-replacement flow rate via (post) replacement pump.

b. *AQUARIUS*:
   i. CVVHF: Pre-replacement and post-replacement modes can be used simultaneously.
   ii. CVVHDF: Only post-replacement mode is possible.

c. *INFOMED:*

	CVVHF	CVVHDF
Flow Rates		
Blood flow	Blood desired flow.	Blood desired flow.
Ultrafiltration (UF) (= fluid removal)	**Weight loss.**	**Weight loss.**
Pre-replacement	(as part of substitution) Manual mode: Set "**Predilution ratio***". Automatic mode: No need to set ratio.	5th **Pump**. If doing pre-replacement only, set UF flow as 0 and use 5th pump for pre-replacement.
Post-replacement	**Substitution** (= pre- + post-replacement). **UF flow** (calculated by machine) = weight loss + substitution.	**UF flow**.
Filtration fraction	Hemoconcentration.	Hemoconcentration.
Pressures		
Access	Arterial.	Arterial.
Return	Venous.	Venous.
Transmembrane (TMP)	TMP hemofilter.	TMP hemofilter.
Filter	Prefilter (before filter).	Prefilter (before filter).
Effluent	—	—
Pressure change across filter	Transfilter (prefilter — venous pressures).	Transfilter (prefilter — venous pressures).
Volumes		
Fluid removed	Weight loss.	Weight loss.
Effluent (UF + replacement + dialysate)	Waste.	Waste.
Dialysate	—	Dialysate.

(*Continued*)

	CVVHF	CVVHDF
Pre-replacement	Predilution.	5th pump.
Post-replacement	Post-dilution.	Post-dilution.

*Pre-dilution ratio refers to the ratio between pre-replacement and post-replacement flow rates.

i. CVVHF: Pre-replacement and post-replacement modes can be used simultaneously.
   - Automatic mode:
     - Substitution rate is set; machine will start as 100% post-replacement.
     - As filter pressure increases, machine will automatically increase pre-replacement % (pre-dilution ratio) up to a maximum of 70%.
   - Manual mode: Pre-dilution ratio is set; maximum is 70%.

ii. CVVHDF:
   - Simultaneous pre- and post-replacement: Set UF flow (post-replacement) and use 5th pump as pre-replacement.
   - Pre-replacement ONLY: Set UF flow (post-replacement) as 0 and use 5th pump as pre-replacement.
   - Post-replacement ONLY: Set UF flow (post-replacement).

d. Fluid removal is automatically performed for replacement pumps and pre-blood/5th/citrate pumps.
   - No need to include these volumes in the UF volume.

D. Dialyzers and Blood Lines

1. Selecting the dialyzer:
   a. Surface area of the dialyzer should be comparable to the body surface area of the patient.
   b. Consider the material or properties of the dialyzer:
      - Avoid blood prime in AN-69 dialyzers.
      - Heparin-coated dialyzer (Oxiris) may be considered in patients with clotting risks.

Body Weight (kg)	Dialyzer	Material	SA (m^2)	Fill Volume (ml)	
				Dialyzer	Dialyzer + Tubing
>8	*Prismaflex HF20*	PAES	0.2	17	60
5–12	*Aquamax HF03* *Infomed* DF-030 (*baby*)	PES PES	0.30 0.30	32 32	96 57
11–20	*Prismaflex M60*	AN-69	0.60	42	93
15–23	*Aquamax HF07* *Infomed DF-080 (child)*	PES PES	0.70 0.76	54 52	 102
21–30	*Prismaflex M100*	AN-69	0.9	75	152
28–42	*Aquamax HF12*	PES	1.2	73	
38–70	*Prismaflex Oxiris* *Infomed DF-140 (adult)*	AN-69 PES	1.5 1.4	109 85	193 185
>70	*Aquamax HF19*	PES	1.9	109	214

SA = surface area; AN-69 = acrylonitrile; PES = polyethersulfone; PAES = polyarylether-sulfone.

2. Blood lines:

PRISMAFLEX	*HF20* *M60*	FV = 60 ml FV = 93 ml
	M100 *Oxiris*	FV = 152 ml FV = 193 ml
AQUARIUS	Aqualine S (<30 kg) Aqualine	64 ml (Q_b 10–200 ml/min) 105 ml (Q_b 30–450 ml/min)
INFOMED	TU-309-05 (baby) TU-301-05 (child) TU-300-24 (adult)	25 ml 50 ml 100 ml

FV = volume of dialyzer + tubings; Q_b = Blood flow rate.

E. Circuit Priming and Preparation for CRKT

I. Selection of priming fluid:

1. Types of priming fluids: 0.9% saline, 5% albumin or packed red cells.

2. Determining which priming fluid to use in non-ECMO circuits:
   a. Consider the patient's ability to tolerate temporary loss of red cell mass and volume overload associated with blood return at circuit termination (in non-blood prime).
   b. Extracorporeal volume (dialyzer + tubing) should not exceed 30% of the patient's blood volume.
      - Calculation of patient's blood volume:
        <10 kg child: 80 ml/kg.
        >10 kg child: 70 ml/kg.
        Adolescent or adult: 60 ml/kg.
   c. Choice of priming fluid is dependent on extracorporeal volume (ECV) in relation to patient's blood volume:
      i. ECV <10% of patient's blood volume: 0.9% saline.
      ii. ECV 10–15% of patient's blood volume:
         - Normal hemoglobin (Hb) and hemodynamically stable: 0.9% saline or 5% albumin.
         - Low Hb (<7 g/dL) or hemodynamically unstable: packed red cells or whole blood.
      iii. ECV >15% of patient's blood volume: packed red cells or whole blood.
   d. Considerations in choice of priming fluid:
      i. 5% albumin prime may decrease ionized calcium due to increased calcium-binding sites in albumin.
      ii. Packed red cells or whole blood:
         - Risk of bradykinin release syndrome with use of AN-69 dialyzers.
         - Repeated blood tranfusions can increase the sensitization risk for future transplants.
         - Use leukocyte-depleted blood or filter.
         - Use blood from the same donor where possible.
3. Priming fluid for CKRT in ECMO circuits:
   a. Use saline prime even for very small patients.
   b. Blood prime is usually not needed because:
      i. Hemodynamics in ECMO patients are usually stable, and even if not, these may be managed by adjusting ECMO settings.
      ii. ECV for CKRT machine is a small percentage of ECMO ECV and patient's blood volume.
      iii. Hb is usually well controlled in ECMO patients.

c. Blood prime may still be given if deemed necessary, in the same way as non-ECMO circuits.

II. Blood prime (for Prismaflex HF20, Fresenius F3, Aquamax HF03, Infomed DF-030):

1. Diluted packed red cells prime:
   a. Whole blood or packed red cells have pH 6.1–6.8, ionized calcium 0.15 mmol/L, and very high potassium levels.
   b. Whole blood (if available) is preferred to packed red cells.
   c. Packed red cells have a hematocrit of about 60% and should be diluted to 30% with sodium bicarbonate 140–150 mmol/L solution.
   d. Dilute packed red cells 1:1 with diluent using a 3-way stopcock or Y connector, drawing the packed red cells and bicarbonate 140–150 mmol/L solution into the circuit simultaneously.
   e. Preparing the solutions:
      i. Obtain leucocyte-depleted packed red cells and draw required volume (50% of the ECV) into a syringe.
      ii. Prepare sodium bicarbonate solution 140–150 mmol/L (50% of ECV) into a second syringe.

Final Volume (ml)	8.4% Sodium Bicarbonate (1 mmol/ml) (ml)	Sterile Water (ml)
80	12	68
60	9	51
50	7	43
40	6	34
20	3	17

      iii. Using a 3-way stopcock or Y connector, connect packed red cells to one end and sodium bicarbonate 140–150 mmol/L solution to the other.
      iv. Connect the third output end to the red access line of the circuit.

f. Priming the machine:
   i. Start "Blood Prime" mode at blood flow 40 ml/min.
   ii. Monitor the speed of infusion of the packed red cells and sodium bicarbonate solution, as both should run at about the same rate so that the blood and bicarbonate solution complete infusion at about the same time.
      - Slow the faster syringe by placing manual resistance to the syringe.
      - Hasten the slow syringe by giving it a manual push.

g. Calcium gluconate should be given with every packed red cell prime regardless of heparin or citrate anticoagulation and patient's baseline calcium level.
   i. Administer 10% calcium gluconate 0.5–1 ml/kg (maximum 10ml) over 5–10 minutes to the patient via a central line.
   ii. Additional calcium gluconate may be needed if ionized calcium is low prior to starting.

2. Closed-circuit dialysis of packed red cells:
   a. Reduces the amount of potassium, citrate and acid given to the patient.
   b. Priming the machine:
      i. Dilute-packed red cells 1:1 with 0.9% saline for priming the circuit.
      ii. Add potassium in dialysate at 2 mmol/L.
      iii. Connect access line to return line.
      iv. Start treatment.
      v. Use a C-clamp if needed to generate pressures, which should be kept <250 mmHg.
      vi. Qd (ml/hour) should be set at ECV (ml) $\times$ 24.
      vii. Qb (ml/min) should be **at least** 3 times of Qd in ml/min, e.g., if Qd = 2 L/hour, Qb should be at least 100 ml/min.
      viii. Bolus heparin at 2 U/ml of ECV, e.g., if the circuit volume is 100 ml, 200 U of heparin is required.
         - Should be deducted from the heparin bolus at the CKRT initiation.
      ix. Duration 10–20 minutes.
         - Irradiated blood may have higher K, so may need longer circuit dialysis time.
      x. Check microelectrolytes (pH, sodium, potassium, ionized calcium) on the "dialyzed" blood prior to connecting to patient.

3. Prime CKRT with 0.9% saline or 5% albumin and give the packed red cells separately to the patient after CKRT is initiated.
   - Not recommended if ECV >15% of patient's blood volume.
4. Bradykinin release syndrome:
   a. Risk is highest in AN-69 dialyzers, especially if packed red cell prime is used.
   b. Clinical features:
      i. Tachycardia.
      ii. Hypotension.
      iii. Vasodilatation.
      iv. Anaphylaxis.
   c. Prevention:
      i. Prime with 5% albumin or 0.9% saline and correct acidosis to pH >7.35 before starting CKRT.
      ii. If blood prime is needed, perform closed circuit dialysis of the packed red cells as above.
      iii. If blood prime is not needed, but patient requires blood transfusion, transfuse packed red cells directly to patient after starting CKRT and correcting patient's blood pH >7.35.

III. Diverting the prime:

1. In very fluid overloaded patients, the prime may be diverted to reduce the additional fluid given to the child.
2. If the calculated volume deficit is greater than 15% of the total blood volume, or greater than the safe fluid loss limit for an individual child, diverting the prime is not recommended.

IV. Correction of electrolytes and acidosis prior to CKRT:

1. In a hemodynamically unstable patient, hypocalcemia and acidosis may aggravate hypotension, especially if blood or albumin prime is used.

2. Correct hypocalcemia and acidosis to ensure hemodynamic stability and maximize cardiac output before starting CKRT.
   a. Check blood gas and microelectrolytes (sodium, potassium, ionized calcium) prior to the start of CKRT.
   b. If blood pH <7.3, give IV sodium bicarbonate infusion 1 mmol/kg (maximum 60 mmol).
      - Use 4.2% sodium bicarbonate infusion in infants.
   c. If baseline ionized calcium <1.1 mmol/L, give 1 ml/kg 10% calcium gluconate over 20 minutes (maximum 10 ml) via a central line.
   d. Start CKRT if blood pH >7.0 and patient is hemodynamically stable.

F. Blood Flow Rate

1. Depends on size of dialysis catheter and best adjusted based on the machine pressures.

	Blood Flow Rate (Q_b) (ml/kg/min)	Typical Ranges (ml/min)
Neonates and infants	10–12 ml/kg/min	<8 kg: 30–80 ≥8 kg: 50–100
Children	4–6 ml/kg/min	100–150
Adolescents	2–4 ml/kg/min	150–250

Note: Maximum Q_b: 400 ml/min/1.73m^2.

   a. Adjust blood flow to achieve the following pressures:
      - Access pressure of 0 to –150 mmHg (ideally closer to 0).
      - Venous return pressures of 0 to +150 mmHg (ideally closer to 0).
   b. In infants, start at 5 ml/kg/min, increasing up to 10–12 ml/kg/min.
      i. If blood prime is used, maximum starting blood flow is 20 ml/min.
      ii. Increase blood flow to the target rate over 5–10 minutes.
2. Filtration fraction should be kept at <20–30% when titrating blood flow.

3. In patients with higher risk of dialyzer clotting (e.g., no anticoagulation), use higher blood flow rates.
4. If using regional citrate anticoagulation, a higher blood flow rate can result in higher citrate infusion and its attendant risks (e.g., citrate toxicity).
5. In patients with very high serum osmolarity, controlled reduction of osmolarity is desired, use lower blood flow rates.
6. Unlike in intermittent hemodialysis (HD), increasing blood flow rates in CKRT does not increase solute clearance as total effluent rate/blood flow rate (Q_{ef}/Q_b ratio) >1.5 cannot be achieved in CKRT.

G. CKRT Dose (Dialysate and Replacement Flow Rates)

1. Definition
   - CKRT dose
     = total effluent rate (Q_{ef})
     = dialysate flow rate (Q_d) + replacement flow rate (Q_r) + ultrafiltration rate (Q_{uf}).
2. CKRT dosing:
   a. Standard dose: 2000–3000 ml/1.73m²/hour (25–30 ml/kg/hour).
   b. Intensive dose: 4000–6000 ml/1.73m²/hour (40–60 ml/kg/hour).
   c. Intensive/high-dose CKRT may be needed in uncontrolled metabolic acidosis, excessive urea or ammonia generation (e.g., metabolic disorders, liver failure), or citrate toxicity.
      - In hyperammonemia set a high CKRT dose.
      - A dose of 8000 ml/1.73m²/hour (up to 90 ml/kg/hour) may reduce ammonia by 70% at 2 hours.
      - A decline in serum ammonia levels should be achieved within the first few hours of CKRT; otherwise, a rapid increase in CKRT dose is required.
      - There is significant clearance of drugs and electrolytes (potassium, magnesium, phosphate) in high-dose CKRT, and these should be monitored and adjusted for.
3. Dialysate and replacement flow rates:
   a. CVVHD: CKRT dose as dialysate flow rate.

b. CVVHDF:
   i. Dialysate flow rate: Two-thirds of CKRT dose.
   ii. Pre-replacement flow rate: One-third of CKRT dose.
c. Keep dialysate flow less than 2–3 times blood flow rate.
d. If there is recurrent circuit clotting, a concurrent post-replacement flow at 50 ml/hour (regardless of patient size) may be added to prevent clotting in the aeration chamber.
e. Dialysate or replacement bags should be changed every 24 hours.

4. Pre-replacement versus post-replacement:
   a. Pre-filter replacement can help prolong circuit lifespan, while post-filter replacement has a higher risk of circuit clotting.
      i. Post-replacement is associated with higher filtration fraction and a higher risk of circuit clotting.
      ii. Pre-replacement is associated with lower filtration fraction and a lower risk of clotting.
   b. Overall, solute clearance with the same blood flow rate is higher with pre-replacement than post-replacement due to longer filter life and less interruption to therapy.
5. Filtration fraction:
   a. Ratio of total filtered fluid across a filter to the rate of plasma entering the filter.

$$\text{Filtration fraction} = \frac{\text{Total filtration rate}}{\text{Plasma flow rate } (Q_p)},$$

$$= \frac{Qr_{(pre)} + Qr_{(post)} + PBP + Q_{uf}}{Q_p + Qr_{(pre)} + PBP},$$

where Q_r = Replacement fluid rate (L/hour)
PBP = Pre-blood pump rate (L/hour)
Q_{uf} = Set UF rate (L/hour)

$$Q_p = \text{Plasma flow rate (L/hour)} = Q_b \times \left(1 - \frac{Hct}{100}\right)$$

Hct = Hematocrit (%)
Q_b = Blood flow rate (L/hour) (note machine Q_b is in ml/min)

b. Machine-specific considerations:
   i. For *PRISMAFLEX*, filtration fraction displayed on machine is calculated using hematocrit entered into machine.
      - Enter patient's hematocrit during setup.
      - Hematocrit should be updated daily on the machine to reflect the patient's actual hematocrit.
   ii. For *INFOMED*, hemoconcentration, interpreted as filtration fraction, is calculated as:

$$\text{Hemoconcentration} = \frac{Q_{uf}}{Q_b + Q_{r(pre)}}$$

c. Monitoring and titration based on filtration fraction:
   i. To decrease the risk of filter clotting:
      - If hematocrit >35% or in post-replacement circuits, keep the filtration fraction ≤20%.
      - If hematocrit <35%, keep the filtration fraction <25%.
   ii. To decrease filtration fraction:
      - Increase blood flow rate.
      - Decrease replacement flow rates (especially post-replacement) and increase dialysate flow rates to maintain similar clearance.
      - Avoid large increases in set hourly UF rates.

H. Ultrafiltration Rate

1. Fluid calculations over a day:
   a. Total UF volume = Total fluid given to patient (e.g., IV fluids, medications) – fluid losses (e.g., gastric losses, drains, urine) + desired fluid balance.
   b. Divide total UF volume over 24 hours to obtain the hourly set UF rate.
2. Aim NET NEGATIVE FLUID rate of 0.5–2 ml/kg/hour or 1–3% of blood volume per hour.
   a. In very fluid overloaded patients, a NET NEGATIVE FLUID volume of 5% of body weight generally results in significant clinical improvement.

b. Maximum daily NET NEGATIVE FLUID volume is 10% of body weight (considered very aggressive and rarely required).

3. In severely fluid overloaded patients with unstable hemodynamics:
   a. Correct acidosis and electrolyte derangements, including hypocalcemia.
   b. Keep NET NEGATIVE FLUID rate at zero till stable hemodynamics, and then slowly start NET NEGATIVE FLUID rate of 0.5–2 ml/kg/h.
   c. If necessary, provide inotropic support to allow for NET NEGATIVE FLUID removal in the first 24–48 hours of CKRT.
4. Monitor filtration fraction as the set UF is changed. Where possible, for ad hoc infusions, remove the volumes within the same hour that it is given.
5. Notes for specific machines:
   a. Replacement fluid volumes need not be added manually into UF volume.
   b. If using citrate-calcium module (Prismocitrate 18/0) in *AQUARIUS* or *PRISMAFLEX*, volumes for citrate and calcium infusions need not be added manually into the UF rate, as this is inbuilt into the program.
   c. Volumes given via the pre-blood pump (*PRISMAFLEX*) or the 5th pump (*INFOMED*) and anticoagulation syringes need not be added manually into the UF.

I. Composition of CKRT Solutions

I. Dialysate fluid composition:

Content	Prismasol B0 (mmol/L)	Biphozyl (mmol/L)
Sodium	140	140
Chloride	109.5	122
Calcium	1.75	0
Potassium	0	4
Magnesium	0.5	0.75
Phosphate	0	1
Bicarbonate	32	22
Lactate	3	0
Theoretical Osmolarity (mOsm/L)	287	290

Note: Warm fluid to 37°C before use.

II. Potassium control:

1. Addition of potassium in PRISMASOL:
   a. If initial serum potassium is ≥5.0 mmol/L, add potassium 3 mmol/L.
   b. If initial serum potassium is <5.0 mmol/L, add potassium 4 mmol/L.
   c. Potassium may be decreased or omitted in:
      i. High potassium production (e.g., tumor lysis syndrome, burns or crush injuries).
      ii. High potassium load from non-CKRT sources, which cannot be easily altered (e.g., total parenteral nutrition, massive transfusion).
      iii. High pre-dialysis serum potassium (e.g., >6–7 mmol/L).
   d. **Do not add potassium into Biphozyl** (used in citrate anticoagulation protocol), which has pre-added potassium 4 mmol/L.
2. Potassium chloride (KCl) versus potassium dihydrogen phosphate (KH_2PO_4):
   a. Use potassium chloride and potassium dihydrogen phosphate together in proportion to avoid hypophosphatemia and hypochloremia.
   b. The ratio of KCl:KH_2PO_4 is approximately 2:1 or 3:1.
   c. In patients with severe hyperphosphatemia (>3 mmol/L), omit phosphate addition in Prismasol for the first few hours.
3. Potassium (K^+) concentrations in concurrent dialysate, pre- and post-replacement solutions should be the same.

Serum Potassium (mmol/L)	To Be Added per 5 L Bag of Prismasol (ml)		Final K^+ Concentration (mmol/L)		
	KCl (7.45%)	KH_2PO_4	KCl	KH_2PO_4	Total K^+
≥5.0	10	5	2	1	3
≥5.0	15	0	3	0	3
<5.0	15	5	3	1	4
<5.0	20	0	4	0	4

4. If there is hypo- or hyperkalemia after starting CKRT, titrate the amount of potassium in non-CKRT sources, e.g., diet, total parental nutrition (TPN) and IV fluids first.

5. If there is refractory hypokalemia (<2.5 mmol/L) or hyperkalemia (>6.0 mmol/L), which can be life-threatening (e.g., cardiac conditions):
   a. Consider increasing the effluent rate by increasing the dialysate rate (preferred) and/or replacement rates.
   b. Consider increasing or decreasing potassium in PRISMASOL dialysate carefully with very frequent monitoring.
      - Up to 10 mmol/L of potassium may be added in the dialysate with **CAUTION**.

III. Glycaemic control:

1. Adjust dextrose delivery in non-CKRT sources, e.g., IV drip, oral intake, acid citrate dextrose A (ACD-A).
2. Dextrose may be added to dialysate if child has refractory hypoglycemia, or in selected metabolic cases:

Dextrose Concentration (%)	Dextrose To Be Added per 5 L Bag (g)	50% Dextrose per 5 L Bag (ml)
0.2	10	20
0.5	25	50
1.0	50	100
1.5	75	150

IV. Sodium control:

1. Hypernatremia (serum sodium >155 mmol/L) or hyponatraemia (serum sodium <125 mmol/L):
   a. Aim to decrease or increase serum sodium by <8–10 mmol/L over 24 hours, especially in chronic hypernatremia or hyponatremia.
   b. Adjust sodium content in IV fluids, TPN, blood products where possible.
   c. Consider CVVHD and alter the sodium concentration in the dialysate.
   d. If refractory:
      i. Consider CVVHDF, adjusting sodium content in dialysate only or dialysate + replacement (pre + post) solutions.

ii. Consider starting with a low CKRT dose, low blood flow rate, and smaller dialyzers, and adjust based on response.

e. To avoid rapid changes in serum sodium: Increase/decrease sodium concentration in dialysate solutions to be about 5 mmol/L above or below serum sodium levels.

f. Sodium content in CKRT solutions may also be increased as part of neuroprotection measures (e.g., head injury cases).

g. Upward adjustment of sodium in Primasol/Biphozyl solutions:

Desired Sodium Concentration In CKRT Solution (mmol/L)	Sodium To Be Added per 5 L Bag (mmol)	20% Sodium Chloride To Be Added per 5 L Bag (ml)
145	25	7.3
150	50	14.7
155	75	22.1
160	100	29.4

Note: Volumes of sodium chloride added are small and will not affect the concentration of other electrolytes in the solution significantly.

h. Downward adjustment of sodium in Prismasol solutions:

Volume of Sterile Water or Dextrose 5% Added per 5 L Bag (ml)	Final Volume per Bag (L)	Final Concentration In Prismasol					
		Na^+	Cl^+	Ca^{2+}	Mg^{2+}	$HCO3^+$	Dextrose*
		(mmol/L)					(%=g/dL)
0	5.00	**140**	110	1.75	0.50	32	0
150	5.15	**136**	106	1.70	0.49	31	0.15
250	5.25	**133**	104	1.67	0.48	30	0.24
350	5.35	**131**	102	1.64	0.47	30	0.33
500	5.50	**127**	100	1.59	0.45	29	0.45
750	5.75	**122**	95	1.52	0.43	28	0.65
1000	6.00	**117**	91	1.46	0.42	27	0.83
1250	6.25	**112**	88	1.40	0.40	26	1.00

*If dextrose 5% is added.

Note: Downward adjustment of sodium should not be performed in Biphozyl solutions as it can decrease the bicarbonate concentration significantly.

V. Magnesium control:

1. Serum magnesium should be monitored at least once daily.
2. If hypomagnesemia is present, give IV 50% magnesium sulfate (2 mmol/ml) 0.2 ml/kg slow IV over 1 hour.

J. Anticoagulation

I. Heparin:

1. Contraindications to heparin:
   a. Coagulopathy: International normalized ratio (INR) >2.0 or activated partial thromboplastin time (aPTT) >53 seconds.
   b. Platelets <80 × 10^9/L.
   c. Recent surgery or invasive procedure.
   d. Confirmed or suspected active bleeding.
   e. Confirmed or suspected heparin-induced thrombocytopenia.
2. Half-life ~30 minutes in normal kidney function and ~90 minutes in kidney failure.
3. Dosing:
   a. Heparin is given pre-filter:
      - Patients <10 kg: Heparin concentration 10 U/ml.
      - Patients >10 kg: Heparin concentration 100 U/ml.
   b. Loading dose: 10–50 U/kg (maximum 1000 U).
   c. Maintenance dose: 5–50 U/kg/hour (maximum 500 U/hour).
4. Monitoring of heparin dosing:
   a. Activated clotting time (ACT): Assesses platelet function, both intrinsic and common pathways, OR
   b. aPTT, OR
   c. Anti-Xa level: Gold standard for titration of heparin.
      - Target is 0.2–0.4 for blood drawn from circuit.
5. Titration of dose:
   a. In patients with very high bleeding risk, consider giving a smaller heparin loading dose (5–10 U/kg) and not to titrate according to aPTT or ACT.
   b. Using **ACT** to guide heparin dosing:
      i. ACT (post-filter) targets:
         - Standard risk: 180–220 seconds.

- High clotting risk: 180–240 seconds.
- High bleeding risk: 150–180 seconds.
- Measure ACT from post-filter blood sample.

ii. At initiation of CKRT if baseline ACT <150 seconds:
- Give heparin bolus 20 U/kg.
- Recheck ACT in 20 minutes.
- Repeat heparin boluses until ACT is >150–180 seconds (maximum 2 repeat boluses).
- Then start heparin infusion at 10 U/kg/hour.

iii. If baseline ACT ≥150 seconds,
- No heparin bolus. Start heparin infusion at 10 U/kg/hour.

iv. During CKRT, adjust heparin according to sliding scale (standard risk):

Post-filter ACT (seconds)	Action
>220	Decrease heparin by 10%
180–220 (target range)	No change
<180	Increase heparin by 10%

v. Monitoring of ACT:
- At each circuit initiation: Check ACT every 30 minutes × 3 or until ACT is stable, hourly × 2, 2-hourly × 2, then 4-hourly if stable.
- After a heparin dose change, check ACT every 30 minutes for 1 hour or until ACT is stable.
- If platelets or packed red cells are given, check ACT at completion of transfusion every 30 minutes for 1 hour.

c. Using aPTT to guide heparin dosing:

i. Measure aPTT from post-filter blood sample.
- Blood taken at CKRT initiation from a catheter locked with heparin may have falsely high aPTT.

ii. aPTT targets:
- Standard risk: 50–70 seconds.
- High clotting risk: 60–90 seconds.
- High bleeding risk: 40–60 seconds.

iii. At initiation of CKRT (standard risk):

Baseline aPTT (seconds)	Bolus Heparin	Maintenance Heparin
Below target range	20 U/kg	20 U/kg/hour
At target range	None	20 U/kg/hour
Above target range*	None	None

*Repeat aPTT in 1 hour and adjust heparin accordingly.

iv. During CKRT, adjust heparin according to sliding scale (standard risk):

aPTT (seconds)	Action
>100	Hold infusion x 1 hour Decrease by 20%
91–100	Decrease by 20%
71–90	Decrease by 10%
50–70 (target range)	No change
41–50	Increase by 10%
<40	Give 20 U/kg bolus Increase by 20%

Note: Sliding scale may be adjusted based on individual patients.

v. Monitoring:
- Adjust heparin according to aPTT at 2 hours and then 4-hourly.
- For infants who had heparin catheter lock prior to CKRT initiation, consider checking aPTT in 30–60 minutes to detect heparin spillage at CKRT setup.

d. If CKRT is disrupted <24 hours, recommence heparin at the last maintenance dose with or without the bolus dose.
e. Consider changing anticoagulation protocol if:
   i. Heparin rate is adjusted 3x within 4 hours.
   ii. Heparin rate is decreased to 0.
   iii. There is bleeding.

6. If required heparin infusion rates are higher than normal, or if there is recurrent circuit clotting, check antithrombin III level.
7. Monitor baseline full blood count daily.

  - If platelet levels fall rapidly, consider heparin-induced thrombocytopenia (1-5%).

8. CKRT in ECMO circuits:
   a. Titrate heparin as per ECMO protocol.
   b. Avoid citrate regional anticoagulation.

II. Citrate anticoagulation:

- See chapter "Regional Citrate Anti-Coagulation In Continuous Kidney Replacement Therapy".

III. No anticoagulation:

1. Consider in patients who have coagulopathy.
2. Circuit lifespan is generally shorter.
3. Decrease clotting risk by using:
   a. Vascular access of the largest possible diameter.
   b. Higher blood flow rates.
   c. CVVHDF with higher pre-filter replacement flow rates, and consider adding a concurrent post-filter replacement of 50 ml/hour.
   d. 0.9% saline flush:
      i. Flush dialyzer with 0.5 times of ECV every 30 minutes.
      ii. For *AQUARIUS*, this may be given via a port before the dialyzer.
         - Volume of the flush has to be added to the UF volume.
      iii. For *INFOMED* and *PRISMAFLEX*, the saline flush can be via a Y connector in the access port of the catheter.
         - Volume of the flush has to be added to the UF volume.

K. Pressure and Alarm Settings

I. Access pressure:

1. *PRISMAFLEX:*
   a. CVVHD(F): Set machine to negative access pressure <–10 mmHg.

   b. ECMO: Set machine to positive access pressure >10 mmHg (maximum 300 mmHg).
2. *AQUARIUS:*
   - Machine is set to access a pressure range from –250 to +350 mmHg.
3. *INFOMED:*
   a. CVVHD(F): Default access pressure settings.
   b. ECMO:
      i. Consider using *INFOMED* in adolescents on atrioaortic venous-arterial (VA) ECMO.
         - High ECMO flows (e.g., 5–7 L/min) coupled to high CKRT blood flows (e.g., 200 ml/min) might push CKRT return pressures to >350 mmHg.
      ii. Set machine to Extended Pressure settings, which will allow the limits of arterial/venous (A/V) pressures to range between –500 and 500 mmHg.
      iii. Connect the arterial transducer to positive port.
      iv. Connect the venous transducer to positive port.
   c. Non-ECMO:
      i. Connect the arterial transducer to negative port.
      ii. Connect the venous transducer to positive port.

II. Pressure ranges:

Pressure	Range (mmHg)	Comments
Access	–50 to –150	Typically negative as blood is "pulled" from vein
Return	+50 to +150	Typically positive as blood is "pushed" back into the vein
Pre-Filter	+100 to +250	Becomes more positive as filter fibers clot
Transmembrane	<0 to >+150	Becomes more positive as filter fibers clot
Effluent	>+50 to –150	Becomes more negative as filter fiber pores block

III. Machine fluid error:

1. Some CKRT machines have a safety feature to avoid excessive fluid volume error.
2. Excess patient fluid loss or gain alarm is set automatically and must be taken into consideration when calculating the fluid balance:
   a. Should be set at about 10% of the estimated blood volume.
   b. *PRISMAFLEX:*
      i. HF20: 60–150 ml over 3 hours (default 60 ml).
      M60: 100–200 ml over 3 hours (default 130 ml).
      M100: 100–300 ml over 3 hours (default 330 ml).
      ii. Consider a higher limit to reduce the chance of circuit termination.
         - 150 ml for patients <30 kg.
         - 200 ml for patients 30–50 kg.
         - 300 ml for patients >50 kg.
      iii. Treatment is discontinued automatically once the alarm limit is reached.
   c. *AQUARIUS:*
      i. Aqualine: 50 ml for each balance alarm.
      Aqualine S: 20 ml for each balance alarm.
      ii. Treatment is discontinued automatically after 5 consecutive alarms.
      iii. To prevent the alarms from setting off if the limits are reached:
         - Set the [Total Fluid Removal] to 10 L.
         - Set the [Time] at 36 hours.
         - If the [Fluid Loss Rate] is set at 0 ml/hour, then the desired [Time] for this setting should not be 0 hours but should be set for the duration of UF cessation.
   d. *INFOMED*
      i. Alarm is generated if there is a fluid balance error of >45 g for *Infomed DF-140* (adult), >15 g for *Infomed* DF-030 (baby), or *Infomed DF-080* (child) from the start of the CKRT.
         - This alarm can be acknowledged and treatment continued.
      ii. The next alarm will sound when there is another additional error of 45 g or 15 g.

iii. Fluid balance error of >5x per hour may potentially be unsafe.
iv. There is no limit to the number of alarms.
  - Treatment will not be discontinued automatically.

3. Machine accuracy for Fluid Removal:
   a. *PRISMAFLEX*: ±30 ml/hour or ±70 ml/3 hours or ±300 ml/24 hours.
   b. *AQUARIUS*: ±50 ml (regular circuits) or ±20 ml (low volume circuits).
   c. *INFOMED*: ±10 ml/hour for pumps and ±6 g for weighing scales.

L. Thermal Regulation

1. Children with body weight <25 kg are at risk of hypothermia due to the larger proportion of blood flow in the ECV.
2. Use radiant warmers, heating blankets or blood warmers, especially for small children.
3. Temperature cannot be used as an indicator of sepsis.

M. Administration of Medications and Blood Products

1. An additional port may be attached via a three-way tap to the return port of the vascular catheter.
2. Where possible, platelets and lipids should not be infused into the return port of the vascular catheter due to high risk of clotting the circuit and vascular catheter.
3. Where possible, avoid administering medications through the circuit because of potential recirculation of blood at the catheter tip.
   - Any infusions given via the circuit may be recirculated and dialyzed out.
4. Volumes for ad hoc infusions of blood products, antibiotics, electrolyte corrections, etc., should ideally be drawn out within the same hour.
5. Adjustment for drug clearance:
   a. Consider fluid overload status, increased metabolic rates, residual kidney clearance, changing kidney function in AKI, and non-kidney clearance.

b. Drugs more likely to be cleared by CKRT:
   - Small molecular weight (<5000 Daltons).
   - Low plasma protein binding (<80%).
   - Low volume of distribution (<1 L/kg of body weight).
   - Limited extrarenal clearance.

c. Inotropes are usually small molecules with low protein binding.
   - Easily cleared by CKRT.
   - An increase in inotrope doses may be required at CKRT initiation, but they often can be reduced after a few hours of CKRT due to improved hemodynamic stability.

d. CKRT is similar to high-flux dialysis in total solute clearance and corresponds to a glomerular filtration rate (GFR) of 10–50 ml/min/1.73m^2.

e. Check *Renal Dose Adjustment Handbook* for individual drugs.

N. Nutrition

1. Protein requirements:
   a. An additional 1–15 g/kg/day or more of protein is needed on top of baseline requirements to account for losses during CKRT.
   b. Total protein intake should be 2.5–3 g/kg/day.
   c. Patients on CVVHD or CVVHDF with high clearance rates, the daily protein intake may be up to 4.0 g/kg/day due to excessive amino acid losses.
2. Caloric intake may be 20–30% above the resting energy expenditure.
3. Maximize phosphorus and magnesium in TPN orders.
4. Water-soluble vitamins are removed in CKRT and should be replaced.

O. Monitoring

1. Hemodynamic monitoring:
   a. Hourly pulse rate, respiratory rate, temperature, and blood pressure.
   b. Strict intake-output chart.

2. Blood parameters:
   a. Microelectrolytes (pH, sodium, potassium, ionized calcium) at 30 minutes × 2, then hourly × 2, 2-hourly × 2, then 4 hourly if stable.
   b. Serum urea, creatinine, phosphate, magnesium 12-hourly.
   c. ACT or aPTT according to anticoagulation protocol.
   d. Hourly blood glucose, then 4-hourly when stable.
      - Consider adding glucose to dialysate if blood glucose <4 mmol/L.
   e. Full blood count daily.

P. Recirculation Procedure

1. Indications for recirculation mode (not limited to these):
   a. Troubleshooting for dialysis catheter, e.g., t-PA instillation.
   b. Scheduled tests or procedures lasting <1 hour (e.g., CT scan).
   c. Code blue.
2. Types of recirculation:
   a. Saline recirculation:
      i. Blood is returned to the patient and saline is recirculated through the circuit.
      ii. Not suitable for infants on circuits with relatively large ECV as they may not tolerate volume load from the blood return and new priming solution.
      iii. May be performed for up to 2 hours.
   b. Blood recirculation:
      i. Blood is not returned to the patient.
      ii. Suitable for infants.
      iii. Maximum 1 hour.
3. Procedure:
   a. May be performed on *PRISMAFLEX*, *AQUARIUS* or *INFOMED*.
   b. Stop dialysate and replacement pumps.
   c. Blood flow should be 100 ml/min.
   d. Stop heparin, ACD-A and/or calcium infusions.
   e. C-clamps may be needed to stabilize machine pressures for successful recirculation.
      - Keep pressures <250 mmHg.

Q. Complications

I. Blood leak:

1. Observe color of UF.
2. If blood leak detected:
    a. Clamp UF line.
    b. **Return blood immediately to the patient**.
    c. Transfuse the patient based on the estimated blood loss.
    d. Check hemoglobin.

II. Clotting of dialyzer:

1. Darkening of color in dialyzer or visible clots are seen.
2. Disconnect and change circuit according to protocol.
3. Increase heparin dose for new dialyzer/hemofilter.
   Note: Increasing the heparin dose to save the clotting dialyzer or filter should not be attempted as this does not reverse the clotting that has already occurred.

III. Accidental disconnection of circuit:

1. Clamp the arterial and venous ports immediately.
2. Do not return blood, as there may be air in the circuit.
3. Transfuse according to the amount of blood loss.

IV. Acute hypotension:

1. Blood pressure low or patient in shock.
2. Clamp UF line and discontinue dialysate infusion.
3. Place patient in Trendelenburg position.
4. Replace volume at 10–20 ml/kg/hour with 5% albumin or plasma.
5. Check fluid balance calculation.

V. Complications in CKRT with ECMO

1. CKRT in VA ECMO: Systemic air emboli.
2. CKRT in VV ECMO: Deposition of fibrin clots from CKRT into the oxygenator (especially if there are frequent CKRT circuit changes) resulting in decreased oxygenator efficiency.

R. Termination of CKRT Circuit

1. Re-assess medication and fluid orders if no prompt re-start of circuit is planned.
2. Return of blood at the end of CKRT:
   a. If the priming fluid was whole blood or packed red cells or the ECV is >15% of patient's blood volume, do not return blood at the end of the CKRT as there is a risk of sudden volume overload with hypertension and pulmonary edema.
      i. If patient is anemic, separate packed red cells (hematocrit ~65%) should be given instead of returning the circuit blood (hematocrit ~30%).
      ii. The return of blood (hematocrit ~30%) will not increase the patient's hemoglobin.
   b. In small children who did not receive a blood prime, return half to two-thirds of circuit volume (maximum 20 ml/kg) at 20 ml/min.
3. Dual circuit change:
   a. In small children who have received a blood prime, consider dual circuit change with 2 simultaneous CKRT machines.
      - This minimizes exposure to blood products.
   b. Connect the return line of the first machine to the access line of the second machine.
      - There may be more alarms related to the machine pressures, and both machines need to be started at the same time
4. CKRT in ECMO circuit:
   a. Blood generally does not need to be returned at the termination of CKRT unless there is a need to increase the volume in the patient or ECMO circuit.
   b. A dual circuit CKRT change is possible.

c. If the patient is decannulated from ECMO and still requires CKRT, a dialysis catheter may be placed at the time of decannulation.

Recommended Reading

1. Ostermann M, Dickie H, Tovey L, Treacher D. (2010) Management of sodium disorders during continuous haemofiltration. *Crit Care* **14**:418. doi:10.1186/cc9002.
2. Flores FX. (2018) Management considerations for the delivery of CRRT in children. In: *Critical Care Nephrology and Renal Replacement Therapy in Children*. Edited by: Deep A, Goldstein SL. pp. 239–250.
3. Brophy P, Khan I, Deep A. (2018) Anticoagulation in CRRT. In: *Critical Care Nephrology and Renal Replacement Therapy in Children*. Edited by: Deep A, Goldstein SL. pp. 251–270.
4. Bunchman TE. (2019) CRRT in a Sick Child. In: *Critical Care Pediatric Nephrology and Dialysis: A Practical Handbook*. Edited by: Sethi SK, Raina R, McCulloch, Bunchman TE. pp. 113–120.

8 Regional Citrate Anti-Coagulation in Continuous Kidney Replacement Therapy

Ng KH, Teo S, Koh LJ and Yap HK

A. Contraindications to Regional Citrate Anticoagulation

1. Severe liver failure.
2. Mitochondrial dysfunction.

B. Regional Citrate Anticoagulation Circuit for Continuous Venovenous Hemodialysis

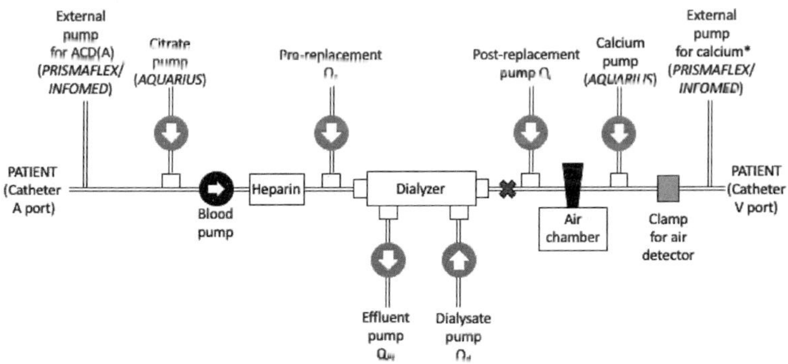

*May also be given via a third port in the catheter or via another central venous catheter.
X: Refers to the site of blood drawn for post-filter calcium.

C. Components of Regional Citrate Anticoagulation

1. Citrate solution:
   a. Acid citrate dextrose A (ACD-A) solution 500 ml.
   b. Given via:
      i. *PRISMAFLEX* or *INFOMED*: A "Y" Luer lock adaptor at the "arterial" port of the catheter or a 3-way stopcock at the "arterial" line, and run through the external IV pump, OR
      ii. *AQUARIUS*: Citrate pump using citrate line set.
2. Biphozyl (calcium-free dialysate/replacement solution):
   a. To avoid hypercalcemia as patients are receiving intravenous (IV) calcium supplementation.
   b. To prevent reversal of the citrate effect in the extracorporeal circuit.
   c. To minimize the amount of citrate and calcium-binding at the level of the dialyzer membrane, hence decreasing the citrate infusion needed.
3. Calcium infusion:
   a. Calcium chloride solution: dilute 80 ml of 10% calcium chloride in 1 L 0.9% saline (to achieve final concentration 56 mmol Ca per L).
   b. This is given EITHER via:
      i. *PRISMAFLEX* or *INFOMED*: A central line separate from the dialysis catheter, or via the third port in a triple-lumen catheter or attaching it to the "Y" Luer lock adaptor or 3-way stopcock at the return port, and attached to an external IV pump, OR
      ii. AQUARIUS: Calcium pump.
4. Avoid using inbuilt machine citrate module in small pediatric patients as this uses Prismocitrate® where the infusion rate is in a fixed ratio to the blood flow rate, making it difficult to titrate.
   - Concentration of citrate in Prismocitrate® is also lower than ACD-A; therefore, infusion volumes required are often too large.

D. Prescription

1. Blood flow rate: Whilst a higher blood flow can improve clearance and decrease filtration rate, it can also increase citrate infusion.

2. Set up the citrate infusion:
   a. At initiation, citrate infusion rate (ml/hour) = 1.5 x blood flow rate (ml/min) (maximum starting infusion rate 270 ml/hour).
      - For example, start citrate at 150 ml/hour if the blood flow rate is 100 ml/min.
   b. If using an AN-69 dialyzer, avoid the use of citrate for the first 15 minutes as it may exacerbate bradykinin release syndrome.
3. Set up the calcium infusion: Run at 40% of the citrate infusion rate.
   - For example, citrate infusion rate = 150 ml/hour, then calcium infusion rate = 60 ml/hour.
4. Fluid removal rate:
   a. Volume of citrate given via citrate pump (*AQUARIUS*), and of calcium via the calcium pump (*AQUARIUS*) will be automatically removed without manual addition into the UF.
   b. If external IV citrate and calcium pumps are used, the citrate and calcium infusion rates need to be added manually into the set UF rate.
5. If using citrate-calcium module (Prismocitrate 18/0) in *AQUARIUS* or *PRISMAFLEX*, the volumes for citrate and calcium infusions are automatically removed from the patient and do not need to be added to the set UF rate.

E. Monitoring

1. Baseline investigations:
   a. Full blood count (FBC).
   b. Blood biochemistry: Urea, electrolytes, creatinine, calcium, phosphate, bicarbonate, uric acid, ionized calcium (iCa^{2+}), magnesium (Mg), glucose.
   c. Arterial blood gas (ABG).
   d. Activated partial thromboplastin time (aPTT).
2. If patient's iCa^{2+} levels <1.1 mmol/L, correct the iCa^{2+} levels as far as possible prior to starting continuous kidney replacement therapy (CKRT).
3. Monitoring:
   a. iCa^{2+} levels: At 30 minutes × 2, then hourly × 2, 2-hourly × 2, and if stable, 4 hourly:
      i. Post-filter iCa^{2+} (drawn from the return line, venous port).

ii. Systemic iCa^{2+} (drawn from patient arterial line or peripheral draw).
iii. If an adjustment is made, repeat iCa^{2+} in 1 hour, then 2–4 hourly.
iv. If the site or tubing for the calcium infusion is changed, then the iCa^{2+} must be checked in 1–2 hours to ensure that the infusion is correct.
v. If blood products are given, the iCa^{2+} levels will need to be checked.

b. ABG and blood glucose 2–6 hourly.
c. Total calcium and measured bicarbonate (not standard bicarbonate) 6 hourly.
d. FBC, urea, creatinine, sodium, potassium, chloride, phosphate, Mg, albumin 12 hourly.

F. Titration of Citrate/Calcium

1. Titrate the citrate infusion according to the citrate sliding scale below:

Post-filter iCa^{2+} (mmol/L)	Citrate Infusion Adjustment	
	> 20 kg	< 20 kg
<0.35	↓ rate by 10 ml/hour	↓ rate by 5 ml/hour
0.35–0.5 (optimum range)	No adjustment	No adjustment
0.5–0.6	↑ rate by 10 ml/hour	↑ rate by 5 ml/hour
>0.6	↑ rate by 20 ml/hour	↑ rate by 10 ml/hour

Note: Notify pediatric nephrologist on call if citrate infusion rate >200 ml/hour.

2. Titrate the calcium infusion according to the calcium sliding scale below:

Patient iCa^{2+} (mmol/L)	Calcium Infusion Adjustment	
	> 20 kg	< 20 kg
>1.3	↓ rate by 10 ml/hour	↓ rate by 5 ml/hour
1.1–1.3 (optimum range)	No adjustment	No adjustment
0.9–1.1	↑ rate by 10 ml/hour	↑ rate by 5 ml/hour
<0.9	↑ rate by 20 ml/hour	↑ rate by 10 ml/hour

Note: Notify pediatric nephrologist on call if calcium infusion rate >200 ml/hour.
If calcium infusion is discontinued, keep the line patent with 0.9% saline at 2 ml/hour.

3. In high volume CKRT, the patient is at risk of acute calcium loss via the circuit, as they are dialyzed against a calcium-free solution.
   a. If systemic iCa^{2+} <0.75 mmol/L, stop citrate infusion for 1 hour.
   b. Monitor post-filter iCa^{2+} during this time as its rise will indicate inadequate anticoagulation of the circuit.
   c. Resume citrate infusion at 30% and bolus with 10 ml/kg of 10% calcium chloride and increase calcium infusion by 10%.
4. Calcium should not be given in non-CKRT intravenous fluids or TPN to avoid interference with the calcium protocols.

G. Complications

1. Metabolic alkalosis:
   a. May occur in patients on regional citrate anticoagulation, especially if >7 days.
      - 1 mmol citrate ≡ 3 mmol bicarbonate.
   b. Etiology:
      i. Gastric losses.
      ii. Acetate base in total parental nutrition (TPN), which converts to bicarbonate.
      iii. Bicarbonate from dialysate.
      iv. Conversion of citrate to bicarbonate in the liver.
   c. If the measured serum bicarbonate is >35 mmol/L and pH >7.45, consider:
      i. Increasing the UF rate by 20–50% (or 200–400 ml/hour) and replacing the UF with either 0.9% saline or 0.45% saline depending on the serum sodium level, OR
      ii. Changing the replacement solution to 0.9% saline solution to provide 30% of the CKRT dose.
         - pH of 0.9% saline is 5.4 and will give enough acid load to the patient to offset the metabolic alkalosis
2. Citrate toxicity ("citrate lock" or "citrate gap"):
   a. Citrate toxicity occurs when the citrate infusion rate exceeds the citrate clearance by dialysis, muscle and hepatic metabolism.
   b. Diagnosed when ratio of total calcium to iCa^{2+} >2.5 mmol/L in the presence of increasing total calcium levels >3.0 mmol/L and decreasing/stable iCa^{2+}.

c. There may be worsening metabolic acidosis with an increasing anion gap.
d. The "citrate lock or gap" refers to the discrepancy between the total and iCa^{2+} and implies the calcium bound to the citrate.
e. Problems with citrate toxicity include:
   i. Hypocalcemia.
   ii. Neuromuscular abnormalities.
   iii. Cardiac abnormalities (prolonged QTc on ECG).
   iv. High anion gap metabolic acidosis (due to free citrate ions) or metabolic alkalosis.
f. Citrate toxicity is most likely to occur in:
   i. Patients with impaired citrate metabolism:
      - Liver impairment with transaminases >1000 IU/L.
      - Cardiogenic shock and lactate concentration >8 mmol/L.
      - Multiorgan failure.
      - Severe hypoxia.
      - Severe sepsis.
   ii. Patients who receive massive blood products containing citrate.
   iii. Young infants and children as they have the highest blood flow rates per kg of body weight, and the citrate infusion is proportional to the blood flow rate.
g. In patients at risk of citrate toxicity, the starting citrate infusion rate may be reduced to 50% of standard rate while maintaining the standard calcium infusion rate.
h. If citrate toxicity occurs, consider the following:
   i. Increase citrate clearance rate by increasing (by 50%) dialysate and/or the replacement rates.
      - Double the dialysate flow rate as a start.
   ii. Reduce the citrate infusion rate, accepting a higher post-filter iCa^{2+} (e.g., 0.45 mmol/L).
   iii. Reduce the blood flow rate so that the citrate infusion can be reduced.
i. Stop the citrate infusion for a minimum of 20 minutes, to 4 hours.
   i. Keep the calcium infusion going at this time.
   ii. Monitor post-filter iCa^{2+}, as its rise will indicate inadequate anticoagulation of the circuit.

iii. Restart the citrate at 50–80% of the original rate when the patient's iCa^{2+} >0.9 mmol/L.
iv. If citrate toxicity persists, consider evaluation for possible hepatic dysfunction.

3. Hyperglycemia:
   a. ACD-A contains 2.45 g/dL of dextrose.
   b. Adjust dextrose from non-CKRT sources.
   c. Consider insulin infusion if needed.
4. Hypernatremia:
   - If serum Na >150 mmol/L, consider changing replacement solution to 0.45% NaCl.
5. Hypomagnesemia:
   - Citrate can bind to Mg and lead to a decrease in Mg levels.
6. Bradykinin release syndrome:
   - In children <10 kg using the AN-69 dialyzers and who require a blood transfusion, stop citrate infusion for the first 15 minutes as it may trigger bradykinin release syndrome.

H. Stopping Dialysis

1. Monitor the venous pressure on the return line to determine imminent clotting.
2. Procedure for ending dialysis:
   a. For elective circuit termination, stop the citrate infusion for 20 minutes before returning the blood.
      - Do not stop the calcium infusion until blood return.
   b. For non-elective circuit termination, stop the dialysis without returning the blood.
      - Remember to stop the citrate and calcium infusions.
3. If the filter clots, stop the citrate and calcium infusions and discontinue dialysis.
4. When restarting after the system has been interrupted due to system clotting, imaging, surgery or filter change, the citrate and calcium infusions should restart at the same rate as when the system was stopped.

I. Composition of CKRT Solutions

Constituent (mmol/L)	Biphozyl	Prismasol B0	ACD-A
Sodium	140	140	224.4
Chloride	122	109.5	
Calcium	0	1.75	
Potassium	4	0	
Magnesium	0.75	0.5	
Phosphate	1	0	
Bicarbonate	22	32	
Lactate	0	3	
Citrate	—	—	112.8
Dextrose	—	—	134 (2.5%)
Volume (ml)	5000	5000	500

Recommended Reading

1. Brophy P, Khan I, Deep A. (2018) Anticoagulation in CRRT. In: *Critical Care Nephrology and Renal Replacement Therapy in Children*. Edited by: Deep A, Goldstein SL. pp. 251–270.
2. Bunchman TE. (2019) CRRT in a Sick Child. In: *Critical Care Pediatric Nephrology and Dialysis: A Practical Handbook.* Edited by: Sethi SK, Raina R, McCulloch, Bunchman TE. pp. 113–120.
3. Davenport A. (2020, updated) Anticoagulation for continuous renal replacement therapy. Edited by: Schwab SJ, Motwani S. *UpToDate ONLINE*. http://www.uptodate_online.com
4. BIPHOZYL: Abbreviated summary of product characteristics.

9 Prolonged Intermittent Kidney Replacement Therapy

Ng KH and Yap HK

A. Definitions

1. Prolonged Intermittent Kidney Replacement Therapy (PIKRT) is sustained low-efficiency dialysis (SLED) that is a hybrid between continuous kidney replacement therapy (CKRT) and intermittent hemodialysis (IHD).
2. Definition of PIKRT:
   a. Duration ≥6 hours, and
   b. Blood flow rate (Qb) ≤3–5 ml/kg/min for patients who are 20–40 kg or ≤150 ml/min for patients who are >40 kg, and
   c. Dialysate flow rate (Qd) ≤2x Qb or up to 300 ml/min.

B. Indications

1. Indications for PIKRT are similar to CKRT:
   a. Poor Pediatric Risk of Mortality (PRISM) scores.
   b. Receiving 1–2 inotropes (children with >2 inotropes should be on CKRT).
   c. Inability to tolerate a rapid UF rate.
   d. Risk of dialysis disequilibrium.
   e. Inability to perform CKRT.
2. Advantages over CKRT:
   a. Lower cost.
   b. Use of less or no anticoagulation and hence decreased risk of bleeding.
   c. Intermittent nature to allow patients scheduled downtime.

3. Advantages over IHD:
   a. Reduced ultrafiltration (UF) rate due to its prolonged duration.
   b. Risk of dialysis equilibrium is less because the lower Qb and Qd result in less rapid osmolar shifts.

C. Prescription

1. Vascular access:
   a. Dialysis catheters are preferred instead of arteriovenous fistulas or grafts (AVF/AVG) because of the risk of needle dislodgement in prolonged dialysis.
   b. However, the use of AVF/AVG is not contraindicated.
2. Modality:
   a. Hemodialysis (diffusive clearance) is the standard.
   b. Hemofiltration (convective clearance) using online generation of replacement fluid may be added to hemodialysis to improve larger molecule clearance. Ultrapure water as per standards should be used.
3. Dialyzers:
   a. May be low-flux or high-flux dialyzers.
   b. Use dialyzers with surface area similar to patient's surface area.
      - In patients at risk of dialysis disequilibrium or further hypotension, a slightly smaller dialyzer (75% of body surface area) with lower KoA may be used.
   c. If convective clearance is performed, high-flux dialyzers are used due to better UF coefficients of >20 ml/mmHg/hour.
4. Priming solution:
   a. Saline or 5% albumin prime.
   b. Blood prime (see chapter "Continuous Renal Replacement Therapy" for criteria).

5. Dialysis machine (single pass) settings:

	Gambro AK96	Gambro AK98	Fresenius 4008	Fresenius 5008
Blood flow (ml/min)	20–500 (adult line) 20–225 (neonatal line)		5–500	30–600
Dialysate flow (ml/min)	300–700	300–700	300, 500, 800	0–1000 (increments of 100)
UF rate (ml/hour)	0–4000	0–4000	1–9990	0–4000 (increments of 10)
Accuracy of UF volume	± 30 ml or ± 1% of reading, whichever is larger	± 50 ml or ± 50ml/hour × passed treatment time (hour) or 2.5% of total UF removed, whichever is larger	± 0.5%	±1%
Dialysate sodium (mmol/L)	130–160	130–150	128–148	125–151
Dry powder concentrate*	Yes	Yes	Bibag	Bibag
Maximum treatment time	10 hours	10 hours	10 hours	Up to 24 hours
Online replacement fluid generation (ml/min)	No	No	Not available	25–600 (two replacement pumps to allow pre- and/or post-dilution)

*Sterile dry powder concentrates should be used instead of liquid bicarbonate concentrate, which predisposes to bacterial growth.

6. Blood flow rate (Qb):
   a. Body weight 20–40 kg: ≤3–5 ml/kg/min.
   b. Body weight >40kg: up to 150 ml/min.
   c. Blood flow may have to be higher if convective clearance is added to ensure filtration fraction <20% or if no anti-coagulation is used to prevent clotting.
7. Dialysis dose:
   a. Dialysate flow rate (Qd):
      i. Aim Qd not more than 2x Qb or lowest possible on the machine.
         - Qd/Qb ratio of 1.6–2 is ideal for dialysate saturation.
         - For patients with body weight <30 kg: maximum Qd 300 ml/min.
      ii. Aim for dose of 20–25 ml/kg/hour or 2000 ml/1.73 m^2/hour for 6–8 hours.
      iii. If high risk of dialysis disequilibrium (urea ≥60 mmol/L), consider co-current dialysate flow.
   b. Replacement flow rate:
      i. Consider pre-filter replacement, especially if there is no anti-coagulation.
      ii. Pre-filter replacement rate of 35 ml/kg/hour, keeping the filtration fraction <20–30%.
   c. UF rate:
      i. Consider starting net negative fluid rate 4–5 ml/kg/hour.
      ii. Most critically ill patients cannot tolerate a net negative rate of 10–12 ml/kg/hour.
8. Duration and frequency:
   a. Duration: 6–18 hours per session (recommended 6–8 hours).
   b. Frequency: At least 3 times a week.
9. Electrolyte considerations:
   a. Dialysate calcium may be low or normal.
      - Correct hypocalcemia if albumin prime is used.
   b. If there is risk of hemodynamic instability, select higher dialysate sodium and normal calcium dialysate.
      - Difference between serum sodium and dialysate sodium should not exceed 10 mmol/L.
   c. Consider using glucose dialysate especially in smaller children.

   d. Correct hypokalemia and hypophosphatemia using oral supplementation or via IV infusion.
10. Thermal regulation:
   a. Increase dialysate temperature to 37.5°C in young infants.
   b. In children with intradialytic hypotension, consider decreasing dialysate temperature slowly by 0.5°C each time, down to 35°C.
11. Drug dosing considerations
   a. Drug clearance is likely at a level between IHD and CKRT.
   b. Antibiotics may be dosed before and after PIKRT.

D. Anticoagulation

1. Heparin protocol:
   a. Heparin loading dose of 10–20 U/kg followed by maintenance of 5–10 U/kg/hour.
   b. Titration according to partial thromboplastin time (PTT):
      i. PTT target may range from 10 seconds above the baseline up to 1.5 times normal (or 40–50 seconds).
      ii. Monitor PTT at 0, 3 and 6 hours after starting.
      iii. Titration according to activated clotting time (ACT):
         - If ACT <150 seconds, bolus heparin 25–50 U/kg (maximum 2,000 U).
         - Check ACT every 30 minutes until stable, then 2 hourly.
         - Maximum of 2 additional heparin boluses can be given to aim ACT 80–220 seconds.
   c. Adjust heparin dose if:
      i. PTT >75 seconds.
      ii. International normalized ratio (INR) >2.
      iii. ACT >275 seconds.
      iv. Platelet count $<50 \times 10^9$/L.
      v. Increased bleeding risk.
2. Enoxaparin protocol (0.01 ml = 1 mg = 100 IU):
   a. Initial bolus: 50–100 IU/kg = 0.5–1 mg/kg.
      - If fibrin rings are found, a further dose of 0.5–1.0 mg/kg may be given.
   b. For patients at risk of thrombosis:
      i. Can increase initial bolus to 0.8–1 mg/kg, OR

ii. Give lower initial bolus of 0.4 mg/kg, followed by a second bolus at 3 hours of 0.4 mg/kg, OR

iii. Give a second dose at half the initial dose.

c. For patients at risk of hemorrhage:
- Keep initial bolus at 0.5 mg/kg.

d. Higher doses may be needed in high flux dialyzers.

e. Administration:

i. High flux dialyzer:
- Preferably administered into the venous limb of the extracorporeal circuit because up to 80% of the drug is cleared if injected into the arterial port before the dialyzer.

ii. Low flux dialyzer:
- No difference in arterial and venous bolus administration.

3. No anticoagulation protocol:

a. Consider in children with thrombocytopenia and bleeding risks.

b. Steps to prevent circuit clotting:

i. Saline flushes at 0.5 times the extracorporeal volume every 30 minutes.
- Volumes of these flushes need to be added to the UF volumes.

ii. Increase the blood flow rate by 20–25%.

iii. Consider adding pre-filter replacement (hemodiafiltration-enabled machines).

E. Monitoring

1. Hemodynamic monitoring:

a. Hourly pulse rate, respiratory rate, temperature, and blood pressure.
- Not necessary for intra-arterial BP monitoring.

b. Strict intake-output chart.

2. Blood biochemistry:

a. Before PIKRT:
- Sodium, potassium, chloride, bicarbonate, urea, creatinine, calcium, phosphate, uric acid, and glucose.

b. During PIKRT:
- Potassium, ionized calcium, and sodium 4 hourly.
- Glucose 2–4 hourly.

   c. After PIKRT:
      - Sodium, potassium, chloride, bicarbonate, urea, creatinine, calcium, phosphate, uric acid, and magnesium.
3. Hematology:
   a. Coagulation screen:
      - PTT at 0, 3 and 6 hours after initiation of dialysis, OR
      - ACT 2 hourly.
   b. Full blood count 1–2× per week.
4. Dialysis dose:
   a. Aim for:
      - Minimum weekly standard Kt/V_{urea} of 2, OR
      - Single pool Kt/V_{urea} of 1.2.
   b. With daily 8 hour sessions, the overall dialysis dose is equivalent to CKRT at 30–35 ml/kg/hour.
5. Nutrition:
   - Amino acid losses can be significant if PIKRT is performed over long periods.

Recommended Reading

1. Rajiv Sinha R, Sethi SK. (2018) Prolonged intermittent renal replacement therapy in children. *Pediatr Nephrol* **33**:1283–1296.
2. Sethi SK, Mittal A. (2020) Pediatric Continuous Renal Replacement Therapy (PCRRT) expert committee recommendation on prescribing prolonged intermittent renal replacement therapy (PIRRT) in critically ill children. *Hemodial Int* **24**:237–251

10 Therapeutic Plasma Exchange

Yap HK, Ng KH, Teo S, Resontoc LP and Prasetyo RV

A. Introduction

1. Plasmapheresis refers to the removal of plasma.
2. Therapeutic plasma exchange (TPE) refers to the exchange of removed plasma with 5% albumin or fresh frozen plasma (given post-filter).
3. TPE is highly efficacious for the removal of pathogenic autoantibodies and substances not usually removed by hemofiltration or high-flux hemodialysis (molecular weight >15000 Da).
4. TPE rapidly removes autoantibodies and immune complexes, unlike immunosuppressive drugs like steroids, which take time to exert an effect.
   - Immunosuppressive therapy only reduces plasma antibody levels by 50% in 21 days.
   - Immunoglobulin G (IgG) has an average molecular weight of >150000 Da and a half-life of approximately 21 days.
5. TPE also modulates the immune system by reducing the T helper type-1:T helper type-2 cytokine ratio.

B. Indications

1. Kidney:
   a. ANCA-associated rapidly progressive glomerulonephritis (RPGN), especially if dialysis dependent or associated with pulmonary hemorrhage.

b. Anti-glomerular basement membrane (GBM) disease, especially if there is pulmonary hemorrhage or RPGN.
c. Thrombotic microangiopathy (TMA):
   i. Infections with severe neurological symptoms:
      - Shiga toxin-producing *Escherichia coli*-hemolytic uremic syndrome (STEC-HUS).
      - *Streptococcus pneumoniae*.
   ii. Complement-mediated (factor H autoantibodies, complement factor gene mutations).
   iii. Lupus nephritis.
d. Thrombotic thrombocytopenic purpura (TTP), in particular, secondary to ADAMTS13 deficiency.
e. Kidney transplantation:
   - Antibody-mediated rejection.
   - Recurrence of focal segmental glomerulosclerosis.
   - Pre-transplant desensitization for ABO incompatibility.

2. Non-kidney:
   a. Acute and chronic inflammatory demyelinating polyradiculoneuropathy.
   b. Demyelinating polyneuropathy with IgG and IgA.
   c. Guillain-Barré syndrome.
   d. Phytanic acid storage disease (Refsum disease).
   e. Myasthenia gravis.
   f. Post-transfusion purpura.

C. Vascular Access

1. Femoral vein or internal jugular vein:
   - Femoral route may reduce the dangers associated with low ionized calcium levels and may be preferred.
   - Use of an internal jugular or subclavian line may increase the risk of cardiac arrhythmia due to the local effect of low ionized calcium on the sinoatrial node.
2. Size of catheters:
   - Catheters <7 F may not support the minimum blood flow of 50 ml/min required and should be used with caution.

Body Weight	Double Lumen
<4kg	6.5–7 F
4–10 kg	8 F
10–20 kg	9–10 F
20–40 kg	10–12.5 F
40–50 kg	12–12.5 F (consider triple-lumen)
>50 kg	12–14.5 F (consider triple-lumen)

D. Plasma Filters and Volume of Extra-corporeal Circuit

1. Fill volumes of the plasma filters and blood lines:

Type	Machine	Model		Fill Vol (ml)
Blood Lines	*AQUARIUS*	Aqualine S (patient <30 kg)		64
		Aqualine N		105
	PRISMAFLEX	TPE 1000 (patient <20kg)		71
		TPE 2000 (patient >20kg)		125
	INFOMED	Baby		25
		Child		50
		Adult		100
Plasma Filters	*AQUARIUS*	P 2S	0.5 m^2	61
	PRISMAFLEX	TPE 1000 (patient <20kg)	0.15 m^2	23
		TPE 2000 (patient >20kg)	0.35 m^2	41
	INFOMED	LF-030 (pediatric)	0.3 m^2	30
		LF-050	0.5 m^2	50

2. Patient's total blood volume (TBV) in liters:
   - <10kg child: 80 ml/kg.
     >10kg child: 70 ml/kg.
     Adolescent or adult: 65 ml/kg (female), 70 ml/kg (male).

3. Avoid extracorporeal volume >15% of patient's TBV.
   - For infants <5 kg, consider manual whole blood exchange instead.
4. Priming solution: 0.9% saline.
   - Consider priming with packed red cells diluted with sodium bicarbonate solution if extracorporeal volume >10–15% of TBV (see chapter "Continuous Kidney Replacement Therapy").

   Note:
   - Give 10% calcium gluconate 1 ml/kg (maximum 10 ml) over 5–10 minutes via a central line if blood prime is performed.
   - Do not return blood if blood prime is performed.

E. Blood Flow Rate

1. Blood flow rate should be kept low so that the transmembrane pressure (TMP) is low (e.g., <75 mmHg) to decrease the risk of hemolysis and filter clotting.
   a. *PRISMAFLEX*: Maintain access transmembrane pressure below the maximum as in the following table:

Blood Flow Q_b (ml/min)	Maximum Access Transmembrane Pressure (TMPa) (mmHg)	
	TPE 1000*	TPE 2000**
50	100	—
100	140	120
160	190	
200	—	171
250	—	193

* Q_b minimum 50 ml/min, maximum 180 ml/min

** Q_b minimum 100 ml/min, maximum 250 ml/min

F. Plasma Exchange Volume

1. For most conditions, standard practice is 1–1.5 plasma volume exchanges per session.

2. Estimated plasma volume (EPV) (ml):
   EPV = (1 – Hct) × (b + cW) or
   EPV = TBV × (1 – Hct/100)
   where TBV = Total blood volume (ml)
   Hct = Hematocrit (%)
   W = Lean body weight (kg)
   b = 1530 (male), 864 (female)
   c = 41 (male), 47.2 (female)
3. Relationship of the plasma exchange volume to plasma removal:

PV Exchanged (Equivalents)	Original Plasma Removed (%)
0.5	39
1.0	63
1.5	78
2.0	92

4. Do not do more than 2 plasma volume exchanges within 24 hours.

G. Plasma Filtration (Replacement) Rate

1. Replacement fluid rate (ml/h):
   a. Should be ~15% of blood flow rate (ml/hour).
      - Keep ≤20% if hematocrit is >35%.
      - Keep ≤25% if hematocrit is <35%.
   b. Keep <50 ml/kg/hour (maximum 2000 ml/hour).
2. *INFOMED*:
   a. Plasma replacement rate is ordered by entering "Plasma/Blood" (= plasma flow:blood flow ratio (%)).
   b. Start Plasma/Blood at 15%.
3. *PRISMAFLEX*:
   a. Blood flow rate should be adjusted to aim a filtration fraction of <20–30%.
   b. The risk of clotting is decreased with a lower filtration fraction.
   c. Filtration fraction can be decreased by:
      - Increasing blood flow.
      - Decreasing replacement fluid rate (increase duration of TPE).

d. Maximum plasma filtration rate based on blood flow:

Blood Flow Q_b (ml/min)	Maximum Plasma Filtration Rate (ml/min)	
	TPE 1000	TPE 2000
50	16	—
100	29	42
160	49	—
200	—	79
250	—	97

e. If no net negative fluid loss is desired, patient plasma loss is entered as "0".

H. Replacement Fluid

1. Types:
   a. Fresh frozen plasma (FFP)
      - Risks of infections, allergy and citrate toxicity.

   b. 5% albumin
      - Less transfusion-related risks, e.g., mild urticaria.
      - Depletion of coagulation factors can occur immediately after plasmaphresis, PT can increase by approximately 30%, and aPTT can double.
      - May be the default replacement fluid in most cases.
2. Indications for full FFP replacement
   a. Prolonged prothrombin time (PT) or activated partial thromboplastin time (aPTT) or active bleeding.
   b. Thrombocytopenia.
   c. Hypofibrinogenemia (<100–150 mg/dL).
   d. Hemolytic-uremic syndrome/TTP.
   e. Surgical procedures 2 to 5 days before or after TPE.
3. Consider replacing the first two-thirds volume as 5% albumin and the last one-third as FFP in multiple TPE sessions over short periods (e.g., daily sessions or multiple alternate-day sessions).

I. Anticoagulation

1. Heparin: A low-dose heparin regime is generally adequate.

Unfractionated Heparin	Loading Bolus (U/kg)	Maintenance Infusion (U/kg/h)	Monitoring
Low dose	>15 kg: 10–20 ≤15 kg: 5–10 (Adult: 1000 U)	5–10 (Adult: 500 U/h)	Keep ACT 150–200 sec
Regular dose	50 (Adult: max 2000 U)	10–50 (Adult: 750 U/h)	Keep ACT 200–250 sec

2. No anticoagulation: In patients with a high risk of bleeding.
3. If FFP is used as replacement fluid, further anticoagulation effect may occur with the citrate present in the FFP (contains 14% citrate by volume.)
4. *PRISMAFLEX*: Rinsing the circuit with heparinized saline prior to starting:
   a. Flush (rinse & prime) with normal saline
   b. Three rinses are required. Add heparin 5000 U or 10000 U into a 1000 ml bag for the second rinse.

J. Schedule

1. Number of sessions and interval between sessions depend on the nature of the pathological substance to be removed.
   - IgM: Only 1–2 sessions are enough to rapidly decrease IgM levels.
   - IgG: 5 plasmapheresis sessions over 7–10 days (one session every 2–3 days) can remove 90% of the initial IgG levels, assuming negligible production of new immunoglobulins.
2. Consider daily TPE in fulminant cases or those with diffuse alveolar hemorrhage, then every 2–3 days for a total of 6–9 procedures.
3. More sessions over a longer period will be needed in conditions where there is continual antibody production.
4. Concurrent immunosuppressive therapy should be given to prevent new immunoglobulin production.

5. Specific conditions such as acquired TTP or anti-GBM mediated disease may require daily sessions.
6. Summary of TPE regimes for kidney diseases:

Diagnosis	Indications	Plasma Exchange Volume	Schedule	Endpoint or Number of Treatments
TTP	In particular, ADAMTS13 deficiency	1–1.5 FFP	Daily	Normal LDH and platelet count
TMA (complement mediated)	Factor H autoantibodies. Complement factor gene mutations	1–1.5 FFP	Daily	Normal LDH and platelet count
TMA (Shiga toxin or *S. pneumoniae*)	Severe neurologic symptoms*	1–1.5 albumin (*S. pneumoniae*) or FFP (Shiga toxin)	Daily	Normal LDH and platelet count
Anti-GBM disease	Especially if pulmonary hemorrhage, dialysis independent RPGN	1–1.5 albumin	Daily or every other day for 2 weeks	Reduction in anti-GBM antibody/ cessation of pulmonary hemorrhage
ANCA associated RPGN	Dialysis dependent or pulmonary hemorrhage	1–1.5 albumin, FFP if pulmonary hemorrhage	Daily or every other day	6–9 treatments
Lupus nephritis	TMA or pulmonary hemorrhage RPGN*	1–1.5 albumin	Daily or every other day	3–6 treatments

(Continued)

(*Continued*)

Diagnosis	Indications	Plasma Exchange Volume	Schedule	Endpoint or Number of Treatments
Post-transplant recurrent FSGS	Proteinuria refractory to escalation of immunosuppressive therapy	1–1.5 albumin/FFP	Daily × 3 then every other day	Minimum 9 treatments or until proteinuria <1 g/day/1.73m^2
Antibody-mediated allograft rejection	Active severe rejection	1–1.5 albumin	Daily or every other day	At least 6 treatments, more if still elevated donor specific antibodies

*No established role of TPE, decision-making should be individualized.

K. Complications

1. The most common side effects are urticaria, paresthesia, leg cramps, nausea, and dizziness.
2. Complications related to vascular access:
   - Hematoma.
   - Pneumothorax.
   - Retroperitoneal bleed.
3. Complications related to the procedure:
   - Hemolysis: Check the effluent bag for a pink or red tinge.
   - Hypotension from externalization of blood in the extracorporeal circuit.
   - Hypotension due to decreased oncotic pressure.
   - Edema formation due to reduced oncotic pressure.
   - Loss of cellular elements (platelets).
   - Ethylene oxide-associated hypersensitivity reaction.
   - Transfusion-related acute lung injury (TRALI).

- Hypocalcemia from citrate toxicity (FFP) or albumin replacement.
- Metabolic alkalosis from citrate toxicity.

Note: Risk of citrate toxicity is increased with hepatic or kidney failure.

4. Complications related to anticoagulation:
   - Bleeding, especially with heparin.

L. Medications

1. To prevent hypersensitivity to albumin or FFP, give 1 hour prior to procedure:
   a. IV or oral diphenhydramine 1.25 mg/kg/dose (25–50 mg).
   b. IV hydrocortisone 4–10 mg/kg/dose (maximum 500 mg) or IV methylprednisolone 1–2 mg/kg/dose.
2. To prevent hypocalcemia:
   a. Correct baseline hypocalcemia if baseline iCa <1.1 mmol/L:
      - IV 10% calcium gluconate (0.22 mmol Ca/ml) 0.5–1 ml/kg over 10 minutes (maximum 20 ml), OR
      - IV 10% calcium chloride (0.7 mmol Ca/ml) 0.2 ml/kg over 10 minutes (maximum 10 ml).
      - Discuss with nephrologist if repeat micro-electrolytes and calcium boluses are required before starting.

   b. Calcium infusion during TPE:
      - IV 10% calcium gluconate (0.23 mmol Ca/ml) 0.1–0.4 ml/kg/hour, OR
      - IV 10% calcium chloride (0.68 mmol Ca/ml) 0.03–0.12 ml/kg/hour.
      - Titrate infusion rates according to micro-electrolyte monitoring during TPE.
      - Less calcium infusion is needed in albumin replacement compared to FFP.

   c. Give calcium through a Y-connector to the return line of the catheter or through a central line.
3. If 5% albumin is used as the replacement fluid:
   a. Potassium should be added to the albumin to avoid hypokalemia.

   b. Start with 4 mmol/L of K^+ in 5% albumin (= 1 ml of 7.45% potassium chloride per 250 ml bottle of albumin).
   c. Titrate according to micro-electrolyte monitoring during TPE.
4. All medications, especially biologicals such as Rituximab and those that are highly protein-bound, should preferably be given after plasmapheresis.
5. Patients receiving angiotensin-converting enzyme inhibitors (ACEi) prior to plasmapheresis are at risk of a severe reaction (bradykinin release) shortly after the start of plasmapheresis, possibly due to inefficient degradation of bradykinin, usually generated during plasmapheresis.
   - Where possible, withhold ACEi at least 24 hours before plasmapheresis.

M. Monitoring

1. Baseline PT/aPTT, full blood count (FBC), iCa, and arterial blood gas (ABG) before starting.
2. Micro-electrolyte monitoring (sodium, potassium, iCa) every 30 minutes during TPE.
   Note: If Y-connector is used for infusion of calcium, then blood should be taken from the arterial port pre-filter (check for recirculation), or preferably a venous cannula, intra-arterial line or capillary blood sampling.
3. Vital signs including heart rate, blood pressure, and oxygen saturation monitoring throughout TPE.
4. Post TPE, check PT/aPTT, FBC, iCa, and ABG.
5. After 5 sessions of plasmapheresis, consider checking blood IgG levels and fibrinogen.
   - If severe infection occurs post-TPE or if blood IgG level is low, a single infusion of intravenous immunoglobulins (IVIG) 500 mg/kg may be given.
   - Cryoprecipitate may be given if fibrinogen level is low.
6. Determine the marker to assess the response to TPE treatment based on the disease.

Recommended Reading

1. Kiprov DD, Sanchez A, Pusey C. (2007) Therapeutic apheresis. In: *Handbook of Dialysis*, 5th edition. Edited by Daugirdas JT, Blake PG, Ing TS. Wolters Kluwer and Lippincott Wiliams & Wilkins. pp. 333–359.
2. Szczepiorkowski ZM, Winters JL, Bandarenko N, Kim HC, Linenberger ML, Marques MB. (2010) Guidelines on the use of therapeutic apheresis in clinical practice — Evidence-based approach from the apheresis applications Committee of the American Society for apheresis. *J Clin Apher* **25**:83–177.
3. Goldstein SL. (2018) Plasmapheresis and total plasma exchange in the PICU. In: *Critical Care Nephrology and Renal Replacement Therapy in Children*. Edited by: Deep A, Goldstein SL. pp. 325–336.
4. Levy-Erez D, Kim HC. (2019) Plasmapheresis in pediatric renal disease. In: *Critical Care Pediatric Nephrology and Dialysis: A Practical Handbook*. Edited by: Sethi SK, Raina R, McCulloch, Bunchman TE. pp. 139–170.
5. Kaplan AA. (2020, updated) Plasmapheresis with hemodialysis equipment. Edited by Schwab SJ, Motwani S. *UpToDate ONLINE*. http://www.uptodateonline.com.
6. Fridey JL, Kaplan AA. (2021, updated) Therapeutic apheresis (plasma exchange or cytapheresis): Indications and technology. Edited by Uhl L, Tirnauer JS. *UpToDate ONLINE*. http://www.uptodateonline.com.

1 Tenckhoff Catheter Insertion and Initial Prescription

Ng KH, Teo S, Koh LJ and Yap HK

A. Tenckhoff Catheter Placement

1. A double-cuffed swan-neck tunneled coiled Tenckhoff catheter with a downward or lateral subcutaneous tunnel configuration should be used:
   a. Children 3–10 kg: Pediatric size catheter.
   b. Children >10 kg: Adult size catheter.
   Note: Single-cuffed catheter may be used in infants <3 kg but there are higher risks of infections and catheter dysfunction.
2. The length of catheter should be carefully discussed with the surgeons, taking into account the future growth of the child.
3. Placement of exit site:
   a. Belt line should be avoided.
   b. In young children, the exit site should be above the diaper line and preferably on the right upper quadrant to allow for gastrostomy on the left.
   c. As far as possible from other exit sites for gastrostomies, colostomies and urostomies.
      - Pre-sternal swan-neck catheter may be considered.
      - Significantly away from the nipples, especially in female infants.
   d. A paramedian fascial or lateral abdominal incision is preferred to avoid hernias and leakage.
   e. Superficial cuff of the catheter should be 1–2 cm from the exit site to reduce risk of cuff extrusion, which is associated with exit site infections.

4. Surgical considerations:
   a. Laparoscopic catheter placement may be performed.
   b. Partial omentectomy should be performed to reduce catheter obstruction.
   c. Elective herniotomy should be considered in male infants with evidence of inguinal or other herniae prior to or during catheter placement.
   d. Skin suture at the exit site should be avoided.
   e. Consider application of fibrin glue, especially if peritoneal dialysis (PD) initiation is expected soon after catheter insertion.
5. Gastrostomy placement:
   a. Gastrostomy insertion prior to or at time of Tenckhoff catheter insertion is preferred to minimize the risk of peritonitis.
   b. Open surgical technique is preferred for patients already on PD, and open or laparoscopic technique for patients not on PD.
      - Open technique reduces the risk of peritonitis by suturing the stomach to the abdominal wall.
   c. Use a rigid gastrostomy tube in the initial period to keep the stomach and abdominal wall apposed until they heal, to prevent leakage of gastric contents in the peritoneal cavity.
   d. Prophylactic antibiotic therapy should be given during gastrostomy placement.
      - Add oral/IV fluconazole prophylaxis in patients at risk of fungal peritonitis (malnourished, immunosuppressed, prolonged or multiple courses of broad-spectrum antibiotics).
   e. Withhold PD for at least 1–4 days after gastrostomy placement in patients on long-term PD.
      - Restart PD with a lower fill volume and increase to maintenance fill volume over 5–7 days.

B. Perioperative Care

1. For all patients planned for catheter insertion, the following measures should be instituted:
   a. Perform Hibiscrub® (4% chlorhexidine gluconate) body wash for at least 1 minute on the day before, and the day of catheter insertion.

- For patients intolerant to chlorhexidine, Octenisan® wash can be used instead.

b. Screen patient and caregivers for *Staphylococcus aureus* nasal carriage (see chapter "Peritoneal Dialysis-Related Catheter Exit Site Infections").

2. Pre-operative laxatives should be given routinely, especially to children who suffer from constipation.
3. Give desmopressin (DDAVP) upon call to operating theater (OT) at a dose of 0.3 mcg/kg (maximum 10 mcg) as a 30-minute intravenous (IV) infusion.
4. Perioperative antibiotic prophylaxis:

   a. Administer IV cefazolin 10 mg/kg (maximum 1 g) within 60 minutes prior to the surgical incision for Tenckhoff catheter, to prevent *Staphylococcus* and *Streptococcus* infections.
      - For patients at high risk of infections or who have had gastrostomy placement during Tenchkoff catheter insertion, administer IV cefazolin for a maximum of 3 days.
      - Alternatively, intraperitoneal cefazolin at 125 mg/L can be given for a total of 3 days, if starting PD immediately post-surgery.

   b. If there is cefazolin allergy, use an alternative antibiotic to cover for *Staphylococcus* and *Streptococcus.*

   c. If there is methicillin-resistant *Staphylococcus aureus* (MRSA) colonization, prophylactic IV clindamycin may be given instead.
      - Routine prophylaxis with vancomycin may cause the development of vancomycin resistance.

   d. If the child has an ileostomy or colostomy, add single dose of IV aminoglycoside for Gram-negative coverage.

C. Post-Tenckhoff Catheter Insertion

1. Check patency and peritoneal leak of the Tenckhoff catheter in the OT by performing at least 5 in-out exchanges with 10 ml/kg dialysate (Dianeal 1.5% with 500 U/L heparin) until the fluid is clear.
   - Attach a transfer set to the Tenckhoff catheter while in the OT.
2. Immobilize the catheter with tape or by dressing securely close to and below the exit site, to minimize movement and traction injury, and to optimise wound healing.

a. The first dressing change should be done only a week after catheter insertion, and then weekly until the third week, or until the wound is well healed (with normal skin around the exit site and no gaping), whichever comes later.
b. Dressing change may be more frequent if the dressing is wet, soiled or leaking. These should only be performed by dialysis nurses.
c. Use chlorhexidine or normal saline for initial dressing changes.
   - Avoid hydrogen peroxide or povidone-iodine.

3. Flush the catheter weekly with 10 ml/kg dialysate (Dianeal 1.5% with 500 U/L heparin) until initiation of PD.
4. Send the peritoneal fluid for cell count (with differentials) and culture:
   a. Weekly with each flush.
   b. At the initiation of PD after the wound has adequately healed at 2–3 weeks.
   c. On days 1, 3 and 5, if immediate initiation of PD is required.
5. If possible, avoid starting PD untill at least 2 weeks after insertion of the catheter, to allow for maximum healing.
6. Topical gentamicin should be applied to the exit site as part of long-term exit-site care.
   - Mupirocin can be used instead if there is nasal *Staphylococcus* aureus carriage or prior *Staphylococcus* catheter-related infections.
7. An X-ray of the abdomen and pelvis should be done before starting PD, to confirm the position of the Tenckhoff catheter tip.
8. Upon initiation of PD, add 250 U/L of intraperitoneal heparin for at least 3 days.

D. Initiation of Automated PD (APD)

I. Fill volume adjustments

1. Increase in fill volume should be based on any symptoms of raised intraperitoneal pressure (abdominal discomfort, gastroesophageal reflux, decreased appetite) or evidence of leak (subcutaneous, hernias).

2. Starting PD immediately or <2 weeks after catheter insertion:
   a. Should be performed only if there is no leak at the exit site and there is a clinical indication to initiate PD early.
   b. Start with manual intermittent PD (hourly cycles) for at least 24–48 hours untill the effluent is clear of gross blood.
      - Monitor closely for leak.
      - Reduce risk of leak by dialyzing only in supine position for several days.
   c. Switch to an automated cycler if the outflow is good.
      - Watch for poor outflow volume, which can lead to high intra-peritoneal pressure (IPP) and leaks.

Post-Insertion Day	Fill Volume (ml/m^2)	
	Patients ≥2 Years	Patients <2 Years (ml/m^2)
1	300	200 (10 ml/kg)
4	500	300 (15 ml/kg)
8	800	400 (20 ml/kg)
10	900	500 (25 ml/kg)
Week 2	1000	600 (30 ml/kg)
Week 3	1100	700 (35 ml/kg)
Week 4	1200	000 (40 ml/kg)

3. Starting PD ≥2 weeks after catheter insertion:
   a. Starting fill volumes:
      - 300 ml/m^2 for children ≥2 years old.
      - 200–300 ml/m^2 for children <2 years old.
   b. Escalation of fill volume:
      - Up to 1100–1200 ml/m^2 over 2 weeks for children >2 years old.
      - Up to 600–800 ml/m^2 over 3–4 months for children <2 years old.
4. Maximum fill volume for APD:
   - ≥2 years old: 1400 ml/m^2 (night), 700–1000 ml/m^2 (day).
   - <2 years old: 600–800 ml/m^2.

Note: At outpatient, the fill volume may be further increased to the maximum fill volume with longer intervals (2–4 weeks) between each increment.

5. IPP may be measured in cases with unexpected outcomes (e.g., symptoms of high IPP when target fill volume has yet to be achieved).
    - IPP ≤13–14 cmH_2O for ≥2 years.
    - IPP ≤8–10 cmH_2O for <2 years.
    - Severe constipation can lead to an increase in IPP.

II. Automated PD Prescription

1. Compute the empirical total therapy volume based on recommended target fill volume (1100–1200 ml/m²) x 5 cycles.
2. Number of exchanges per day:

$$\text{Number of exchanges} = \frac{\text{Empirical total therapy volume (ml)}}{\text{Current fill volume (ml)}}.$$

3. Minimum duration per cycle is 1 hour, but may be shorter in tidal PD.
4. For infants, dwell times are initially 30–60 minutes, and PD is performed manually.
5. Initial dialysis duration with low fill volume may be 20–24 hours, but this will decrease to 10–12 hours as the fill volume increase.
6. Aim for the lowest glucose concentration that allows for adequate ultrafiltration.
7. Adjust dialysis based on the ultrafiltrate volume and clearance (urea, potassium, acid-base, and phosphate).

E. Continuous Ambulatory PD Prescription (CAPD)

1. When initiating CAPD, the fill volumes increments are similar to APD.
    - The increase in fill volume for day dwells may be slower due to higher IPP when patient is upright during the day.
2. Maximum fill volume:
    - ≥2 years old: 1000 ml/m² (day) and 1200 ml/m² (night).
    - <2 years old: 600–800 ml/m².

3. Usually, 3–5 exchanges are performed per day, with dwells of 4–6 hours during the day and a long overnight dwell.

F. Complications

1. Effluent containing blood and/or fibrin:
   a. Administer intraperitoneal heparin 500–1000 U/L.
   b. If effluent is very bloody:
      - Consider flushes every 1–3 days until the effluent is clear.
      - Initiate PD with manual PD; avoid using automated cycler initially.
   c. Discontinue heparin when the effluent is clear of blood and fibrin.
2. Leakage of dialysate:
   a. Confirm leak by checking for glucose in the leaked fluid by using a dipstick.
   b. Ensure the connections are secure and that there are no cracks in the catheter.
   c. If the leakage is from the exit site or into the subcutaneous tissue:
      i. Stop PD for at least 2 weeks.
      ii. Administer IV cefazolin for at least 5 days or until the leak has stopped.
      iii. If PD has to be restarted within 2 weeks, use a low fill volume of 200–300 ml/m^2 for 2 weeks.
         - Intraperitoneal cefazolin may be used, instead of IV, for a minimum of 5 days following the leak.
      iv. Check PD fluid for cell count and culture upon diagnosis of leak, when peritonitis is clinically suspected, and at re-initiation of PD.
         - Treat for peritonitis if cell count is abnormal.
3. Hematoma in the catheter tract:
   - Treat with oral cephalexin for 2 weeks.
4. Catheter migration:
   a. Suspect when the drainage is poor, or if the patient has flank pain during drain.
   b. Check position of catheter tip on X-Ray.

c. Give oral laxatives. Consider fleet enema if the catheter tip is still not in the pelvis.
d. If catheter remains malpositioned, refer to surgeons to re-position the catheter.

Recommended Reading

1. Watson AR, Gartland C; European Paediatric Peritoneal Dialysis Working Group. (2001) Guidelines by an Ad Hoc European Committee for Elective Chronic Peritoneal Dialysis in pediatric patients. *Perit Dial Int* **21**:240–244.
2. Ha IS, Lai WM. (2005) Continuous ambulatory peritoneal dialysis (CAPD) and automated peritoneal dialysis (APD). In *Practical Paediatric Nephrology. An Update of Current Practices*. Edited by: Chiu MC, Yap HK. Medcom Limited. pp. 267–272.
3. Warady BA, Bakkaloglu S, Newland J, Cantwell M, Verrina E, Neu A, Chadha V, Yap HK, Schaefer S. (2011) Consensus guidelines for the prevention and treatment of catheter-related infections and peritonitis in pediatric patients receiving peritoneal dialysis: 2011 Update. *Perit Dial Int* **32**:S32–S86.
4. Verrina E, Harshman LA. (2021) Technical aspects and prescription of peritoneal dialysis in children. In: *Pediatric Dialysis*, 3rd edition. Edited by: Warady BA, Alexander SR, Schaefer F. Springer. pp. 193–228.

2 Long-Term Peritoneal Dialysis Prescription

Yap HK, Ng KH, Teo S and Koh LJ

A. Modalities of Long-Term Peritoneal Dialysis (PD)

1. Chronic ambulatory PD (CAPD):

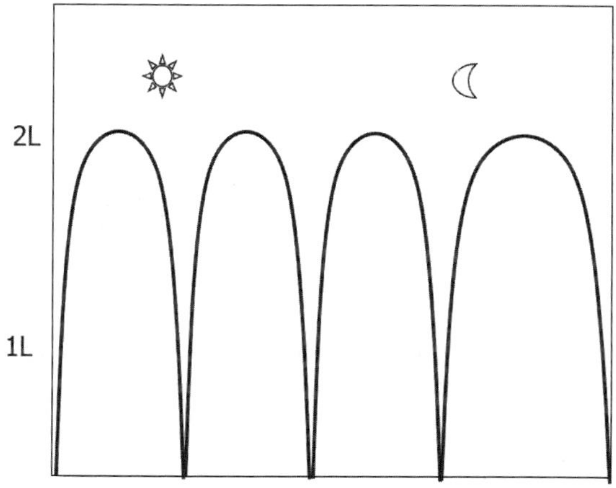

- 3–4 daytime exchanges, 4–5 hourly.
- Long night exchange over 6–9 hours.

2. Automated PD (APD)

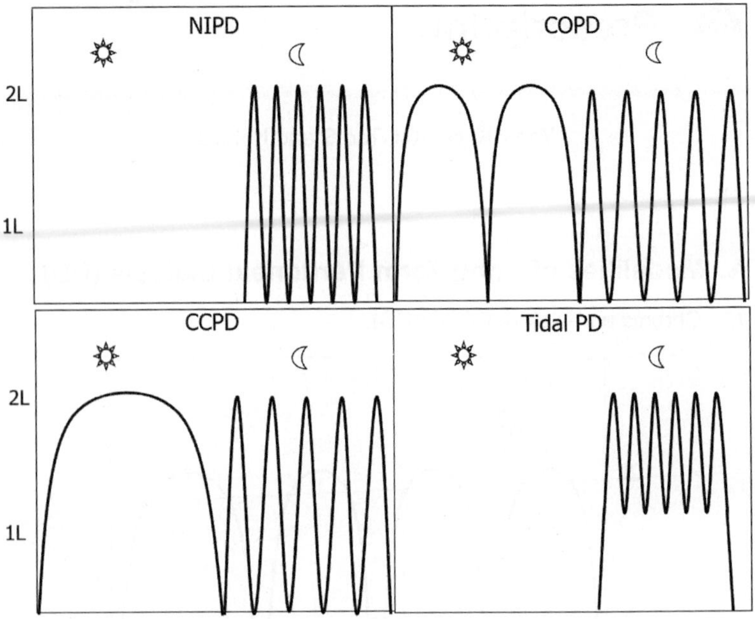

a. Nocturnal intermittent PD (NIPD):
   - 5–10 exchanges over at least 10 hours in the night.
   - No day dwell.
b. Continuous cycling PD (CCPD)
   - 5–10 exchanges over at least 10 hours in the night.
   - Adequate day dwell to increase solute clearance.
c. Continuous optimized PD (COPD)
   - 5–10 exchanges over at least 10 hours in the night.
   - Adequate day dwell with an extra day exchange.
d. Tidal PD:
   - Only a percentage (usually 50–80%) of the total volume of dialysate is exchanged at each cycle.
   - Advantage of optimizing treatment time when catheter drainage is slow towards the end of each drain.

3. The selection between CAPD and APD should be according to the lifestyles and preferences of patients and their families, as well as the cost, logistics and available expertise.

B. Physiology of Peritoneal Membrane Transport

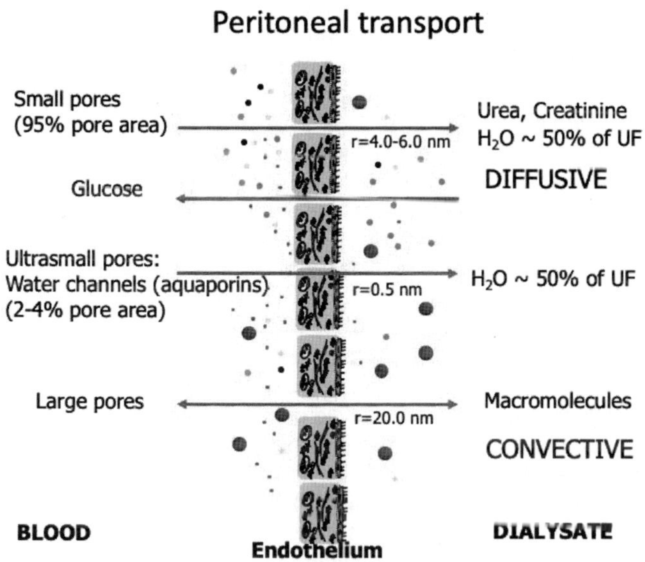

1. Solute and water transport across the peritoneal membrane occurs through three types of pores according to the three-pore model:
   a. Large pores (3% of pore area): Transport of macromolecules like albumin.
   b. Small "paracellular" pores (95% of pore area): Transport of small solutes, including sodium and water.
   c. Ultra-small aquaporins (2% of pore area): Transport of only water.
2. Solute transport by diffusion:
   a. Diffusion occurs through the small pores.

b. Rate of solute diffusion depends on:
   - Solute concentration gradient between blood and dialysate: Maintained by exchanging the dialysate in the abdomen as often as feasible.
   - Molecular weight of the solute: Smaller molecules (e.g., urea, creatinine) diffuse more rapidly than larger molecules (e.g., "middle" molecules, proteins).
   - Effective surface area and permeability of peritoneal membrane: Determined by the peritoneal vascular mesenteric perfusion and density of functional pores of the perfused capillaries.

3. Ultrafiltration (UF):
   a. UF is the movement of water across the peritoneal membrane.
   b. UF depends on:
      - Transmembrane pressure (hydrostatic and osmotic pressure across the membrane).
      - Effective peritoneal membrane surface area and its hydraulic permeability.
      - Lymphatic absorption.
   c. Hydrostatic pressure is often of minor importance except when intraperitoneal pressures are exceedingly high.
   d. Glucose exerts its crystalloid osmotic effect through aquaporins, but this is quickly lost as glucose gets absorbed into the blood.
   e. Icodextrin exerts its colloid osmotic effect mainly through small pores, and this is more sustained over prolonged periods of time.
   f. Principles of water transport:
      i. Aquaporins allow sodium-free water transport, while small pores allow for both sodium and water transport.
      ii. Sodium sieving is observed during the initial 30–90 minutes of a dwell with a glucose solution.
         - Osmotic gradient over the aquaporins is high, thus inducing sodium-free water transport from the plasma to the dialysate and decreasing the dialysate sodium concentration.
         - Subsequently, the increased sodium concentration difference between the dialysate and the plasma results in enhanced diffusive transport of sodium and water over the small pores, therefore, increasing the dialysate sodium concentration.

iii. Rapid exchanges can result in significant sodium sieving, resulting in hypernatremia, thirst, fluid overload, and hypertension.
iv. Water movement during a dwell with icodextrin:
- Sodium and water transport predominantly via small pores because they are much more abundant than aquaporins.
- No sodium sieving effect.
- Icodextrin is therefore useful when there is poor function of aquaporins.

4. Solute transfer by convection:
   a. Convective mass transfer occurs when water moves from capillaries to a peritoneal cavity down a pressure gradient, dragging dissolved solutes along with it, a process known as solvent drag.
   b. The large pores facilitate solvent drag.
   c. Convective transport of a solute depends on the amount of fluid removed by UF and membrane permeability, expressed by the sieving coefficient.
   d. In PD, the contribution of convection to solute removal is limited for small molecules, but is significant for middle-size molecules.

C. Goals of PD Prescription

1. Achieve adequate ultrafiltration.
2. Perform blood purification of solutes (small molecules like urea, and middle molecules).

D. Components of PD Prescription

1. Fill volume:
   a. CAPD:
      i. Initial volume: 300 ml/m^2 per exchange (200 ml/m^2 per exchange in infants).
      ii. Increase to 800–1000 ml/m^2 per daytime exchange and 1000–1200 ml/m^2 per night-time. Maximum volume is 2 L.
      iii. In infants, fill volume should not exceed 800 ml/m^2, as they have lower tolerance threshold for intraperitoneal pressure.

b. APD:
   i. For ≥2 years old, target night fill volume is 1000–1200 ml/m², up to 1400 ml/m² (maximum 2.5 L).
      - Fill volume for day dwell is 50–70% of night fill volume.
   ii. For <2 years old, the day target fill volume is 600–800 ml/m².

2. Dwell times:
   a. Dwell time is determined in part by the solute transporter status of the peritoneal membrane, measured by the peritoneal equilibration test (PET).
      - Short dwells favor UF and urea clearance.
      - Long dwells favor creatinine and phosphate clearance and may decrease UF.
   b. Younger children require shorter dwell times.
   c. APD: Each cycle should be ≥1 hour.
      - If the dwell time is too short, there may be a problem with sodium sieving.
   d. CAPD: Each day cycle is 3–6 hours.
   e. Dwell times will determine the number of cycles and PD duration.

3. Fluid composition:
   a. The lowest glucose concentration possible should be used.
   b. Choice of PD fluids with reduced glucose degradation products (GDP) content is preferred whenever possible, to reduce local and systemic toxicity.
   c. Correction of metabolic acidosis is superior with pH-neutral bicarbonate-based fluids, compared with a single chamber, acidic, lactate-based solutions.
   d. Icodextrin may be used once daily during the long dwell in children with insufficient ultrafiltration; however, ultrafiltration may not be as successful in young children.
      - A minimum fill volume of 550 ml/m² should be used.
   e. Low calcium-containing solutions should be used in patients at risk of hypercalcemia.
   f. Consider bicarbonate-based solutions in patients with infusion pain.

E. Types of PD Fluids

1. Composition of PD fluids:

	Dianeal®	Physioneal 40®	Balance®	Extraneal®
Sodium (mmol/L)	132	132	134	132
Chloride (mmol/L)	95	95	100.5	96
Calcium (mmol/L)	1.25/1.75	1.25/1.75	1.25/1.75	1.75
Magnesium (mmol/L)	0.25	0.25	0.5	0.25
Glucose (%)	1.5/2.5/4.25	1.36/2.27/3.86	1.5/2.3/4.25	0 (7.5% Icodextrin)
Osmolarity (mosm/L)	344/395/483	344/395/483	356/399/509	284
Lactate (mmol/L)	40	15	35	40
Bicarbonate (mmol/L)	0	25	0	0
pH	5.5	7.0	7.0	
Glucose degradation products (at medium glucose concentrations):				
Formaldehyde (µmol/L)	6.8 ± 0.2	3.4 ± 0	<3.3	3.6 ± 0.7
3-deoxy-glucosone (DG) (µmol/L)	167 ± 0.3	93.3 ± 5.0	17.6 ± 0.3	7.5 ± 0.4
3,4-dideoxy-glucosone-3-ene (DGE) (µmol/L)	11.3 ± 0.5	14.3 ± 2.5	<2.4	<2.4

2. Addition 10% calcium chloride to convert Low Calcium Dianeal to Normal Calcium Dianeal (5 L bag):
   Calcium content in low calcium Dianeal: 1.3 mmol/L
   Calcium content in normal calcium Dianeal: 1.8 mmol/L
   Amount of calcium ions (Ca^{2+}) to be added to 1 L: (1.8 – 1.3) mmol = 0.5 mmol/L
   For every 5 L bag, the amount of Ca^{2+} to be added: (0.5 × 5) mmol = 2.5 mmol.

10 ml of 10% calcium chloride ($CaCl_2$) contains 7 mmol Ca^{2+} and 14 mmol Cl^-.
Amount of 10% $CaCl_2$ (ml) to be added per 5 L bag: (2.5 × 10) ÷ 7 = 3.6 ml.

F. General Principles

1. The fill volume should be increased as tolerated by the patient first (target 1000–1200 ml/m^2, maximum 1400 ml/m^2), before increasing the number of exchanges.
2. Use of NIPD with no daytime dwell can be considered in patients who are clinically well, whose combined dialysis prescription and residual kidney function exceed the target solute clearance and who are without evidence of hyperphosphatemia, hyperkalemia, hypervolemia, or acidosis.
3. Daytime dwell in CCPD is recommended to maximize middle molecule clearance, phosphate clearance, and ultrafiltration volume.
   - Ensure an adequate day dwell of at least 50–70% of the full fill volume.
4. CAPD may be inadequate in children with poor residual kidney function, and in infants on a liquid diet.
5. Sodium and fluid restriction is recommended to maintain euvolemia rather than increasing the glucose concentration of the dialysate. Diuretics may be prescribed in patients with residual kidney function.

Recommended Reading

1. Twardowski ZJ. (2006) Pathophysiology of peritoneal transport. *Contrib Nephrol* **150**:13–19.
2. van Biesen W, Heimburger O, Krediet R, Rippe B, La Milia V, Covic A, Vanholder R; the ERBP Working Group on Peritoneal Dialysis. Evaluation of peritoneal membrane characteristics: A clinical advice for prescription management by the ERBP working group. *Nephrol Dial Transplant* **25**:2052–2062.
3. Schmitt CP, Bakkaloglu SA, Klaus G, Schröder C, Fischbach M. (2011) Solutions for peritoneal dialysis in children: Recommendations by the European Pediatric Dialysis Working Group. *Pediatr Nephrol* **26**:1137–1147.
4. Chua A, Warady BA. (2020, updated) Chronic peritoneal dialysis in children. Edited by: Niaudat P, Kim MS. *UpToDate ONLINE*. http://www.uptodateonline.com.
5. Verrina E, Harshman LA. (2021) Technical aspects and prescription of peritoneal dialysis in children. In: *Pediatric Dialysis*, 3rd edition. Edited by: Warady BA, Alexander SR, Schaefer F. Springer. pp. 193–228.

3 Tidal Peritoneal Dialysis

Ng KH and Yap HK

A. Principles:

1. Tidal peritoneal dialysis (TPD) is a form of automated peritoneal dialysis (PD) in which partial drainage of the dialysate is performed during each tidal exchange.

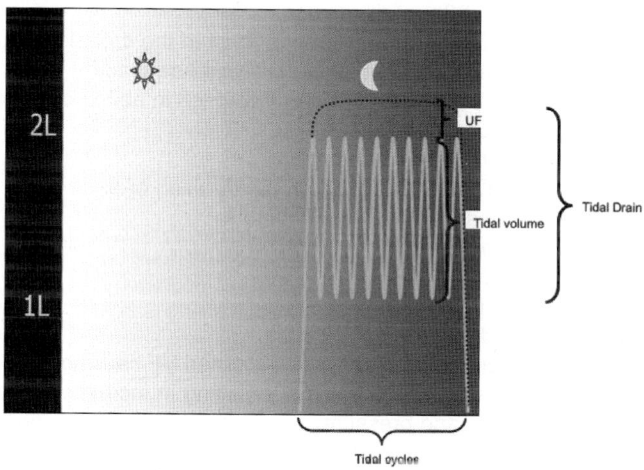

2. TPD is ~20% more effective than conventional PD in terms of both solute clearance and ultrafiltration (UF) because:
   a. Amount of dialysate fluid used is higher.
   b. The time for (slow) drainage is reduced, as the tidal drain volume can be adapted to the drainage profile of the catheter, resulting

in more contact time between dialysate and peritoneal membrane.

B. Indications:

1. Pain at the beginning of inflow and/or the end of drain.
2. Slow catheter drainage or frequent low-drain alarms, to optimize effective treatment time so as to increase the clearance or UF.
3. To increase solute clearance (controversial).

C. Tidal Prescription:

1. Fill volume: 1100–1400 ml/m^2.
2. Tidal percentage:
   - Generally 40–90% of fill volume.
   - Best determined by the transition point in the catheter drainage profile (see chapter "Peritoneal Dialysis Adequacy").
   - Tidal% = [(Fill volume – volume of fluid left in abdomen at break-point)/fill volume]*100%.
3. Therapy time: Minimum 10 hours.
4. Number of tidal cycles is based on the duration of each cycle:
   - Duration of each cycle: 15–50 minutes.
   - Inflow: 2–6 minutes.
   - Dwell: 10–40 minutes.
   - Drain: 2–6 minutes.
5. Number of full drains:
   - Full drains are needed to avoid undrained UF causing a progressive rise in residual PD volume, resulting in increased intraperitoneal volume and pressure.
   - A full drain may be prescribed at every third or more tidal cycle.
   - There should be at least one full drain at the end of the PD.
   - For catheters with poor outflow, too many full drains can result in frequent low-drain alarms.
6. Expected UF:
   - Defined as the predicted UF expected for the entire PD session.

- Tidal drain = (expected UF/number of tidal cycles) + tidal%*fill volume.
- If the expected UF is set too high, low-drain alarms may occur during tidal drains.
- If the expected UF is set too low, there is a risk of rising intraperitoneal pressure due to undrained UF volume.

7. Last fill volume:
   - Long day dwell to further improve clearance or UF.
8. Total volume:
   - (Fill volume × total number of full drains) + (tidal% × fill volume × number of tidal cycles) + Last fill.
9. Glucose concentration: Lowest glucose concentration needed for adequate UF.

Recommended Reading

1. Kathuria P, Twardowski ZJ. (2000) Automated peritoneal dialysis. In: *Peritoneal Dialysis*. Edited by: Gokal R, Khanna R, Krediet R, Nolph K. Kluwer Academic Publishers Netherlands. pp. 444–445.
2. Ha IS, Lai WM. (2005) Continuous ambulatory peritoneal dialysis and automated peritoneal dialysis. In: *Practical Paediatric Nephrology*. Edited by: Chiu MC, Yap HK. Medcom Limited Hong Kong. pp. 270–271.
3. Heimbürger O, Blake PG. (2015) Apparatus for peritoneal dialysis. In: *Handbook of Dialysis*, 5th edition. Edited by: Daugirdas JT, Blake PB, Ing TS. Wolters Kluwer Health New Delhi. pp. 408–424

4 Peritoneal Dialysis Adequacy

Ng KH, Koh LJ and Yap HK

A. Goal-directed Peritoneal Dialysis

1. Peritoneal dialysis (PD) should be prescribed based on care goals established between the child, family, and the medical team in order to maintain quality of life and minimize symptoms.

B. Assessment of PD Adequacy

1. Patient-reported outcome measures:
   - Symptoms.
   - Quality of life.
   - Cognitive development, school attendance, and performance.
2. Fluid status.
   - Weight, blood pressure.
   - Clinical examination, including jugular venous pressure assessment.
   - Bioimpedance spectroscopy.
   - Left ventricular hypertrophy and cardiac function.
   - N-terminal pro-brain natriuretic peptide.
3. Nutrition status:
   - Appetite, dietary evaluation.
   - Anthropometric measurements, height velocity, pubertal status.
   - Blood biochemistry: Potassium, phosphate, bicarbonate, albumin, and pre-albumin.
   - Normalised protein catabolic rate.

4. Solute clearance:
   - Blood biochemistry: Potassium, phosphate.
   - Kt/V_{urea}, creatinine clearance (C_{Cr}).
5. Residual kidney function (RKF):
   - Renal Kt/V_{urea} or K_r urea.
6. Other aspects:
   - Mineral bone disease.
   - Anemia.
   - Metabolic status, including hyperlipidemia and hyperglycemia.

C. Peritoneal Membrane Function Tests

1. Types:
   a. Standard peritoneal equilibration test (PET).
   b. Modified PET:
      - For a better assessment of ultrafiltration (UF) capacity, the standard PET may be modified to use 4.25% or 3.86% glucose solution.

   c. Accelerated Peritoneal Examination (APEX) time.
2. Aims:
   a. To optimize dialysis prescription with respect to peritoneal membrane properties, namely:
      - Small solute clearance.
      - Middle molecule clearance.
      - UF capacity.
      - Inflammatory status (peritoneal protein loss).

   b. To evaluate the evolution of peritoneal membrane function over time.
3. Peritoneal Equilibration Test:
   a. Most widely used test, primarily small solute transport.
      - Does not evaluate UF capacity.

   b. Recommended test exchange fill volume is scaled to body surface area (BSA) based on an age independent relationship between BSA and peritoneal membrane surface area:
      - Fill volume 1000–1100 ml/m² to a maximum of 2 L.
      - Dialysate glucose concentration 2.5% or 2.27%.

- Use of fill volumes, which are too small, can result in a falsely higher transporter status due to "geometry of diffusion".
- However, the usual fill volume of the patient may be used as it reflects the actual situation.

Note: The PD solutions used for the dwell(s) of the preceding night should be the same as the PET.

c. Measurements:

	Time (hour)	Glucose (mmol/L)	Creatinine (mmol/L)	Urea (mmol/L)	Phosphate (Optional) (mmol/L)
Serum	2	√	√	√	√
Dialysate	0	√	√	√	√
Dialysate	2	√	√	√	√
Dialysate	4	√	√	√	√

Note: D/P phosphate may be added into the standard PET to allow for dialysis adjustments for improved phosphate clearance.

d. Creatinine, urea and phosphate: Ratios of dialysate to plasma solute levels (D/P) at 2 and 4 hours are calculated:
   - D/P of 1.0 means that the dialysate has the same concentration of solutes as the plasma, or it is 100% equilibrated.

e. Glucose: Ratios of dialysate glucose concentration to the dialysate glucose concentration at time 0 (D/D_0) at 2 and 4 hours are calculated:
   - D/D_0 glucose of 0.59 means that 59% of the 0-hour dialysate glucose is still in the peritoneum, or 41% of the dialysate glucose has been absorbed from the peritoneum.

f. Peritoneal membrane transporter status is defined by the 4-hour D/P creatinine and D/D_0 glucose:

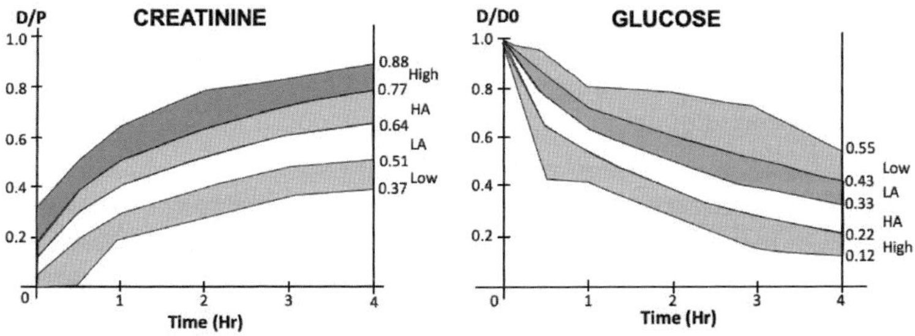

Transporter Status	4-hour D/P Creatinine	4-hour D/D_0 Glucose
High (H)	0.77–0.88	0.12–0.21
High average (HA)	0.64–0.76	0.22–0.32
Low average (LA)	0.51-0.63	0.33–0.42
Low (L)	0.37–0.50	0.43–0.55

g. D/P urea is not used to characterize transporter status as it shows far less variability between patients than D/P of larger molecules.

h. Sequestration of PD fluid due to intraabdominal adhesions can lead to a false interpretation of a high transporter status (pseudo-high transporter).
   - Sequestrated fluid will have high creatinine and low glucose content.
   - Mixture of PET fluid with the sequestrated volume will result in high D/P creatinine and low D/D_0 glucose ratios.
   - Can be suspected from the catheter drainage profile.

4. Modified PET:
   a. Same procedure as standard 4-hour PET except that a 4.25% or 3.86% glucose solution is used.

b. Use of different glucose dialysate in PET does not significantly affect D/P creatinine or D/D_0 glucose ratios; hence, there is minimal impact on transporter status characterizations.

c. Measurements are performed in accordance with the table below:

	Time (hour)	Glucose (mmol/L)	Creatinine (mmol/L)	Urea (mmol/L)	Sodium (mmol/L)	Phosphate (Optional) (mmol/L)
Serum	2	√	√	√	√ P_{Na}	√
Dialysate	0	√	√	√	√ (D_0Na)	√
Dialysate	1				√ ($D_{60}Na$)	
Dialysate	2	√	√	√		√
Dialysate	4	√	√	√		√

d. Provides additional information on sodium dip:
- Occurs in the first phase of a glucose solution dwell as a result of sodium sieving.
- Indirect indicator of free water transport and osmotic conductance to glucose.
- Requires a 60-minute dwell of 4.25% or 3.86% glucose and measurement of dialysate sodium at 0-minute (D_0Na) and 60-minute ($D_{60}Na$).
- Sodium dip at 60 minutes (mmol/L) = $\Delta D_{60}Na = D_0Na - D_{60}Na$
- Considered as decreased if $\Delta D_{60}Na$ is <5 mmol/L.

5. Accelerated Peritoneal Examination (APEX) time:

a. Proposed to be the optimal dwell time in terms of UF capacity and solute clearance.

b. APEX time is the time point at which the falling D/P urea curve intersects the rising D/D_0 glucose curve.

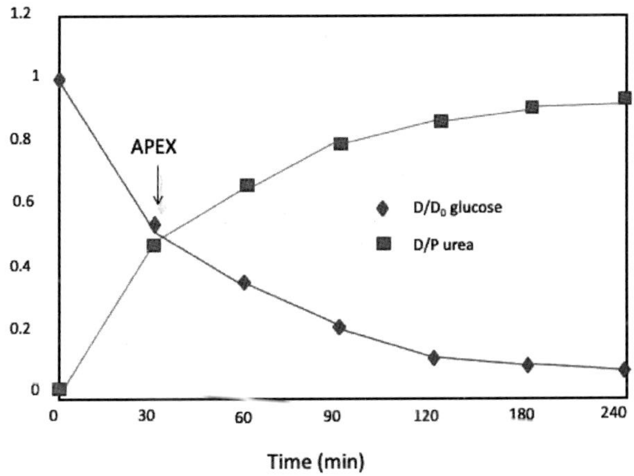

c. To optimize phosphate clearance, dwell time should approximately be the time at which D/P phosphate = 0.6 or 4 times the APEX time.

D. Catheter Drainage Profile

1. This can be assessed by plotting a drain volume curve over time.

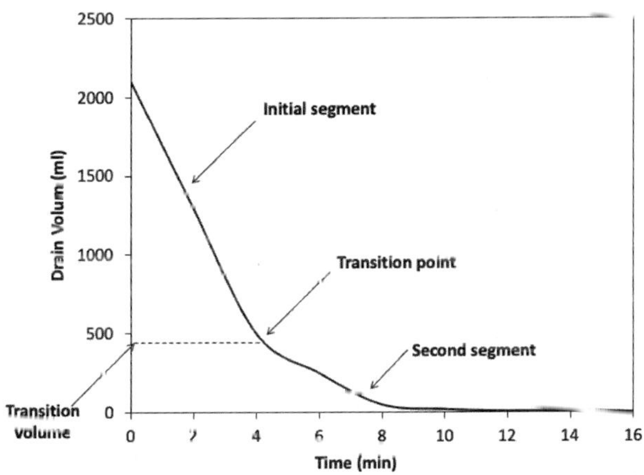

2. Drain volume is estimated by weighing the drainage bag and subtracting it from the initial fill volume.
3. Drainage of the last portion takes more time than the bulk of the fluid.
4. The transition point is the point when the slope changes on the graph.
   a. After the transition point, there is insufficient contact of the dialysate with the peritoneal membrane resulting in no more solute or fluid clearance.
   b. If this period is long, it can result in significant loss of treatment time, especially in APD.
5. This loss of treatment time can be avoided by allowing the cycler to stop drainage after the "transition point", where a new fill can start.
   - This corresponds to the tidal % in tidal dialysis.

E. PD Adequacy Parameters

1. Solute clearance:
   a. Estimating total body water (V) (L), with height (Ht) in cm, weight (Wt) in kg, and age in years:
      i. Morgenstern equation (age ≤23 years)
         - Males: $V = 0.10*(Ht*Wt)^{0.68} - (0.37*Wt)$
         - Females: $V = 0.14*(Ht*Wt)^{0.64} - (0.35*Wt)$
      ii. Watson equation (age >23 years)
         - Males: $V = 2.447 + 0.3362*Wt + 0.1074*Ht - 0.09516*Age$
         - Females: $V = -2.097 + 0.2466*Wt + 0.1069*Ht$
      iii. Estimation of weight (Wt):
         - Use actual weight on test day minus day dwell.
         - If severely malnourished, use ideal weight to estimate V.
         - For obese patients, the formula is as follows:
           Adjusted Wt = (Ideal Wt for Ht) + 25%*[Actual Wt – Ideal Wt] where 25% represents the percentage of body fat tissue that is metabolically active.
   b. Estimating BSA using the Gehan and George equation:
      - $BSA\ (m^2) = 0.0235*Wt^{0.51456}*Ht^{0.42246}$.
   c. Total small solute clearance measured as Kt/V_{urea}:
      i. Kt/V_{urea} is the sum of:

- Renal Kt/V_{urea} ($K_r t/V_{urea}$) based on 24-hour urine collection if residual urine volume >100 ml/day, AND
- Peritoneal Kt/V_{urea} ($K_p t/V_{urea}$) based on 24-hour collection of total drained effluent volume.

ii. Calculation of total weekly Kt/V_{urea} ($K_t t/V_{urea}$):

- Weekly total renal $K_r t/V_{urea}$

$$= \frac{24\text{-hour urine volume (L)} * \frac{U_{urea}}{P_{urea}} * 7}{V\ (L)}$$

- Weekly total peritoneal $K_p t/V$

$$= \frac{24\text{-hour effluent volume (L)} * \frac{D_{urea}}{P_{urea}} * 7}{V\ (L)}$$

- Weekly total $K_t t/V = K_p t/V + K_r t/V$
  where:
  U_{urea} = Urine urea concentration (mmol/L)
  P_{urea} = Plasma urea concentration (mmol/L)
  D_{urea} = 24-hour effluent urea concentration (mmol/L)
  24-hour effluent volume = Total therapy volume + UF + initial drain + manual drain

d. RKF refers to the estimated glomerular filtration rate (eGFR) and is measured as the average of the renal urea clearance (K_r urea) and renal C_{Cr} based on a 24-hour urine collection and corrects for secretion of creatinine in urine when GFR is low.

- RKF (ml/min/1.73m²)

$$= \frac{K_r \text{ urea (ml/min)} + \text{renal } C_{Cr} \text{ (ml/min)}}{2} * \frac{1.73}{BSA\ (m^2)},$$

where

$$K_r \text{ urea (ml/min)} = \frac{U_V * \frac{U_{urea}}{P_{urea}}}{1440}$$

$$\text{Renal } C_{cr} \text{ (ml/min)} = \frac{U_V * \frac{U_{creat}}{P_{creat}}}{1440}$$

BSA = Body surface area (m^2)
U_v = Volume of 24-hour urine collected (ml)
U_{urea} = 24-hour urine urea concentration (mmol/L)
P_{urea} = Plasma urea concentration (mmol/L)
U_{creat} = 24-hour urine creatinine concentration (μmol/L)
P_{creat} = Plasma creatinine concentration (μmol/L)

- 24-hour urine volume ≤100 ml is considered negligible.
- If the patient micturates ≤3 times a day, collect 48-hour urine.

e. Calculation of total weekly C_{Cr} (L/week/1.73m^2):

- Weekly RKF (L/week/1.73m^2)

$$= \frac{K_r \text{ urea (ml/min)} + \text{renal } C_{Cr} \text{ (ml/min)}}{2*1000} * 7 * \frac{1.73}{\text{BSA } (m^2)}.$$

- Weekly peritoneal C_{Cr} (L/week/1.73m^2)

$$= \frac{D_{creat}}{P_{creat}} * 24\text{-hour effluent volume (L)} * 7 * \frac{1.73}{\text{BSA } (m^2)}.$$

- Total weekly C_{Cr} = weekly RKF + weekly peritoneal C_{Cr}, where

$$K_r \text{ urea (ml/day)} = \frac{U_{urea}}{P_{urea}} * Uv$$

$$\text{Renal } C_{cr} \text{ (ml/day)} = \frac{U_{creat}}{P_{creat}} * Uv$$

BSA = Body surface area (m^2)
U_v = Volume of 24-hour urine collected (ml)
U_{urea} = 24-hour urine urea concentration (mmol/L)
P_{urea} = Plasma urea concentration (mmol/L)
U_{creat} = 24-hour urine creatinine concentration (μmol/L)
P_{creat} = Plasma creatinine concentration (μmol/L)
D_{creat} = 24-hour effluent creatinine concentration (μmol/L)

f. Targets:

i. $K_t t/V_{urea}$:

- Patients with RKF (renal $K_r t/V_{urea}$ >0.1/week): Minimal "delivered" weekly dose of total (peritoneal and kidney) $K_t t/V_{urea}$ ≥1.7.
- Patients without RKF or for those in whom RKF cannot be measured accurately: Minimal "delivered" dose of weekly peritoneal $K_p t/V_{urea}$ ≥1.7.

ii. Creatinine clearance (C_{Cr}):
- There is no clear evidence for using clearance equations other than Kt/V_{urea} to evaluate PD adequacy.
- May be considered in children on APD.
- Aim for the ratio of weekly $K_t t/V_{urea}$:total weekly C_{Cr} (L/week/1.73m^2) to be at least 1:30.

iii. If symptoms, nutrition and fluid status are all controlled, PD prescription need not be changed to improve Kt/V or C_{cr}.

2. Ultrafiltration:
   a. Dietary fluid and salt indiscretion is the most common cause of fluid overload, and this should be addressed first.
   b. Definition of UF failure:
      - Children: UF volume <150 ml/m^2 after a 4-hour dwell with 1000–1100 ml/m^2 of 2.5% or 2.27% glucose solution.
      - Adults: UF volume <400 ml after a 4-hour dwell with 2 L of 4.25% or 3.86% glucose solution.
3. Normalized protein catabolic rate (nPCR):
   a. Takes into account both the protein catabolic rate and protein losses per kg body weight.
      - Estimation of dietary protein intake.
   b. Modified Borah equation for children:
      - Urine nitrogen appearance (UNA) (g/day)

$$= \left[U_V * U_{urea} * \frac{2.808}{100}\right] + \left[24\text{-hour effluent volume (L)} * D_{urea} * \frac{2.808}{100}\right].$$

      - PCR (g/day) = [6.49*UNA] + [0.294*V] + [$U_{protein}$*U_v] + [$D_{protein}$*24-hour effluent volume (L)].
      - $\text{nPCR (g/kg/day)} = \frac{\text{PCR}}{\text{body weight in kg}}$,

      where
      U_v = Volume of 24-hour urine collected (L)
      U_{urea} = 24-hour urine urea concentration (mmol/L)
      D_{urea} = 24-hour effluent urea concentration (mmol/L)
      V = Total body water (L)
      $U_{protein}$ = 24-hour urine total protein concentration (g/L)
      $D_{protein}$ = 24-hour effluent total protein concentration (g/L)
   c. Bergstrom equation for adults:
      - nPCR (g/kg/day) = 15.1 + [6.95*UNA] + [$U_{protein}$*U_v] + [$D_{protein}$*24-hour effluent volume (L)] .

- $\text{nPCR (g/kg/day)} = \dfrac{\text{PCR}}{\text{body weight in kg}}$,

  where

  $U_{protein}$ = 24-hour urine total protein concentration (g/L)

  U_v = Volume of 24-hour urine collected (L)

  $D_{protein}$ = 24-hour effluent total protein concentration (g/L)

d. Target:
   - This is according to the suggested dietary intake for protein in children on PD (see chapter "Recommended Dietary Intake in Children with Chronic Kidney Disease"), plus 0.28 g/kg/day in infants to 0.1 g/kg/day in adolescents to compensate for the peritoneal losses.

F. Assessment for Inadequate Dialysis

1. The patient's clinical status should be reviewed at least monthly.
   - PD should render the patient free of signs and symptoms of uremia.
2. Clinical signs of inadequate dialysis include:
   a. Uncontrolled hypertension or hypervolemia.
   b. Cardiomyopathy.
   c. Hyperphosphatemia or excessive calcium-phosphorus product.
   d. Overt uremia with pericarditis or pleuritis.
   e. Repeated hyperkalemic episodes.
   f. Clinical or biochemical signs of malnutrition or poor growth.
   g. Poor school performance.
3. Factors contributing to inadequate dialysis include:
   a. Non-adherence to diet and fluid.
   b. Non-adherence with PD prescription.
   c. Decline of RKF.
   d. Poorly functioning PD catheter with complications such as malposition.
   e. Change in peritoneal membrane characteristics due to:
      - Increase in effective peritoneal surface area due to neo-angiogenesis and sclerosis.

- Decrease in effective surface area due to extensive intra-abdominal adhesions.

f. Inappropriate fill volumes, which may be too high or too low.

g. Inappropriate dwell times for membrane transport characteristics.

4. Peritoneal membrane function tests should be performed:
   a. At least 4 to 8 weeks after initiation of PD and yearly subsequently.
   b. Repeat testing in the setting of inadequate dialysis, overhydration or malnutrition especially where clinical events may have altered membrane transport characteristics, including:
      - Repeated peritonitis (should only be performed at least one month after a peritonitis episode).
      - Abdominal surgery.
5. Measurements of dialysis adequacy should be performed:
   a. At least 4 to 8 weeks after initiation of dialysis.
   b. At least 6-monthly.
   c. At least 1 month after a peritonitis episode, if there is clinical evidence of inadequate dialysis, overhydration or malnutrition.
6. RKF should be evaluated 3-monthly in patients with RKF defined as:
   - Renal K_rt/V_{urea} >0.1/week OR
   - Renal urea clearance (K_r urea) >0.2 ml/min/1.73m^2.

G. Adjustment of Dialysis Prescription

1. Fill volumes should be optimized first as this maximizes the effective peritoneal surface.
2. Dwell times according to solute transporter status:
   a. Low and LA transporters do better with large fill volumes and longer dwell times to allow for adequate solute clearance while maintaining UF.
   b. HA and high transporters do better with shorter dwell times to allow for adequate UF while maintaining solute clearance.
      - Efficiency of removal of small solutes increases with increase in number of exchanges in intermittent flow PD and contact time between dialysate and the peritoneal membrane as seen in tidal PD.

Transporter Status	Predicted		Dialysis Recommendations
	UF	Solute Clearance	
High	Poor	Adequate	• Shorten dwell times, e.g., NIPD • CAPD: Avoid long dwells; shorter dwells may be required. • Icodextrin in long dwells.
High average	Adequate	Adequate	• Standard dose PD or CCPD
Low average	Good	Adequate	• Standard dose PD or CCPD.
		Inadequate	• COPD. • Reduce number of dwells (lengthen dwell times).
Low	Excellent	Inadequate	• COPD. • Use larger volumes. • Reduce number of dwells (lengthen dwell times). • Hemodialysis.

CAPD: Chronic ambulatory PD
NIPD: Nocturnal intermittent PD
CCPD: Continuous cycling PD
COPD: Continuous optimized PD

3. Change in transporter status over time:
   a. There is increasing vasculopathy and neo-angiogenesis of the peritoneal membrane resulting in increased effective surface area.
   b. D/P ratios and transporter status generally will increase with time.
   c. The RKF will decrease with time, and the dialysis UF and clearance will have to correspondingly increase.
   d. To increase PD clearance, consider:
      - Increase in total therapy volume.
      - Addition of day dwells.
      - Use of a mid-day exchange in APD (COPD).
4. Middle molecule clearance:
   - In children on APD who have minimal RKF, a day dwell is recommended, even if small solute clearance is above target.

5. Phosphate clearance in PD:
   a. Phosphate binders are often required in patients with an adequate protein diet.
      - Optimize phosphate binders and dietary phosphate intake before considering adjusting dialysis to optimize phosphate clearance.
   b. In PD patients who remain hyperphosphatemic despite the use of phosphate binders, the PD prescription can be modified:
      i. In high transporters, increase the total therapy volume and number of cycles.
      ii. In HA, LA and low transporters, consider longer dwells and increasing PD duration.
      iii. For patients on nightly APD, consider addition of a day dwell, a mid-day exchange, or conversion to CAPD.
      iv. Increase convective clearance by increasing UF.
      v. Measure D/P phosphate ratio in standard or modified PET.
         - Optimal dwell time for phosphate clearance is the time when D/P phosphate is 0.5–0.6.
6. UF:
   a. Rapid exchanges of glucose solutions can result in significant sodium sieving, resulting in hypernatremia, thirst, fluid overload, and hypertension.
      - Most pronounced with rapid exchanges of high glucose solutions in a low transporter because sodium sieving increases with increasing glucose concentration and decreases with diffusive transport rate and the duration of the dwell.
   b. When UF is poor, exclude catheter malfunction, fluid leaks, and sequestration first.

c. Add icodextrin to improve UF:
   - Consider fill volume of at least 550 ml/m^2.
   - Icodextrin reabsorption may occur, especially in younger children.

H. Other Aspects to Improve Dialysis Adequacy

1. Preservation of RKF is important in dialysis care:
   a. Avoid nephrotoxic insults, in particular, aminoglycosides, nonsteroidal anti-inflammatory drugs, and radiological contrast.

b. Avoid acute kidney injury due to dehydration.
c. Avoid and promptly treat urinary tract infections.
d. Use diuretics to maximize urinary salt and water excretion.
e. Avoid hypercalcemia and hyperphosphatemia.
f. Consider angiotensin-converting enzyme inhibitors or angiotensin receptor blockers in hypertensive patients with RKF.
   - Temporarily discontinue during episodes of dehydration.

2. Maintain euvolemia:
   a. Salt and fluid restriction.
   b. Use of diuretics in patients with RKF.
3. Maintain dietary protein intake at 100% of the suggested dietary intake for an ideal body weight plus an allowance for dialytic protein and amino acid losses.
4. Other aspects:
   a. Lipid monitoring yearly and consider statins or ezetimibe.
   b. Monitoring of fasting glucose 6 monthly and use the lowest dextrose concentration in dialysate where possible.

Recommended Reading

1. Warady BA, Alexander SR, Hossli S, Vonesh E, Geary D, Watkins S, Salusky IB, Kohaut EC. (1996) Peritoneal membrane transport function in children receiving long-term dialysis. *J Am Soc Nephrol* **7**:2385–2391.
2. Fishbach M, Lahlou A, Eyer D, Desprez P, Geisert J. (1996) Determination of individual ultrafiltration time (APEX) and purification phosphate time by peritoneal equilibration test: Application to individual peritoneal dialysis modality prescription in children. *Perit Dial Int* **16**(Suppl 1):S557–S560.
3. Peritoneal Dialysis Adequacy Work Group. (2006) Clinical practice guidelines for peritoneal dialysis adequacy. *Am J Kidney Dis* **248**(Suppl 1):S98–S129.
4. Van Biesen W, Heimburger O, Krediet R, Rippe B, La Milia V, Covic A, Vanholder R; ERBP working group on peritoneal dialysis. (2010) Evaluation of peritoneal membrane characteristics: A clinical advice for prescription management by the ERBP working group. *Nephrol Dial Transplant* **25**:2052–2062.
5. Schaefer F. (2017) Ultrafiltration failure in children undergoing chronic PD. In: *Pediatric Dialysis Case Studies*. Edited by: Warady BA, Schaefer F, Alexander SR. Springer. pp. 83–88.
6. Warady BA, Schaefer F, Bagga A, Cano F, McCulloch M, Yap HK, Shroff R. (2020) Prescribing peritoneal dialysis for high-quality care in children. *Peritoneal Dialysis International* **40**:333–340.
7. Brown EA, Blake PG, Boudville N, Davies S, Arteaga J, Dong J, Finkelstein F, Foo M, Hurst H, Johnson DW, Johnson M, Liew A, Moraes T, Perl J, Shroff R, Teitelbaum I,

Wang AY, Warady B. (2020) International Society for Peritoneal Dialysis practice recommendations: Prescribing high-quality goal-directed peritoneal dialysis. *Peritoneal Dialysis International* **40**:244–253.
8. Verrina EE, Harshman LA. (2021) Technical aspects and prescription of peritoneal dialysis in children. In: *Pediatric Dialysis*, 3rd edition. Edited by Warady BA, Alexander SR, Schaefer F. Springer. pp. 193–228.

5 Management of Abdominal Pain During Peritoneal Dialysis

Yap HK and Ng KH

A. Etiology

1. Dialysate:
   - Acidic pH (5.2–5.5) of conventional lactate dialysate.
   - Extreme temperatures of dialysate.
   - High glucose concentration in hypertonic dialysate.
   - Expired dialysate with high concentrations of glucose degradation products.
2. Catheter:
   - Malposition: Tip of Tenckhoff catheter impinging on peritoneum or bowel wall.
   - Too rapid inflow or outflow rates in automated peritoneal dialysis (PD).
3. Peritoneal cavity:
   - Peritonitis.
   - Adhesions in peritoneal cavity or encapsulating peritoneal sclerosis.
   - Accidental infusion of air (referred shoulder pain).
   - Too rapid increment of fill volume at initiation of PD.
   - "Dry" abdomen (no last fill).

B. Management

1. Pain during inflow:
   a. Initial steps:

i. Peritonitis must be excluded; send effluent fluid for cell count and cultures.
ii. Perform manual dialysis exchange to assess the degree of discomfort, its relation to inflow and outflow, as well as completeness, color and clarity of effluent fluid.
iii. Check for inadequate drain prior to the next fill resulting in inadvertent excessive dialysate in the peritoneal cavity:
   - Machine or catheter malfunction.
   - Fluid sequestration related to adhesions.
   - Inadequate tidal outflow in tidal PD prescription.
   - Inappropriate machine alarm settings.
iv. Ensure dialysate solution is not expired and is correctly warmed.
v. Avoid using 4.25% dextrose dialysate as the heater bag (if possible).
vi. Abdominal X-Ray to determine location of the catheter tip.
vii. Try changing body position during infusion.

b. If initial steps are unsuccessful, consider the following:
   i. For patients who are new to peritoneal dialysis, avoid too rapid increment of fill volumes.
   ii. Decrease the infusion rate if this is adjustable in the automated cycler.
   iii. Perform modified tidal dialysis with tidal cycles at 85–90% of full fill volume.

c. For refractory inflow pain, consider the following:
   i. Laparoscopic adjustment or replacement of the catheter if malposition is the likely cause.
   ii. Check the intraperitoneal pressure (IPP), as IPP >18 cmH_2O can cause abdominal pain and decrease in lung vital capacity.
      - Optimal IPP in children >2 years: ≤13–14 cmH_2O.
      - Optimal IPP in children <2 years: ≤8–10 cmH_2O.
   iii. Add sodium bicarbonate (2–4 mmol/L) to dialysate.
   iv. Add 1% lidocaine (50 mg per 2 L exchange) to dialysate before infusing.
   v. Use more biocompatible dialysate with lower glucose degradation products and higher pH (7–7.4).
   vi Discontinue PD.

2. Pain during outflow:
   a. Peritonitis must be excluded by sending effluent fluid for cell count and cultures.
   b. Perform modified tidal dialysis with tidal cycles at 85–90% of full fill volume.
   c. Decrease the outflow rate either by modifying the machine settings or by partially occluding the outflow dialysis tubing manually during the outflow.

Recommended Reading

1. Schmidt RJ. (2019, updated) Non-infectious complications of continuous peritoneal dialysis. Edited by Golper TA, Motwani S. *UpToDate ONLINE*. http://www.uptodateonline.com.

6 Peritoneal Dialysis-Related Catheter Exit Site Infections

Ng KH, Liu ID, Kakar S and Yap HK

A. Diagnosis of Peritoneal Dialysis Catheter Exit Site Infections

1. Exit site scoring system (International Society of Peritoneal Dialysis [ISPD] Pediatric Guidelines 2012):

Indication	0	1	2
Swelling	No	Exit site only (<0.5 cm)	Including part of or the entire tunnel
Crust	No	<0.5 cm	>0.5 cm
Erythema	No	<0.5 cm	>0.5 cm
Pain on pressure	No	Slight	Severe
Discharge	No	Serous	Purulent

2. Exit-site infection (ESI):
   - Exit site score of ≥2 in the presence of a pathogenic organism, OR
   - Exit site score of ≥4, regardless of culture results, OR
   - Any purulent discharge from the exit site, with or without erythema, OR
   - Severe acute erythema without purulent discharge in the absence of recent trauma to the exit site or allergic skin reactions.
3. Tunnel infection:
   - Exit site score of ≥6, OR
   - Erythema, odema, induration, or tenderness along the subcutaneous portion of the catheter, with or without purulent drainage from the exit site.

4. Colonization:
   - Positive culture from an exit site that does not satisfy ESI or tunnel infection criteria, especially in the absence of discharge.

B. Evaluation of Exit Site

1. Clinical features:
   a. Mild erythema, skin induration, or increased crust formation alone may not represent an infection.
      - May occur after catheter placement, mild trauma, or allergic reactions.
      - Regular exit site reviews should be performed to assess the progression.
      - Exit site care should be escalated.

   b. Acute ESI:
      - Pain, induration, redness with a diameter ≥13 mm.
      - Exuberant granulation tissue.
      - Duration of infection <4 weeks.

   c. Chronic ESI:
      - Liquid external discharge.
      - Exuberant granulation tissue.
      - Duration of inflammation >4 weeks.
      - No pain, induration or redness.

   d. External cuff infection without ESI:
      - Expression of intermittent or chronic discharge (either spontaneously or after cuff pressure).
      - Normal-appearing exit site.

2. Investigations:
   a. Exit site swab for Gram stain and culture.
      - Swabs should not be performed if there is no discharge, as any positive culture may just imply colonization.

   b. Ultrasound scan of catheter tunnel (to look for fluid collections) if:
      - Marked induration or tenderness over the tunnel tract.
      - Drainage from the exit site after milking the tract.
      - Mass palpable over tunnel tract.
      - ESI or tunnel infections refractory or resistant to treatment.

- During or after antibiotics treatment for tunnel abscess to assess the response to therapy.

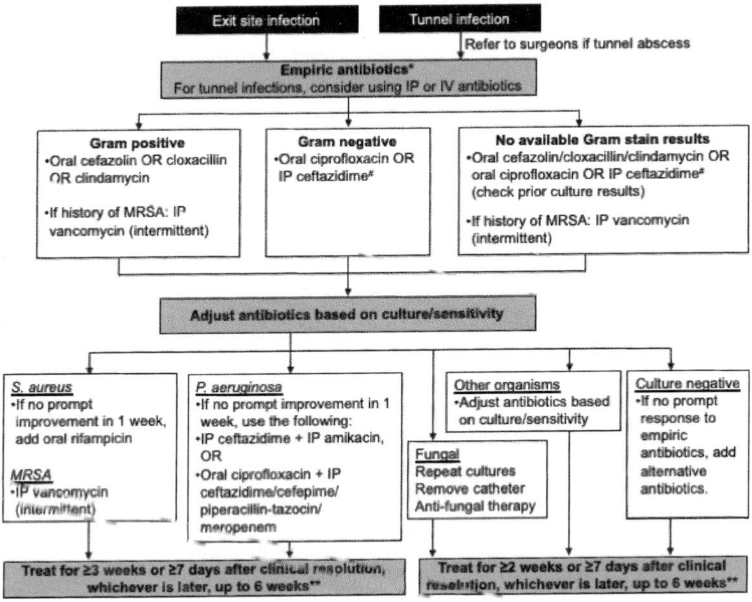

*May be adjusted based on previous cultures.
#Can be continuous or intermittent dosing.
**Add oral nystatin or oral fluconazole if antibiotic duration >3 weeks.

C. Treatment of ESI or Tunnel Infections

1. Empiric therapy:
   a. Start empiric antibiotics once a diagnosis of exit site or tunnel infection is made, without need for culture confirmation.
   b. Empiric anti-microbial therapy depends on the Gram stain and history of recent catheter-related infections or peritonitis.
   c. Empiric oral antibiotics are acceptable for ESI and mild tunnel infections.
      - Tunnel infections, especially if severe, may also be treated with intraperitoneal (IP) or intravenous (IV) antibiotics.

d. Gram-positive organisms:
   i. Start oral cefazolin or cloxacillin as first-line, or clindamycin if there is allergy.
   ii. If there is a history of methicillin-resistant *Staphylococcus aureus* (MRSA) infection, start empirical IP vancomycin (intermittent dosing 15–30 mg/kg every 5–7 days, aiming serum vancomycin level at 15–20 μg/ml before redosing).
e. Gram-negative organisms:
   i. Start oral ciprofloxacin or IP ceftazidime (continuous or intermittent dosing).
   ii. If there is a history of multi-resistant *Pseudomonas aeruginosa* infection, start on IP ceftazidime and oral ciprofloxacin.
f. Yeast: Add empiric treatment with an echinocandin.
   i. IV anidulafungin 2–4 mg/kg/day loading dose then 1–2 mg/kg/day OR
   ii. IV caspofungin 70 mg/m^2/day loading dose (maximum dose 70 mg) then 50 mg/m^2 daily (maximum dose 50 mg) OR
   iii. IV micafungin 2–4 mg/kg/day (maximum dose 100 mg).
g. No available Gram stain results:
   i. Start oral cefazolin/cloxacillin/clindamycin OR oral ciprofloxacin OR IP ceftazidime, guided by prior culture results (if available).
   ii. If there is a history of MRSA, start IP vancomycin.

2. Definitive therapy:
   a. Antibiotics should be adjusted based on the culture and sensitivity results.
   b. *Staphylococcus aureus* infections:
      i. If no prompt improvement within 1 week, add oral rifampicin.
      ii. If MRSA is confirmed, treat with IP vancomycin or oral linezolid.
      iii. Tunnel abscess can occur.
   c. *Pseudomonas aeruginosa* infections:
      i. If no prompt improvement within 1 week, change to IP ceftazidime with IP amikacin, or oral ciprofloxacin with another IP anti-pseudomonal antibiotic (ceftazidime, cefepime, piperacillin-tazocin, or meropenem).
      ii. Treatment response occurs only in about 50%.
      iii. Tunnel abscess can occur.

   d. Fungal infection:
      i. Treat according to culture sensitivity.
      ii. Remove PD catheter and convert to hemodialysis.
   e. Negative culture results and no prompt response to empirical antibiotics:
      i. Repeat swab cultures, including fungal smear/culture, acid-fast bacilli smear and culture.
      ii. Change or add antibiotics.
3. Duration of treatment:
   a. For all infections, antibiotics should be given for at least 7 days after complete clinical resolution of infection, up to 6 weeks.
   b. For *Staphylococcus aureus* or *Pseudomonas aeruginosa*:
      - ESI: At least 3 weeks.
      - Tunnel infections: At least 4 weeks.
   c. For other bacteria:
      - ESI: At least 2 weeks.
      - Tunnel infections: At least 2–4 weeks.
4. Other considerations:
   a. Use of oral ciprofloxacin:
      - If the patient is on concomitant treatment with sevelamer, calcium, oral iron, sucralfate, magnesium aluminum antacids, give ciprofloxacin 2 hours prior to these, as chelation interactions may reduce fluoroquinolone absorption.
   b. Add oral nystatin or oral fluconazole if antibiotic duration >3 weeks.
      - Continue anti-fungal therapy for one more week after antibiotics are stopped.
5. Adjunctive therapy:
   a. Clean the exit site twice a day with chlorhexidine.
   b. Apply 0.1% gentamicin cream or 2% mupirocin ointment at the exit site.
   c. Remove granulation tissue, if any, by cauterization with silver nitrate.
   d. Immobilize the catheter and protect from trauma.
6. Monitoring:
   a. Exit site review should be performed at least weekly to assess for resolution.

   b. In tunnel fluid collections, repeated ultrasound scans will aid in assessing response to therapy.
7. Resistant infection:
   a. Defined by
      i. No clinical improvement after 1 week of therapy OR
      ii. Lack of complete resolution after 6 weeks of antibiotics.
   b. Evaluation
      i. Check compliance to antibiotics.
      ii. Repeat cultures if earlier cultures were unreliable.
      iii. Examine for cuff extrusion, which may require cuff shaving.
         - Continue antibiotic treatment after cuff shaving.
      iv. If still refractory or recurrent, remove the dialysis catheter.

D. Tenckhoff Catheter Removal

1. Tenckhoff catheter removal prevents the progression to peritonitis and risk of prolonged antibiotic treatment leading to fungal peritonitis.
2. Indications for catheter removal include:
   a. Concurrent or subsequent development of peritonitis with the same organism, suggesting a biofilm along the catheter (especially for *Staphylococcus aureus* and *Pseudomonas aeruginosa*).
   b. No clinical improvement after 2 weeks of therapy.
   c. No complete resolution after 4 weeks of therapy.
   d. Fungal ESI or tunnel infection.
   e. Tunnel abscess.
   f. Resistant or relapsing ESI with the same organism after 3 courses of antibiotics.
3. Perioperative antibiotics should continue for at least 1 week after catheter removal.
4. The new catheter may be inserted at the same time as removal of the old catheter, or subsequently at a separate surgery.
5. The new catheter should be inserted only if:
   a. There is no peritonitis.
   b. Peritonitis has been treated for at least two weeks (peritoneal fluid cell count <100 /μL and no symptoms).

E. Prevention of ESI

1. Clean the exit site daily with normal saline, povidone-iodine or chlorhexidine.
2. Exit site dressing:
   a. Use nonocclusive dressing (such as gauze).
   b. Use hypoallergenic dressing and tapes in patients with contact dermatitis.
3. Apply topical gentamicin to the exit site daily.
   a. Topical gentamicin is effective against Gram-positive and Gram-negative organisms, but is associated with increased risk of anti-microbial resistance.
   b. Use topical mupirocin instead in patients with recurrent or refractory *Staphylococcus aureus* carriage or infections, or if there is previous infection with multi-resistant bacteria.
      - Topical mupirocin may cause increased risk of pseudomonas infections.
      - Excessive amounts of topical mupirocin directly on polyurethane or silicone catheter can cause catheter erosion.
4. Immobilize the catheter securely to prevent traction injury.
5. Avoid contact with pets to prevent zoonotic infection.
6. Screen for *Staphylococcus aureus* nasal carrier status:
   a. This should be performed:
      i At first Tenckhoff catheter insertion (for the patient and caregiver(s)).
      ii. At every Tenckhoff catheter replacement (for the patient only).
      iii. If there is *Staphylococcus aureus* catheter-related infection or peritonitis (patient and caregiver).
   b. If nasal swab is positive:
      i. Apply nasal 2% mupirocin 3 times a day for 7 days and then repeat nasal swab twice at the end of treatment.
         - A person is deemed "negative" if both swabs are negative.
         - In refractory cases, apply 2% mupirocin nasal ointment for 5 days every month till Tenckhoff catheter is removed.
      ii. Apply prophylactic 2% mupirocin at the catheter exit site till Tenckhoff catheter is removed.

Recommended Reading

1. Twardowski ZJ, Prowant BF. (1997) Current approach to exit-site infections in patients on peritoneal dialysis. *Nephrol Dial Transplant* **12**:1284–1295.
2. Li PK, Szeto CC, Piraino B, Bernardini J, Figueiredo AE, Gupta A, Johnson DW, Kuijper EJ, Lye WC, Salzer W, Schaefer F, Struijk DG; International Society for Peritoneal Dialysis. (2010) Peritoneal dialysis-related infections recommendations: 2010 update. *Perit Dial Int* **30**:393–423.
3. Warady BA, Bakkaloglu S, Newland J, Cantwell M, Verrina E, Neu A, Chadha V, Yap HK, Schaefer F. (2012) Consensus guidelines for the prevention and treatment of catheter-related infections and peritonitis in pediatric patients receiving peritoneal dialysis: 2012 update. *Perit Dial Int* **32**(Suppl 2):S32–86.
4. Burkart JM, Bleyer A. (2020, updated) Peritoneal catheter exit-site and tunnel infections in peritoneal dialysis in adults. Edited by: Golper TA, Motwani S, Chen W. *UpToDate ONLINE*. http://www.uptodateonline.com.

7 Peritonitis in Pediatric Peritoneal Dialysis

Dela Cruz DC, Resontoc LP, Ng KH and Yap HK

A. Definition of Terms

Recurrent peritonitis	An episode that occurs within 4 weeks of completion of therapy of a prior episode but with a different organism.
Relapsing peritonitis	An episode that occurs within 4 weeks of completion of therapy of a prior episode with the same organism or 1 sterile episode (includes 2 culture-negative infections occurring within 4 weeks of completion of the prior episode).
Repeat peritonitis	An episode that occurs more than 4 weeks after completion of therapy of a prior episode with the same organism.
Refractory peritonitis	Failure of the effluent to clear, defined as white blood cell (WBC) count <100/μl, after 5 days of appropriate antibiotics.
Catheter-related peritonitis	Peritonitis in conjunction with an exit site or tunnel infection with the same organism or 1 site sterile.

B. Doctors On-Call: What to Do?

1. Suspect peritonitis in a patient on peritoneal dialysis (PD) presenting with cloudy peritoneal effluent with or without:
   - Fever.
   - Abdominal pain.
   - Chills and rigors.
   - Anorexia.
   - Vomiting.
   - Abdominal distention.
   - Septic shock (late).

2. Review the child immediately.
3. Have a high index of suspicion.
4. Monitor vital signs and stabilize the child if necessary.
5. Inform the pediatric nephrologist-on-call who will activate the dialysis nurse.
6. Careful inspection of the catheter exit site and tunnel.
7. Septic workup:
   a. Full blood count (FBC).
   b. C-reactive protein ± procalcitonin.
   c. Serum urea, creatinine, sodium, potassium, chloride, bicarbonate, calcium, phosphate and uric acid.
   d. Liver function test: Total protein, albumin, alanine aminotransaminase (ALT), aspartate aminotransferase (AST) and bilirubin.
   e. Blood culture.
   f. Exit site culture if there is discharge.
   g. PD effluent: Dipstick for leukocyte esterase, WBC count with differential, Gram stain and bacterial culture.

   Note: Trace the PD effluent cell count within 4–6 hours of admission.

   h. Abdominal X-Ray or ultrasound if a bowel source is suspected.
8. Start empiric intraperitoneal (IP) antibiotics immediately.

C. Diagnosis of Peritonitis

1. Clinical Features:
   a. Cloudy PD effluent:

Differential Diagnosis of Cloudy Effluent
Culture-positive infectious peritonitis
Infectious peritonitis with sterile cultures
Chemical peritonitis
Eosinophilia of the effluent
Hemoperitoneum
Malignancy (rare)
Chylous effluent (rare)
Specimen taken from "dry" abdomen

b. Abdominal pain
   - Degree of pain is dependent on the type of organism.
   - Less with coagulase-negative *Staphylococcus* (CoNS).
   - Greater with *Streptococcus*, Gram-negative rods, *Staphylococcus aureus.*

   Note: Abdominal pain and fever are too non-specific in children.

2. Empiric diagnosis of peritonitis should be made if:
   a. PD effluent WBC count >100/μL with >50% neutrophils in dialysate with a dwell time of at least 2 hours.
   b. If the dialysate has been instilled for 1–2 hours, the presence of >50% neutrophils, even if WBC count is <100/μL is still highly suggestive of peritonitis.
   c. In children with systemic or abdominal symptoms but with clear effluent, a second sample should be obtained with a dwell of at least 2 hours.
3. PD effluent collection for culture:
   a. Initial sample is usually optimal for the evaluation of patients on automated peritoneal dialysis (APD) with day dwell or continuous ambulatory peritoneal dialysis (CAPD) (dialysate should have dwelt for at least 2 hours).
   b. If there is no day dwell for APD patients, then a fill volume of at least 10–20 ml/kg should be instilled for at least 1–2 hours.
   c. Inject at least 10–20 ml of PD effluent into each blood culture bottle (aerobic and anaerobic).
   d. PD effluent sample must be delivered to the laboratory immediately.
      - If the time of transport is >1 hour, refrigerate fluid at 4°C.
   e. A negative culture does not exclude peritonitis (31% of pediatric peritonitis episodes have negative cultures).

D. Empiric Initial Treatment

1. Start empiric IP antibiotic therapy immediately once the PD effluent is positive for leukocytes on the dipstick or if the clinical features are highly suggestive.
   a. IP dosing of antibiotics is preferable to intravenous dosing since IP dosing results in very high local levels of antibiotics.

b. Continuous IP dosing is preferred over intermittent IP dosing, except for aminoglycosides and glycopeptides (vancomycin).

2. Selection of initial therapy according to:
   a. Severity of symptoms.
   b. Peritonitis history.
   c. Patient's risk profile — history of infections and colonization pattern.
   d. Local pattern of distribution of causative organisms and their antibiotic susceptibilities (antibiogram).
3. Drug delivery and stability:
   a. Vancomycin, aminoglycosides, and cephalosporins can be mixed in the same dialysis solution bag (≥1 L volume) without loss of bioactivity (but not in the same syringe).
   b. Aminoglycosides should not be added to the same dialysate bag with penicillins because of chemical incompatibility.
   c. Stability of antibiotics in dextrose-containing dialysis solution:
      - Vancomycin (25 mg/L) is stable for 28 days in dialysis solution stored at room temperature.
      - Gentamicin (8 mg/L) is stable for 14 days but the duration of stablity is reduced by admixture of heparin.
      - Cefazolin (500 mg/L) is stable for at least 8 days at room temperature or 14 days if refrigerated, and is not influenced by addition of heparin.
      - Ceftazidime (125 mg/L) is stable for 4 days at room temperature or 7 days refrigerated, and concentrations of 200 mg/L are stable for 10 days if refrigerated.
      - Cefepime is stable in dialysate solution for 14 days if the solution is refrigerated.
4. Dialysis adjustments:
   a. Initial flushing of the peritoneal cavity several times with dialysate reduces abdominal pain.
   b. Fill volume may be reduced slightly (<25%) during the initial 24–48 hours of therapy in patients with significant abdominal discomfort.
      - Alteration in IP antibiotic concentration is not needed because the high antibiotic levels are above the minimum inhibitory concentration (MIC) of susceptible organisms.
      - Fill volume should subsequently be increased to prevent underdialysis.

c. IP Heparin 500–1000 U/L should be added until effluent becomes clear.

d. For those on routine APD with short dwells, the dwell time should be increased to 4 hours (3–6 hours) until PD effluent WBC count is <100/μL for 3 consecutive days.
   - If PD effluent WBC count <100/μL for 3 consecutive days and the child is asymptomatic, revert to APD regime with a full day dwell.

5. Algorithm for empiric antibiotic treatment:

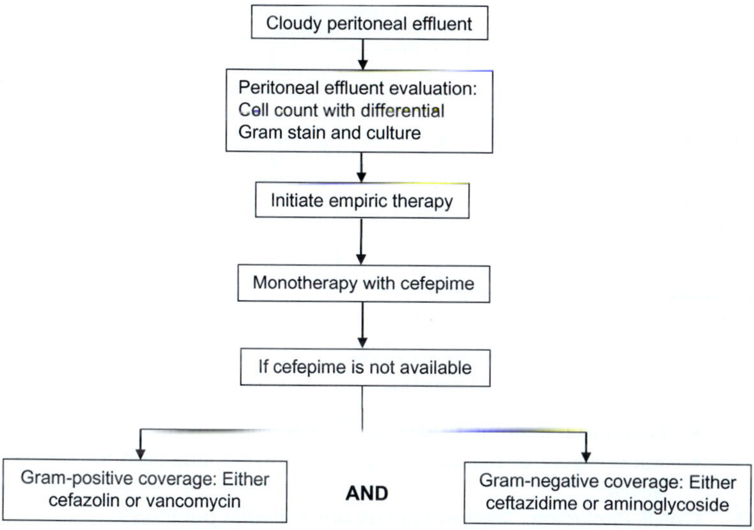

- If the center-specific resistance rate of *Staphylococcus aureus* isolates to methicillin exceeds 10%, or the patient has a history of methicillin-resistant *Staphylococcus aureus* (MRSA) infection or colonization, glycopeptide (vancomycin or teicoplanin) should be added to cefepime or replace cefazolin for Gram-positive coverage.
- Glycopeptide can also be considered if the patient has a history of severe allergy to penicillins and cephalosporins.

I. Gram-positive peritonitis:

1. Algorithm:

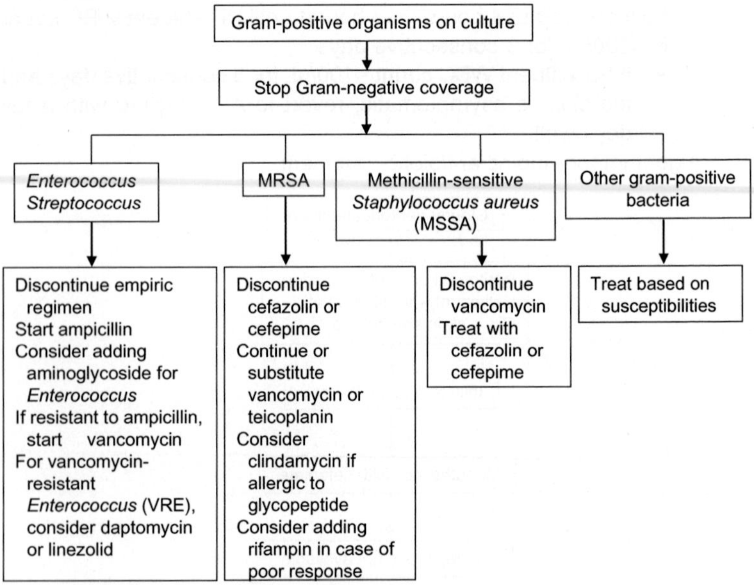

- Rifampicin is not indicated for CoNS.
- Vancomycin or teicoplanin, or clindamycin indicated for MRSA/ MRSE.

2. CoNS (including *Staphylococcus epidermidis*) peritonitis:
   a. Primarily due to touch contamination.
   b. Mild form of peritonitis responding to antibiotic therapy.
   c. Relapsing peritonitis suggests colonization of the intra-abdominal portion of the catheter with biofilm and is best treated with replacement of the catheter once the effluent clears with antibiotics.
   d. Duration of treatment is 2 weeks for first peritonitis and 3 weeks for relapsing or repeat CoNS peritonitis.
3. Streptococcal and enterococcal peritonitis:
   a. Streptococcal and enterococcal peritonitis tend to be severe and are best treated with IP ampicillin, cefazolin, or cefepime.
   b. Enterococcal infections may be due to touch contamination or from the gastrointestinal tract.

c. For *Enterococcus* sp., an aminoglycoside may be added to ampicillin, penicillin or glycopeptide for synergistic effect if the species is susceptible.
   - For IP penicillins, aminoglycoside is added as intravenous (IV) drug due to IP incompatibility.
   - For IP glycopeptides, aminoglycosides can be added as IP in the same dialysate bag.

d. Vancomycin-resistant *Enterococcus* (VRE) is often associated with recent hospitalization and prior antibiotic therapy, especially vancomycin and cephalosporins.
   - Linezolid or daptomycin should be used to treat VRE peritonitis.

e. Duration of treatment is 2 weeks for streptococcal peritonitis and 2–3 weeks for enterococcal peritonitis.

4. *Staphylococcus aureus* peritonitis:
   a. *Staphylococcus aureus* causes severe peritonitis, often due to a catheter infection.
   b. For infections that show little or no response by 48 hours, rifampicin may be added.
   c. Catheter-related peritonitis is unlikely to respond to antibiotic therapy without catheter removal.
   d. If MRSA is present, the patient must be treated with either vancomycin or teicoplanin, or clindamycin if the patient is allergic to glycopeptides.
   e. If vancomycin-resistant *Staphylococcus aureus* peritonitis develops, linezolid must be used.
   f. Duration of treatment is 3 weeks.

5. Recommended antibiotics listed in the preferred order and length of therapy:

Organism	Recommended Antibiotic	Length of Therapy
Staphylococcus aureus		
Methicillin-resistant	Vancomycin or Teicoplanin (Clindamycin if allergic)	3 weeks
Methicillin-sensitive	Cefazolin or Cefepime	3 weeks
CoNS	Cefazolin or Cefepime or Clindamycin or Vancomycin or Teicoplanin	2 weeks

(*Continued*)

(*Continued*)

Organism	Recommended Antibiotic	Length of Therapy
Enterococcus sp.	Ampicillin or Cefazolin or Cefepime or Vancomycin or Teicoplanin	2–3 weeks
Vancomycin-resistant	Ampicillin or Linezolid	2–3 weeks
Streptococcus sp.	Ampicillin or Cefazolin or Cefepime	2 weeks

II. Gram-negative peritonitis:

1. Algorithm:

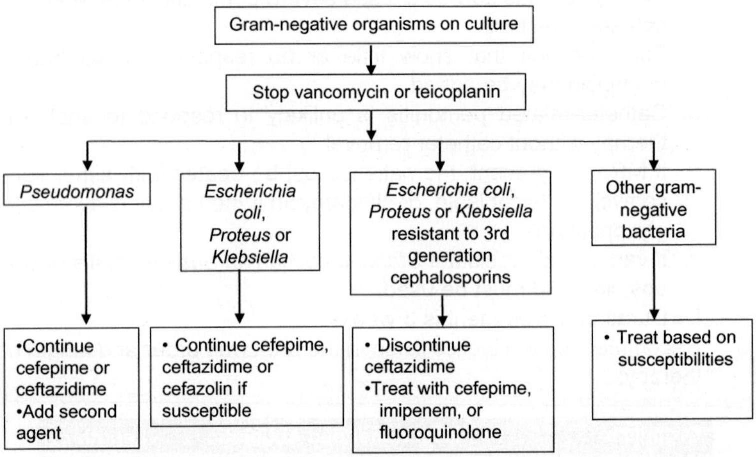

a. If cefazolin plus aminoglycoside are used for empiric therapy, the aminoglycoside should be discontinued if the organism is susceptible to a less toxic antibiotic, provided that the causative bacteria is not *Pseudomonas* sp.
   - Aminoglycoside monotherapy is not routinely recommended for maintenance therapy because of the risk of ototoxicity and nephrotoxicity.

2. *Pseudomonas aeruginosa* peritonitis:
   a. If concomitant *Pseudomonas* exit site infection, removal of the catheter is required.
   b. Two antibiotics are always needed:
      - An oral quinolone or aminoglycoside can be given as second agent together with ceftazidime or cefepime.
   c. Duration of treatment is 3 weeks.
   d. Every effort to avoid *Pseudomonas aeruginosa* peritonitis should be made by replacing the catheter in recurrent, relapsing or refractory exit site infections with *Pseudomonas aeruginosa*.
   e. Following catheter removal, antibiotics must be continued for 2 weeks while the patient is on hemodialysis.
3. Other single Gram-negative microorganisms:
   a. If a single Gram-negative organism such as *Escherichia coli*, *Klebsiella* sp. or *Proteus* sp. is isolated, the antibiotic used is based on sensitivities, safety and convenience.
   b. Ceftazidime or cefepime may be indicated based on *in vitro* sensitivity testing.
   c. Use of cefazolin alone requires caution.
   d. Duration of treatment for *Stenotrophomonas* peritonitis is 3 weeks.
4. Recommended antibiotics listed in order of preference and length of therapy:

Organism	Recommended Antibiotic	Length of Therapy
Escherichia coli, *Klebsiella* sp.	Cefepime or Cefazolin or Ceftazidime or Ceftriaxone or Cefotaxime	2 weeks
Resistant to third-generation cephalosporins	Imipenem or Cefepime or Fluoroquinolone	3 weeks
Enterobacter, *Citrobacter*, *Serratia* and *Proteus* spp.	Cefepime or Ceftazidime or Imipenem	2–3 weeks
Acinetobacter sp.	Cefepime or Ceftazidime or Imipenem	2–3 weeks

(*Continued*)

(*Continued*)

Organism	Recommended Antibiotic	Length of Therapy
Pseudomonas sp.	Cefepime or Ceftazidime or Piperacillin or Ticarcillin or Imipenem + Aminoglycoside or Fluoroquinolone	3 weeks
Stenotrophomonas maltophilia	Trimethoprim-sulfamethoxazole or Ticarcillin-clavulanic acid	3 weeks

III. Polymicrobial peritonitis:

1. Multiple enteric organisms:
   a. Ultrasound and/or CT scan to identify intra-abdominal pathology.
   b. Therapy of choice is metronidazole in combination with ampicillin and ceftazidime or an aminoglycoside.
   c. Remove the catheter.
2. Multiple Gram-positive organisms:
   a. The source is most likely contamination or catheter infection.
   b. Generally responds to antibiotic therapy.

IV. Culture-negative peritonitis:

1. Continue initial empiric antibiotics for 2 weeks if initial PD effluent culture remains sterile at 72 hours, provided there are resolution of symptoms and signs AND adequate decrease in PD effluent WBC count >50% after 48–72 hours.
   - Discontinue empiric aminoglycoside to avoid toxicity, and switch to ceftazidime for Gram-negative coverage.
2. If no clinical improvement, perform the following tests with PD effluent:
   - Cell count with differential, gram stain.

- Bacterial culture (add 20 ml of PD effluent per blood culture bottle).
- Fungal smear and culture (for lipid-dependent yeast and other fungi).
- Acid-fast bacilli smear and culture (*Mycobacteria* including atypical mycobacteria).

3. If the initial fungal and acid-fast bacilli smears are negative and there is no clinical improvement, consider special culture techniques for the isolation of unusual or fastidious organisms:
   - *Legionella.*
   - *Campylobacter.*
   - *Ureaplasma.*
   - Slow-growing bacteria.
   - Enteroviruses.
4. If there is inadequate improvement by 5 days, catheter removal should be strongly considered.

V. Fungal peritonitis:

1. Catheter removal is indicated immediately once fungal peritonitis is confirmed.
   - Several in/out flushes of PD fluid prior to catheter removal may be performed to aid in decreasing the fungal load.
2. Anti-fungal therapy is based on species identification and MIC:
   a. Empiric therapy:
      - Fluconazole (most *Candida* sp.).

   b. Alternative drugs:
      - Triazoles, e.g., voriconazole or posaconazole (filamentous fungi such as *Aspergillus* sp.).
      - Echinocandins, e.g., caspofungin, micafungin, anidulafungin (*Aspergillus* sp. and non-responding non-albicans *Candida* sp.).
3. Following removal of catheter, therapy should continue for ≥2 weeks after a complete resolution of clinical symptoms.
4. In invasive *Candida* bloodstream infections, therapy should continue for 2 weeks after a negative culture is obtained.

VI. Mycobacterial peritonitis:

1. Diagnosis should be considered in any patient with:
   a. Prolonged failure to thrive.
   b. Prolonged symptoms despite antibiotic therapy.
   c. Relapsing or refractory peritonitis with negative bacterial culture.
2. Treatment:
   a. *Mycobacterium tuberculosis*: Start with 4 drugs.

Antibiotic	Length of Therapy
Rifampicin (IP)	12 months
Isoniazid	12 months
Pyrazinamide	3 months
Ofloxacin	3 months

      i. Supplement with Pyridoxine 50–100 mg/day.
      ii. Rifampicin dialysate levels are low if given orally due to its high molecular weight.
      iii. Ethambutol is not recommended because of the high risk of optic neuritis in kidney failure.
      iv. Streptomycin is generally avoided because of the risk of ototoxicity.
   b. Non-tuberculous Mycobacteria:
      i. Treat according to sensitivity, in consultation with the infectious disease physician.
      ii. Antibiotics include IP amikacin (limited duration), oral clarithromycin, and oral clofazimine.
      iii. Dual agents may be required for a prolonged period of 9–12 months.
3. Consider catheter removal if inadequate improvement after 5 days.
4. Consider reinsertion of the catheter after 6 weeks of anti-mycobacterial therapy.

VII. Relapsing peritonitis

1. Relapsing peritonitis is strongly associated with PD technique failure.

2. Empiric therapy should be re-initiated with consideration of the susceptibilities of the prior bacteria.
3. Post-empiric antibiotic therapy is guided by *in vitro* susceptibility results.
4. Avoid cefazolin monotherapy as it is less effective against biofilm formation, compared to glycopeptides or antibiotic combinations.
5. Intraluminal instillation of fibrinolytic agent (urokinase 1500–5000 IU/ml or recombinant tissue plasminogen activator 1 mg/ml) should be considered in relapsing peritonitis not explained by an extraluminal cause like tunnel infection or intra-abdominal abscess.

E. Intraperitoneal Antibiotic Dosing Recommendations

1. Continuous dosing:
   a. Preferred because it allows for constant local antibiotic concentrations.
   b. Recommended for beta-lactam antibiotics and cephalosporins.
   c. For APD, do continuous 4-hourly cycles (6 cycles in 24 hours).
2. Intermittent dosing:
   a. Recommended for vancomycin, teicoplanin and aminoglycosides.
      - Avoid intermittent administration of beta-lactam antibiotics and cephalosporins, especially if there is residual kidney function, because drug level monitoring is not possible.
   b. Efficacy and safety depend on dialysate flow rate, which alters drug absorption and elimination.
   c. Drugs should be administered over ≥6 hours in the night dwell for CAPD or in the day dwell for APD.
   d. Drugs should be administered in one exchange per day.
      i. Glycopeptides are usually dosed every few days, and this is based on drug monitoring every 2–5 days (first drug level should be checked within 2–4 days of the first dose).
      ii. Re-dosing should occur when blood level is <15–30 mg/L for vancomycin and <8 mg/L for teicoplanin in intermittent therapy.
      iii. Aminoglycoside blood trough levels should be monitored in intermittent therapy to prevent ototoxicity.

- Amikacin trough level: <8 mcg/ml (usually 1–4 mcg/ml).
- Gentamicin trough level: <1 mcg/ml.

3. IP drug doses are based on a fill volume of 1100 ml/m^2.
   a. If using a smaller fill volume, increase antibiotic concentration to ensure the antibiotic mass per bag is equivalent to that delivered in 1100ml/m^2 fill volume.
   b. Minimum fill volume is 300 ml/m^2 for children and 200 ml/m^2 for infants.
4. In patients with residual kidney function (defined as urine output >100 ml/day), increase the doses of drugs with renal clearance by 25%.
5. Intraperitoneal antibiotic dosing:

Anti-microbial	Continuous Therapy (All Exchanges)		Intermittent Therapy (1 Exchange Per Day)
	Loading	Maintenance	
Glycopeptides			
Vancomycin	1000 mg/L	25 mg/L	Loading: 30 mg/kg Repeat dosing: 15 mg/kg every 3–5 days (maximum 2–3 g)
Teicoplanin	400 mg/L	20 mg/L	15 mg/kg every 5–7 days
Cephalosporins			
Cefazolin	500 mg/L	125 mg/L	20 mg/kg
Cefepime	500 mg/L	125 mg/L	15 mg/kg
Cefotaxime	500 mg/L	250 mg/L	30 mg/kg
Ceftazidime	500 mg/L	125 mg/L	20 mg/kg
Aminoglycosides			
Amikacin	25 mg/L	12 mg/L	2 mg/kg
Gentamicin/ Netilmycin/ Tobramycin	8 mg/L	4 mg/L	Anuric: 0.6 mg/kg Non-anuric: 0.75 mg/kg
Penicillins			
Ampicillin	—	125 mg/L	—
Quinolones			
Ciprofloxacin	50 mg/L	25 mg/L	—

(*Continued*)

Anti-microbial	Continuous Therapy (All Exchanges)		Intermittent Therapy (1 Exchange Per Day)
	Loading	Maintenance	
Anti-fungal			
Fluconazole	—	—	6–12 mg/kg every 24–48 hours (maximum daily 400 mg)
Others			
Clindamycin	300 mg/L	150 mg/L	—
Aztreonam	1000 mg/L	250 mg/L	—
Imipenem-cilastin	250 mg/L	50 mg/L	—
Meropenem	—	—	1 g
Piperacillin/ Tazobactam	4 g/0.5 g*	1 g/0.125 g*	—

*For adult-sized patients with at least 2 L exchange volume only.

6. Oral and IV antibiotic dosing for bacterial peritonitis:

Anti-microbial	Route	Dose	Maximum Dose
Anti-bacterial			
Linezolid	Oral	<5 years: 30 mg/kg/day, in 3 doses 5–11 years: 20 mg/kg/day, in 2 doses ≥12 years: 600 mg/dose 12 hourly	600 mg/dose
Metronidazole	Oral	30 mg/kg/day, in 3 doses	1.2 g daily
Rifampicin[#]	Oral	10–20 mg/kg/day, in 2 doses	600 mg /dose
Anti-fungal			
Fluconazole	IV, oral	6–12 mg/kg every 24–48 hours	400 mg daily
Caspofungin	IV	70 mg/m^2 on Day 1 50 mg/m^2 daily	70 mg daily 50 mg daily

[#]Should be used in combination with other anti-microbials.

F. Duration and Evaluation of Treatment

1. Daily assessment:
   a. Improvement of clinical symptoms and signs.
   b. Degree of PD effluent cloudiness.
   c. PD effluent cell count and differentials till WBC count <100/μL for 3 consecutive days.
2. Response to therapy:
   a. Decrease in PD effluent WBC count by >50% after 72 hours of treatment.
   b. Improvement in clinical status after 72 hours of treatment.
3. Disease Severity Score (DSS)
   - Improvement in DSS: Reduction in the DSS to <2.

Score	Interpretation
Pain (0–3)	
0	None
1	Moderate pain or nausea not requiring specific therapy
2	Severe pain, usually requiring analgesic therapy, or vomiting
3	Peritonitic pain with tense abdomen, or paralytic bowel, or both
Fever (0–2)	
0	<37.5°C
1	37.5–38.9°C
2	>38.9°C
Total (0–5)	Sum of scores for pain and fever

4. Lack of initial response to treatment is predictive of subsequent relapsing peritonitis.
5. If there is no response to therapy after 48–72 hours of empiric antibiotics:
   a. Adjust the antibiotics based on the culture sensitivity.
   b. Use a continuous antibiotic dosing regime instead of intermittent dosing, except for vancomycin, teicoplanin and aminoglycosides.
   c. Ensure the antibiotic dose is adjusted for smaller fill volumes, and residual kidney function.
   d. For susceptible organisms, add a second antibiotic:
      i. CoNS, *Staphylococcus epidermidis or Staphylococcus aureus*: Add rifampicin.

- Rifampicin should not be used as monotherapy due to the risk of resistance.

ii. Gram-negative infections: Consider adding aminoglycosides if susceptible.

e. Assess for catheter tunnel infection by clinical evaluation and ultrasonography.

f. Consider Tenckhoff catheter removal (especially for *Staphylococcus aureus* or *Pseudomonas* sp. peritonitis).

6. Duration of treatment should be counted from the first day the PD effluent WBC count decreases consistently to below 100/μL.

I. PD catheter removal and replacement:

1. Indications:

Approach	Indication	Timing of Catheter Re-insertion
Prompt removal of PD catheter and conversion to HD (temporary or permanent)	• Refractory bacterial peritonitis. • Fungal peritonitis. • Exit site infection or tunnel infection in conjunction with peritonitis with the same organism (mainly *Staphylococcus aureus* and *Pseudomonas aeruginosa*, except CoNS).	• At least 2–3 weeks. • At least 2–3 weeks. • After 2–3 weeks.
Simultaneous catheter removal and replacement	• Relapsing or refractory exit site infection or tunnel infection (including *Pseudomonas aeruginosa*). • Relapsing peritonitis (especially for *Staphylococcus aureus* and CoNS).	
Relative indications for catheter removal	• Repeat peritonitis. • Mycobacterial peritonitis. • Peritonitis with multiple enteric organisms (intra-abdominal pathology or abscess).	• After 2–3 weeks. • After 6 weeks. • Depends on clinical course; at least 2–3 weeks.

2. Simultaneous catheter removal and replacement:
   a. Infected catheter is removed, and a new catheter is inserted simultaneously in the opposite quadrant.
   b. Performed only after PD effluent WBC count <100/μl.
   c. Antibiotics should be continued for 1–2 weeks after the surgery.

II. Adjunctive therapy:

1. Consider intravenous immunoglobulin (500 mg/kg) in small children with hypogammaglobulinemia and sepsis and sepsis, and in selected immunosuppressed patients with recurrent or refractory peritonitis.

G. Prevention of PD-associated Peritonitis:

1. Oral nystatin (10000 U/kg daily) or IV/oral fluconazole (3–6 mg/kg every 24–48 hours, maximum 200 mg) may be given during the entire antibiotic course to reduce fungal peritonitis risk if:
   a. Anti-bacterial treatment is expected to be prolonged (>3 weeks).
   b. Prior recent prolonged or broad-spectrum antibiotic usage.
   c. Frequent bacterial peritonitis.
   d. Immunosuppressed or malnourished state.
2. Prophylactic anti-microbial therapy:
   a. Prior to invasive dental procedures that involve manipulation of gingival tissue or periapical region of teeth, or perforation of the oral mucosa:
      i. Dental extractions.
      ii. Dental implant placement.
      iii. Endodontic "root canal" instrumentation.
      iv. Periodontal surgery.
      v. Professional scaling or tooth cleaning.

Situation	Agent	Dose	Maximum dose
Standard general prophylaxis	Amoxicillin	20 mg/kg PO	2 g
Unable to take oral medications	Ampicillin	50 mg/kg IM/IV	2 g

(*Continued*)

Situation	Agent	Dose	Maximum dose
Allergy to penicillin	Clindamycin or Azithromycin or Clarithromycin	20 mg/kg PO 15 mg/kg PO 4 mg/kg PO	600 mg 500 mg 500 mg
Allergy to penicillin and unable to take oral medications	Clindamycin or Cefazolin or Ceftriaxone	20 mg/kg IV 25 mg/kg IV 50 mg/kg IM/IV	600 mg 1 g 1 g

IM, intramuscular; PO, per oral.
Note: Give antibiotics 30–60 minutes before the dental procedure.

b. Prior to genitourinary, gastrointestinal (GI) or obstetric procedures:
   i. Types of procedures:
      - Colonoscopy or oesophagogastroduodenoscopy (OGD).
      - Placement of intrauterine device.
      - Cervical biopsy or hysteroscopy.
      - Pelvic examination.
      - Papanicolaou (Pap) smear.
      - Intrauterine device (IUD) placement.
   ii. PD effluent should be drained completely before the procedures.
   iii. Duration of dry abdomen (no PD) after the procedure:
      - Endoscopy without biopsy or polypectomy: 1 day.
      - Endoscopy with biopsy or polypectomy: 3 days.
      - IUD placement: 3 days.
      - Pelvic examination/Pap smear: None.
   iv. Increase PD for 3 days prior to the procedure by increasing duration and/or number of cycles so that PD may be withheld for 1–3 days after the procedure without the need for interim hemodialysis.
   v. Give antimicrobial prophylaxis 30–60 minutes before the procedure:

Procedure	Drug	IV Dose	Maximum Dose
Upper GI procedures a) Uncomplicated OGD	None	—	—
b) High-risk procedures (esophageal stricture dilatation, treatment of varices, ERCP, and PEG)	Cefazolin or Clindamycin or Vancomycin (if high risk for MRSA)	25 mg/kg 10 mg/kg 10 mg/kg	2 g 600 mg 1 g
Other GI or genitourinary procedures (e.g., colonoscopy, hysteroscopy)	Cefazolin + Metronidazole or Cefoxitin/cefotetan or Clindamycin + Aztreonam	25 mg/kg 10 mg/kg 30–40 mg/kg 10 mg/kg 30 mg/kg	2 g 1 g 2 g 600 mg 2 g

ERCP = endoscopic retrograde cholangiopancreatography; PEG = percutaneous endoscopic gastrostomy.

c. At the PD catheter placement (see chapter "Tenckhoff Catheter Insertion and Initial Prescription").
d. Following accidental contamination (see chapter "Tenckhoff Catheter Contamination and Breaks in Technique").

3. Root cause analysis, involving patients, caregivers, nurses, doctors, and social workers, should be performed for each peritonitis episode.
4. Structured training and re-training programs are important in preventing subsequent peritonitis.

Recommended Reading

1. Warady BA, Bakkaloglu S, Newland J, Cantwell M, Verrina E, Neu A, Chadha V, Yap HK, Schaefer S. (2012) Consensus guidelines for the prevention and treatment of catheter-related infections and peritonitis in pediatric patients receiving peritoneal dialysis: 2012 Update. *Perit Dial Int* **32**:S32–S86.
2. Piraino B, de Arteaga J, Fan S, Figueiredo AE, Fish DN, Goffin E, Kim YL, Salzer W, Struijk DG, Teitelbaum I, Johnson DW. (2016) ISPD peritonitis recommendations: 2016 update on prevention and treatment. *Perit Dial Int* **36**(5):481–508.
3. Neu AM, Warady BA, Schaefer F. (2021) Infectious complications of peritoneal dialysis in children. In: *Pediatric Dialysis*, 3rd edition. Edited by: Warady BA, Alexander SR, Schaefer F. Springer. pp. 265–290.

8 Tenckhoff Catheter Contamination and Breaks in Technique

Hussain NH, Ng KH and Yap HK

A. Introduction

1. Types of contamination:
   a. "Dry contamination": Contamination distal to a closed transfer set clamp, but the tubing and dialysate bag are not leaking.
   b. "Wet contamination":
      - Leak in the dialysate bags.
      - Leak in the tubing distal to an open clamp.
      - Leak in the tubing proximal to a closed clamp.
      - Contamination while peritoneal dialysis (PD) fluid was being infused.
2. Causes of contamination:
   a. Touch contamination.
   b. Tear or stress mark on catheter, dialysis tubing or dialysate bags.
   c. Contamination of the catheter with stools from diapers.
3. After bacterial contamination of the peritoneal cavity, the incubation period for most organisms is about 12–48 hours.
   - Antibiotics should be instituted promptly to prevent peritonitis.

B. Management of "Dry Contamination"

1. Patient should come to the hospital immediately.
2. Change the transfer set.
3. Antibiotics are not required as risk of infection is low.
4. Monitor closely for evidence of peritonitis.

5. Patient to return if there is fever, abdominal pain, or cloudy PD fluid.
6. Perform root-cause analysis for the contamination.

C. Management of "Wet Contamination"

I. Immediate management by the patient

1. Patient should clamp Tenckhoff (TK) catheter between abdomen and leak with the emergency clamp.
2. End PD if it is ongoing.
3. Patient should come to the hospital immediately.

II. Immediate in-center management

1. Examine carefully for tear or stress marks on the TK catheter.
2. If there is a tear/stress mark on TK catheter, proceed to Protocol A.
3. If there is no tear/stress mark on the TK catheter, or if there is a tear/stress mark on the transfer set, proceed to Protocol B.
4. **Protocol A**:
   a. Cover tear or stress area with povidone-iodine soaked gauze.
   b. Perform 2 scrubs with povidone-iodine, each 1 minute, at the connection between the transfer set and titanium connector.
   c. Remove contaminated transfer set.
   d. Perform 2 scrubs with povidone-iodine (each 1 minute) at the titanium connector.
   e. Remove the titanium and soak it in povidone-iodine solution for 5 minutes.
   f. Proceed to scrub with povidone-iodine at the tear site.
   g. Cut any stress mark or tear proximal to the tear site.
   h. Scrub the cut end with povidone-iodine.
   i. Re-attach the titanium connector to the cut end of the TK catheter.
   j. Drain residual PD fluid, then perform 3 flushes with dialysate.
   k. Send initial drain or PD fluid for cell count, Gram stain, and culture.

l. Start intraperitoneal (IP) antibiotics: Dwell loading dose for 4–6 hours, followed by maintenance dose for 3–5 days.
  - Cefazolin loading 500 mg/L, maintenance 125 mg/L (if urine output >100 ml/day, increase loading and maintenance doses by 25%).
  - If there is prior methicillin-resistant *Staphylococcus aureus* (MRSA) colonization or infection, use vancomycin instead.
  - A second antibiotic (e.g., ceftazidime) may be added if high infection risk and recent Gram-negative bacteria infections.
  - Keep the same automated PD regime except the last fill is the full fill volume.
  - If low infection risks, consider 3 days of IP cefazolin, followed by 2 days of oral cephalexin.

m. If "wet" contamination of TK catheter with stools from diapers:
  - Administer prophylactic IP cefazolin with IP ceftazidime.
  - Alternatively, IP cefepime may be used.

5. **Protocol B**:
   a. Perform 2 scrubs with povidone-iodine (each 1 minute) at the connection between the transfer set and titanium connector.
   b. Remove contaminated transfer set.
   c. Connect the new transfer set.
   d. Continue with Step j in Protocol A.

III. Subsequent management

1. Patient to return if there is fever, abdominal pain, or cloudy PD fluid.
2. Subsequent antibiotic therapy is directed by culture results.
3. Return on the sixth day for repeat PD fluid cell count and culture.
4. Perform root-cause analysis for the contamination.

Recommended Reading

1. Burkart JM. (2020, updated) Risk factors and prevention of peritonitis in peritoneal dialysis. Edited by: Golper TA, Motwani S. *UpToDate ONLINE.* http://www.uptodateonline.com.

9 Noninfectious Complications of Peritoneal Dialysis

Ng KH, Inamdar P, Qader MA, Teo S and Yap HK

A. Pericatheter Leak

1. Defined as any moisture, identified as dialysate, appearing around the peritoneal dialysis (PD) catheter.
2. Early leak:
   a. Occurs within 30 days of PD catheter insertion.
   b. Presents as moisture around the exit site.
3. Late leak:
   a. Occurs after 30 days of PD catheter insertion.
   b. Presents as:
      - Subcutaneous swelling.
      - Weight gain.
      - Peripheral or genital edema.
      - Apparent ultrafiltration failure.
4. Risk factors for pericatheter leakage:
   a. High dialysate volume.
   b. Weak abdominal wall after multiple surgeries.
   c. Immediate initiation of PD.
   d. PD catheter insertion in the midline.
5. Diagnosis:
   a. For external leak:
      i. Check glucose concentration of the leaked fluid by dipstick.
      ii. Icodextrin solutions may test positive for glucose if a glucose dehydrogenase pyrroloquinolinequinone method is used.
   b. For a subcutaneous leak:
      i. Ultrasound of abdominal wall.
      ii. Computerized tomography (CT) peritoneography:

- Mixture of contrast material (1 ml/kg nonionic contrast) and dialysate (30 ml/kg) instilled after drainage of the peritoneal cavity.
- CT is then performed and may be repeated at 1 and 4 hours.
- Drain the mixture after the procedure is completed.

iii. T2 weighted magnetic resonance imaging (MRI) with empty and filled abdominal cavity.

iv. Peritoneal scintigraphy:
- Dose of 2–10 mCi of ^{99m}Technetium-macroaggregated human albumin (^{99m}Tc-MAA) is injected into a dialysate bag and instilled into the peritoneal cavity via the indwelling PD catheter.
- Appropriate exchange volume and tonicity are adjusted according to individual requirements.
- After infusion of labeled dialysate, obtain an initial set of images in the supine position.
- Take multiple projections (anterior, lateral, posterior, and oblique) to distinguish an abdominal wall leak from the PD fluid posteriorly.
- The patient should ambulate or (if nonambulatory) be made to roll from side to side.
- Take images subsequently at regular time intervals, with most leaks being detected in 2–6 hours.
- Delayed scans (24–48 hours later) are advocated in small leaks or initially equivocal studies.

6. Management of pericatheter leakage:
   a. Stop PD for at least 2 weeks.
   b. Administer IV cefazolin for at least 5 days or until the leak has stopped.
   c. If PD has to be restarted within 2 weeks, use low fill volume 200–300 ml/m^2 for 2 weeks.
      - Intraperitoneal cefazolin may be used instead of IV for a minimum of 5 days following the leak.
   d. Check PD fluid for cell count and culture at diagnosis of the leak when peritonitis is clinically suspected and at re-initiation of PD.
      - Treat for peritonitis if cell count is abnormal.

   e. Surgical repair of deep cuff or a catheter replacement may be required (rare).
7. Prevention of pericatheter leak:
   a. Surgical techniques:
      - A paramedian fascial or lateral abdominal incision is preferred to avoid hernias and leakage.
      - Ensure proper implantation of the deep Dacron cuff of the catheter into the rectus muscle and sheath.
      - Apply fibrin glue in the tunnel, especially if PD initiation is expected soon after catheter insertion.
      - Avoid insertion through a previous PD catheter site.
   b. Avoid using catheter for at least 2 weeks after insertion.
      - If PD is necessary prior to 2 weeks, start with low fill volumes and hourly cycles.
   c. Use of abdominal isometric contraction exercises to strengthen weak abdominal muscles to prevent late leaks.

B. PD Catheter Outflow Failure

1. Definition:
   - Incomplete recovery of the instilled dialysate.
2. Etiology:
   a. Intraluminal catheter occlusion:
      - Fibrin.
      - Thrombus.
   b. Extraluminal catheter occlusion:
      - Constipation/obstipation.
      - Catheter malposition.
      - Catheter migration.
      - Omental wrapping.
      - Adhesions.
      - Catheter kinking.
      - Catheter abutment.
   c. Tip entrapment in peritoneal pockets.

3. Clinical approach:
   a. History and physical examination:
      i. Onset of outflow failure:
         - Immediately post-catheter placement: Kinking.
         - Within days of catheter placement: Malposition.
         - Several weeks later: Omental occlusion.
      ii. Evaluate for constipation.
      iii. Look for blood-stained dialysate or fibrin in the dialysate:
         - History of menses.
      iv. Localized abdominal wall bulging may suggest:
         - Subcutaneous leak.
         - Intra-abdominal adhesions resulting in pocket formation.
      v. Careful examination of hernial sites.
      vi. Prior history of abdominal surgeries, including Mitrofanoff surgery.
      vii. Previous peritonitis may suggest possible loculation.
   b. Perform a manual in/out flush of 10–30 ml/kg and a catheter drainage profile (see chapter "Peritoneal Dialysis Adequacy") to determine if there is accompanying inflow failure and the severity of the outflow failure.
      - Inflow failure indicates intraluminal obstruction by fibrin or thrombus.
   c. Imaging:
      i. Abdominal X-Ray to look for the catheter tip position.
         - Tip of the PD catheter must be located within the pelvis.
         - A lateral view may be necessary to identify a subcutaneous and intraperitoneal catheter kink.
      ii. Abdominal ultrasound, CT peritoneography, abdominal MRI, or peritoneal scintigraphy if a subcutaneous leak is suspected.
4. Prevention:
   a. Appropriate catheter selection:
      i. Coiled catheters are less likely to migrate.
      ii. Adequate catheter length.
      iii. Optimal surgical technique:
         - Catheter tip should be placed deep in the pelvis.
         - Laparoscopic placement of the catheter is superior to open surgical placement in terms of catheter migration.
         - Routine empiric omentectomy.

- Laparoscopic adhesiolysis may be done for high-risk patients who had previous complicated abdominal surgeries.

5. Management of extraluminal obstruction:
   a. Laxatives (oral, suppositories or enema) to treat constipation.
      i. Catheter tips that have migrated to the left upper quadrant may spontaneously reposition as peristalsis favors downward movement of the catheter on the left side.
      ii. Spontaneous repositioning of a catheter that has migrated into the right upper quadrant is less likely as peristalsis favors continued upward movement of the catheter on this side.
   b. Changing the patient's position during drain.
   c. Fluoroscopically guided manipulation:
      - Insert a device such as a malleable rod, guidewire, cannula, or tip-deflecting wire into the catheter to redirect or reposition the catheter tip into a more favorable position.
   d. Surgical repositioning (laparoscopy or open surgery).
6. Management of intraluminal catheter obstruction:
   a. Eliminate kinks or remove clamps on transfer set and catheter.
   b. Infuse heparinized dialysate or normal saline with a 50 ml syringe using moderate pressure ("push and pull" maneuver).
   c. Instillation of fibrinolytic agent:
      i. Urokinase:
         - Dose: 1500 U/ml in intraluminal volume (catheter + transfer set).
            - Dilute urokinase (60000 U per vial) in 40 ml of 0.9% saline.
            - Inject the diluted urokinase into the effluent sampling bag:
              16.5 ml for 42-cm curved swan neck catheter (catheter 2.5 ml + transfer set 2 ml + effluent line 12 ml).
              17 ml for 62-cm curved swan neck catheter (catheter 3 ml + transfer set 2 ml + effluent line 12 ml).
            - Using gravity, run in the diluted urokinase into the PD catheter.
            - Dwell the diluted urokinase for 1–4 hours and then drain.
            - This process can be repeated once if the catheter remains blocked.

- Consider increasing urokinase dose up to 2500–5000 U/ml in refractory or recurrent cases, up to once daily for 3 days.
  - Dilute 60000 U of urokinase in 12–24 ml of 0.9% saline.
  - Inject the diluted urokinase into the effluent sampling bag if the volume of diluted urokinase is large enough, OR
  - Inject the diluted urokinase directly into the catheter (catheter + transfer set volume) without using the effluent bag, if the volume of the diluted urokinase is insufficient.

ii. Recombinant tissue plasminogen activator (t-PA, Alteplase™):
- Available as 2 mg per vial.
- Dilute to 1 mg/ml using 0.9% saline, and draw up a volume equivalent to the intraluminal volume (catheter lumen + transfer set).
- Inject the diluted t-PA into the PD catheter using sterile technique.
- Allow to dwell for 1–2 hours, or till the next PD.
- Aspirate t-PA from the catheter lumen using the 10 ml syringe.
- This should be followed by rapid in/out exchanges with reduced fill volumes using dialysate with heparin (1000 U/L dialysates).
- t-PA instillation may be repeated if the catheter remains occluded.

7. Surgery
   a. Laparoscopy with adhesiolysis.
   b. Open surgical repositioning of the catheter or replacement.
   c. Partial omentectomy or omentopexy.

C. Hernia

1. Sites:
   - Inguinal, umbilical, patent processus vaginalis, prior incision sites, obturator, foramen of Morgagni.

2. Risk factors:
   a. Neonates and infants due to patent processus vaginalis and higher intra-abdominal pressure.
   b. Previous laparotomies.
3. Clinical features:
   a. Painless swelling or disfigurement at the hernial site with or without mild discomfort.
   b. Abdominal wall or genital (labial or scrotal) swelling from PD fluid leak.
   c. Complicated hernias present as:
      - Tender lump.
      - Recurrent Gram-negative peritonitis.
      - Bowel obstruction or perforation from strangulation or incarceration of the bowel, especially if hernia is small.
   d. Obturator hernia may present as paresthesia or hyperesthesia of the anteromedial aspect of the thigh.
   e. Hernia through foramen of Morgagni may present as right-sided chest pain or right hypochondrial pain.
4. Diagnosis:
   a. In case of a diagnostic dilemma, CT or MRI peritoneography.
   b. Peritoneal scintigraphy is used in patients allergic to contrast dye or where MR peritoneography is not available.
5. Prevention:
   a. Use of a double-cuffed catheter and placement of the deep cuff in the intramuscular location.
   b. Laparoscopic catheter placement.
   c. Keeping intra-peritoneal pressure at ≤12–14 cmH_2O.
   d. Elective herniotomy should be considered in male infants with evidence of inguinal or other hernias prior to or during catheter placement.
   e. Avoidance of constipation, especially in the early post-operative period.
6. Treatment:
   a. Most hernias require surgical repair.
   b. Maintain on low volume nocturnal PD.

D. Hydrothorax

1. Almost always on the right side (50–90% of cases) due to patent foramen of Morgagni.
2. Clinical presentation:
   a. Asymptomatic effusion detected on chest radiograph.
   b. Symptomatic:
      - Dyspnea beginning shortly after start of PD (50% within 30 days) and progressively worsens as the dialysis continues despite efficient ultrafiltration.
      - Chest pain.
      - Hypotension.
   c. Inadequate ultrafiltration.
3. Investigations:
   a. Chest X-Ray to detect pleural effusion.
   b. Pleural tap with simultaneous measurement of glucose, protein, and lactate dehydrogenase:
      - High pleural fluid glucose content >22 mmol/L or pleural fluid to serum glucose concentration gradient >2.8 mmol/L).
      - Low protein concentration <1 g/dL.
      - Leukocyte count <100/μL (predominantly mononuclear cells).
      - Lactate dehydrogenase <100 IU/L.
   c. MRI or CT peritoneography if required.
4. Management:
   a. First line of treatment is temporary cessation of PD, or frequent small volume exchanges with avoidance of supine dwells can be attempted.
   b. Therapeutic thoracocentesis should be performed if there is massive hydrothorax and the patient has severe dyspnea or cardiovascular instability.
   c. With persistent or recurrent hydrothorax, pleurodesis using talc, autologous blood, or tetracycline may be considered.
   d. If this fails, diaphragmatic repair by videothoracoscopic surgery or open surgery can be considered.

E. Hemoperitoneum

1. Definition:
   - Presence of blood in PD fluid.
2. Etiology:
   a. Menstrual bleeding:
      i. Retrograde menstruation.
         - May start a few days before menstrual bleed.
      ii. Endometriosis.
      iii. Mid-cycle bleed associated with ovulation.
   b. Catheter-related:
      i. Post-catheter insertion or manipulation.
      ii. Trauma or strenuous exercise.
   c. Bleeding disorder or anticoagulation therapy.
   d. Intra-abdominal pathology:
      i. Hemorrhagic luteal cyst.
      ii. Ruptured cysts — ovarian, hepatic or renal.
      iii. Ectopic pregnancy.
      iv. Splenic rupture or infarct.
      v. Malignancy, including liver carcinomatosis and renal cell carcinoma.
      vi. Ruptured hepatic or renal cyst.
      vii. Acute or chronic pancreatitis.
      viii. Sclerosing peritonitis and peritoneal calcification.
      ix. Vascular catastrophe.
3. Indications for further evaluation:
   a. Fever, pain, tenderness or guarding of the abdomen, which may indicate a surgical emergency.
   b. Persistent hemoperitoneum.
4. Investigations:
   a. PD fluid cell count, culture and sensitivity.
   b. PD fluid hematocrit >2% suggests intraperitoneal pathology.
   c. PD fluid amylase levels >50 U/L suggests an intra-abdominal process.
   d. Abdominal imaging by ultrasound, CT or MRI.
      - Intravenous contrast agents should be avoided in patients with residual kidney function.
   e. Isotope labeled red blood cell scan may be required in persistent undiagnosed bleeding.
   f. Angiography may occasionally be required.

5. Management:
   a. Reassurance when the cause is benign, like menstrual bleed.
   b. Rapid flushes and instillation of heparin in the dialysate to prevent catheter clots.
   c. Infusion of cool dialysate (at room temperature).
   d. Surgical intervention as indicated.

F. Intestinal Perforation

1. Intestinal perforation can occur:
   a. At the time of catheter implantation because of direct injury.
   b. Weeks to months after placement because of bowel erosion.
2. Presentation:
   a. Feculent or bloody dialysate.
   b. Dialysate retention.
   c. Diarrhea occurring after dialysate instillation associated with very high glucose concentration in the stool.
   d. Peritonitis with multiple enteric organisms.
3. Management:
   a. Stop PD.
   b. Intravenous antibiotic covering enteric organisms.
   c. Surgical removal of catheter and bowel repair.

Recommended Reading

1. Zorzanello MM, Fleming WJ, Prowant BE. (2004) Use of tissue plasminogen activator in peritoneal dialysis catheters: A literature review and one center's experience. *Nephrol Nurs J* **31**:534–537.
2. McCormick BB, Bargman JM. (2007) Noninfectious complications of peritoneal dialysis: Implications for patient and technique survival. *J Am Soc Nephrol* **18**:3023–3025.
3. Schmidt RJ. (2019, updated) Noninfectious complications of continuous peritoneal dialysis. Edited by Golper TA, Motwani S. *UpToDate ONLINE*. http://www.uptodateonline.com.
4. Bakkaloglu SA, Sethna CB. (2021) Noninfectious complications of peritoneal dialysis in children. In: *Pediatric Dialysis*, 3rd edition. Edited by: Warady BA, Alexander SR, Schaefer F. Springer NY. pp. 291–314.

10 Approach to Encapsulating Peritoneal Sclerosis

Teo S, Ng KH and Yap HK

A. Definition

1. Encapsulating peritoneal sclerosis (EPS) is a clinical syndrome that continuously, intermittently or repeatedly presents with symptoms of intestinal obstruction due to adhesions of a diffusely thickened peritoneum.
2. Symptoms of bowel obstruction must be accompanied by evidence of peritoneal membrane thickening that causes encapsulation of the bowel, documented either at laparotomy or on radiological investigations (ultrasonography or computed tomography [CT] scan).

B. Risk Factors

1. Duration on peritoneal dialysis (PD):
   - Risk of occurrence after 5 years of PD is about 0.6–6.6%.
2. Type of dialysate:
   - High glucose concentration.
   - Glucose degradation products.
   - Acidic pH.
3. Peritonitis.
4. Cessation of PD.
   - EPS may develop up to 5 years after stopping PD.
5. Post kidney transplantation.
   - Use of profibrotic calcineurin inhibitors.
6. Ultrafiltration failure and high peritoneal solute transport rate.

C. Diagnostic Evaluation

1. Clinical Features:
   a. Signs of ileus:
      - Appetite loss.
      - Nausea.
      - Vomiting.
      - Abdominal fullness.
      - Abdominal pain.
      - Absent bowel sounds.
      - Diarrhea or constipation.
      - Weight loss.

   b. Signs of Inflammation:
      - Elevated temperature.
      - Ascites.
      - General fatigue.
      - Weight loss.

   c. Signs of peritoneal adhesions:
      - Bloody dialysate.
      - Ascites.
      - Abdominal discomfort.
      - Abdominal mass.

2. Investigations:
   a. Blood Investigations:
      i. Full blood count: Anemia.
      ii. Liver panel: Hypoalbuminemia.
      iii. C-reactive Protein: Elevated.

   b. Peritoneal Equilibration Test (PET):
      i. Associated with progressive transport defects:
         - High peritoneal membrane transport state.
         - Loss of ultrafiltration capacity.

   c. Radiology:
      i. Plain abdominal film:
         - Dilated small-bowel loops.
         - Air-fluid level in the small bowel.
         - Peritoneal calcifications.

ii. Ultrasound:
- Fixed, rigid bowel loops with ineffective peristaltic contractions.
- Dilated fixed loops matted together and tethered posteriorly.
- Intraperitoneal echogenic strands.
- Trilaminar appearance of the bowel wall.
- Echogenic "sandwich appearance" of the peritoneal membrane.

iii. CT scan:
- Adherent, dilated bowel loops.
- Variable diameter of bowel segments with bowel luminal narrowing.
- Thickened intestinal wall and peritoneal membrane.
- Increased mesenteric fat density.
- Air-fluid level.
- Entrapped fluid collection.
- Peritoneal calcification.

3. Stages of EPS (Nakamoto, 2005):

Stage		Findings
1	Pre-EPS	Asymptomatic with mild ascites and no inflammation. Ultrafiltration failure. Fast transport status.
2	Inflammation period	Symptomatic with nausea and diarrhea consistent with partial encapsulation of the bowel and intestinal swelling. Mild inflammation with fibrin exudation is present: • Elevated C-reactive protein. • Leukocytosis.
3	Encapsulating or progressive period	Symptoms of bowel obstruction due to formation of the fibrous cocoon causing encapsulation: • Obstipation, nausea and vomiting. • Abdominal mass. Mild to severe inflammation: • Bloodstained effluent. • Ascites.
4	Ileus or complete period	Complete bowel obstruction caused by thickening of the encapsulating fibrous cocoon: • Anorexia. • Abdominal mass. Little or no inflammation present.

D. Management

1. Discontinuation of PD:
   a. Stop PD as soon as diagnosis is made.
   b. Remove Tenckhoff catheter.
2. Nutritional Support:
   a. Indications:
      i. Malnutrition.
      ii. Peri-operatively until gut function recovers.
   b. Can be enteral or parenteral.
3. Drug therapy (no definitive conclusion as to its effectiveness, as EPS can still occur post kidney transplant despite immunosuppression):
   a. Prednisolone:
      i. Decreases the inflammation that precedes encapsulation.
      ii. Dosage:
         - 0.5–1 mg/kg/day for the first month.
         - 0.25–0.5 mg/kg/day for the second and third months.
         - 5–10 mg/day to continue for at least 1 year.
         - Prolong the high dose of prednisolone in a clinically responding patient with a persistently elevated C-reactive protein.
   b. Tamoxifen:
      i. Selective estrogen receptor modulator with antifibrotic properties
      ii. Inhibits the production of transforming growth factor (TGF)-β by fibroblasts.
      iii. Adult dosage: 10–40 mg/day for at least 3 months.
         - If there are signs of clinical improvement, continue for at least 1 year.
      iv. Side effects:
         - Hot flushes
         - Nausea
         - Fatigue
         - Risk of venous thrombosis.
4. Surgery:
   a. Peritonectomy and careful enterolysis ± Noble plication (suturing of intestines to each other to prevent obstruction)

b. Indications:
   i. Complete bowel obstruction.
   ii. Bowel perforation or haemoperitoneum.
   iii. Failed medical therapy.
   iv. Immediate continuation of corticosteroid therapy to prevent recurrence of EPS.

E. Prevention

1. Avoidance of risk factors:
   a. Use of biocompatible PD fluids with neutral pH, low concentrations of glucose degradation products.
   b. Implement measures to reduce the risk of peritonitis.
2. Early detection and management of pre-EPS stage:
   a. Do PET yearly to identify patients at risk of EPS:
      i. After 5 years of PD.
      ii. Evidence of changing peritoneal transport characteristics following:
         - Repeated episodes of peritonitis.
         - Following abdominal surgery.
   b. If there is evidence of ultrafiltration failure, or an increase in dialysate/plasma (D/P) urea ratio to the high average transport range on the PET, check the inflammatory markers and perform a CT scan of the abdomen to look for early signs of EPS.
   c. If there is evidence of persistent inflammation and at least one radiological feature of EPS, consider changing patient to hemodialysis.

Recommended Reading

1. Nakamoto H. (2005) Encapsulating peritoneal sclerosis — A clinician's approach to diagnosis and medical treatment. *Perit Dial Int* **25 Suppl 4**:S30–38.
2. Guest S. (2009) Tamoxifen therapy for encapsulating peritoneal sclerosis: Mechanism of action and update on clinical experience. *Perit Dial Int* **29**:252–255.
3. Honda M, Warady BA. (2010) Long-term peritoneal dialysis and encapsulating peritoneal sclerosis in children. *Pediatr Nephrol* **25**:75–81.
4. Korte MR, Sampimon DE, Betjes MGH, Krediet RT. (2011) Encapsulating peritoneal sclerosis: The state of affairs. *Nat Rev Nephrol* **7**:528–538.

5. Stefanidis CJ, Shroff R. (2014) Encapsulating peritoneal sclerosis in children. *Pediatr Nephrol* **29**:2093–2103.
6. Moinuddin Z, Summers A, Van Dellen D, Augustine T, Herrick SE. (2015) Encapsulating peritoneal sclerosis — a rare but devastating peritoneal disease. *Front Physiol* **5**:470 doi:10.3389/fphys.2014.00470.
7. Brown EA, Bargman J, van Biesen W, Chang MY, Finkelstein FO, Hurst H, Johnson DW, Kawanishi H, Lambie M, de Moraes TP, Morelle J, Woodrow G. (2017) Length of time on peritoneal dialysis and encapsulating peritoneal sclerosis — position paper for ISPD: 2017 update. *Perit Dial Int* **37**:363–374.

1 Live Donor Evaluation

Koh LJ, Sinnathamby A, Teo S, Chhabra M, Ng KH and Yap HK

A. Donor Criteria

1. Donor must be ≥21 years old.
2. Baseline kidney function normal within the preceding 6 months, or at the time of admission.

B. Clinical Evaluation

1. History and physical examination, including blood pressure on at least 2 occasions.
2. Significant past medical history.
   a. Hypertension.
   b. Diabetes mellitus.
   c. Ischemic heart disease.
   d. Tuberculosis (TB) infection.
   e. Creutzfeldt–Jakob disease (CJD).
   f. Smoking history.
      - Donors who smoke should be advised to quit at least 4 weeks before donation.
3. Family history of TB infection or CJD.
4. Travel history to malarial-endemic region.
5. Social history of high-risk behaviors:
   a. Recreational drugs.
   b. High-risk sexual behavior.
   c. Alcoholism.

C. Investigations

1. Blood:
   a. Full blood count.
   b. Urea, creatinine, sodium, potassium, chloride, bicarbonate, calcium, phosphate, and uric acid.
   c. Liver function test.
   d. Fasting lipid including total cholesterol, triglycerides, low-density lipoprotein (LDL)-cholesterol, and high-density lipoprotein (HDL)-cholesterol.
   e. Fasting blood glucose.
   f. Glycated hemoglobin (HbA1c).
   g. Thyroxine level (T_4) and thyroid-stimulating hormone (TSH).
   h. Infection screen:
      i. Human immunodeficiency virus serology (HIV Ag/Ab Combo Test).
      ii. Hepatitis B surface antigen (HBsAg).
      iii. Hepatitis B virus serology (anti-hepatitis Bs antibody and total anti-hepatitis B core antibody).
      iv. Hepatitis C virus serology.
      v. Treponemal test for syphilis.
      vi. Epstein–Barr virus serology.
      vii. Cytomegalovirus serology.
      viii. TB testing if positive contact history or living in high endemic area.
         - Interferon-gamma release assay (TB Quantiferon or TB Spot test).
2. Urine tests:
   a. Urine microscopy and culture.
   b. 24-hour creatinine clearance.
   c. Urine albumin:creatinine ratio and 24-hour urinary albumin excretion.
3. Cardiac evaluation:
   a. Electrocardiogram (ECG).
   b. Chest X-Ray.
4. Uroradiological evaluation:
   a. Computed Tomography (CT) angiogram.
   b. ^{99m}Dimercaptosuccinic acid (DMSA) scan.

   c. Renal angiogram (if CT angiogram does not delineate renal vessels well).
5. Tissue typing:
   a. ABO, Rh.
   b. HLA class I, II.
   c. Recipient-donor T- and B-cell direct crossmatch:
      i. Anti-human globulin (AHG)-enhanced to detect IgG antibodies (warm antibodies reactive at 37°C).
      ii. Dithiothreitol (DTT) to detect IgM antibodies (cold antibodies reactive at 5°C).
      Note: Crossmatch must be negative on the recipient serum obtained at least 2 weeks after last blood transfusion or peritonitis episode. For live donor transplant, this should be negative within 1 month of the transplant surgery.
   d. Recipient-donor T- and B-cell flow cytometric crossmatch.
   Note: Crossmatch must be done within 1 month of the transplant.
6. Tests to be repeated 1 week before the kidney transplant:
   a. HIV–1/2 Ag/Ab Combo.
   b. HBsAg.
   c. Anti-hepatitis Bs antibody and total anti-hepatitis B core antibody.
   d. Hepatitis C virus serology.
   e. Treponemal test for syphilis.
   f. Nucleic acid tests:
      - HIV.
      - Hepatitis B virus.
      - Hepatitis C virus.
   g. Dengue nucleic acid test (to be done 48–72 hours before transplant).
   h. Zika virus nucleic acid test (plasma and urine) (to be done 48–72 hours before transplant).
   i. Chikungunya nucleic acid test (to be done 48–72 hours before transplant if clinically indicated).
   j. SARS-CoV-2 nucleic acid amplification (to be done 48–72 hours before transplant).
   k. Nucleic acid tests:
      - HIV.
      - Hepatitis B virus.
      - Hepatitis C virus.

D. Counseling and Psychosocial Evaluation

1. Psychiatric evaluation.
2. Ethics Committee evaluation.
3. For recipients with genetic kidney disease, genetic testing should be performed for donors, and donors should receive genetic counseling for:
   a. Risk of disease recurrence in the recipient.
   b. Risk of kidney impairment post-donation in the donor related to risk alleles which may not be fully recognized currently.
4. For highly sensitized kidney transplantation (e.g., ABO blood group or HLA incompatible), the donor and recipient should be informed of treatment options such as kidney paired donation and incompatibility management strategies.
5. Counseling for post-donation care and follow-up.

E. Exclusion for Donation

1. Donors with IgA nephropathy.
2. Donors with genetic diseases who have:
   - A (likely) pathogenic allele in dominant (autosomal or X-linked) disease.
   - Proven mutation in mitochondrial genes (e.g., MELAS syndrome).
3. Donors with diabetes.
4. Donors with active malignancy.
5. Donors who are pregnant at the time of transplant surgery.

Recommended Reading

1. Lentine KL, Kasiske BL, Levey AS, Adams PL, Alberú J, Bakr MA, Gallon L, Garvey CA, Guleria S, Li PK, Segev DL, Taler SJ, Tanabe K, Wright L, Zeier MG, Cheung M, Garg AX. (2017) KDIGO Clinical practice guideline on the evaluation and care of living kidney donors. *Transplantation* **101**(8S Suppl 1):S1–S109.
2. MOH. (2018) Manual on organ donation and transplantation. Ministry of Health Singapore.
3. Mandelbrot DA, Reese PP, Garg N, Thomas CP, Rodrigue JR, Schinstock C, Doshi M, Cooper M, Friedewald J, Naik AS, Kaul DR, Ison MG, Rocco MV, Verbesey J, Hladunewich MA, Ibrahim HN, Poggio ED. (2020) KDOQI US commentary on the 2017 KDIGO clinical practice guideline on the evaluation and care of living kidney donors. *AJKD* **75**:299–316.

2 Pre-Transplant Evaluation of Potential Recipient

Koh LJ, Ng KH, Teo S, Lau PYW and Yap HK

A. Goal of Evaluation

1. The main goal of evaluating a pediatric kidney transplant recipient is to reduce post-transplant complications and improve the patient and allograft's survival.
2. The potential kidney transplant recipient must be evaluated to determine if he or she is a suitable candidate in terms of both the underlying medical problems and tissue compatibility.
3. Areas of assessment:
   a. Pre-existing medical conditions, including complications of chronic kidney disease (CKD).
   b. Risk for post-transplant infections.
   c. Risk of recurrent disease.
   d. Immunological risk for allograft rejection.

B. Contraindications to Kidney Transplantation

1. Active infections, in particular, tuberculosis.
2. Active hepatitis, in particular, hepatitis B and C.
3. Chronic liver disease with bridging fibrosis or cirrhosis.
4. Active malignancy.
5. Non-kidney disorders with significantly shortened life expectancy.
6. Patient or caregivers unable to cope with post-transplant care as documented by active and ongoing treatment nonadherence.
7. Active substance abuse.
8. Reversible kidney failure.
9. Uncontrolled psychiatric disease.

10. Uncontrolled systemic diseases including:
    a. Systemic lupus erythematosus (SLE).
    b. Anti-neutrophil cytoplasmic antibodies (ANCA)-associated vasculitis.
    c. High levels of circulating anti-glomerular basement membrane (GBM) antibodies.
    d. Primary hyperoxaluria.
11. Active peptic ulcer disease.

C. Important Points in the History

1. Underlying kidney disease, especially those with risk of recurrence, such as focal segmental glomerulosclerosis, hemolytic-uremic syndrome, SLE, primary hyperoxaluria, C3 glomerulopathy.
2. Kidney biopsy findings.
3. Associated systemic diseases: Seizure disorders, SLE, congenital heart disease, bronchial asthma, cytopenias, peptic ulcer disease, liver disease.
4. Known or suspected genetic conditions.
5. Complications of CKD and dialysis, including hypertension, anemia and mineral bone disease (control and medications).
6. History of urological abnormalities, including bladder dysfunction and urological surgery.
7. Thrombotic risk:
    a. Previous history of thrombotic events, including thrombosis at hemodialysis catheter sites or arteriovenous fistula.
    b. Nephrotic syndrome.
8. Infectious risk:
    a. Recent history of dengue infection in the past 3 months.
    b. Previous coronavirus disease 2019 (COVID-19) infection or contact with high-risk individuals.
    c. Close contact history of tuberculosis and treatment.
    d. Any history of unprotected sex or intravenous drug use.
9. History of drug allergy and adverse reactions, including latex allergy (especially for patients with neurogenic bladder).
10. History of malignancy, treatment and disease-free period.
11. Smoking history.

12. Immunization history and immune status:
    a. BCG.
    b. Diphtheria, tetanus, pertussis, poliomyelitis.
    c. Hepatitis B.
    d. Hemophilus influenza type B (Hib).
    e. Measles.
    f. Mumps.
    g. Rubella.
    h. Varicella zoster.
    i. Pneumococcus.
    j. Meningococcus.
    k. Human papillomavirus (after the age of 9 years).
    l. Hepatitis A (optional).
    m. Influenza.
    n. Severe acute respiratory syndrome coronavirus 2 (SARS-CoV2).
    o. Japanese B encephalitis (endemic regions).
13. Sensitization risk:
    a. Previous blood and platelet transfusions.
        - If blood transfusion is required, leucocyte-free packed cells should be given.
    b. Previous transplants.
    c. Previous pregnancies.

D. Physical Examination

1. Size of child: weight and height centiles, body mass index.
2. Blood pressure.
3. Cardiovascular status.
4. Pulmonary status.
5. Spinal deformities.
6. Abdominal masses.
7. Neurological status.
8. Pubertal status.
9. Developmental assessment.

E. Investigations

1. Blood investigations:
   a. Full blood count.
   b. Urea, creatinine, sodium, potassium, chloride, bicarbonate.
   c. Calcium, phosphate, alkaline phosphatase.
   d. Uric acid.
   e. Fasting lipid profile:
      - Total cholesterol
      - Low-density lipoprotein (LDL) cholesterol
      - High-density lipoprotein (HDL) cholesterol
      - Triglycerides.
   f. Total protein, albumin.
   g. Alanine aminotransaminase (ALT), aspartate aminotransferase (AST), gamma-glutamyltranspeptidase (GGT), bilirubin.
   h. Fasting blood glucose.
   i. Parathyroid hormone (iPTH).
   j. Prothrombin time (PT) and partial thromboplastin time (PTT).
   k. Thyroxine (T4) and thyroid-stimulating hormone (TSH).
   l. Serum immunoglobulins (IgG, IgM, IgA).
   m. Immunodeficiency workup (if history of recurrent infections).
   n. Infection screen:
      i. Human immunodeficiency virus serology (HIV Ag/Ab combo test).
      ii. Hepatitis B surface (HBs) antigen.
      iii. Hepatitis B virus serology:
         - Anti-HBs antibody.
         - Anti-hepatitis B core antibody (anti-HBc total).
      iv. Hepatitis C virus serology (anti-HCV antibody).
      v. Hepatitis E virus serology (if the patient has transaminitis).
      vi. Epstein–Barr virus serology:
         - Anti-viral capsid antigen (VCA) IgG.
      vii. Cytomegalovirus serology (anti-CMV IgG).
      viii. Treponemal test for syphilis.
      ix. Measles, mumps, rubella, varicella-zoster IgG.
      x. Nucleic acid testing within 1 month preceding the transplant:

- HIV.
- Hepatitis B.
- Hepatitis C.

xi. SARS-CoV2 nucleic acid testing at 1 week and 3 days prior to the transplant.

o. Serum complements C3 and C4.
p. Anti-double stranded DNA antibody levels (for patients with SLE).
q. Thrombophilia screen (for live-donor transplant recipients):
   i. Anti-cardiolipin IgG and IgM*.
   ii. Anti-β2-glycoprotein-1 IgG and IgM*.
   iii. Lupus anti-coagulant*.
   iv. Protein C.
   v. Protein S.
   vi. Factor V Leiden factor.
   vii. Anti-thrombin III.

   *Annually for patients with SLE on the deceased donor waiting list.

2. Urine investigations:
   a. Urine microscopic examination.
   b. Urine culture.
   c. Residual urine volume and 24-hour urine protein excretion.
3. Chest X-Ray.
4. Electrocardiogram (ECG).
5. 2-D Echocardiogram.
6. Tuberculosis screen if positive contact history or living in high endemic area:
   a. Tuberculin skin test in patients aged <2 years.
   b. Interferon-gamma release assay in patients aged ≥2 years:
      - TB T-spot test (preferred in immunocompromised patients).
      - TB Quantiferon (less sensitive in immunocompromised patients).
7. Tissue typing:
   a. ABO blood group.
   b. Preformed anti-HLA cytotoxic antibodies (panel reactive antibodies by flow) (for transplant recipients on the deceased donor waiting list).
   c. HLA-A, B, C typing.
   d. HLA-DR, DP, DQ typing.

e. Recipient-donor T- and B-cell direct crossmatch:
   i. Anti-human globulin (AHG)-enhanced to detect IgG antibodies (warm antibodies reactive at 37ºC).
   ii. Dithiothreitol (DTT) to detect IgM antibodies (cold antibodies reactive at 5ºC).

   Note:
   i. Crossmatch must be negative on recipient serum obtained at least 2 weeks after the last blood transfusion or peritonitis episode.
      - For live donor transplant, this should be negative within one month of the transplant surgery.
   ii. False positive B-cell crossmatch may occur after anti-CD20 antibody treatment.

f. Recipient-donor T- and B-cell flow cytometric crossmatch:

   Note:
   i. Crossmatch must be done within 1 month of the transplant.
   ii. Pronase treatment is essential, especially for B-cell flow crossmatch positive tests.
      - Proteolytic enzyme-removing Fc receptors from the surface of T- and B-cells.
      - Pronase treatment improves the sensitivity of both B- and T-cell crossmatch.
      - No false positives for T-cell crossmatch.
      - Decreases false positives for B-cell crossmatch due to pre-existing antibodies on the surface of recipient B-cells, including anti-CD20 antibodies (post-Rituximab treatment).

g. Donor-specific antibody levels.

8. Urological evaluation if a structural abnormality is present:
   a. Ultrasound of kidneys and bladder.
   b. Micturating cystourethrogram (MCU).
   c. Urodynamics if dysfunctional bladder is suspected.

   Note:
   - Mitrofanoff and augmentation cystoplasty should be performed at least 3 months before the transplant.
   - Corrective surgery for vesicoureteric reflux grades III–V should be performed at least 3 months before the transplant surgery, with repeat MCU.

9. Esophagogastroduodenocopy for patients aged ≥18 years, or with symptoms suggestive of peptic ulcer disease.
   - Resolution of lesions should be confirmed by endoscopy prior to transplantation.
10. Ultrasound scan of blood vessels:
    a. Common internal and external iliac vessels and femoral vessels.
    b. Lower abdominal aorta and inferior vena cava if weight <15 kg.
    c. Neck veins if history of previous central line insertion.

F. Further Assessment

1. Psychosocial and psychiatric evaluation:
   - Adherence assessment, education and counseling.
2. Neurocognitive assessment in children who progressed to kidney failure before the age of 5 years.
3. Dental clearance.
4. Referral for evaluation by transplant surgical team.

G. Considerations for Pre-transplant Native Nephrectomies

1. Severe refractory hypertension.
2. Intractable urinary tract infection associated with high-grade vesicoureteric reflux.
3. High risk of Wilms' tumor in children with X-Y gonadal dysgenesis and kidney failure (Denys–Drash syndrome).
4. Persistent nephrotic syndrome with associated complications due to hypercoagulability.

Recommended Reading

1. Vaidya S, Cooper TY, Avandsalehi J, Barnes T, Brooks K, Hymel P, Noor M, Sellers R, Thomas A, Stewart D, Daller J, Fish JC, Gugliuzza KK, Bray RA. (2011) Improved flow cytometric detection of HLA alloantibodies using pronase: Potential implications in renal transplantation. *Transplantation* **71**:422–428.

2. Yap HK. (2005) Renal transplantation: Pre-operative/post-operative care and transplant immunosuppression. In: *Practical Paediatric Nephrology. An Update of Current Practices*. Edited by: Chiu MC, Yap HK. Medcom Limited. pp 314–325.
3. MOH. (2018) Manual on organ donation and transplantation. Ministry of Health Singapore.
4. McDonald RA. (2019, updated) Kidney transplantation in children: General principles. Edited by Niaudet P, Kim MS. UpToDate ONLINE. http://www.uptodate.com.
5. Chadban SJ, Ahn C, Axelrod DA, Foster BJ, Kasiske BL, Kher V, Kumar D, Oberbauer R, Pascual J, Pilmore HL, Rodrigue JR, Segev DL, Sheerin NS, Tinckam KJ, Wong G, Balk EM, Gordon CE, Earley A, Rofeberg V, Knoll GA. (2020) Summary of the Kidney Disease: Improving Global Outcomes (KDIGO) clinical practice guideline on the evaluation and management of candidates for kidney transplantation. *Transplantation* **104**:708–714.

3 Management of Highly Sensitized Kidney Transplant Recipient

Koh LJ, Teo S, Ng KH, Lau PYW and Yap HK

A. HLA Sensitization

I. Human Leukocyte Antigens (HLA)

1. Certain regions of the major histocompatibility complex (MHC) molecule appear to be immunogenic.
   a. Class I molecules: Corresponds to the antigenic region encoded by exons 2 and 3 of the alpha chain.
   b. Class II molecules: Corresponds to the antigenic region encoded by exon 2 of the beta chain for the HLA-DR molecules and exon 2 of the alpha and beta chains for HLA-DQ and DP.
2. Serologic antigen equivalents (serotypes): MHC molecules that share similar antigenic epitopes and therefore appear serologically identical.
3. HLA mismatches refer to an HLA antigen found on the cells of the donor allograft but not in the recipient.
   - The greater the mismatch, the higher the likelihood of developing an allograft rejection.
4. Molecular typing allows for higher resolution typing of all loci (HLA-A, HLA-B, HLA-C, HLA-DRB1, HLA-DRB3, HLA-DRB4, HLA-DRB5, HLA-DQA, HLA-DQB, and HLA-DPB).

Serological Typing	Sequence-specific Primers (SSP) Typing	Sequence-specific Oligonucleotide Probes (SSOP) Typing	Sequence-based Typing (SBT) or Sanger Sequencing	Next-generation Sequencing (NGS)
HLA-A1	A*01:01	A*01:01	A*01:01:01	A*01:01:01

Note: 1st field = HLA allele group
2nd field = Unique HLA protein
3rd field = Alleles with synonymous nucleotide substitutions (similar amino acid sequence)

II. Anti-HLA antibodies

1. Specificity of anti-HLA antibodies:
   a. Private specificities: Unique to a particular HLA molecule or a limited group or family of closely related alleles.
   b. Public specificities: Shared by more than one HLA molecule.
   c. Public epitopes are responsible for cross-reactivity observed in HLA alloantiserum and are grouped into major cross-reactive groups (CREG).
   d. Screening of potential transplant recipients is used to ensure a true negative crossmatch with the intended donor by:
      - Accounting for all relevant antibodies, and
      - Avoiding a false positive crossmatch with clinically irrelevant antibodies.
2. Types of anti-HLA antibodies:
   a. IgG antibodies:
      i. IgG warm antibodies reactive to HLA Class I antigens (on both T and B cells) at 37°C are the most important.
      ii. IgG antibodies reactive to HLA Class II antigens (on B cells).
   b. IgM antibody characterized by reactivity at 4°C, which is removed by heating at 55°C or by treatment with dithiothreitol (DTT).
      - IgM antibody is often an autoantibody and can be ignored.
   c. IgG antibodies detected by sensitization or crossmatch assays are generally considered to reflect true sensitization against HLA.

d. T cell-negative/B cell-positive reaction can be due to:
   i. Presence of only preexistent HLA Class II antibody, OR
   ii. Presence of low titers of preexistent HLA Class I antibody as B cells express HLA Class I antigen at a level quantitatively greater than on T cells.
e. T cell-positive/B cell-negative reactions are the most likely results from a non-HLA antibody as Class I antigen is expressed on both T and B cells.
f. Complement fixation:
   i. Complement fixing antibodies are considered cytotoxic and likely to be of clinical importance.
   ii. Non-complement fixing antibodies may not be cytotoxic and therefore, the clinical significance is unclear.

III. Determination of HLA sensitization:

1. Panel reactive antibody (PRA):
   a. PRA (%) is an estimate of the likelihood of a positive crossmatch to a pool of potential donors.
   b. PRA is assessed at regular intervals whilst on a transplant waiting list.
      - Reported as historical (the highest value recorded on previous testing) and as current PRA.
   c. Measurement of PRA:
      i. Complement-dependent lymphocytotoxicity (CDC) assay used for HLA antibody screening.
         - Patient's serum is incubated separately with B cells (HLA Class II) and T-cells (HLA Class I) from panels of donors.
         - Results expressed as the percentage of panel cells killed by the serum: Panel-reactive antibodies (PRA).
         - Detects high-affinity antibodies that efficiently activate complement.
         - IgM autoantibodies can cause false positive results with 100% PRA binding.
         - Adsorption of antibodies on autologous cells can remove the antibodies and render the serum negative.
      ii. Anti-human globulin (AHG)-enhanced cytotoxicity:

- A single IgG antibody may not bind the complement as easily as multiple IgG antibodies in close proximity.
- AHG increases C1q binding by providing more Fc regions for C1q to bind, hence mimicking multiple IgG binding in close proximity.
- Cytotoxicity assay can be enhanced by adding AHG to the microcytotoxicity plate after adding the patient's serum and before adding complement.

iii. ELISA assay:
- Uses micro-test trays containing known HLA, to which potential recipient serum is added.
- More rapid than the CDC assay.

iv. Multiplexed particle-based flow cytometric (Luminex) assay (Flow PRA):
- More sensitive assay to detect low levels of anti-HLA antibodies.
- Does not require complement binding.
- Patient's serum is incubated with a set of HLA flow beads, and fluorescently-labeled anti-human IgG antibodies are used to detect the anti-HLA antibodies in the serum.

2. Donor-specific antibodies (DSA):
   a. Single antigen bead assay:
      i. Using affinity-purified HLA antigens coated on microparticles or beads.
      - Patient's serum is incubated with a mixture of beads, and fluorescently labeled anti-human IgG antibodies are used to detect the anti-HLA antibodies in the serum.

      ii. Detects both complement and non-complement activating antibodies.
      iii. DSAs can be identified if donor HLA typing is known.

Anti-HLA Antibodies	Standardized Fluorescent Intensity (SFI)	Mean Fluorescent Intensity (MFI)
Strong binding	>200000	>10000
Moderate binding	100000 to 200000	5000 to 10000
Weak binding	50000 to <100000	2500 to <5000
Negative	<50000	<2500

*MFI = SFI/20.

3. Pre-transplantation crossmatch:
   a. Performed to evaluate for any evidence of preformed antibodies with specificity for the potential donor that could lead to hyperacute or acute antibody-mediated rejection (AMR).
   b. Fresh serum should be used for the final crossmatch.
   c. Timing of crossmatch:
      i. Within 1 month of transplant.
      ii. To repeat if there is an interval potential sensitization event (e.g., blood product transfusion, peritonitis or IgG antibody infusion).
   d. Virtual crossmatch:
      i. Compares the anti-HLA antibody screen to the HLA type of the donor, looking for preformed DSA.
      ii. Molecular methods of HLA typing (SSOP, SSP or NGS) are important for the specificity of virtual crossmatching.
      iii. Positive virtual crossmatch is determined by the accepted MFI threshold.
      iv. Under-recognition of shared epitopes or CREGs of DSAs can result in false negative virtual crossmatching.
      v. There are limitations in the loci of antigen beads, which may lead to under-recognition of a DSA of a rare antigen.
      vi. Presence of a historical DSA may indicate an immunologic memory against the donor antigen.
   e. CDC crossmatch.
      i. Similar to the CDC test used to define PRA.
         - Performed using wells containing donor cells, rather than a pool of lymphocytes.
         - Potential recipient serum is added, along with rabbit complement, and cytotoxicity is determined after administration of a vital dye.
         - The test is done in dilutions to rule out prozone effect (false negative reaction due to high antibody titers) and to help estimate the magnitude of the immunologic reaction.
         - IgM autoantibodies can cause false positive CDC crossmatch test results.
         - False positive B-cell antibodies may be seen in patients treated with anti-CD20 antibody (Rituximab), which may still be present in the serum.

- Presence of non-HLA anti-lymphocyte antibody not present on allograft tissue, and this can be excluded by testing the patient's sera against their own lymphocytes (autocrossmatch).

ii. AHG-enhanced crossmatch:
- Performed to detect low levels of IgG anti-HLA antibodies.

iii. DTT-treated crossmatch:
- Used to eliminate IgM autoantibodies by reducing the disulfide bonds present in IgM antibodies.
- Also eliminates IgM alloantibodies.
- IgM alloantibodies are rare and may be associated with hyperacute rejection in isolated cases.
- DTT-positive crossmatch indicates the presence of IgG alloantibodies.

iv. Pronase treatment of donor cells:
- Pronase is a non-specific peptidase that preferentially digests Fc receptors and other cell surface proteins on lymphocytes without substantially destroying HLA molecules under certain conditions.
- Pretreating donor cells with pronase reduces non-specific binding of recipient serum to donor lymphocytes, thus decreasing the incidence of false positive reactions on the CDC crossmatch.

f. Flow cytometry crossmatch (FCXM):

i. Very sensitive crossmatch test detecting very low levels of circulating anti-HLA antibodies:
- T-cell FCXM is particularly useful in sensitized and re-transplantation candidates whose antibody levels have fallen but who can mount a rapid memory response on challenge.
- May potentially result from a non-HLA antibody.

ii. Potential for false positive reactions:
- Caused by non-specific immunoglobulin binding to lymphocyte immunoglobulin Fc receptors.
- Persistence of anti-CD20 antibodies in the serum in patients treated with Rituximab may cause a false positive reaction.

iii. Pronase treatment of donor cells:
   - Pre-treating donor cells with pronase reduces non-specific binding of recipient serum to donor lymphocytes decreasing the incidence of false positive reactions on FCXM.

B. Sensitized Patients

1. High risk:
   a. Flow cytometry PRA >30%, with a history of sensitizing events, including blood transfusions and previous transplants.
   b. T-cell CDC crossmatch positive at >1:2 dilution.
   c. (+/–) B-cell CDC IgG crossmatch positive at >1:2 dilution.
   d. T-cell FXCM positive with a mean flow-channel shift of >225 (normal background number ≤50).
   e. (+/–) B-cell FXCM positive (IgG) with a mean flow-channel shift of >225 and DSA flow cytometry MFI >5000.
   f. Donor-specific antibodies relative intensity scale (DSA-RIS) ≥17 at transplantation:

Points	Strength of DSA
0	No DSA
2	Each weak DSA (MFI 2500–5000)
5	Each moderate DSA (MFI 5000–10000)
10	Each strong DSA (MFI>10000)

   g. Presence of other antibodies such as angiotensin II receptor antibodies, anti-endothelial cell antibodies, and MHC Class I polypeptide-related sequence A (MICA).
2. Moderate risk:
   a. T-cell FCXM positive but T-cell CDC crossmatch negative.
   b. B-cell CDC IgG crossmatch positive at 1:2 dilution.
   c. B-cell IgG FCXM positive (mean flow-channel shift >225).
   d. Donor-specific antibodies (DSA): Flow cytometry mean fluorescent intensity (MFI) >5000 with DSA-RIS <17.

3. Prediction of AMR based on the relationship between DSA and FCXM following desensitization:

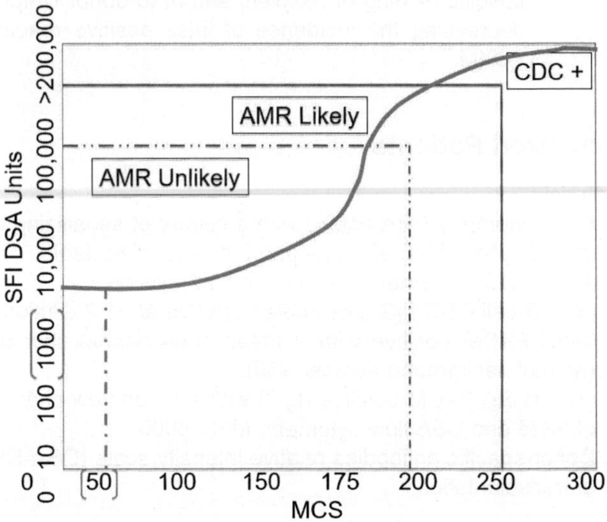

C. Desensitization Protocol

I. Live-donor transplant recipient:

1. Moderate risk:
   a. Intravenous immunoglobulin (IVIG) 2 g/kg (maximum 140 g) monthly for 3 months.
      - Volume infused has to be removed in those on dialysis, especially if hypertensive.
      - May be necessary to give the total dose over 2 days.
   b. Repeat DSA titers and/or FCXM crossmatch (with Pronase treatment) after completing the course.
      - Course can be repeated if the patient is still in the moderate risk category.

c. At transplant:
    - IVIG 1 g/kg dose within 72 hours of live-donor transplant (2 g/kg if the patient has not received the 3-monthly doses).

2. High risk:
    a. Consider alternate donor or paired kidney exchange.
    b. Desensitization of recipient prior to transplant:
        i. IVIG 2 g/kg (maximum 140 g) on Day 0 and Day 30.
        ii. IV Rituximab 375 mg/m2 (maximum 1 g) on Day 7.
            - Pre-medication according to Rituximab protocol.
        iii. Repeat DSA titers and/or FCXM crossmatch (with Pronase treatment) after completion of the course.
        iv. Proceed with the transplant if desensitization is successful.
    c. At transplant:
        - IVIG 1 g/kg dose within 72 hours of the live-donor transplant.
        - Combination of IVIG and Rituximab required because of the inability of Rituximab to deplete CD20-negative plasma cells that continue to produce DSAs and mediate graft injury.

II. Deceased-donor transplant recipient:

1. Transplant recipient on waiting list with high PRA:
    - Consider modulating PRA levels with IVIG 2 g/kg (maximum 140 g) monthly for 3 months followed by repeat PRA levels.
2. Moderate risk:
    a. IVIG 2 g/kg (maximum 140 g) within 72 hours of the deceased-donor transplant.
    b. IV Rituximab 375 mg/m^2 (maximum 1 g) on Day 7.
        - Pre-medication according to Rituximab protocol.
    c. Repeat DSA titers on Day 30 before IVIG.
    d. IVIG 2 g/kg (maximum 140 g) on Day 30.

III. *Risk assessment and management based on crossmatch results:*

Crossmatch					Interpretation	Management
DSA	FCXM		CDC			
	T	B	T	B		
+	+	+/−	+	+/−	• High risk.	• Transplant contraindicated unless DSA can be reduced with desensitization protocols and crossmatch becomes negative.
+	+	+/−	−	−	• Moderate risk. • Non-complement fixing DSA.	• Monthly IVIG 2g/kg for 3 months, then • Repeat DSA and FCXM. • If proceed with transplant, IVIG 1g/kg at transplant.
+	−	+	−	+	• Moderate risk of AMR (Class II Ab). • False positive from monoclonal/ polyclonal antibodies. • Weak, low titer Class I Ab.	• Monthly IVIG 2g/kg for 3 months, then • Repeat DSA and FCXM • If proceed with transplant, IVIG 1g/kg at transplant.
+	−	−	−	−	• Different samples used for DSA versus crossmatch. • False positive: o Overcalling (MFI threshold too low). o HLA typing not specific. o High background.	• Repeat DSA. • Consider higher resolution HLA typing.

(*Continued*)

Crossmatch					Interpretation	Management
DSA	FCXM		CDC			
	T	B	T	B		
−	+	+/−	+	+/−	• High risk. • Non-HLA IgG. • Drug interference. • Antibodies to allele not tested by HLA panel. • Different serum samples. • False negative HLA antibody test.	• Transplant contraindicated. • Repeat FCXM and CDC, if Rituximab, ATG or IVIG given within 4 weeks. • Repeat DSA if serum for DSA was done on the historical sample, or if there was an interval sensitizing event.
−	−	−	+	+/−	• IgM antibody.	• Repeat CDC with DTT or pronase treatment.
−	+	+/−	−	+/−	• Moderate risk. • Non-complement fixing HLA antibody. • Low-level IgG non-HLA antibody. • False negative DSA test.	• Repeat DSA. • If still negative, test for non-HLA IgG (autocrossmatch).

Recommended Reading

1. Vo AA, Lukovsky M, Toyoda M, Wang J, Reinsmoen NL, Lai CH, Peng A, Villicana R, Jordan SC. (2008) Rituximab and intravenous immune globulin for desensitization during renal transplantation. *N Engl J Med* **359**:242–251.
2. Jordan SC, Pescovitz MD. (2006) Presensitization: The problem and its management. *Clin J Am Soc Nephrol* **1**:421–432.
3. Jordan SC, Reinsmoen N, Peng A, Lai CH, Cao K, Villicana R, Toyoda M, Kahwaji J, Vo AA. (2010) Advances in diagnosing and managing antibody-mediated rejection. *Pediatr Nephrol* **25**:2035–2045.
4. Vo AA, Sinha A, Haas M, Choi J, Mirocha J, Kahwaji J, Peng A, Villicana R, Jordan SC. (2015) Factors predicting risk for antibody-mediated rejection and graft loss in highly human leukocyte antigen sensitized patients transplanted after desensitization. *Transplantation* **99**: 1423–1430.

5. Sethi S, Choi J, Toyoda M, Vo A, Peng A, Jordan SC. (2017) Desensitization: Overcoming the immunologic barriers to transplantation. *J Immunol Res* **2017**:6804678. doi:10.1155/2017/6804678.
6. Kim IK, Choi J, Vo A, Kang A, Steggerda J, Louie S, Haas M, Mirocha J, Cohen JL, Pizzo H, Kamil ES, Jordan SC, Puliyanda D. (2017) Risk factors for the development of antibody-mediated rejection in highly sensitized pediatric kidney transplant recipients. *Pediatr Transplant* **21**(8): doi:10.1111/petr.13042.
7. Yeung M. (2020, updated) Kidney transplantation in adults: Overview of HLA sensitization and crossmatch testing. Edited by: Brennan DC, Lam AQ. *UpToDate ONLINE*. http://www.uptodateonline.com.

4 Peri-operative Management of Pediatric Renal Transplantion Recipient

Koh LJ, Teo S and Yap KH

A. Pre-operative Management

1. Pre-operative laboratory investigations:
   a. Full blood count (FBC).
   b. Prothrombin time (PT) and partial thromboplastin time (PTT).
   c. Sodium, potassium, chloride, bicarbonate, urea, creatinine, calcium, phosphate, and uric acid.
   d. Intact parathyroid hormone levels (iPTH).
   e. Ionized calcium, magnesium.
   f. Liver function test.
   g. Infection screen (should be done 0–4 weeks prior to transplant).
      i. Treponemal test for syphilis.
      ii. Human immunodeficiency virus serology (HIV Ag/Ab combo test).
      iii. Hepatitis Bs antigen.
      iv. Hepatitis B virus serology (anti-HBs, anti-HBc total).
      v. Hepatitis C virus serology.
      vi. Nucleic acid testing:
         - HIV.
         - Hepatitis B.
         - Hepatitis C.
      vii. SARS-CoV-2 DNA quantification 1 week (Day –7) and 2 days (Day –2) prior to transplant.
   h. Chest X-Ray

i. Electrocardiogram (ECG).
j. 2-D echocardiogram (in the last 3 months).
k. Urine protein:creatinine ratio (if non-oliguric).
l. Urine microscopy.
m. Urine culture and sensitivity.
n. Group and match 4 units of leukocyte-filtered packed red blood cells (RBCs).
o. Nasal swab.
p. Exit site swab.
q. Blood for cytomegalovirus (CMV) PCR and Epstein–Barr virus (EBV) PCR (EBV-negative recipient).

2. Transfuse with leukocyte-filtered packed-RBC if hemoglobin (Hb) <6 g/dL.
   Do not over-transfuse Hb >10 gm/dL.
3. Dialysis orders:
   a. Peritoneal dialysis (PD)
      - Individual normal PD regime to drain completely prior to surgery.
      - Do not ultrafiltrate excessively.
      - Send PD fluid for cell count and culture.
   b. Hemodialysis (HD)
      - Regular HD 1 day prior to transplant.
      - Do not ultrafiltrate excessively.
4. Repeat sodium, potassium, chloride, bicarbonate, urea, creatinine, phosphate, calcium, and uric acid post-dialysis.
5. Vital signs monitoring: 4-hourly temperature, pulse rate, respiratory rate, and blood pressure.
6. Strict input/output chart. Aim to keep the patient slightly overhydrated.
7. Refer to anesthetist.
8. Inform transplant surgeons for consent on admission.

B. Intraoperative Management:

1. Set central venous pressure (CVP) line, especially for patients <30 kg body weight.
   - Keep CVP 15–20 cm H_2O before release of vascular clamps.
   - Keep CVP 10–15 cm H_2O after surgery.

2. Set intra-arterial line.
3. At the time of vascular anastomosis:
   a. IV furosemide 1–2 mg/kg.
   b. IV 20% mannitol:
      - 0.5 g/kg (live-donor transplant).
      - 1.0 g/kg (deceased donor transplant).
4. Use 5% Dextrose + 0.45% saline or 0.9% saline drip without adding potassium.
5. If adult donor kidney is used, **infuse** leukocyte-filtered whole-blood (especially if Hb <10 g/dL), or 5% albumin before release of vascular clamp, in a volume estimated to perfuse the kidney:
   - 70-kg donor: 300 ml.
   - 50-kg donor: 150–200 ml.

   Watch for signs of inadequate intravascular volume, e.g., tachycardia, hypotension.
6. Consider a **dopamine infusion 3–5 μg/kg/min** (maximum dose 10 μg/kg/min) if the systolic blood pressure (BP) cannot be maintained >100 mm Hg despite adequate volume infusion (CVP >15–20 cm H_2O).
   - Avoid phenylephrine and ephedrine.
7. **Call for urgent Doppler kidney ultrasound** if:
   a. No urine output is established following vascular anastomosis in a live-donor transplant.
   b. Urine flow decreases significantly or ceases after closure of the abdominal incision.

C. Post-operative Management:

1. **Fluid and electrolyte orders:**
   a. Insensible loss: 5% Dextrose 500 ml/m²/day.
   b. Urine output replacement: Replace ml for ml urine output with 0.45% saline.
   c. Naso-gastric drainage replacement. Replace ml for ml with 0.45% saline + 10 mmol 7.45% potassium chloride per 500 ml.

   Note: Keep CVP 10–15 cm H_2O.

   Do not use Dextrose in replacement of (b) or (c), as this will cause hyperglycaemia, glycosuria and osmotic diuresis.

d. Aim for a urine output of between 100–200 ml/hour: Replace urine output ½-hourly to hourly with 0.45% saline ml for ml for the first 3–5 days, especially in young patients <30 kg body weight and those with a thrombotic risk.
e. Subsequently, decrease urine output replacement by replacing ml for ml for first 200 ml, then 50–75% replacement with 0.45% saline in excess of 200 ml.
f. If urine output remains good, reduce urine replacement to 50–75% of the hourly output, maintaining flow at 50–100 ml/hour or >2 ml/kg/hour.
g. Subsequently, switch to maintenance requirements (estimated based on the daily urine output).
    - Should target at least 2.5 L/m²/day.

2. **Urinary catheter:**
    a. Foley catheter to free drainage for 3–5 days.
    b. If urine contains copious clots and urine flow stops abruptly:
        - Irrigate catheter gently with 20 ml 0.9% saline.
        - Inform the transplant surgeon.
3. **Monitoring:**
    a. Hourly temperature, pulse rate, blood pressure, oxygen saturation (SaO_2).
    b. Hourly input/output chart.
    c. Daily weight.
4. **Blood pressure control:**
    a. Keep systolic BP >100 mm Hg even in small children in the first 24 hours after surgery.
        - If the systolic BP remains low despite adequate volume replacement, consider dopamine infusion 3–5 μg/kg/min (maximum dose 10 μg/kg/min).
    b. If hypertensive, consider use of glyceryl trinitrate (GTN) infusion or labetalol infusion.
        - Add amlodipine if hypertension is sustained post-transplant.
        - Avoid use of angiotensin-converting enzyme (ACE) inhibitors in the immediate post-transplant period when the serum creatinine is high.
5. **Laboratory investigations:**
    a. Sodium, potassium, chloride, bicarbonate, urea, creatinine, calcium, phosphate, uric acid, ionized calcium 6-hourly till stable kidney function.

b. Daily FBC, sodium, potassium, chloride, bicarbonate, urea, creatinine, calcium, phosphate, uric acid, and magnesium.
c. Urine microscopy, urine culture three times per week for the first week, followed by twice per week until ureteric stent is removed.
d. Daily trough tacrolimus or 2-hour cyclosporine levels.
e. Urine protein:creatinine ratio daily for the first week, then three times a week for the first month in patients at risk of recurrent focal segmental glomerulosclerosis.
f. Liver function and Gamma-glutamyltransferase (GGT) twice per week for the first week, then weekly.
g. Drug pharmacokinetics (area under the curve) pre-discharge:
   - Mycophenolate.
   - Tacrolimus or cyclosporine.

6. **Baseline imaging:**
   a. Baseline kidney ultrasound and Doppler scan on Day 1 or immediate post-operation if there is poor urine output.
   b. Baseline isotope renal allograft scan (MAG3 scan) and if there are clinical problems or abnormal findings on Doppler kidney ultrasound.
7. **Antibiotics:**
   a. IV cephazolin (convert to oral cefaclor/cefuroxime) at therapeutic dose, until removal of the urinary catheter.
   b. Oral cefaclor/cefuroxime at prophylactic dose until removal of the ureteric stent.
8. **Prophylactic heparinization:**
   a. Consider in patients with a thrombotic risk:
      - Persistent nephrotic state.
      - Anti-phospholipid syndrome.
      - Previous recurrent thrombosis.
      - Abnormal thrombophilic screen: protein-C, protein-S, antithrombin III, Factor V (Leiden factor).
      - Technical, e.g., small donor renal artery, atherosclerotic plaques.
   b. Start on intravenous heparin infusion:
      i. Loading dose: 50 U/kg (maximum dose 1000 U).
      ii. Maintenance dose: 10–50 U/kg/hour (maximum dose 500 U/hour).

iii. Monitor aPTT 6 hourly. Keep aPTT between 30 and 40 seconds. After dose change, repeat aPTT in an hour. Keep aPTT between 30 and 40 seconds.
- If aPTT >45 seconds, withhold heparin for one hour, then restart at 10% less per hour and re-check in an hour.
- If aPTT <30 seconds, bolus with 10 Units/kg, and increase the infusion by 10%.

iv. Monitor platelet count daily, especially if the patient is on anti-thymocyte globulin.

v. Continue for at least 2 weeks post-transplant. Consider changing to subcutaneous enoxaparin (1 mg = 100 U) (0.5 mg/kg daily) in patients requiring longer-term heparinization (high risk of thrombosis).

vi. Consider changing to aspirin 3–5 mg/kg (maximum 100 mg) daily or dipyridamole 1–2 mg/kg 8-hourly in patients with no evidence of thrombosis.

D. Possible Management Problems:

1. Abrupt cessation of urine flow after good urine output established:

Consider:

a. Blockage of Foley catheter
- Gently irrigate the Foley catheter with 20–30 ml sterile 0.9% saline and note return.
- Apply minimal pressure on irrigation as bladder has suture line.
- Foley catheter may need to be changed if continually blocked with clots. Inform the pediatric surgeon before catheter change.

b. Hypovolaemia
- Look for signs of third spacing.
- Check pulse, postural BP, CVP.
- Treat with 10–20 ml/kg 0.9% saline or 5% albumin.

c. Allograft rejection
- Consider accelerated acute rejection.
- MAG3 scan is useful to distinguish rejection from urinary extravasation.

d. Urinary extravasation
   - Check drainage from abdominal drain for urea and creatinine and compare with levels in bladder urine.
   - Consider MAG3 to detect urinary leak.

e. Acute tubular necrosis (ATN)
   - Consider if no urine output from outset.
   - MAG3 scan to look for cortical retention without bladder accumulation. Radioisotope accumulation is uniform in ATN and patchy in allograft rejection.

f. Acute bleeding from anastomosis or arterial embolization post-transplantation.
   - Perform Doppler ultrasound and MAG3 scan, followed by angiogram if necessary.

2. Rejection:

a. Usually appears at Day 7 post-operatively.

b. Signs/symptoms:
   i. Fever.
   ii. Malaise.
   iii. Hypertension.
   iv. Allograft tenderness and swelling.
   v. Oliguria.
   vi. Weight gain.

   Note: Signs may be masked, especially fever and allograft tenderness in a patient on cyclosporine or tacrolimus.

c. Perform kidney ultrasound to look for:
   i. Allograft swelling.
   ii. Perinephric and peri-pyramidal edema resulting in increased pyramidal prominence (squaring).
   iii. Decreased pyramidal prominence in the later stage.

3. Post-operative fever:

a. Exclude bacterial infection and CMV infection.

b. If temperature >38°C, perform:
   i. FBC.
   ii. C-reactive protein (CRP).
   iii. Urine microscopy and urine culture.
   iv. Blood culture.
   v. PD fluid cell count and culture if signs suggestive of peritonitis.
   vi. Blood for CMV IgM, IgG titers, and CMV PCR.

vii. Blood for EBV serology (VCA IgG and IgM) and EBV PCR.
viii. Respiratory multiplex PCR and COVID-19 PCR if respiratory symptoms present.
ix. Chest X-Ray.
x. Arterial blood gas if tachypnea present.

c. Consider allograft rejection.

4. Allograft dysfunction (rising serum creatinine):

a. Consider:
i. Pre-renal causes, e.g., hypovolemia.
ii. Urinary tract obstruction.
iii. Urinary extravasation.
iv. Acute tubular necrosis.
v. Arterial anastomotic leak or thrombosis.
vi. Acute allograft rejection.
vii. Cyclosporine or tacrolimus nephrotoxicity.
viii. Acute pyelonephritis.
ix. Lymphocele.
x. CMV infection.

b. Perform kidney ultrasound and power Doppler to look for
i. Resistive index (RI) and arterial and venous flow patterns.
ii. Pelvicalyceal and ureteric dilatation.
iii. Fluid collections.
iv. Evidence of acute rejection.

c. Check tacrolimus trough or 2-hour cyclosporine levels.

d. If indicated, perform:
i. MAG3 scan or MRU.
ii. Kidney biopsy.

5. Hypophosphatemia

a. Due to high iPTH acting on normal renal tubules.

b. Phosphate replacement: 2 mmol/kg/day given 4–8 hourly.
Phosphate solution: Na_2HPO_4
Na : 5.75 mmol/5 ml
PO_4 : 3.51 mmol/5 ml
Watch for diarrhea.

c. Calcitriol 10–40 ng/kg/day or 1-alpha calcidol 0.05 μg/kg/day up to a maximum of 1 μg/day.

6. **Hypomagnesemia**
   a. Tubulopathy associated with calcineurin inhibitors, especially with tacrolimus.
   b. Associated renal tubular acidosis and hypophosphatemia.
   c. Treatment:
      i. Intravenous magnesium (Mg) replacement:
         - 50% Mg sulphate 0.2 ml/kg/dose (= 0.4 mmol/kg/dose = 10 mg/kg/dose) over 2 hours given BD (maximum dose 10 ml).
         - Watch for signs of hypermagnesemia: Facial flushing, loss of deep tendon reflexes, hypotension, atrioventricular block.
      ii. Maintain on oral GNC® Mg: (250 mg = 10.3 mmol Mg):
         - Watch for diarrhea.
      iii. Consider amiloride in patients with refractory hypomagnesemia.

E. Management of Tenckhoff Catheter:

1. Pre-transplant cap off transfer tubing after draining fluid (heparinized PD fluid left in transfer tubing).
2. Flush Tenchkoff catheter weekly using 10 ml/kg up to 500 ml dialysate.
   Note: Add heparin 250–500 U/L into bag if fibrin is present
3. If cultures are required, use 500-ml bag to do a flush, followed by dwell of 20 minutes, and drain. Obtain culture and cell count from drain bag.
4. Consider removal of Tenckhoff catheter at time of ureteric stent removal if allograft function is excellent.

Recommended Reading

1. Salvatierra O Jr, Millan M, Concepcion W. (2006) Pediatric renal transplantation with considerations for successful outcomes. *Semin Pediatr Surg* **15**:208–217.
2. MOH. (2018) Manual on organ donation and transplantation. Ministry of Health.

5 Sequential Immunosuppression Protocol for Kidney Transplantation

Yap HK, Lau PYW, Teo ST, Ng KH, Chhabra M and Koh LJ

A. General Principles

1. Goal of immunosuppression in kidney transplantation:
   a. Prevent acute rejection.
   b. Minimize drug side effects.
2. Immunosuppression should be highest during the first 3 months post-transplantation as the risk of acute rejection is greatest, followed by gradual tapering to a maintenance level by 6–12 months.

B. Immunosuppressive Agents

1. Types of immunosuppressive drugs:
   a. Antibody induction agents:
      - Interleukin (IL)-2 receptor antibody: Basiliximab (Simulect®).
      - Anti-thymocyte globulin (ATG).
   b. Glucocorticoids:
      - Prednisolone (PNL).
      - Methylprednisolone (MP).
   c. Calcineurin inhibitor (CNI):
      - Cyclosporine (CsA).
      - Tacrolimus (Tac).
   d. Purine synthesis inhibitor:
      - Azathioprine (AZA).
      - Mycophenolate mofetil (MMF).

   e. Mammalian (mechanistic) target of rapamycin inhibitors (mTORi):
      - Sirolimus (SRL).
      - Everolimus (EVL).
2. Choice of immunosuppressive drugs depends on:
   a. Immunological risk:
      - Degree of sensitization (donor-specific antibody titers).
      - Degree of human leukocyte antigen (HLA) mismatch.
      - Previous acute rejection episodes.
      - ABO incompatibility.
      - Previous kidney transplantation.
   b. Risk of recurrent disease.
3. Choice of induction protocol:
   a. Basiliximab is preferred in low immunological risk patients (unsensitized).
   b. ATG can be considered for high immunological risk patients.

C. Pre-operative Immunosuppression

I. 3 Days before transplant (Day –3):

- MMF 600 mg/m^2/dose BD.

II. Day before transplant (Day –1):

1. PNL 2 mg/kg OM.
2. Continue MMF.
3. CsA PO 5 mg/kg between 6 and 12 hours before transplant (maximum 800 mg) OR Tac PO 0.1 mg/kg between 6 and 12 hours before transplant (maximum 10 mg).

D. Peri-operative Immunosuppression

I. Antibody induction:

1. Basiliximab (SIMULECT®):
   a. Dose: 12 mg/m^2/dose.
      - Body weight <30 kg = 10 mg.
      - Body weight ≥30 kg = 20 mg.

b. Duration: Days 0 and 4.
c. Infuse over 30 minutes.
d. Consider switching to ATG protocol if there is slow graft function in the immediate post-operative period.
   - Defined by urine output ≤0.5 ml/kg/hour.
   - To be initiated by 12 hours post-transplant.

2. ATG (see chapter "Anti-thymocyte Globulin for Kidney Transplantation" for the infusion protocol):
   a. Dose for Rabbit ATG (Thymoglobulin®):
      - IV 1 mg/kg/day for 3 days (total 3 mg/kg).
   b. Titrate dose (increase or decrease dose by 20%) to a maximum dose of 1.5 mg/kg/dose:
      - Aim for absolute lymphocyte count 0.1–0.2 × 10^9/L or CD3 levels <1%.
      - Hold ATG if platelet count <50 × 10^9/L.
   c. Treat for a maximum of 5 days.

II. Immunosuppressive protocol on day of transplant (Day 0):

1. Pre-operative:
   a. IV MMF 600 mg/m^2 12 hours starting 2 hours before going to operating theater (OT) OR
      IV AZA 2 mg/kg at induction of anesthesia.
   b. Basiliximab on call to OT.
2. Intra-operative:
   a. IV MP 10 mg/kg (maximum 500 mg) at induction of anesthesia.
   b. IV cephazolin:
      BW <10 kg: 250 mg.
      BW 10–30 kg: 500 mg.
      BW >30 kg: 1000 mg.

E. Post-operative Immunosuppression

I. Immunosuppressive regimen post-transplant:

1. Continue MMF starting 12 hours after the pre-transplant dose.
2. Continue IV MP daily in accordance with the tapering schedule.

3. Start CNI 8–12 hours after anastomosis provided urine output >0.5 ml/kg/hour:
   - Sublingual Tac 0.07 mg/kg/dose BD OR
   - Oral CsA 4 mg/kg/dose BD.
4. Basiliximab on day 4.

II. Glucocorticoids:

1. While on ATG:

Period	GC Dose
Day 1	IV MP 10 mg/kg 1 hour before ATG dose to a maximum of 250 mg
Day 2	IV MP 1 mg/kg or a minimum of 20 mg
Day 3	IV MP 0.5 mg/kg or a minimum of 20 mg
Day 4	Oral PNL 0.5 mg/kg or a minimum of 20 mg

2. PNL + MMF/AZA + CNI protocol:

Period	GC Dose	
Day 1	IV MP 2 mg/kg.	
Day 2	IV MP 2 mg/kg or oral PNL 2 mg/kg/day (maximum 80 mg/day given as BD dose).	
Days 3–5	IV MP 1.75 mg/kg or PNL 1.75 mg/kg/day (maximum 70 mg/day given as BD dose).	
Days 5–6	PNL 1.2 mg/kg/day (maximum 70 mg given as BD dose).	
Day 7	PNL 1 mg/kg/day (maximum 60 mg OM).	
Week 1–4	BW ≤30 kg BW >30 kg	Decrease PNL by 2.5 mg weekly to a dose of 0.3 mg/kg/day or 5 mg OM minimum. Decrease PNL by 2.5–5 mg weekly to a dose of 0.3 mg/kg/day.
Week 5–8	BW ≤30 kg BW >30 kg	Decrease PNL by 1 mg weekly till dose is 0.25 mg/kg/day or 3 mg OM minimum. Decrease PNL by 2.5–5 mg weekly till dose is a minimum of 5 mg OM.

(Continued)

(*Continued*)

Period	GC Dose	
Week 9–12	BW ≤30 kg	Decrease PNL by 1 mg weekly till dose is 0.2 mg/kg/day.
	BW >30 kg	Continue PNL 5 mg OM.
6 months to >1 year	Prepubertal	Change to alternate day regimen at 0.2 mg/kg/EOD **if there is no rejection after 6 months for those on Tac and after 1 year for those on CsA**, increasing/decreasing alternate day dose by 2.5 mg until total dose is given EOD.
	Postpubertal	Keep PNL dose at 5 mg OM. Consider alternate day 0.2 mg/kg/EOD or 10 mg EOD maximum if kidney function is stable after 2 years.

III. Azathioprine (AZA):

1. While on ATG:
   a. Start AZA at 1 mg/kg if total white count normal.
   b. After stopping ATG, increase dose to 2 mg/kg (maximum dose 120 mg OM).
2. PNL + AZA + CNI protocol:
   a. Consider genotyping thiopurine S-methyltransferase (TPMT) and nucleoside diphosphate linked moiety X-type motif 15 (NUDT15) first before starting AZA.
   b. Start AZA at 2 mg/kg if total white count is normal.
   c. Dose titration:
      - Hold dose if absolute neutrophil count <2.0 × 10^9/L or total white count <3.0 × 10^9/L.
      - Reduce dose by 50% if total white count <4.0 × 10^9/L.
   d. Long-term maintenance dose: 1.5–2 mg/kg/day.
      - Lower dose of 1.5 mg/kg/day if creatinine >200 μmol/L.
   e. Do not use allopurinol in combination with AZA.
   f. Monitor:
      - Full blood count (FBC) weekly during the first month, 2x/month between the second and third month and monthly thereafter.
      - Liver function test monthly for the first year, then 3-monthly.

IV. Mycophenolate mofetil (MMF):

1. Dosing (dependent on immunosuppression protocol):
   a. While on ATG:
      - Dose: 15 mg/kg 12 hourly or 300 mg/m^2 12 hourly while on ATG.
      - Increase dose after stopping ATG.

   b. PNL/MMF/CsA:
      - Dose: 600 mg/m^2/dose 12 hourly (15–23 mg/kg/dose 12 hourly).
      - Maximum dose: 1 g 12 hourly.

   c. PNL/MPA/Tac:
      - Dose: 300 mg/m^2/dose 12 hourly (8–12 mg/kg/dose 12 hourly).
      - Maximum dose: 500 mg 12 hourly.
2. Dose adjustment:
   a. Required for abnormal kidney function.
   b. Drug is not removed by hemodialysis.
   c. Omit if absolute neutrophil count $<1.5 \times 10^9$/L.
   d. Take drug on an empty stomach (1 hour before food or 2 hours after food).
3. Common side effects: (see chapter "Immunosuppressive Medications")
   a. Neutropenia (especially at 1–6 months), anemia, thrombocytopenia (rare).
   b. Gastritis, peptic ulceration, abdominal colic, diarrhea, gastrointestinal hemorrhage, and perforation.
      - Start famotidine prophylactically at 0.5–1 mg/kg/day once nightly or a divided dose 12 hourly (maximum 40 mg) OR
      - Rabeprazole 0.5–1.0 mg/kg once nightly or divided dose 12-hourly (maximum 40 mg).
      - Consider changing to Myfortic® if gastrointestinal side effects persist.
4. Monitor:
   a. FBC weekly during the first month, 2x/month between the second and third month and monthly thereafter.
   b. Serum amylase levels 6-monthly, and serum lipase levels when serum amylase levels are elevated.
   c. Serum mycophenolate levels when side effects present. Trough levels range from 2 to 4 mg/L.

d. Mycophenolic Acid (MPA) pharmacokinetics study:
- See chapter "Immunosuppressive Medications" for formula.
- To be done before discharge post-transplant.

5. Drug interactions:
   a. Aciclovir and ganciclovir increase MPA levels.
   b. Antacids decrease MPA levels.
   c. Do not administer drugs simultaneously.
6. Formulation switch:
   - MMF (CellCept®) to enteric-coated mycophenolate sodium (Myfortic®):
     250 mg (CellCept®) ≡ 180 mg (Myfortic®).
     500 mg (CellCept®) ≡ 360 mg (Myfortic®).

V. *Tacrolimus (Tac):*

1. Dosing:
   a. While on ATG:
      i. Start Tac 2 days prior to end of ATG therapy.
      ii. Rapid escalation of Tac dose to achieve desired levels by the end of ATG protocol.
   b. Basiliximab induction protocol:
      i. Oral Tac 0.07 mg/kg/dose BD to start 12 hours after anastomosis-provided urine output >0.5 ml/kg/hour.
      ii. If nil by mouth, give sublingual Tac (open capsule and place powder under the tongue).
      iii. Do not administer oral Tac within 2 hours before or after antacids, cholestyramine or colestipol.
   c. IV Tac:
      i. If unable to attain target Tac levels, give IV Tac 0.075–0.1 mg/kg/day as a continuous infusion at a concentration of 0.004–0.002 mg/ml in 5% dextrose or normal saline to attain desired levels (steady state 15–25 µg/L).

ii. Use polyolefin or glass sets (PVC and polyurethane contra-indicated).
iii. On converting IV to oral Tac, start recommended oral dose and reduce IV infusion by 50%.
   - **PO intake = 3–4 × IV dose.**
   - Check trough Tac levels at 12 hours.
   - Wean off IV infusion once trough level is within target range.

2. Drug monitoring:
   a. Maintain Tac levels at:

Period Post-transplant	Tac Trough Level (μg/L)
First 2 weeks	10–12
2 weeks to 3 months	8–10
4–6 months	7–9
>6 months	5–7 (minimum 4)

   b. If desired Tac levels cannot be achieved, consider adding diltiazem or fluconazole.
   c. If creatinine increases by 25% and Tac nephrotoxicity is suspected, reduce Tac dose by 20% to determine if this is the cause.
   d. Tac pharmacokinetics study:
      i. See chapter "Immunosuppressive Medications" for AUC formula.
      ii. Do Tac pharmacokinetics study before discharge.
      iii. Maintain AUC at:

Period Post-transplant	AUC (μg-h/L)
0–1 months	175–250
1–3 months	100–175
>3 months	75–100

e. Adjusted whole blood Tac levels based on hematocrit (Hct):

	Adjusted Hct 0.35		**Measured Hct**				
			0.2	0.25	0.3	0.4	0.45
Adjusted Tac Levels	2	**Measured Tac level**	1.2	1.4	1.7	2.3	2.6
	3		1.7	2.2	2.6	3.4	3.8
	4		2.3	2.9	3.4	4.6	5.1
	5		2.9	3.6	4.3	5.7	6.4
	6		3.5	4.3	5.2	6.8	7.7
	7		4.1	5.1	6.0	8.0	8.9
	8		4.7	5.8	6.9	9.1	10.2
	9		5.2	6.5	7.7	10.3	11.5
	10		5.8	7.2	8.6	11.4	12.8
	11		6.4	7.9	9.5	12.5	14.1
	12		7.0	8.7	10.3	13.7	15.3
	13		7.6	9.4	11.2	14.8	16.6
	14		8.2	10.1	12.1	15.9	17.9
	15		8.8	10.8	12.9	17.1	19.2

Reference: https://www.kidney.wiki/quick-references/tacro-calculator

i. Measured Tac level at the measured Hct has the same plasma concentration as the adjusted Tac level at the adjusted Hct.
ii. Tac is generally measured as total concentrations in whole blood, whereas only the unbound concentration in plasma is pharmacologically active.
iii. Low Hct results in lower whole blood exposure and can be incorrectly interpreted as increased apparent clearance of Tac from whole blood, while the plasma concentrations and clearance remain unchanged.

3. Tac interactions (see chapter "Immunosuppressive Medications"):
   - High doses of glucocorticoids used in early post-transplant period (first month) affect Tac levels due to upregulation of the cytochrome P450 3A and intestinal P-glycoprotein systems.

4. Side effects (see chapter "Immunosuppressive Medications"):
   a. Majority of the side effects are early within initiation of therapy, with the incidence decreasing over time, often responding to a reduction in dosage.
   b. Neurological side effects may respond to a reduction in dosage with a delay between blood levels and symptoms.
   c. Monitor for electrolyte and acid-base abnormalities as these may require supplementation or treatment:
      i. Hypomagnesemia: Replace with GNC magnesium.
      ii. Renal tubular acidosis type 4: Replace with sodium bicarbonate.
      iii. Hyperkalemia: Aggravated by concurrent use of renin-angiotensin system blockers (RASBs), trimethoprim and co-trimoxazole.
   d. Glucose intolerance and new-onset diabetes after transplantation (NODAT):
      i. Occurs more frequently in the first month post-transplant.
      ii. Monitor the following weekly for the first 3 months, then 3-monthly for 1 year:
         - Fasting or 2-hour post-prandial blood glucose.
         - Glycated hemoglobin (HbA1c).
      iii. May require hypoglycemic agents or insulin.
   e. Increased risk of infections, especially in seronegative recipients:
      - Cytomegalovirus (CMV).
      - Epstein–Barr virus (EBV): EBV-associated lymphoproliferative disorders occur in up to 6.2%, especially in primary EBV infection from donor kidney with seroconversion 5–36 weeks after transplantation.
      - BK virus nephropathy.
5. Tacrolimus conversion protocols:
   a. CsA to Tac conversion:
      i. Reduce CsA dose by 50% and start Tac at full dose (0.1–0.15 mg/kg Q12 hourly).
      ii. Monitor Tac levels and discontinue CsA once desired Tac levels are achieved.
   b. Conversion to prolonged-release formulations:

i. Advagraf (Tacrolimus prolonged-release formulation) dosing:
   - 0.2–0.3 mg/kg/day as single daily dose to achieve target trough levels.

ii. Conversion dose from oral Tac (immediate-release capsules) 6 months post-transplant:
   - If Tac level ≥6 μg/L, convert 1:1 as total daily dose.
   - If Tac level <6 μg/L, convert 1:1.1 as total daily dose.

iii. Monitoring:
   - Check trough Tac levels post-conversion Days 3, 7 and 14.
   - Takes about 1 week to achieve pre-conversion Tac levels, so avoid adjusting dose before 1 week unless the level is lower than the target or desired Tac level.

iv. If Tac level is very high or in the toxic range:
   - Stop the daily dose for 1–2 days and monitor trough levels daily, until levels have returned to an acceptable range.
   - Re-introduce Advagraf at an appropriately reduced dose (about two-thirds of previous dose).

v. If the patient has missed a dose:
   - Dose may be taken up to 14 hours after the scheduled time without the risk of overexposure (i.e., for a missed 8 am dose, take by 10 pm).
   - Beyond the 14-hour time frame, wait until the usual scheduled time the following morning to take the next regular daily dose.

vi. If the patient is on diltiazem, this should be converted to once-daily dosing at 1–3 mg/kg (maximum 360 mg) to be taken together with the Advagraf.

VI. Cyclosporine (CsA):

1. Dosing:
   a. While on ATG:
      i. Start CsA 2 days prior to end of ATG therapy.
      ii. Continue ATG until desired levels of CsA are achieved.

b. Basiliximab induction protocol:
   i. Oral CsA 8 mg/kg/day 8–12 hourly to start 12 hours after anastomosis-provided urine output >0.5 ml/kg/hour.
   ii. If nil by mouth, give IV CsA continuous infusion 2–3 mg/kg/day, increasing to 3–4 mg/kg/day to attain desired levels (steady state 150–175 μg/L).
   iii. Maintain parent CsA levels at:

Period Post-transplant	Trough Level (μg/L)	C2 Levels (μg/L)
0–1 months	225–250	1500–2000
2 months	200–225	1500
3 months	200–225	1300
4–6 months	200–225	1100
7–12 months	150–200	900
>1 year	125–150	800

2. CsA drug monitoring:
   a. CsA pharmacokinetics study to determine average concentration (C_{AV}):
      i. See chapter "Immunosuppressive Medications" for formula.
      ii. CsA pharmacokinetics study to be done prior to discharge post-transplant.
   b. Maintain C_{AV} at:
      i. PNL + AZA + CsA protocol:

Period Post-transplant	C_{AV} Level (μg/L)
0–1 months	476–500
1–6 months	451–475
6–12 months	426–450
> 1 year	400–425

ii. PNL + MMF + CsA:

Period Post-transplant	C_{AV} Level (μg/L)
0–1 months	450–475
1–6 months	425–450
6–12 months	400–425
> 1 year	375–400

3. Dose conversion:
   a. On converting IV to oral CsA, start the recommended oral dose and reduce IV infusion by 50%.
   b. Check trough CsA at 8 or 12 hours (depending on the 12-hourly or 8-hourly dosing interval).
   c. Wean off IV infusion once trough level is within target range.
   d. IV dose (mg/kg/day) = 0.4 × "Full Oral Dose".
4. Dose adjustment:
   a. Use diltiazem 15–30 mg 8–12 hourly to modulate CsA levels (diltiazem increases CsA levels), increasing by 15 mg/dose until a maximum of 60 mg 8–12 hourly.
      - If levels are still low, consider changing diltiazem to fluconazole 3 mg/kg/day single dose (maximum 100 mg daily).
   b. After 1 month, reduce CsA dose by 1 mg/kg/week till 6 mg/kg/day, maintaining desired trough levels.
   c. After 6 months, reduce CsA dose by 1 mg/kg/month till 4–5 mg/kg/day, maintaining desired trough levels.
   d. After 1 year, consider 12-hourly dosing of CsA for those who are on TDS dosing interval.
   e. To perform CsA pharmacokinetics study before and after adjustment.
   f. If creatinine increases by 25% and CsA nephrotoxicity is suspected, reduce CsA dose by 20% to determine if this is the cause.
5. Oral solution may be mixed with milk, chocolate milk, orange juice, or apple juice.
6. CsA interactions and side effects — see chapter "Immunosuppressive Medications".

VII. Sirolimus (SRL):

1. Start only after 1-month post-transplant as there is an increased risk of:
   a. Kidney arterial and venous thrombosis resulting in graft loss (black box warning).
   b. Poor wound healing.
   c. Do not use in combination with CsA as there is an increased risk of thrombotic microangiopathy.
2. Dosing:
   a. Children:
      i. Loading dose on Day 1: 3–5 mg/m^2/day divided every 12 hours.
      ii. Initial maintenance dose: 3 mg/m^2/day divided every 12 hours to achieve target levels.
      iii. Maintenance dose: 3 mg/m^2/day divided every 12 hours.
      iv. SRL dosages should be adjusted to maintain trough concentrations within desired range with a maximum daily dose of 40 mg/day.
      v. SRL serum concentrations should be checked earlier than 7 days after starting SRL due to pharmacokinetic differences.
      vi. New SRL dose = (current dose) x (target concentration/current concentration).
      vii. If large dose increase is required, consider loading dose calculated as: (new maintenance dose – current maintenance dose) × 3.
      viii. If required dose is >40 mg/day (due to loading dose), divide over 2 days.
   b. Adolescents <40 kg:
      i. Loading dose on Day 1: 3 mg/m^2/day divided every 12 hours.
      ii. Maintenance dose: 1 mg/m^2/day divided every 12 hours or daily to achieve target levels.
   c. Adolescents ≥40 kg:
      i. Loading dose on Day 1: 6 mg daily.
      ii. Maintenance dose: 2 mg daily to achieve target levels.
      iii. Dosage should be adjusted at intervals of 7–14 days to account for the long half-life of SRL.

3. Drug levels:
   a. PNL + MPA + SRL:
      - Keep SRL levels at 5 µg/L (maximum 6–7 µg/L).
   b. PNL + SRL + Tac:
      - Early post-transplant period: Keep SRL+Tac levels at 10 µg/L.
      - Late post-transplant period >1 year: Keep SRL+Tac levels between 7 and 8 µg/L.

   Note: SRL can increase Tac clearance in children leading to lower trough levels. Tac only slightly decreases SRL clearance.
4. Steroid-tapering protocol similar to PNL + MMF + Tac.
5. Can be taken with water or orange juice.
   - Should not be mixed with grapefruit juice.
6. Side effects (see chapter "Immunosuppressive Medications"):
   a. Poor wound healing:
      i. SRL should not be used absolutely in the first 2 weeks post-transplant.
      ii. Obesity is a significant risk factor.
      iii. Minimizing/avoiding corticosteroids can significantly reduce the risk of delayed wound healing.
   b. Hematologic complications:
      i. Reversible neutropenia occurs within 2 weeks of starting the drug.
      ii. Thrombocytopenia is dose-related.
      iii. Combination of MMF and SRL associated with increased incidence of anemia.
   c. Proteinuria:
      i. Proteinuria may be controlled with RASBs, together with reduction in SRL dose.
      ii. Consider stopping SRL if proteinuria >1 g/day/1.73m^2.
      iii. Do not start SRL if proteinuria >0.8 g/day/1.73m^2.
   d. Mouth ulcers, especially when using MMF and SRL combination:
      - Can be treated with clobetasol, a potent topical steroid.

VIII. Everolimus (EVL):

1. Dosing:
   a. Starting dose: 0.8 mg/m^2 BD (adult 0.75 mg BD, maximum 1.5 mg BD).

b. Start only after 1-month post-transplant as there is an increased risk of:
   - Kidney arterial and venous thrombosis resulting in graft loss (black box warning).
   - Poor wound healing.

2. Drug levels:
   a. PNL + EVL + Tac:
      i. Early post-transplant period <1 year:
         - Keep EVL + Tac levels at 10 μg/L.
         - Keep EVL levels at 4–6 μg/L (therapeutic range: 3–8 μg/L).
      ii. Late post-transplant period ≥1year:
         - Keep EVL + Tac levels between 7 and 8 μg/L.
         - Keep EVL levels at 3–5 μg/L.
      iii. Takes about 4–5 days to achieve EVL levels.
   b. PNL + EVL + CsA:
      i. Early post-transplant period <1 year.
      ii. Keep EVL levels at 4–6 μg/L (therapeutic range: 3–8 μg/L).
      iii. Late post-transplant period ≥1year.
      iv. Keep EVL levels at 3–5 μg/L.
   c. Keep CsA levels as follows:

Period Post-transplant	Trough Level (μg/L)
1–6 months	75–100
7–12 months	50–100
>12 months	50–75

   d. CsA affects EVL clearance and vice versa, therefore, CsA and EVL should be dosed at the same time so as to avoid variations in drug trough levels.
   e. It is important to monitor EVL blood concentrations, when CsA dosing is reduced and when switching CsA formulations (tablets versus suspension).
      Note: Tablet form of CsA is preferred, as it has been validated in studies.
   f. Prior to dose reduction of CsA, it should be ascertained that steady-state EVL trough concentration is at least 3 μg/L and EVL concentrations should be monitored after CsA dose reduction.

3. Steroid-tapering protocol similar to PNL + MMF + Tac protocol and PNL + MMF + CsA protocol.
4. Can be taken with water or orange juice, but not grapefruit juice.
5. Side effects (see section on SRL and chapter "Immunosuppressive Medications").

F. Immunodeficiency

1. Check serum immunoglobulin levels pre-transplant in particular:
   a. Patients with previous intractable nephrotic syndrome in which preemptive transplant is being considered.
   b. Patients who had been given anti-CD20 monoclonal antibody in the past 6 months.
2. If serum IgG is low, give IVIG 500 mg/kg.
   - Consider monthly IVIG 500 mg/kg if serum IgG continues to remain low.

G. Antimicrobial Prophylaxis

I. CMV prophylaxis:

CMV status	ATG	IVIG	IV Ganciclovir	Valganciclovir
Negative donor to negative recipient* + blood transfusion	Y/N	N		3 months
Positive donor to positive recipient	Y	N		3 months
Positive donor to positive recipient	N	N		3 months
Negative donor to positive recipient	Y	N		3 months
Negative donor to positive recipient	N	N		3 months
Positive donor to negative recipient	Y	Y	10 days	6 months (depending on lymphocyte count to prolong to 1 year)

(*Continued*)

CMV status	ATG	IVIG	IV Ganciclovir	Valganciclovir
Positive donor to negative recipient	N	Y		6 months
Negative donor to negative recipient on mTORi	Y	N		3 months

*Arrange for CMV-negative blood products if possible to avoid ganciclovir.

1. Immunosurveillance for high-risk recipients:
   a. CMV PCR for "positive donor to negative recipient" on:
      - Day 1, then
      - Weekly for Month 1, then
      - Biweekly for Month 2, then
      - Monthly for 1 year.

   b. CMV PCR for "positive donor to positive recipient" on:
      - Day 1, then
      - Monthly for 1 year.
2. Antiviral prophylaxis:
   a. IV Ganciclovir (prophylactic dose):

Creatinine Clearance ($ml/min/1.73m^2$)	Dose	Frequency
>70	5 mg/kg/dose	24-hourly
50–69	2.5 mg/kg/dos	24-hourly
25–49	1.5 mg/kg/dose	24-hourly
10–24	0.625 mg/kg/dose	24-hourly
<10	0.625 mg/kg/dose	3x/week (dose after hemodialysis)

   b. Valganciclovir (prophylactic dose):
      i. 1 capsule = 450 mg.
      ii. Dosing in children should be based on body surface area (BSA) and kidney function.

iii. Recommended dosage:

Creatinine Clearance ($ml/min/1.73m^2$)	Dose Adult (Pediatric)	Frequency
≥60	900 mg (15 mg/kg/dose)	OD
40–59	450 mg	OD
25–39	450 mg	EOD
10–24	450 mg	Twice weekly
<10	100 mg suspension	3×/week (dose after hemodialysis)

OR

Pediatric dosing equivalent to 900 mg/dose (4 months to 16 years old)

$= 900/125 \times BSA \times GFR$ ($ml/min/1.73m^2$)

$= 7 \times BSA \times GFR$ ($ml/min/1.73m^2$)

(Ettenger *et al.*, 2003)

Note: If calculated GFR exceeds 150 $ml/min/1.73m^2$, then a maximum calculated GFR of 150 $ml/min/1.73m^2$ should be used in the equation.

c. Start antiviral prophylaxis within 48–72 hours after transplantation.

d. Antiviral drug dosing should not be adjusted down due to leukopenia or pancytopenia as suboptimal dosing may be associated with increased risk of clinical failure and/or resistance.

- If there is neutropenia (absolute neutrophil count $<1.0 \times 10^9/L$), consider giving granulocyte-colony stimulating factor (GCSF) till absolute neutrophil count $\geq 1.5 \times 10^9/L$.

e. Drug interactions:

Nephrotoxic Drugs	Abnormal Kidney Function
Imipenem, cilastatin sodium	Seizures
Pentamidine, pyrimethamine, flucytosine, co-trimoxazole, amphotericin B	Hematological side effects

3. Intravenous immunoglobulin (IVIG):

a. Preparations:

IVIG Preparation	Purification	Sugar	Osmolarity* (mOsm/kg)	CMV Titer (Paul-Ehrlich U/ml)	Equivalent dose to ≥35 Paul-Ehrlich U/ml
Gammagard (5%*)	Solvent-detergent	Glucose 20 g/L	636 mOsm/L	35–45	500 mg/kg/dose
Intragam (6%)	Solvent-detergent	Maltose 10 g/dL	Isotonic (actual osmolarity unknown)	No data	650 mg/kg/dose
Flebogamma (5%)	Cold alcohol fractionation, PEG precipitation, ion exchange chromatography	D-sorbitol	240–350 mOsm/L	32–34	650 mg/kg/dose
Intratect	Octanoic acid, solvent-detergent and nanofiltration	Glycine 270–330 mmol/L	280–350 (supplied <320) mOsm/kg	25	700 mg/kg/dose
Octagam (high CMV titre)	Solvent-detergent	Maltose 10g/dL	310–380 mOsm/kg	66	500 mg/kg/dose
Megalotect CP	Octanoic acid, solvent-detergent and nanofiltration	Glycine 270–330 mmol/L	280–350 (supplied <320) mOsm/kg	100	50 mg/kg/dose

*IVIG preparations with high osmolarity are contraindicated in transplantation.

b. IVIG dose equivalent:
   - Weekly × 2 doses, then
   - Alternate weeks for 5 more doses for a total of 12 weeks (Weeks 1, 2, 4, 6, 8, 10, and 12), followed by
   - Single dose at Week 16.

c. Megalotect CP®:
   - Alternate weeks for 6 doses (Weeks 1, 3, 5, 7, 9, and 11), followed by
   - Single dose at Week 16.

d. Start within 24–72 hours post-transplantation.

e. Adjust dose for comparable CMV antibody titers of ≥35 Paul-Ehrlich Units/ml.

II. EBV prophylaxis:

Risk Factors		Recommended Prophylaxis		
EBV Status	**ATG**	**CMV HypIG†**	**IV Ganciclovir**	**Valganciclovir**
Negative donor to Negative recipient + blood transfusion (leukocyte filtered)	Y	Y (single dose)		
Positive donor to Positive recipient	Y	Y (single dose)		3 months
Negative donor to Positive recipient	Y	Y (single dose)		3 months
Positive donor to Negative recipient	Y/N	Y	10 days	6 months (Prolong to 1 year if lymphopenic)

*CMV HypIG: CMV hyperimmune globulin.

1. Immunosurveillance for high-risk recipients:
   a. Seronegative recipient:
   - Monthly EBV PCR for the first year, 3-monthly for the second year, then 6-monthly till seroconversion, then yearly.
   - Monthly liver panel, GGT for the first 6 months, then 3-monthly up to 1-year post-transplant.

b. Seropositive recipient:
   - 3-monthly EBV PCR for the first year, then yearly.

2. CMV hyperimmune globulin (Megalotect CP®):
   a. Seropositive recipient or seronegative recipient receiving blood transfusion:
      - Single dose: 50 mg/kg/dose (1 ml/kg/dose)
   b. Seronegative recipient with seropositive donor:
      - Megalotect CP® 50 mg/kg/dose (1 ml/kg/dose) 2 weekly starting 24–72 hours after transplantation, for a total of 6 doses (Weeks 1, 3, 5, 7, 9, and 11), followed by
      - Single dose at Week 16.

III. *Pneumocystis jirovecii pneumonia prophylaxis:*

1. Co-trimoxazole oral 3 mg/kg/dose alternate day for:
   a. 3 months from D4.
   b. 6 months for those who received Rituximab as part of the desensitization protocol.
   c. 12 months for those who received mTORi for maintenance therapy.
2. Check glucose-6-phosphate dehydrogenase (G6PD) status and use aerosolized pentamidine 300 mg monthly (via a Respigard nebulizer) in G6PD-deficient patients.
3. Dapsone 2 mg/kg daily (maximum 100 mg) for patients who are allergic to co-trimoxazole.

IV. *Antibiotic prophylaxis for urinary catheter and D-J stent:*

1. IV cephazolin converting to oral cefaclor or cephalexin until urinary catheter is removed.
2. IV cephazolin cover during removal of D-J stent.

V. *Fungal prophylaxis:*

1. Nystatin oral for 1 month.
   - Dose: 250000 U 8 hourly.

2. Consider oral fluconazole if *Candida* sp. is isolated.
   a. Dose: 3 mg/kg/day (maximum dose: 100 mg daily).
   b. Check CNI levels due to drug interactions.

VI. BK virus monitoring:

1. Monitor blood BK virus DNA PCR monthly for the first 9 months then 3-monthly for the first 2 years post-transplant.
2. Screening should be considered for any patient with unexplained graft dysfunction.

Recommended Reading

1. Alloway R, Steinberg S, Khalil K, Gourishankar S, Miller J, Norman D, Hariharan S, Pirsch J, Matas A, Zaltzman J, Wisemandle K, Fitzsimmons W, First MR. (2007) Two years postconversion from a Prograf-based regimen to a once-daily tacrolimus extended-release formulation in stable kidney transplant recipients. *Transplantation* **83**:1648–1651.
2. Hill P, Cross NB, Barnett AN, Palmer SC, Webster AC. (2017) Polyclonal and monoclonal antibodies for induction therapy in kidney transplant recipients. *Cochrane Database Syst Rev* 1(1):CD004759. doi:10.1002/14651858.CD004759.pub2
3. Mincham CM, Wong G, Teixeira-Pinto A, Kennedy S, Alexander S, Larkins N, Lim WH. (2017) Induction therapy, rejection, and graft outcomes in pediatric and adolescent kidney transplant recipients. *Transplantation* **101**:2146–2151.
4. Metz DK, Holford N, Kausman JY, Walker A, Cranswick N, Staatz CE, Barraclough KA, Ierino F. (2019) Optimizing mycophenolic acid exposure in kidney transplant recipients: Time for target concentration intervention. *Transplantation* **103**:2012–2030. Erratum in: *Transplantation* **103**(2019):e390.
5. Hahn D, Hodson EM, Hamiwka LA, Lee VW, Chapman JR, Craig JC, Webster AC. (2019) Target of rapamycin inhibitors (TOR-I; sirolimus and everolimus) for primary immunosuppression in kidney transplant recipients. *Cochrane Database Syst Rev* **12**(12):CD004290. doi:10.1002/14651858.CD004290.pub3
6. McDonald RA. (2021, updated) Kidney transplantation in children: Immunosuppression. Edited by: Niaudat P, Kim MS. *UpToDate ONLINE*. http://www.uptodateonline.com.

6 Anti-Thymocyte Globulin for Kidney Transplantation

Teo S, Lau PYW and Yap HK

A. Preparations

1. Thymoglobulin® (Sanofi Genzyme):
   - Immunosuppressant gamma globulin obtained by immunization of rabbits with human thymocytes.
2. ATGAM® (Pfizer, Pharmacia & Upjohn Co):
   - Immunosuppressant gamma globulin primarily monomeric IgG from hyperimmune serum of horses immunized with human thymic lymphocytes.
3. Potency of anti-thymocyte globulin (ATG): Rabbit > horse.

B. Indications

1. Induction therapy in kidney transplantation.
2. Treatment of acute rejection.

C. Dose

I. Induction therapy for transplant immunosuppression:

1. Rabbit ATG (Thymoglobulin®):
   a. IV 1 mg/kg/day for 3 days (total: 3 mg/kg).
   b. Titrate dose (increase or decrease dose by 20%) to a maximum dose of 1.5 mg/kg/dose:
      - Aim for absolute lymphocyte count 0.1–0.2 × 10^9/L or CD3 levels <1%.
   c. Treat for a maximum of 5 days.

2. Horse ATG:
   - IV 15 mg/kg/day IV for 5–14 days.
3. First dose of ATG should be administered within 24 hours before or after transplantation, or even during induction.

II. Rejection therapy:

1. Rabbit ATG (Thymoglobulin®):
   - IV 1.5 mg/kg/day for 2–7 days (cumulative dose 10.5 mg/kg).
2. Horse ATG:
   - IV 10–15 mg/kg/day for 14 days.

D. Administration

1. Test dose:
   a. Intradermal rabbit (1 µg) or horse (5 µg) ATG 0.1 ml of a 1:1000 dilution.
   b. Control 0.1 ml normal saline.
   c. Positive reaction: Wheal and/or erythema greater than 10 mm.
   d. Observe every 15–20 minutes for 1 hour.
2. ATG infusion:
   a. Dilute ATG 1 mg/ml in normal saline.
      - Do **not** use dextrose solutions as low salt concentrations can cause precipitation.
   b. Give over 4–12 hours (do not exceed 24 hours in diluted form).
   c. Give ATG through a central line or vascular access if possible to minimize phlebitis and thrombosis.
   d. Use an in-line filter with a pore size of 0.2–1.0 micron to prevent inadvertent administration of any insoluble material.
3. Pre-medication:
   a. Diphenhydramine 1mg/kg/dose (25–50 mg) orally or IV.
   b. Paracetamol 10–15 mg/kg/dose.
   c. Give dose of IV methylprednisolone 1–2 mg/kg 1 hour prior to ATG.

4. Precautions:
    a. Greatest toxicity is bone marrow suppression.
    b. Stop treatment if the following occur:
        i. Symptoms of anaphylaxis.
        ii. Thrombocytopenia: Platelet count $<50 \times 10^9$/L.
        iii. Leukopenia: Total white blood cell count $<2.0 \times 10^9$/L.
            - Should have no effect on absolute neutrophil count.
    c. Inadvertent overdose of rabbit ATG (Thymoglobulin®) >5 mg/kg/day may induce leucopenia and thrombocytopenia.
    d. Prolonged use >3 weeks increases the risk of severe infections and risk of lymphoma.

E. Adverse Effects

1. Anaphylaxis:
    a. Symptoms: Urticaria, angioedema, hypotension, respiratory distress, wheeze, cough, chest pain.
    b. Stop infusion immediately.
    c. Administer IM 0.01 ml/kg of **1:1000** solution of adrenaline × 3 doses 20 minutes apart if required, OR
    IV 0.05–0.1 ml/kg/dose of **1:10000** solution.
2. Hemolysis:
    a. Symptoms: Pallor, dark/red urine, chest pain, back pain, flank pain.
    b. IV packed red blood cell transfusion.
    c. If oliguric, consider the following:
        i. IV hydration with normal saline to correct for maintenance +5% deficit.
        ii. Correction of metabolic acidosis with sodium bicarbonate and alkalinize the urine.
        iii. IV furosemide 1–2 mg/kg.
        iv. Severe and unremitting hemolysis may require discontinuation of therapy.
3. Thrombocytopenia:
    - Usually transient.

Recommended Reading

1. Lexicomp Inc. (n.d.) Antithymocyte globulin (rabbit derived, Thymoglobulin): Drug information Lexicomp®. *UpToDate ONLINE*. http://www.uptodate.com.
2. Lexicomp Inc. (n.d.) Antithymocyte globulin (horse derived, Atgam): Drug information Lexicomp®. *UpToDate ONLINE*. http://www.uptodate.com.

7 Megalotect CP® (Human Cytomegalovirus Immunoglobulin) Infusion Protocol

Lim SH, Teo S and Yap HK

A. Preparation Forms

1. Ampoules with 10 ml (1000 U).
2. Ampoules with 50 ml (5000 U).

B. Indications

1. Treatment and prophylaxis of clinical cytomegalovirus (CMV) disease in kidney transplant recipients.
2. Treatment and prophylaxis of Epstein–Barr virus (EBV)-associated post-transplant lymphoproliferative disorder (PTLD).

C. Contraindications

1. Selective IgA deficiency.
2. Hypersensitivity to excipients such as glycine.

D. Dosing

1. 100 units PEI (1 ml) per kg/dose.
2. 1 ml contains:

- Human plasma protein 50 mg (96% IgG against CMV).
- 5% protein solution with glycine stabilizer.

E. Route of Administration

1. Megalotect CP® is administered intravenously.
   a. Solution should be warmed to room or body temperature prior to administration.
   b. Do not use solutions that are cloudy or have a deposit.
2. Infusion rate:
   a. Run at 0.08 ml/kg/hour during the first 10 minutes.
   b. Increase as tolerated every half-hour by doubling the rate up to a maximum of 0.8 ml/kg/hour if no adverse reactions.
   c. Do not exceed 60 ml/hour.

F. Monitoring

1. Pulse rate, respiratory rate, blood pressure, SpO_2:
   - Every 10 minutes for the first hour, then
   - Half-hourly till end of infusion.
2. Temperature hourly.
3. Patients should be observed for at least 2 hours after completion of infusion.

G. Adverse Effects

1. Symptoms:
   a. Headache.
   b. Fever.
   c. Vomiting.
   d. Allergic reactions.
   e. Nausea.
   f. Arthralgia.
   g. Back pain.
   h. Hypotension.

2. If adverse effects occur:
   a. Slow down infusion rate or stop infusion until effects subside.
   b. If reactions occur consider giving:
      i. Paracetamol 10–15 mg/kg (maximum 1 g) for fever and chills.
      ii. IV Hydrocortisone 4–10 mg/kg (maximum 500 mg).
      iii. IV Diphenhydramine 1 mg/kg (maximum 50 mg).
   c. Inform the Physician-In-Charge if the above occurs.

Recommended Reading

1. Megalotect CP® Product Insert.

8 Routine Outpatient Monitoring of Transplant Recipient

Koh LJ, Yap HK, Qader MA, Teo S and Lau PYW

A. Frequency of Monitoring Post-transplant

1. Frequency of routine follow-up after discharge from hospital:
   a. 3 times a week in Month 1 post-transplant.
   b. 2 times a week in Month 2.
   c. Weekly in Month 3.
   d. Every 2 weeks in Months 4 to 6, then monthly thereafter.
2. At every visit, clinical parameters including weight, height, body surface area, body mass index (BMI), pulse rate, and blood pressure (BP) should be recorded.
3. Annual ophthalmologic evaluation to screen for:
   a. Cataracts in transplant recipients on long-term steroid protocol.
   b. Maculopathy in transplant recipients with systemic lupus erythematosus on hydroxychloroquine.
   c. Diabetic retinopathy in transplant recipients with diabetes mellitus.

B. Routine Investigations

1. Graft function monitoring:
   a. Blood biochemistry including urea, creatinine, sodium, potassium, chloride, and bicarbonate.
   b. Urine protein:creatinine ratio and/or albumin:creatinine ratio, 24-hour urine protein excretion, and/or albumin excretion.
   c. Creatinine clearance and estimated glomerular filtration rate (eGFR).

   d. Donor-specific antibody (DSA) titers.
   e. Doppler ultrasound of the transplant kidney.
2. Drug level monitoring:
   a. Trough tacrolimus/sirolimus/everolimus.
   b. Cyclosporin 2 hours post-dosing (C2 levels).
   c. Mycophenolate area under the curve (AUC).
3. Hematological disease monitoring:
   a. Full blood count (hemoglobin, differential white count, platelets).
   b. Iron profile.
4. Liver function test:
   a. Albumin.
   b. Alanine aminotransferase.
   c. Aspartate aminotransferase.
   d. Gamma-glutamyltransferase (GGT).
   e. Alkaline phosphatase.
   f. Lactate dehydrogenase.
5. Transplant bone disease:
   a. Calcium, phosphate.
   b. Magnesium.
   c. Parathyroid hormone (PTH).
   d. 25-hydroxycholecalciferol (25-OH D3).
   e. Urine calcium:creatinine ratio.
6. Infectious disease monitoring:
   a. Urinalysis (microscopy and sediment examination) and culture
   b. Nucleic acid amplification technique (NAT) for cytomegalovirus (CMV), Epstein–Barr virus (EBV), and BK virus.
   c. Human immunodeficiency virus (HIV) antibody/antigen combination test (HIV Ab-Ag) and NAT.
   d. Hepatitis B surface antigen (HBsAg), anti-hepatitis B surface antibody (anti-HBs Ab), and hepatitis B virus (HBV) NAT.
   e. Anti-hepatitis C antibody (anti-HCV Ab) and hepatitis C (HCV) NAT.
7. New-onset diabetes mellitus after transplant (NODAT):
   a. Fasting and/or 2-hour postprandial blood glucose.
   b. Glycated hemoglobin (HbA1c).
8. Cardiovascular disease risk screening:
   a. Fasting lipid profile.
   b. Uric acid.

c. Ambulatory blood pressure (ABP) monitoring.
d. Echocardiography.

9. Cancer screening:
   a. Post-transplant lymphoproliferative disorder (PTLD) and malignant change in acquired cystic disease in native kidneys (renal cell carcinoma):
      - Ultrasound abdomen (hepatobiliary system and native kidneys).
   b. Skin cancers:
      - Total body skin examination.
   c. Genital cancers (in sexually active recipients):
      - Papanicolaou (Pap) smear in females.
10. Screening for recurrence of primary disease:
   a. Focal segmental glomerulosclerosis (FSGS)
      - Urine protein:creatinine ratio or 24-hour urine protein excretion.
   b. IgA nephropathy:
      - Urinalysis for hematuria.
      - Urine protein:creatinine ratio or 24-hour urine protein excretion.
   c. Anti-neutrophil cytoplasmic antibody (ANCA)-associated vasculitis:
      - Urinalysis for hematuria.
      - Urine protein:creatinine ratio or 24-hour urine protein excretion.
   d. Anti-glomerular basement membrane (anti-GBM) disease:
      - Urinalysis for hematuria.
      - Urine protein:creatinine ratio or 24-hour urine protein excretion.
   e. Lupus nephritis:
      - Urinalysis for hematuria.
      - Urine protein:creatinine ratio or 24-hour urine protein excretion.
      - Serum complements C3 and C4.
      - Anti-dsDNA antibody.

C. Monitoring Schedule of Transplant Recipient

Screening Test or Evaluation	Screening Intervals By Time After Transplantation				
	Month 1	Month 2–3	Month 4–6	Month 7–12	>Month 12
Clinical Parameters					
Pulse rate, BP, height, weight, BMI	Each clinic visit				
Graft Function Monitoring					
Creatinine and eGFR	3 times/ week	1–2 times/ week	2-weekly	Monthly	Monthly to 2-monthly
Urea, sodium, potassium, chloride, bicarbonate	3 times/ week	1–2 times/ week	2-weekly	Monthly	Monthly to 2-monthy
Creatinine clearance	Yearly				
Urine protein: creatinine ratio and/or albumin: creatinine ratio	Once	Monthly to 3-monthly			
24-hour urine protein and/or albumin	Yearly				
DSA	6–12 monthly				
Doppler ultrasound transplanted kidney	Once	Yearly			
Drug Level Monitoring					
Tacrolimus/ sirolimus/ everolimus trough level	3 times/ week	1–2 times/ week	2-weekly	Monthly	Monthly to 2-monthly

(Continued)

(*Continued*)

Screening Test or Evaluation	Screening Intervals By Time After Transplantation				
	Month 1	Month 2–3	Month 4–6	Month 7–12	>Month 12
Cyclosporin C2 level	3 times/ week	1–2 times/ week	2-weekly	Monthly	Monthly to 2-monthly
Mycophenolate AUC	Once before discharge	Optional			
Hematological Disease Monitoring					
Full blood count	2–3 times/ week	1–2 times/ week	2-weekly	Monthly	Monthly to 2-monthly
Iron panel	Once	3-monthly			
Liver Function Test					
Liver panel	Weekly	Monthly			Monthly to 2-monthly
GGT	Once	Monthly			Monthly to 2-monthly
Transplant Bone Disease Monitoring					
Calcium and phosphate	Weekly	Monthly			Monthly to 2-monthly
Magnesium	Weekly	Monthly			Monthly to 2-monthly
PTH	Once	3 monthly if abnormal after transplant or eGFR <60 ml/min/1.73m^2			
25-OH D3		3 monthly			
Urine calcium: creatinine ratio	Once	6 monthly if on vitamin D therapy			
Infectious Disease Monitoring					
Urine microscopy and sediment examination	2 times/ week till DJ stent removal	Monthly for patients with neurogenic bladder, vesicoureteric reflux, and recurrent urinary tract infection			

(*Continued*)

Screening Test or Evaluation	Screening Intervals By Time After Transplantation				
	Month 1	Month 2–3	Month 4–6	Month 7–12	>Month 12
Urine culture	2 times/ week till DJ stent removal	Monthly for patients with neurogenic bladder, vesicoureteric reflux, and recurrent urinary tract infection			
CMV NAT	Weekly for Month 1 then 2 weekly for Month 2 then monthly for seronegative recipients				Yearly
	Monthly for seropositive recipients				
EBV NAT	Monthly for seronegative recipients				3-monthly for first 2 years then 6-monthly till sero-conversion, then yearly
	3-monthly for seropositive recipients				Yearly
BKV NAT	Monthly for first 9 months			3-monthly for first 2 years, then yearly	
HBsAg and anti-HBs Ab	Month 1, Month 3 and Month 12				Yearly
Anti-HCV Ab	Month 12				
HIV Ag-Ab	Month 12				
HBV, HCV, HIV NAT	Month 1 and Month 3				Continue monitoring if the respective screening tests positive

(*Continued*)

(Continued)

Screening Test or Evaluation	Screening Intervals By Time After Transplantation				
	Month 1	Month 2–3	Month 4–6	Month 7–12	>Month 12
New-onset Diabetes Risk Screening					
Fasting and/or 2-hour post prandial plasma glucose	Weekly		3-monthly		6-monthly
HbA1c	Weekly		3-monthly		6-monthly
Cardiovascular Disease Risk Screening					
Fasting lipid profile	Once after 3 months		6-monthly		
Uric acid	Once after 3 months		6-monthly		
Ambulatory BP	Yearly				
Echocardiogram	Yearly				
Cancer Screening					
Ultrasound abdomen	Yearly				
Skin examination	Yearly				
Pap smear	Yearly for first 3 years if sexually active, then 3-yearly subsequently				
Recurrence of Primary Disease Monitoring					
FSGS	Daily for the first week then 3x/week		Weekly for 3 months then monthly		3-monthly
IgA nephropathy	Once		3-monthly		6-monthly
Lupus nephritis	Once		3-monthly		
ANCA-vasculitis	Once		3-monthly		6-monthly
Anti-GBM disease	Once		3-monthly		Yearly
Ophthalmologic Screen					
Eye evaluation	Yearly				

Recommended Reading

1. KDIGO. (2009) KDIGO clinical practice guideline for the care of kidney transplant recipients. *Am J Transplant* **9**(Suppl 3):Si–S155.
2. KDIGO. (2010) Managing your adult patients who have a kidney transplant-based on select guidelines from KDOQI US commentary on the 2009 KDIGO practice guideline for the care of kidney transplant recipients. *Am J Kidney Dis* **56**:189–218.
3. MOH. (2018) Manual on organ donation and transplantation. Ministry of Health Singapore.
4. Green M, Blumberg EA, Danziger-Isakov L, Huprikar S, Kotton CN, Kumar D. (2019) Foreword: 4th edition of the American Society of Transplantation Infectious Diseases guidelines. *Clin Transplant* **33**:e13642.
5. Chandraker A, Yeung MY. (2021, updated) Kidney transplantation in adults: Overview of care of the adult kidney transplant recipient. Edited by: Brennan DC, Lam AO. *UpToDate Online.* http://www.uptodateonline.com.

9 Management of Recurrent Primary Idiopathic Focal Segmental Glomerulosclerosis Post Kidney Transplant

Koh LJ, Yap HK, Lau PYW, Ng KH and Teo S

A. Introduction

1. Useful Definitions:

Primary idiopathic FSGS	Sporadic presentation of FSGS, likely associated with permeability factor or loss of inhibition to permeability factor.
Primary non-idiopathic FSGS	FSGS related to a known cause: a. Genetic forms, including syndromic FSGS. b. Viral infections. c. Drugs: • mTOR inhibitors. • Bisphosphonates. • Anabolic steroids. • Interferon.
Secondary FSGS	Related to hyperfiltration injury due to loss of functioning renal parenchyma: a. Reduced renal mass. b. Hypertension. c. Reflux nephropathy. d. Severe obesity. e. Drugs and toxins resulting in nephron loss. f. Ischemia-reperfusion injury. g. Chronic rejection. h. Recurrent glomerular disease other than FSGS.

(*Continued*)

	i. Renal artery stenosis. j. Thrombotic microangiopathy. k. Diabetic nephropathy.
Recurrent FSGS (rFSGS)	a. Heavy proteinuria: • Urine protein/creatinine ratio (UPCR) ≥0.1 g/mmol in a previously anuric patient. • Urinary total protein excretion >1 g/day/1.73m^2. • Hypoalbuminemia <25 g/L in a previously anuric patient. • Increase of UPCR ≥0.1 g/mmol in a patient with proteinuria prior to transplant. b. Biopsy showing FSGS pattern of injury in the allograft.
Remission	a. Loss of edema. b. Remission of proteinuria: • UPCR <0.02 g/mmol. • Urinary total protein <0.3 g/day/1.73m^2 or <4 mg/m^2/hour. • First void urine dipstick negative/trace for 3 consecutive days.
Early recurrence	Within 48 hours of transplant.
Late recurrence	After 1 month post-transplant.

2. Recurrence risk in primary idiopathic FSGS post-transplant is 30–50%.
3. Graft loss has been reported in up to 50% of kidney transplants with rFSGS.
4. In patients who have graft loss due to rFSGS, there is up to an 80% chance of developing recurrent disease in the subsequent allografts.

B. Pre-transplant Risk Assessment of Recurrence of FSGS

I. Risk factors:

1. Genetically proven FSGS:
   a. Recipients with only a single heterozygous pathogenic variant in autosomal recessive genes are considered not to have genetic

disease and hence have the same risk of recurrence as that of idiopathic FSGS.

- Exceptions are heterozygous carriers of p.R229Q variant in the *NPHS2* gene, as this mutation exerts a dominant negative effect.

b. Genetic FSGS generally has a very low risk of recurrence post-transplant, with few exceptions, such as:
   - Truncating gene mutations in *NPHS1* (Fin-major) with the development of anti-nephrin antibodies post-transplant.
   - Truncating gene mutations in collagen IV genes with the development of anti-glomerular basement membrane antibodies post-transplant.

c. If (likely) pathogenic genetic variant(s) is/are identified in the recipient, screen potential related donors for the genetic variant(s).
   i. Donors with a single heterozygous pathogenic variant in autosomal recessive genes are eligible to donate, except for:
      - Those with a single heterozygous p.R229Q variant of the *NPHS2* gene as there is an increased risk of recurrence in the transplant kidney.
      - Those with pathogenic variants in *COL4A5*, *COL4A3* and *COL4A4*.

   ii. Donors with a likely pathogenic variant in a dominant gene should be excluded as potential donors.

2. Higher risk in non-genetically proven FSGS (may include a small proportion of as-yet-unidentified genetic FSGS) if:
   a. Younger age of disease onset.
   b. Being of European origin.
   c. Rapid disease progression.
   d. Initial steroid sensitivity with late steroid resistance.
   e. History of recurrence in a prior allograft (up to 80% risk of recurrence in the second allograft).
3. Histologic features suggesting a higher recurrence risk:
   - Presence of mesangial hypercellularity with few sclerotic glomeruli.

II. Choice of donor:

1. In first transplants, living or deceased donors can be used.

2. Allografts from donors >40 years old increase the risk of rFSGS.
3. Deceased donor allografts are recommended in patients who have experienced disease recurrence in their prior transplants.

C. Diagnostic Approach

1. Post-transplant monitoring for proteinuria in patients with primary idiopathic FSGS:
   a. UPCR within 24 hours of transplant, then daily for the first week, then 3× a week for 3 weeks, then weekly for 3 months, then monthly post-transplant for the first year, then 3-monthly subsequently.
   b. 24-hour urinary protein excretion if abnormal UPCR.

   Note: Native proteinuria may mask rFSGS and may require unilateral or bilateral nephrectomy before transplant.
2. Perform kidney biopsy if there is suspicion of rFSGS:
   a. 7 days post-transplant if there is delayed graft function when oliguria or anuria results in difficulty quantifying proteinuria.
   b. Any occurrence of significant proteinuria within 2 years of transplant.

   Note: Biopsy sample should include juxtamedullary tissue.
3. Histological features:

Histological Change	Timing (Relative to Proteinuria)
Normal appearance	Early
Early FSGS with foam cell change, endocapillary cellularity, or podocyte hyperplasia	Mid
Late focal sclerosing lesions	Late
Collapsing FSGS, arterial and artoriolar narrowing	Rapid course

4. Exclude other causes of primary non-idiopathic FSGS or secondary FSGS, especially in patients with late recurrence of disease.
   a. History of medications, in particular, mTOR inhibitors.
   b. Acute rejection.
   c. Arterial hypertension.

d. Ischemia-reperfusion injury.
e. Interstitial fibrosis/tubular atrophy.
f. Check for associated viral infections by polymerase chain reaction (PCR):
   i. Parvovirus B19.
   ii. Cytomegalovirus (CMV).
   iii. Epstein–Barr virus (EBV).
   iv. BK virus (BKV).
   v. Hepatitis C virus.
   vi. Human immunodeficiency virus (if risk factors are present).

D. Treatment of Recurrent Primary Idiopathic FSGS

I. Treatment of viral infections:

1. Viral infections should be excluded and treated prior to institution of specific treatment for rFSGS occurring after 48 hours post-transplant.
2. High dose intravenous gammaglobulin (IVIG) 1–2 g/kg should be given as empiric treatment for parvovirus-associated FSGS.
   - Avoid IVIG preparations with high osmolality.
3. Specific treatment of other viral infections should be instituted following a definitive diagnosis.

II. Plasmapheresis (PE):

1. Early initiation in patients is associated with higher remission rates.
2. Indicated in patients with rFSGS:
   a. Protein excretion of >1 g/day/1.73m^2 or UPCR ≥0.1 g/mmol within 1 year of transplantation.
   b. Refractory to escalation of immunosuppressive therapy.
3. Vascular access:
   a. Hemodialysis catheter in the right internal jugular vein is preferred.
   b. Heparin lock preferred over citrate lock due to prothrombotic risk.

   c. If arteriovenous fistula present, consider use only if central line access not possible.
   d. Do not run infusions via arteriovenous fistula.
4. Protocol:
   a. Plasma exchanges: 1–1.5× plasma volume.
   b. Frequency:
      i. Daily for 3 days, then
      ii. 3× per week for 2 weeks for a total of 9 exchanges.
   c. Replacement fluid:
      i. 5% albumin.
      ii. If plasma fibrinogen is low, use fresh frozen plasma.
   d. Give IVIG 0.5 g/kg at the end of the PE cycle or if there is hypogammaglobulinemia.
5. Consider repeating the PE cycles until proteinuria <1 g/day/1.73m^2.
6. Stop PE if there is no response after 36 plasma exchanges (4 cycles).

III. High dose steroids:

1. Oral prednisolone 60 mg/m^2 for at least 4 weeks before considering tapering the steroid dose if proteinuria has improved to <1 g/day/1.73m^2.
   - Do not taper to alternate-day steroids as this may result in a relapse.
2. Consider monthly IV methylprednisolone pulse 10 mg/kg × 3 doses if plasmapheresis is unavailable.

IV. High dose calcineurin inhibitor (CNI) therapy:

1. Increase dose of CNI to achieve high levels:
   a. Cyclosporine (CsA): Trough level >200 µg/L or C2 level 1500–2000 µg/L.
   b. Tacrolimus (Tac): Trough level of 12–15 µg/L.
2. CsA protocol:
   a. Intravenous CsA:
      i. IV bolus infusion over 2 hours: 2–3 mg/kg/dose 8–12 hourly (50% of oral dosing), aiming for target trough levels as above OR

ii. If continuous infusion 2–3 mg/kg/day, increasing to 3–4 mg/kg/day to attain steady-state levels of 150–175 μg/L.
iii. Duration of IV CsA: 14 days

b. Oral CsA 6–8 mg/kg/day increasing up to 25 mg/kg/day to achieve target levels above.
   - Conversion from IV dose: 2.5 × IV dose (mg/kg/day).

c. Taper CsA to standard post-transplant dose once remission is achieved.

3. Tac protocol:
   a. Increase Tac dose to achieve high trough levels.
   b. Taper Tac to standard post-transplant dose once remission is achieved.

V. *Anti-CD 20 monoclonal antibody:*

1. Check hepatitis B serology prior to administration.
2. Rituximab:
   a. Consider giving rituximab if:
      i. Plasmapheresis is unavailable or contraindicated (4 weekly doses).
      ii. Early rFSGS within 48 hours post-transplant (2 doses given 1 week apart).
      iii. Patient has not gone into remission after the first 9 doses of PE (2 doses given 1 week apart).
      iv. FSGS recurrence occurs after stopping plasmapheresis.
   b. Dose of rituximab: 375 mg/m^2.
   c. PE should be withheld for 48 hours following each rituximab infusion to prevent drug removal.
3. Obinutuzumab:
   a. Consider giving obinutuzumab if patient has:
      i. Known anti-rituximab antibodies.
      ii. Failed to respond to Rituximab.
   b. Dose: 1 g /1.73m^2 (maximum 1 g), 2 doses given 1 week apart.
   c. Withhold PE for 48 hours following each obinutuzumab infusion.

4. Consider repeating the dose if the patient relapses or if CD19 counts recover.

VI. Cytotoxic T-lymphocyte-associated Antigen 4-immunoglobulin (CTLA-4-Ig):

1. Third-line after plasmapheresis and rituximab or obinutuzumab.
   - Consider in patients with B7-1 (CD80) positive immunostaining on kidney biopsy.
2. Abatacept:
   a. Intravenous dosing: 10 mg/kg to a maximum of 1 g × 2 doses given 2 weeks apart.
   b. If the patient is still proteinuric, give a third dose in 2 weeks, then monthly till there is a response.
3. Dose of belatacept:
   a. Induction: 10 mg/kg to a maximum of 1 g × 2 doses given 2 weeks apart.
   b. Maintenance: IV 5 mg/kg monthly (plus or minus 3 days) starting 2 weeks after the induction dose.
4. Avoid abatacept or belatacept in patients who are EBV serology negative as there is a high risk of primary EBV infection.

E. General Management

1. Fluid management:
   a. Avoid intravascular hypovolemia to ensure perfusion to transplant kidney (especially in the first week of transplant) as there is a high risk of thrombosis.
   b. Consider restricting fluid to insensible losses + urine output.
2. Anti-proteinuric agents:
   a. Avoid use of angiotensin-converting enzyme inhibitors (ACEi) or angiotensin receptor blockers (ARBs) in the first month post-transplant to avoid decreasing perfusion to graft.
   b. Avoid the use of combination of ACEi and ARB.

3. Lipid-lowering agents:
   a. Start on statins to control hypercholesterolemia.
   b. Rosuvastatin in combination with CNI has the lowest risk of rhabdomyolysis.
   c. Simvastatin has the highest risk of rhabdomyolysis.
   d. Monitor hepatic transaminases and creatine kinase monthly for the first 3 months, then 3-monthly.
4. Anti-thrombotic prophylaxis:
   a. Indications:
      i. When serum albumin <25 g/L, consider warfarin or low molecular weight heparin.
      ii. When serum albumin is persistently between 25 and 30 g/L, consider low dose aspirin.
   b. Warfarin:
      - Dose: 0.2 mg/kg starting dose followed by 0.05–0.2 mg/kg daily.
      - Keep international normalized ratio (INR) between 2 and 2.5.
   c. Low molecular weight heparin (subcutaneous):
      i. Enoxaparin:
         - Dose: 0.5 mg/kg/dose 12 hourly (maximum dose 40 mg).
         - Dose reduction for abnormal kidney function:
           eGFR 10–29 ml/min/1.73m^2: 70% of dose.
           eGFR <10 ml/min/1.73m^2: 50% of dose given once a day.
           Note: Monitor anti-Xa levels 4–5 hours post-dose (do not exceed 1.0 U/ml).
      ii. Tinzaparin:
         - Dose: 50 U/kg daily.
   d. Aspirin:
      - Dose: 3–5 mg/kg/day (maximum 100 mg).
5. Infection prophylaxis:
   a. Close surveillance for viral infections: CMV, EBV and BKV PCR:
      - Day 1 of treatment, then
      - Monthly for 6 months, then
      - 3-monthly for one year.

b. *Pneumocystis jirovecii* prophylaxis for 3 months after anti-CD20 antibody infusion.
   i. Co-trimoxazole oral 3 mg (TMP)/kg/dose alternate day, OR
   ii. Aerosolized pentamidine 300 mg monthly (via Respigard nebulizer) in glucose-6-phosphate dehydrogenase (G6PD)-deficient patients, OR
   iii. Dapsone 2 mg/kg daily (maximum 100 mg) for patients who are allergic to co-trimoxazole.
c. Fungal prophylaxis:
   i. Oral nystatin for 1 month at a dose of 250000 U 8 hourly.
   ii. Consider oral fluconazole if *Candida* sp. is isolated.
      - Dose: 3 mg/kg/day (maximum dose 100 mg daily).
      - Check Tac/CsA levels due to drug interactions.

F. Prevention of Recurrence Post-transplant

1. In patients with graft loss due to rFSGS, the second allograft should be from a deceased donor.
2. No interventions have been proven to prevent rFSGS in the allograft.
3. Preventative strategy for second allograft:
   a. Prophylactic PE:
      I. 1.5 plasma volume exchanges
      ii. 3× weekly for 2 weeks:
         - Beginning 1 week prior to living donor transplant OR
         - Within 1 day of deceased donor transplant.
   b. Rituximab 375 mg/m^2 peri-operatively or immediately after transplant followed by a second dose after 1 week.
      - PE should be withheld for 48 hours following each rituximab infusion.

G. Algorithm for Management of rFSGS

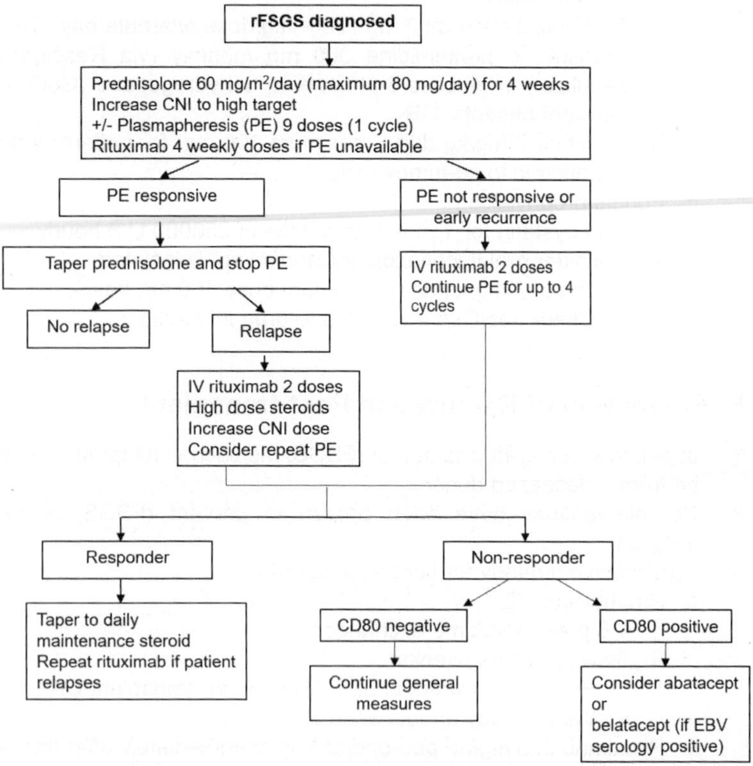

Recommended Reading

1. Leroy S, Guigonis V, Bruckner D, Emal-Aglae V, Deschênes G, Bensman A, Ulinski T. (2009) Successful anti-TNFalpha treatment in a child with posttransplant recurrent focal segmental glomerulosclerosis. *Am J Transplant* **9**:858–861.
2. Vincenti F, Charpentier B, Vanrenterghem Y, Rostaing L, Bresnahan B, Darji P, Massari P, Mondragon-Ramirez GA, Agarwal M, DiRusso G, Lin CS, Garg P, Larsen CP. (2010) A phase III study of belatacept-based immunosuppression regimens versus cyclosporine in renal transplant recipients (BENEFIT study). *Am J Transplant* **10**:535–546.

3. Yu CC, Fornoni A, Weins A, Hakroush S, Maiguel D, Sageshima J, Chen L, Ciancio G, Faridi MH, Behr D, Campbell KN, Chang JM, Chen HC, Oh J, Faul C, Arnaout MA, Fiorina P, Gupta V, Greka A, Burke GW 3rd, Mundel P. (2013) Abatacept in B7-1-positive proteinuric kidney disease. *N Engl J Med* **369**:2416–2423.
4. Kang HG, Ha IS, Cheong HI. (2016) Recurrence and treatment after renal transplantation in children with FSGS. *Biomed Res Int* **2016**:6832971.
5. Chadban SJ, Ahn C, Axelrod DA, Foster BJ, Kasiske BL, Kher V, Kumar D, Oberbauer R, Pascual J, Pilmore HL, Rodrigue JR, Segev DL, Sheerin NS, Tinckam KJ, Wong G, Knoll GA. (2020) KDIGO clinical practice guideline on the evaluation and management of candidates for kidney transplantation. *Transplantation* **104(4S1 Suppl 1)**:S11–S103.
6. Alachkar N, Brennan DC, Kaplan AA, Kwoh CH. (2019, updated) Kidney transplantation in adults: Focal segmental glomerulosclerosis in the transplanted kidney. Edited by: Murphy B, Lam AQ. *UpToDate ONLINE*. http://www.uptodateonline.com.
7. McDonald RA. (2020, updated) Kidney transplantation in children: Complications. Edited by: Niaudet P, Kim MS. *UpToDate ONLINE*. http://www.uptodateonline.com.
8. Weber LT, Tönshoff B, Grenda R, Bouts A, Topaloglu R, Gülhan B, Printza N, Awan A, Battelino N, Ehren R, Hoyer PF, Novljan G, Marks SD, Oh J, Prytula A, Seeman T, Sweeney C, Dello Strologo L, Pape L. (2020) Clinical practice recommendations for recurrence of focal and segmental glomerulosclerosis/steroid-resistant nephrotic syndrome. *Pediatr Transplant* **25**(3):e13955. doi:10.1111/petr.13955.

10 Management of Transplant Rejection

Lau PYW, Chhabra M, Teo S and Yap HK

A. Classification of Kidney Allograft Rejection

Type of Rejection	Time	Cause	Humoral	Cellular
Hyperacute	Minutes to hours	Preformed anti-donor antibodies and complement	+++	–
Accelerated	Days	Reactivation of sensitized cells	++	+
Acute Cellular Vascular	Days to weeks	Primary activation of T-cells	 + +++	 +++ +
Chronic	Months to years	Both immunogenic and non-immunogenic factors	++	+?

B. Diagnosis of Transplant Rejection

1. Clinical manifestations:
   a. Timing:
      - Most acute rejection episodes occur within the first 6 months after transplantation.
      - Rejection after 12 months is usually due to noncompliance or over-aggressive reduction in immunosuppression.

   b. Acute rise in serum creatinine:
      - Relatively late in the development in the course of a rejection episode because most children are transplanted with an adult-sized kidney with a large kidney functional reserve compared to body size.

- Usually indicates the presence of significant histological change.

c. Development of hypertension with low-grade fever is one of the earliest and most sensitive signs of acute rejection in children.
   - Any increase in creatinine accompanied by hypertension in children should be considered an acute rejection unless proven otherwise.

d. Decreased urine output.

e. Pyuria.

f. New or worsening proteinuria.

g. Fever, graft pain and/or tenderness, and graft swelling are currently uncommon with modern immunosuppressive regimens, which include calcineurin inhibitors unless immunosuppression is completely discontinued.

2. Diagnostic imaging:

a. Kidney ultrasound findings suggestive of acute rejection include:
   - Graft enlargement.
   - Obscured corticomedullary differentiation.
   - Decreased echogenicity of the renal sinus.
   - Thickened urothelium.
   - Prominent hypoechoic medullary pyramids.
   - Increased or decreased cortical echogenicity.

b. Kidney Doppler ultrasound finding of an elevated resistive index (RI).
   - RI = [peak systolic velocity (PSV) – end-diastolic velocity]/PSV
   - RI >0.9 is a non-specific finding since increases in RI can also be due to ureteral obstruction, renal vein occlusion, pyelonephritis, and calcineurin inhibitor toxicity.

c. Dynamic nuclear medicine imaging (^{99m}Tc-MAG3 renogram) suggestive of acute rejection include:
   - Decreased perfusion.
   - Delayed transplant visualization.
   - Poor parenchymal uptake.
   - High background activity because of decreased clearance.

   Note: In acute tubular necrosis where there is preservation of renal blood flow relative to glomerular filtration, dynamic renogram shows good perfusion on the first phase images, with preserved concentration during the second phase by the transplant, followed by poor excretion into the collecting system and the bladder during the third phase.

3. Kidney biopsy:
   a. Kidney allograft biopsy with conventional histological examination is the gold standard for diagnosing acute rejection.
   b. Diagnosis of antibody-mediated rejection is typically associated with positive immunostaining for C4d and/or immunoglobulin in peritubular capillaries.
   c. Kidney biopsy should be performed before treating acute allograft rejection unless the biopsy will substantially delay treatment.
   d. It is recommended to give an intravenous infusion of desmopressin (DDAVP) 0.3 μg/kg one hour before the kidney biopsy in children with allograft dysfunction to correct any potential bleeding tendency.
4. Serologic evidence of donor-specific antibody (DSA):
   a. DSA may be pre-formed (in sensitized recipients) or develop *de novo* post-transplantation.
   b. Types of DSA:
      - DSAs to HLA antigens are best characterized in the pathogenesis of antibody-mediated rejection (ABMR).
      - Antibodies against non-HLA molecules expressed on graft endothelium are increasingly recognized as pathogenic.
   c. In the presence of graft dysfunction, detection of significant levels of DSA is highly predictive for the diagnosis of ABMR.

Anti-HLA Antibodies	Standardized Fluorescent Intensity (SFI)	Mean Fluorescent Intensity (MFI)
Strong binding	>200000	>10000
Moderate binding	100000 to 200000	5000 to 10000
Weak binding	50000 to <100000	2500 to <5000
Negative	<50000	<2500

*MFI = SFI/20

d. Detection of DSA in the absence of graft dysfunction or histological changes is not diagnostic for ABMR, but overall is associated with increased risk of ABMR and graft loss.
e. Characteristics of DSA that have been associated with poorer outcomes among patients with ABMR:
   i. Peak DSA MFI >5000.
   ii. C1q-binding or C3d-binding DSA.
   iii. IgG3 immunodominant DSA.
      - DSA IgG subclass testing not validated for clinical use yet.
   iv. *De novo* DSA associated with poorer outcomes compared to pre-existing DSA.

5. Molecular techniques for the detection of endothelial cell dysfunction are being developed to identify rejection more sensitively than histological or serological markers (C4d staining/DSA), which may be absent in some cases of ABMR:
   a. Microarray analysis of RNA transcripts extracted from endothelial cells in allograft tissue has been used to examine patterns of gene expression consistent with ABMR.
   b. Assessment of percentage of donor-derived cell-free DNA (dd-cf-DNA) in the recipient plasma is emerging as a non-invasive correlate of graft injury due to ABMR or microvascular inflammation, and in the case of ABMR, may precede the development of DSA.
      - dd-cf DNA <1% supports the absence of active rejection (negative predictive value 84–96% depending on the assay).

C. Histopathological Classification of Transplant Rejection

I. Revised Banff 2017 Grading System (with updates in 2019):

1. Acute Banff scores:
   a. Quantitative criteria for interstitial inflammation ("i") score:
      - i0: No inflammation or in <10% of unscarred cortical parenchyma.
      - i1: Inflammation in 10–25% of unscarred cortical parenchyma.

- i2: Inflammation in 26–50% of unscarred cortical parenchyma.
- i3: Inflammation in >50% of unscarred cortical parenchyma.

b. Quantitative criteria for tubulitis ("t") score:
- t0: No mononuclear leukocytes in tubules.
- t1: Foci with 1–4 mononuclear leukocytes/tubular cross-section (or 10 tubular cells).
- t2: Foci with 5–10 mononuclear leukocytes/tubular cross-section (or 10 tubular cells).
- t3: Foci with >10 mononuclear leukocytes/tubular cross-section or the presence of two or more areas of tubular basement membrane destruction accompanied by i2/i3 inflammation and t2 tubulitis elsewhere.

c. Quantitative criteria for intimal arteritis ("v"):
- v0: No arteritis.
- v1: Mild-to-moderate intimal arteritis in at least one arterial cross-section.
- v2: Severe intimal arteritis with at least 25% luminal loss in at least one arterial cross-section.
- v3: Transmural arteritis and/or arterial fibrinoid change and medial smooth muscle necrosis with lymphocyte infiltrate in vessel.

d. Quantitative criteria for early allograft glomerulitis ("g") score:
- g0: No glomerulitis.
- g1: Segmental or global glomerulitis in <25% of glomeruli.
- g2: Segmental or global glomerulitis in 25–75% of glomeruli.
- g3: Segmental or global glomerulitis in >75% of glomeruli.

e. Quantitative criteria for peritubular capillaritis ("ptc"):
- ptc0: At least one leukocyte in <10% of cortical peritubular capillaries and/or maximum number of leukocytes <3.
- ptc1: At least one leukocyte cell in ≥10% of cortical peritubular capillaries with 3–4 leukocytes in most severely involved peritubular capillaries.
- ptc2: At least one leukocyte in ≥10% of cortical peritubular capillaries with 5–10 leukocytes in most severely involved peritubular capillaries.
- ptc3: At least one leukocyte in ≥10% of cortical peritubular capillaries with >10 leukocytes in most severely involved peritubular capillaries. The extent of PTC inflammation should be documented as focal (10–50%) or diffuse (>50%).

f. Quantitative criteria for C4d score:
   - C4d0: No staining of peritubular capillaries and medullary vasa recta (0%).
   - C4d1: Minimal C4d staining (>0 but <10% of peritubular capillaries and medullary vasa recta).
   - C4d2: Focal C4d staining (10–50% of peritubular capillaries and medullary vasa recta).
   - C4d3: Diffuse C4d staining (>50% of peritubular capillaries and medullary vasa recta).

2. Chronic Banff scores:
   a. Quantitative criteria for interstitial fibrosis ("ci"):
      - ci0: Interstitial fibrosis in up to 5% of cortical area.
      - ci1: Interstitial fibrosis in 6–25% of cortical area (mild interstitial fibrosis).
      - ci2: Interstitial fibrosis in 26–50% of cortical area (moderate interstitial fibrosis).
      - ci3: Interstitial fibrosis in >50% of cortical area (severe interstitial fibrosis).
   b. Quantitative criteria for tubular atrophy ("ct"):
      - ct0: No tubular atrophy.
      - ct1: Tubular atrophy in up to 25% of the area of cortical tubules (mild tubular atrophy).
      - ct2: Tubular atrophy involving 26–50% of the area of cortical tubules (moderate tubular atrophy).
      - ct3: Tubular atrophy involving >50% of the area of cortical tubules (severe tubular atrophy).
   c. Quantitative criteria for vascular fibrous intimal thickening ("cv"):
      - cv0: No chronic vascular changes.
      - cv1: Vascular narrowing of up to 25% luminal area by fibrointimal thickening.
      - cv2: Vascular narrowing of 26–50% luminal area by fibrointimal thickening.
      - cv3: Vascular narrowing of >50% luminal area by fibrointimal thickening.
   d. Quantitative criteria for double contour ("cg"):
      - cg0: No glomerular basement membrane (GBM) double contours by light microscopy (LM) or electron microscopy (EM).
      - cg1a: No GBM double contours by LM but GBM double contours (incomplete or circumferential) in at least three

glomerular capillaries by EM, with associated endothelial swelling and/or subendothelial electron-lucent widening.
- cg1b: Double contours of the GBM in 1–25% of capillary loops in the most affected nonsclerotic glomerulus by LM; EM confirmation is recommended if EM is available.
- cg2: Double contours affecting 26–50% of peripheral capillary loops in the most affected glomerulus.
- cg3: Double contours affecting >50% of peripheral capillary loops in the most affected glomerulus.

e. Peritubular capillary basement membrane multilayering score ("ptcml") (requires electron microscopy, stated as NA if not performed):
- pctml0: Not meeting below criteria.
- pctml1: ≥7 basement membrane layers in the most affected PTC and ≥5 layers in two additional PTCs.

3. Acute and chronic Banff Scores:

a. Quantitative criteria for total inflammation ("ti"):
- ti0: No, or trivial interstitial inflammation (<10% of total cortical parenchyma).
- ti1: 10–25% of total cortical parenchyma inflamed.
- ti2: 26–50% of total cortical parenchyma inflamed.
- ti3: >50% of total cortical parenchyma inflamed.

b. Quantitative criteria for inflammation in areas of interstitial fibrosis and tubular atrophy (i-IFTA score):
- i-IFTA0: No inflammation or <10% of scarred cortical parenchyma.
- i-IFTA1: Inflammation in 10–25% of scarred cortical parenchyma.
- i-IFTA2: Inflammation in 26–50% of scarred cortical parenchyma.
- i-IFTA3: Inflammation in >50% of scarred cortical parenchyma.

c. Quantitative criteria for tubulitis in area of cortex with interstitial fibrosis and tubular atrophy (t-IFTA score):
- t-IFTA0: No mononuclear leucocytes per tubular cross-section.
- t-IFTA1: 1–4 mononuclear leukocytes per tubular cross-section or 10 tubular epithelial cells in most severely involved tubule.

- t-IFTA2: 5–10 mononuclear leukocytes in most severely involved tubule.
- t-IFTA3: >10 mononuclear leukocytes in most severely involved tubule.

4. Other descriptive lesions of uncertain significance, not included in the Banff 2017 classification:
   a. Quantitative criteria for mesangial matrix increase ("mm"):
      - mm0: No more than mild mesangial matrix increase in any glomerulus.
      - mm1: At least moderate mesangial matrix increase in up to 25% of non-sclerotic glomeruli.
      - mm2: At least moderate mesangial matrix increase in 26–50% of non-sclerotic glomeruli.
      - mm3: At least moderate mesangial matrix increase in >50% of non-sclerotic glomeruli.
   b. Quantitative criteria for arteriolar hyalinosis ("ah"):
      - ah0: No Periodic acid-Schiff (PAS)-positive hyaline arteriolar thickening.
      - ah1: Mild to moderate PAS-positive hyaline thickening in at least 1 arteriole.
      - ah2: Moderate to severe PAS-positive hyaline thickening in >1 arteriole.
      - ah3: Severe PAS-positive hyaline thickening in many arterioles.
   c. Alternative quantitative criteria for hyaline arteriolar thickening ("aah"):
      - aah0: No typical lesions of calcineurin inhibitor-related arteriolopathy.
      - aah1: Replacement of degenerated smooth muscle cells by hyaline deposits in only 1 arteriole, without circumferential involvement.
      - aah2: Replacement of degenerated smooth muscle cells by hyaline deposits in >1 arteriole, without circumferential involvement.
      - aah3: Replacement of degenerated smooth muscle cells by hyaline deposits with circumferential involvement, independent of the number of arterioles involved.

II. Revised Banff 2017 classification (with updates in 2019):

1. Normal or non-specific changes.
2. Antibody-mediated rejection (ABMR):
   a. Active ABMR (all 3 features must be present for diagnosis):
      i. Histologic evidence of acute tissue injury, including one or more of the following:
         - Microvascular inflammation (g score >0 and/or ptc score >0), in the absence of recurrent or *de novo* glomerulonephritis, although in the presence of acute T-cell mediated rejection (TCMR), borderline infiltrate, or infection, ptc ≥1 alone is not sufficient and g must be ≥1.
         - Intimal or transmural arteritis (v score >0).
         - Acute thrombotic microangiopathy, in the absence of any other cause.
         - Acute tubular injury, in the absence of any other apparent cause.
      ii. Evidence of current/recent antibody interaction with vascular endothelium, including at least one of the following:
         - Linear C4d staining in peritubular capillaries or medullary vasa recta (C4d2 or C4d3 by immunofluorescence on frozen sections, or C4d>0 by immunohistochemistry on paraffin sections).
         - At least moderate microvascular inflammation (sum of g and ptc scores ≥2), in the absence of recurrent or *de novo* glomerulonephritis, although in the presence of acute TCMR, borderline infiltrate or infection, ptc ≥2 alone is not sufficient, and g must be ≥1.
         - Increased expression of gene transcripts/classifiers in the biopsy tissue strongly associated with AMR, if thoroughly validated.
      iii. Serologic evidence of donor-specific antibodies (DSA to HLA or other antigens):
         - C4d staining or expression of validated transcripts/classifiers as noted in criterion (ii) may substitute for DSA.
         - Thorough DSA testing, including testing for non-HLA antibodies if HLA antibody testing is negative, is strongly advised whenever criteria 2(a)(i) and 2(a)(ii) are met.

b. Chronic active AMR (all 3 features must be present for diagnosis):
   i. Morphologic evidence of chronic tissue injury, including one or more of the following:
      - Transplant glomerulopathy (TG) (cg >0), if no evidence of chronic thrombotic microangiopathy or chronic recurrent/*de novo* glomerulonephritis; includes changes evident by EM alone (cg1a).
      - Severe peritubular capillary basement membrane multilayering (ptcml1; requires EM).
      - New onset arterial intimal fibrosis, excluding other causes; leukocytes within the sclerotic intima favor chronic AMR if there is no prior history of TCMR, but are not required.
   ii. Identical to criterion 2(a)(ii) for active AMR above.
   iii. Identical to criterion 2(a)(iii) for active AMR above, including strong recommendation for DSA testing whenever criteria 2(b)(i) and 2(b)(ii) are met.
      - Biopsies meeting criterion 2(b)(i), but not criterion 2(b)(ii) with current or prior evidence of DSA (post-transplant) may be stated as showing **chronic AMR**.
      - Remote DSA should not be considered for diagnosis of chronic active or active AMR.

c. Chronic (inactive) AMR:
   i. cg >0 and/or severe ptcml (ptcml1).
   ii. Absence of criterion 2(a)(ii) of current/recent antibody interaction with the endothelium.
   iii. Prior documented diagnosis of active or chronic active AMR and/or documented prior evidence of DSA.

d. C4d staining without evidence of rejection (all 4 features must be present for diagnosis):
   i. Linear C4d staining in peritubular capillaries (C4d2 or C4d3 by immunofluorescence on frozen sections, or C4d >0 by immunohistochemistry on paraffin sections).
   ii. Histologic criteria for active or chronic active AMR, e.g., criterion 2(a)(i) or 2(b)(i), not met.
   iii. No molecular evidence for active and chronic active AMR, e.g., criterion 2(a)(ii) or 2(b)(ii).
   iv. No acute or chronic active TCMR or borderline changes.

3. Borderline (suspicious) for acute TCMR:
   a. Foci of tubulitis (t1, t2 or t3) with mild interstitial inflammation (i1), or mild (t1) tubulitis with moderate-severe interstitial inflammation (i2 or i3).
   b. No intimal or transmural arteritis (v = 0).
4. T-cell mediated rejection (TCMR):
   a. Acute TCMR (Grade):
      IA. Cases with significant interstitial infiltration (>25% of parenchyma affected, i2 or i3) and foci of moderate tubulitis (t2) involving 1 or more tubules, not including tubules that are severely atrophic.
      IB. Cases with significant interstitial infiltration (>25% of parenchyma affected, i2 or i3) and foci of severe tubulitis (t3) involving 1 or more tubules, not including tubules that are severely atrophic.
      IIA. Cases with mild to moderate intimal arteritis (v1), with or without interstitial inflammation and/or tubulitis.
      IIB. Cases with severe intimal arteritis (v2), with or without interstitial inflammation and/or tubulitis.
      III. Transmural arteritis and/or arterial fibrinoid necrosis of medial smooth muscle with accompanying mononuclear cell intimal arteritis (v3), with or without interstitial inflammation and/or tubulitis.
   b. Chronic active TCMR (Grade):
      IA. Interstitial inflammation involving >25% of the sclerotic cortical parenchyma (i-IFTA2 or i-IFTA3) and >25% of the total cortical parenchyma (ti2 or ti3) with moderate tubulitis (t2 or t-IFTA2) involving 1 or more tubules, not including severely atrophic tubules; other known causes of i-IFTA should be ruled out.
      IB. Interstitial inflammation involving >25% of the sclerotic cortical parenchyma (i-IFTA2 or i-IFTA3) and >25% of the total cortical parenchyma (ti2 or ti3) with severe tubulitis (t3 or t-IFTA3) involving 1 or more tubules, not including severely atrophic tubules; other known causes of i-IFTA should be excluded.

II. Chronic allograft arteriopathy (arterial intimal fibrosis with mononuclear cell inflammation in fibrosis and formation of neointima).
   - May also be a manifestation of chronic active or chronic AMR or mixed AMR/TCMR.

D. Treatment of Acute Cellular Rejection

I. First rejection:

1. Pulse glucocorticoids (GC):
   a. High intravenous (IV) doses of GC reverse about 60–70% of first acute rejections.
   b. IV methylprednisolone (MP) 10 mg/kg/dose (maximum 1 g) given over 30–60 minutes for 3 days.
      - Give IV furosemide 0.5–2.0 mg/kg (depending on kidney function) prior to the MP infusion.
   c. Change to oral prednisolone (PNL) after completing the pulse GC:
      - Start PNL at 0.5–1 mg/kg/day and taper over 2 weeks to the previous level.
   d. High maintenance doses of PNL are not indicated.
   e. A successful response to treatment is achieved when there is decrease in serum creatinine to within 10% of the baseline creatinine (before rejection) during the first 5–7 days of treatment.
   f. Steroid-resistance: Lack of improvement in the plasma creatinine concentration defined as ≥Day 0 creatinine level after 7 days following institution of anti-rejection treatment.
   g. Repeat kidney biopsy is warranted in steroid-resistant rejections, and second-line antibody therapy is advised.
2. Anti-thymocyte globulin (ATG) treatment:
   a. ATG is effective for the management of first acute rejection.
      - Can reverse about 90% of first rejections.
   b. Indications:
      i. First-line option (in addition to pulse MP) for TCMR Banff grade ≥IIB, or for first episode of rejection unresponsive to pulse MP.

   ii. Considered in TCMR Banff grade ≥IB with severe allograft dysfunction, especially in the first year post-transplant.
  c. Dose: Rabbit ATG (Thymoglobulin®) 1.5 mg/kg day for a total dose of 5–10.5 mg/kg depending on the severity of Banff grading:
   - Grade 1B: 1.5 mg/kg daily for 2 days or 3 mg/kg single dose.
   - Grade 2A/B: 1.5 mg/kg daily for 3–5 days.
   - Grade 3: 1.5 mg/kg daily for 5–7 days.
  d. Titrate dose (increase or decrease dose by 20%) to achieve absolute lymphocyte count 0.1–0.2 × 10^9/L or CD3 levels <1%.
  e. Reduce the dose of mycophenolate by 50% while on ATG.
  f. Antimicrobial prophylaxis and viral surveillance are recommended following treatment with ATG (see Section G).
3. Intensification of maintenance immunosuppressive agents (see Section F).
4. Monitoring response to treatment:
  a. Serum creatinine daily during inpatient treatment with pulse GC and/or ATG.
  b. After discharge, monitor serum creatinine weekly until it has returned to baseline level (prior to the episode of rejection) or until it plateaus at a new baseline level, after which routine monitoring of kidney function can resume.

II. Recurrent and/or refractory rejection:

1. Pulse GC:
  a. For clinically mild and less severe rejection episodes.
  b. Repeated courses of steroids may be effective in reversing acute rejections.
   - Do not exceed more than 2 courses of pulse GC therapy, after which consider antibody treatment.
2. Antibody treatment (ATG):
  a. Indicated for rejection episodes that are steroid-resistant.
  b. Start antibody treatment early if the kidney function is deteriorating rapidly.
  c. Second course of depletional antibodies can be given in selected patients, and long-term graft function can be achieved in 40–50% of such patients.

d. Risk-benefit ratio of the severity and the potential reversibility of rejection must be weighed against the risk for infection and malignancy, particularly if the two courses are given close together.

III. Late rejections:

1. Late rejection is one that occurs more than 3–4 months after transplantation and may be a first, or more frequently, a recurrent rejection.
2. Late rejection may occur:
   a. As a result of inadequate immunosuppression (commonly in nonadherent patients)
   b. Despite adequate immunosuppression.
3. Late rejections are often a prelude to chronic rejection and accelerated graft loss, and the histologic findings are often mixed.
4. Treatment with pulse GC is more likely to be successful in late rejections associated with nonadherence.

E. Treatment of Antibody-Mediated Rejection

I. Clinical phenotypes:

Timing	Early Acute (≤30 Days Post-transplant)	Late (>30 Days Post-transplant)	
DSA	Preexisting DSA (or non-immunologically naïve)	Preexisting DSA	*De novo* DSA
Histology	Banff 2017 active AMR Usually C4d+ TMA often present	Banff 2017 active or chronic active AMR May be Cd4±	Banff 2017 active or chronic active AMR May be Cd4± Concomitant TCMR often present

(Continued)

(Continued)

Timing	Early Acute (≤30 Days Post-transplant)	Late (>30 Days Post-transplant)	
Clinical presentation	Abrupt allograft dysfunction correlating with increased DSA MFI or titer usually 7–10 days post-transplant	± Allograft dysfunction and proteinuria	± Allograft dysfunction and proteinuria
Pathophysiology	Memory B-cell response	Pre-existing plasma cell response	Under-immunosuppression
Prognosis	Graft loss within days if not treated	Graft loss within months to years	Graft loss within months to years
Features associated with reduced allograft survival	Pre-transplant crossmatch (+T-AHG-CDC+ or high-flow cytometric crossmatch)	Histological: ▪ Banff cg >0 lesion ▪ Degree of IFTA ▪ Concomitant TCMR ▪ Banff cv score >0 ▪ Cd4 positivity Clinical: ▪ Proteinuria ▪ Allograft dysfunction ▪ Years post-transplant ▪ Patient nonadherence ▪ Immunosuppression reduction DSA characteristics: ▪ C1q-positive DSA ▪ High DSA MFI or titer and pre-transplant crossmatch ▪ Anti-class II DSA	

II. Clinical and pathologic recognition of AMR:

1. Rising creatinine.
2. High resistive index on graft kidney Doppler ultrasound.

3. Inflammatory changes on allograft biopsy.
4. Positive C4d.
    - Up to 60% of chronic AMR may be C4d negative.
5. Positive DSA:
    - Pre-existing.
    - *De novo*.

III. Treatment of active AMR with mild clinical features:

1. Clinical and pathological criteria:
    a. Allograft dysfunction.
    b. Associated with risk factors for AMR:
        i. DSA positivity.
        ii. History of sensitization.
        iii. Previous transplants and transfusions.
    c. Biopsy:
        i. Focal C4d+ staining.
        ii. Minimal pathologic features:
            - Acute tubular necrosis (ATN)-like minimal changes.
            - Absence of microvascular inflammation, arteritis and thrombotic microangiopathy.
2. Treatment protocol:
    a. IV MP 10 mg/kg × 3 days.
    b. IVIG 2 g/kg (maximum 140 g) on Day 1, then repeat on Days 30–60.
    c. IV Rituximab 375 mg/m^2/dose on Day 2.

IV. Treatment of active AMR with severe clinical features:

1. Clinical and pathological criteria:
    a. Rapid cessation of kidney function post-transplant.
    b. Associated with DSA positivity.
    c. Biopsy:
        i. Diffuse C4d+ staining.
        ii. Evidence of capillary and/or glomerular inflammation with thrombosis (thrombotic microangiopathy).

2. Treatment protocol:
   a. IV MP 10 mg/kg × 3 days.
   b. Early plasmapheresis to remove antibodies and other inflammatory mediators.
      i. Daily, or alternate day × 6 on Days 1, 3, 5, 7, 9, and 11 based on DSA titer, with albumin and fresh frozen plasma replacement.
      ii. Each session consists of 1.5-plasma volume removal.
   c. IVIG 2 g/kg (maximum of 140 g) is given on Day 12 at the completion of plasmapheresis.
   d. IV Rituximab 375 mg/m^2 is given on Day 13 following completion of plasmapheresis and IVIG.
3. If the allograft biopsy shows concurrent histologic evidence of both AMR and acute TCMR (Banff grade ≥2A), ATG should be added to the above treatment regime.
   - 3 doses of ATG 1.5 mg/kg/dose can be given on Days 2, 4 and 6.
4. Response to therapy:
   a. Most patients with active AMR with a successful response to anti-rejection therapy will demonstrate improvement in serum creatinine within 7 days of treatment.
   b. If there is no improvement in serum creatinine after completing the above treatment regime, a repeat kidney allograft biopsy should be performed.
   c. If repeat kidney biopsy shows evidence of persistent active AMR, second-line agents can be used as rescue therapy.
5. Second-line agents:
   a. Consider IV Eculizumab 1–4 doses (see chapter "Eculizumab (Anti-C5 Monoclonal Antibody) Therapy for Complement-Mediated Injury").
      - If patient has not had meningococcal vaccine, immunize on Day 1 and give antibiotic prophylaxis for at least 2 weeks.
   b. Other treatment options: Bortezomib.

V. Treatment of chronic active AMR:

1. Goals of therapy:
   a. Stabilize kidney function, proteinuria and histological injury score.

   b. Reduce DSA titers.
   c. Optimize baseline immunosuppression therapy and treat any concomitant TCMR.
   d. Minimize drug toxicity.
2. Treatment protocol:
   a. IV MP 10 mg/kg × 3 days.
   b. IVIG 1 g/kg given weekly × 4 doses.
   c. IV Rituximab 375 mg/m^2 is given on Day 30.
   d. If DSA remains high despite the IVIG treatment, consider using Tocilizumab:
      i. IV Tocilizumab 8 mg/kg monthly for 6 months.
      ii. Screen for tuberculosis with a chest X-Ray and Mantoux test prior to institution of Tocilizumab treatment.

VI. Monitoring of response:

1. Monitor:
   a. Serum creatinine daily during active treatment, then weekly till the new baseline is reached, then 2-weekly for 1 month, then monthly.
   b. Proteinuria at least monthly.
   c. DSA after treatment course and subsequently monthly for 3 months, then 3–6-monthly.
2. Patients are considered to have successful reversal of AMR if all of the following parameters are met within 3 months of treatment:
   a. Decrease in serum creatinine to within 20–30% of baseline level.
   b. Decrease in proteinuria to baseline level.
   c. Decrease in immunodominant DSA >50%.
   d. Resolution of changes associated with AMR on repeat biopsy.
3. For chronic AMR, monitor:
   a. Blood pressure and proteinuria at each clinic visit.
   b. Bone health 1–3 monthly depending on stage of chronic kidney disease: Calcium, phosphate, vitamin D, alkaline phosphatase, parathyroid hormone.
   c. Blood glucose, glycated hemoglobin (HbA1c) and lipid levels at least 6-monthly.

F. Intensification of Baseline Immunosuppression

1. Change to oral PNL after completing the pulse GC:
   - Start PNL at 0.5–1 mg/kg/day and taper over 2 weeks to the previous baseline dose.
2. Check if the patient is receiving adequate doses of Tac or mycophenolate (MPA) and adjust the dose accordingly.
   a. Target higher Tac trough levels (5–7 μg/L) in patients whose tacrolimus trough levels are in the lower range (3–5 μg/L).

Period Post-transplant	Tac Trough Level (μg/L)
First 2 weeks	10–12
2 weeks to 3 months	8–10
4–6 months	7–9
>6 months	5–7 (minimum 4)

   b. Consider doing Tac pharmacokinetic studies (see chapter "Immunosuppressive Medications" for AUC formula):

Period Post-transplant	AUC (μg-h/L)
0–1 months	175–250
1–3 months	100–175
>3 months	75–100

   c. In patients on cyclosporine (CSA), switch to Tac (see chapter "Sequential Immunosuppression Protocol for Kidney Transplantation").
   d. Check adequacy of MPA levels (see chapter "Immunosuppressive Medications" for AUC formula):
      - Target MPA AUC 30–60 mg-h/L.

G. Immunosurveillance/Prophylaxis for Opportunistic Infection

I. Viral monitoring:

1. CMV surveillance is recommended following ATG treatment:

a. CMV PCR for "positive donor to negative recipient" on:
   - Day 1, then weekly for Month 1, biweekly for Month 2, and then monthly for 1 year.

b. CMV PCR for "positive donor to positive recipient" on:
   - Day 1, then monthly for 1 year.

2. EBV surveillance is recommended following ATG treatment:
   a. Seronegative recipient.
      - Monthly EBV PCR for the first year, 3-monthly for the second year, 6-monthly till seroconversion, then yearly.
      - Monthly liver panel, GGT for the first 6 months, then 3-monthly up to 1-year post-transplant.
   b. Seropositive recipient:
      - 3-monthly EBV PCR for the first year, then yearly.
3. Monitor for polyomavirus-associated nephropathy in all patients treated for rejection:
   - BK virus PCR on Day 1 and monthly thereafter for 9 months, then 3-monthly for 2 years post-rejection treatment.

II. Antimicrobial prophylaxis:

1. CMV prophylaxis for patients who receive ATG:
   a. Oral valganciclovir:
      - For 6 months in donor CMV-positive, recipient CMV negative (D+R–).
      - For 3 months in recipient CMV-positive (R+).
   b. Consider the addition of immunoglobulin as an adjunct to antiviral prophylaxis.
   c. Dosing regimen (see chapter "Sequential Immunosuppression Protocol for Kidney Transplantation").
2. *Pneumocystis jirovecii* pneumonia prophylaxis:
   a. Prophylaxis duration:
      - 3 months for patients treated with ATG or Rituximab.
      - 6 months for those who received both ATG and Rituximab.
      - 12 months for those who received mTOR inhibitor for maintenance therapy.
   b. Dosing options:
      - Co-trimoxazole oral 3 mg/kg/dose on alternate days.

- Check glucose-6-phosphate dehydrogenase (G6PD) status and use aerosolized pentamidine 300 mg monthly (via Respigard nebulizer) in G6PD-deficient patients.
- Dapsone 2 mg/kg daily (maximum 100 mg) for patients who are allergic to co-trimoxazole.

3. Fungal prophylaxis for patients receiving ATG
   a. Nystatin oral for 1 month.
      - Dose: 250000 U 8 hourly.
   b. Consider oral fluconazole if *Candida* sp. is isolated.
      - Dose: 3 mg/kg/day (maximum dose 100 mg daily).
      - Check CNI levels due to drug interactions.

H. Cessation of Therapy

1. The decision to stop therapy in recurrent rejection is difficult but important and is determined by the overall clinical status of the patient.
2. Cessation of therapy is recommended in the following situations:
   a. A concurrent infectious process represents undue risk with further intensification of immunosuppression.
   b. There is no evidence of response following an intense course of treatment with agents such as ATG, nor evidence of ABMR on repeat biopsy (which would dictate an alternate treatment regiment); there should not be apparent extenuating etiologies for continued kidney failure.
   c. Repeat kidney biopsy shows nonviable kidney tissue.
      - If there is little evidence of a reversible process, the risk of infection and malignancy resulting from high-dose immunosuppression probably outweighs any benefit.

Recommended Reading

1. Vo AA, Lukovsky M, Toyoda M, Wang J, Reinsmoen NL, Lai CH, Peng A, Villicana R, Jordan SC. (2008) Rituximab and intravenous immune globulin for desensitization during renal transplantation. *N Engl J Med* **359**:242–251.
2. Jordan SC, Reinsmoen N, Peng A, Lai CH, Cao K, Villicana R, Toyoda M, Kahwaji J, Vo AA. (2010) Advances in diagnosing and managing antibody-mediated rejection. *Pediatr Nephrol* **25**:2035–2045.

3. Pape L, Becker JU, Immenschuh S, Ahlenstiel T. (2015) Acute and chronic antibody-mediated rejection in pediatric kidney transplantation. *Pediatr Nephrol* **30**:417–424.
4. Haas M, Loupy A, Lefaucheur C, Roufosse C, Glotz D, Seron D, Nankivell BJ, Halloran PF, Colvin RB, Akalin E, Alachkar N, Bagnasco S, Bouatou Y, Becker JU, Cornell LD, Duong van Huyen JP, Gibson IW, Kraus ES, Mannon RB, Naesens M, Nickeleit V, Nickerson P, Segev DL, Singh HK, Stegall M, Randhawa P, Racusen L, Solez K, Mengel M. (2018) The Banff 2017 Kidney Meeting Report: Revised diagnostic criteria for chronic active T cell-mediated rejection, antibody-mediated rejection, and prospects for integrative endpoints for next-generation clinical trials. *Am J Transplant* **18**:293–307.
5. Loupy A, Haas M, Roufosse C, Naesens M, Adam B, Afrouzian M, Akalin E, Alachkar N, Bagnasco S, Becker JU, Cornell LD, Clahsen-van Groningen MC, Demetris AJ, Dragun D, Duong van Huyen JP, Farris AB, Fogo AB, Gibson IW, Glotz D, Gueguen J, Kikic Z, Kozakowski N, Kraus E, Lefaucheur C, Liapis H, Mannon RB, Montgomery RA, Nankivell BJ, Nickeleit V, Nickerson P, Rabant M, Racusen L, Randhawa P, Robin B, Rosales IA, Sapir-Pichhadze R, Schinstock CA, Seron D, Singh HK, Smith RN, Stegall MD, Zeevi A, Solez K, Colvin RB, Mengel M. (2020) The Banff 2019 Kidney Meeting Report (I): Updates on and clarification of criteria for T cell- and antibody-mediated rejection. *Am J Transplant* **20**:2318–2331.
6. Brennan DC, Malone A. (2020, updated) Treatment of acute T-cell mediated (cellular) rejection of the renal allograft. Edited by: Legendre C, Vella, J, Lam AQ. *UpToDate ONLINE.* http://www.uptodateonline.com.
7. Djamali A, Brennan DC. (2020, updated) Prevention and treatment of antibody-mediated rejection of the renal allograft. Edited by: Legendre C, Lam AQ. *UpToDate ONLINE.* http://www.uptodateonline.com.
8. Brennan DC, Alhamad T, Malone A. (2020, updated) Clinical features and diagnosis of acute renal allograft rejection. Edited by: Legendre C, Lam AQ. *UpToDate ONLINE.* http://www.uptodateonline.com.
9. Cooper JE. (2020) Evaluation and treatment of acute rejection in kidney allografts. *Clin J Am Soc Nephrol* **15**:430–438.
10. Schinstock CA, Mannon RB, Budde K, Chong AS, Haas M, Knechtle S, Lefaucheur C, Montgomery RA, Nickerson P, Tullius SG, Ahn C, Askar M, Crespo M, Chadban SJ, Feng S, Jordan SC, Man K, Mengel M, Morris RE, O'Doherty I, Ozdemir BH, Seron D, Tambur AR, Tanabe K, Taupin JL, O'Connell PJ. (2020) Recommended treatment for antibody-mediated rejection after kidney transplantation: The 2019 Expert Consensus from the Transplantation Society Working Group. *Transplantation* **104**:911–922.

11 Management of Cytomegalovirus Disease in Kidney Transplantation

Lau PYW, Arias-Briones AR, Teo S, Koh LJ and Yap HK

A. Definitions

1. Cytomegalovirus (CMV) infection is defined by the presence of CMV replication regardless of symptoms, and is considered present if one or more of the following findings is noted:
   a. Seroconversion with the appearance of anti-CMV IgM antibodies.
   b. Fourfold increase in pre-existing anti-CMV IgG titers.
   c. CMV antigenemia assay (pp65).
   d. Detection of CMV-DNAemia or CMV-RNAemia by molecular techniques.
   e. Isolation of the virus in cultures of the throat, buffy coat, or urine (CMV viremia).

   Note: Infection can be asymptomatic or symptomatic (CMV disease).
2. CMV disease is defined by CMV infection accompanied by clinical signs and symptoms:
   a. CMV syndrome defined by the detection of CMV in the blood and at least 2 of the following:
      - Fever ≥38°C for at least 2 days.
      - New or increased malaise or fatigue.
      - Leukopenia or neutropenia on 2 separate measurements.
      - 5% atypical lymphocytes.
      - Thrombocytopenia.
      - Hepatic aminotransferases increase to 2x the upper limit of normal.

   b. Tissue-invasive CMV disease including:
      - Hepatitis.

- Pneumonitis.
- Pancreatitis.
- Enteritis and/or colitis.
- Meningoencephalitis.
- Chorioretinitis.
- Myocarditis.
- Nephritis.

Note: For proven or definite tissue-invasive CMV disease, there must be documentation of CMV in the tissues by virus isolation, rapid culture, histopathology, immunohistochemistry, or DNA hybridization.

3. Refractory CMV infection:
   a. Proven or definite:
      - CMV DNAemia or antigenemia increasing (>10 times increase in blood CMV DNA from baseline viral load) after at least 2 weeks of appropriately dosed antiviral treatment.
   b. Probable:
      - Viral load persistence (blood CMV titers at the same level, or <10 times of the baseline viral load) after at least 2 weeks of appropriately dosed antiviral treatment.
4. Refractory CMV disease:
   a. Proven or definite:
      - Worsening signs and symptoms, or progression to end-organ disease after at least 2 weeks of appropriately dosed antiviral treatment.
   b. Probable:
      - Lack of improvement in clinical signs and symptoms after at least 2 weeks of appropriately dosed antiviral treatment.
5. Resistant CMV:
   - Presence of viral genetic alteration that confers reduced susceptibility to one or more antiviral drugs

B. Risk Factors

1. Pre-transplant risk stratification: Donors and transplant recipients should be tested for baseline CMV immune status using CMV-IgG serology prior to transplant.
   a. High risk: Donor positive/recipient negative.

b. Intermediate risk: Donor positive or negative/recipient positive.
c. Low risk: Donor negative/recipient negative.
   - *De novo* CMV infection occurs in 7% of patients in the first year post-transplant.

2. Prolonged cold ischemia time.
3. Leukopenia and lymphopenia.
4. Immunosuppressive state, particularly lymphocyte-depleting agents such as anti-thymocyte globulin (ATG) and alemtuzumab or high doses of maintenance immunosuppressive drugs.
5. Other concurrent infections such as bacteremia, invasive fungal disease, and Epstein–Barr virus-associated post-transplant lymphoproliferative disease (PTLD).

C. Laboratory Investigations

I. Diagnosis of CMV infection:

1. Consider CMV infection as an etiologic agent in the context of chronic allograft nephropathy of unexplained cause.
2. CMV serology (IgG or IgM):
   a. High IgM or four-fold increase of IgG in immunocompetent host indicates acute or recent infection.
   b. Standard test to screen transplant candidates and potential donors for previous exposure to CMV to determine the risk category of post-transplant CMV disease and the type of CMV prevention strategy.
   c. Limited utility in diagnosis of CMV infection post-transplant due to the inability to mount an antibody response because of immunosuppression.
      - May be used after transplant to determine ongoing susceptibility amongst CMV-seronegative recipients.

   d. False positives may be seen in passive transfer of CMV antibodies following a recent blood transfusion of blood products or IV immunoglobulin, or from transplacental transfer of maternal CMV-IgG antibodies.

3. Molecular tests:
   a. Performed by semiquantitative polymerase chain reaction (PCR) or quantitative nucleic acid testing (QNAT) assays.
   b. CMV viral load is higher in whole blood than in plasma.
      - Serial CMV monitoring should use one sample type, either plasma or whole blood.
   c. CMV QNAT informs on viral load:
      i. High CMV viral load is associated with tissue-invasive disease.
      ii. Tissue-invasive disease can be diagnosed by:
         - CMV QNAT in bronchoalveolar lavage (BAL) fluid: CMV pneumonia.
         - CMV QNAT in cerebrospinal fluid (CSF): Central nervous system CMV disease.

      Note: CMV QNAT of urine should not be used for diagnosis and surveillance of CMV-positive recipients.
      iii. Negative or low CMV viral load despite tissue-invasive disease can occur due to CMV disease compartmentalization, in particular, CMV retinitis and some cases of gastrointestinal CMV disease without systemic dissemination.
      iv. The faster the CMV viral load rises, the higher the risk of CMV disease.
   d. CMV RNA is indicative of active CMV replication.
4. CMV antigenomia assay in peripheral blood leukocytes (neutrophils):
      i. pp65 antigen has good sensitivity but limited utility in leukopenic patients.
      ii. Main disadvantage is the need to process the clinical sample within a few hours due to the short lifespan of neutrophils.
5. Viral culture:
   a. From blood (buffy coat), bronchoalveolar lavage (BAL), or tissue biopsy.
   b. Turnaround time is too slow for clinical decision-making and supplanted by molecular tests.
6. Histopathology:
   a. Helps to confirm the diagnosis of tissue-invasive CMV disease, especially if the clinical suspicion of CMV disease is high despite a negative molecular test or pp65 antigenemia.
   b. Kidney biopsy may help to differentiate tissue-invasive disease from concomitant graft rejection.

II. Evaluation of tissue-invasive disease:

1. Full blood count.
2. Erythrocyte sedimentation rate.
3. C-reactive protein.
4. Liver panel: Albumin, alanine aminotransaminase (ALT), aspartate aminotransferase (AST), gamma-glutamyltranspeptidase (GGT), and bilirubin.
5. Kidney function assessment: Urea, creatinine, sodium, potassium, chloride, and bicarbonate.
6. Chest X-Ray.
7. Ophthalmology screen.

III. Risk stratification of CMV disease:

1. Absolute lymphocyte count and CD4+/CD8+ T-cell subsets.
2. Total IgG levels.
   - Hypogammaglobulinemia is associated with CMV disease.
3. Nonspecific (mitogen-stimulated) T-cell immune responses.
4. CMV-specific CD8+ and/or CD4+ T cell immunity, e.g., interferon-gamma release assay, enzyme-linked immunosorbent spot (ELISPOT) assay.

D. Treatment

I. Ganciclovir/Valganciclovir:

1. For mild-to-moderate CMV disease, oral valganciclovir and IV ganciclovir are equally effective initial therapies.
2. Antiviral treatment of CMV disease should be continued until the following criteria are met:
   a. Resolution of clinical symptoms AND
   b. Virologic clearance below a threshold-negative value based on weekly laboratory monitoring (e.g., at least two consecutive negative weekly CMV PCR) AND
   c. Minimum 2 weeks of antiviral treatment.
3. IV ganciclovir is recommended initial treatment for:
   a. Severe or life-threatening CMV disease.
   b. Patients with very high viral load.
   c. Patients with questionable gastrointestinal absorption.

Note: Daily IV Ganciclovir should be given for a minimum of 2 weeks at a full dose adjusted for kidney function.

4. Can consider switching IV ganciclovir to oral valganciclovir at treatment doses once there is adequate clinical and virologic control.
5. Antiviral drug dosing should not be adjusted down due to leukopenia or pancytopenia as suboptimal dosing may be associated with an increased risk of clinical failure and/or resistance.
   - If there is neutropenia (absolute neutrophil count $<1.0 \times 10^9$/L), consider giving granulocyte-colony stimulating factor (GCSF) till an absolute neutrophil count of $\geq 1.5 \times 10^9$/L.
6. Antiviral drug dosing should be adjusted based on kidney function.
   a. IV Ganciclovir (treatment dose):

Creatinine Clearance (ml/min/1.73m^2)	Dose	Frequency
>70	5 mg/kg/dose	12 hourly
50–69	2.5 mg/kg/dose	12 hourly
25–49	2.5 mg/kg/dose	24 hourly
10–24	1.25 mg/kg/dose	24 hourly
<10	1.25 mg/kg/dose	3×/week (dose after hemodialysis)

   b. Valganciclovir (treatment dose):
      i. 1 capsule = 450 mg.
      ii. Dosing in children should be based on body surface área (BSA) and kidney function.
      iii. Recommended dosage:

Creatinine Clearance (ml/min/1.73m^2)	Dose Adult (Pediatric)	Frequency
≥60	900 mg (30 mg/kg/dose)	BD
40–59	450 mg	BD
25–39	450 mg	OD
10–24	450 mg	EOD
<10	200 mg suspension	3×/week (dose after hemodialysis)

OR

Pediatric dosing equivalent to 900 mg/dose (4 months to 16 years old)

= 900/125 × BSA x GFR (ml/min/1.73m^2)

= 7 × BSA × GFR (ml/min/1.73m^2)

(Ettenger *et al.*, 2003)

Note: If calculated GFR exceeds 150 ml/min/1.73m^2, then a maximum-calculated GFR of 150 ml/min/1.73m^2 should be used in the equation.

II. Second-line treatment for refractory and resistant CMV infection and disease:

1. Evaluate possible causes for refractory CMV infection:
   a. An overly immunosuppressed state, including the absence or deficiency of CMV-specific T-cell immunity.
   b. Sub-therapeutic antiviral drug concentrations.
   c. Resistance to ganciclovir or other antiviral drugs.
2. Perform genotypic assay to detect UL97 and UL54 mutations.
   a. Ganciclovir-resistant CMV isolates with UL97-only mutations remain susceptible to foscarnet and cidofovir.
   b. Ganciclovir-resistant CMV with UL54 mutation is more likely to be cross-resistant to cidofovir.
3. Management strategies include:
   a. Doubling the dose of IV Ganciclovir (10 mg/kg BD for normal kidney function) while waiting for genotypic resistance testing results in non-severe CMV disease.
   b. Switching to IV Foscarnet as empiric treatment of severe CMV disease or when UL97 Ganciclovir-resistance is detected.
   c. Adding CMV hyperimmune globulin or high-dose intravenous immunoglobulin (IVIG) as an adjunct to antiviral drugs.
   d. Switching to mammalian target of rapamycin inhibitor (mTORi)-containing immunosuppressive regimen may be an option due to reportedly lower risk of CMV disease in these patients.
   e. Other therapeutic options:
      - Cidofovir.
      - Maribavir (ongoing clinical trial for the treatment of refractory and resistant CMV).

- Letermovir (off-label use).
- Adoptive transfer of CMV-specific T-cells.

4. Forscanet:
   a. Second-line treatment for UL-97 mutant ganciclovir-resistant CMV infection or disease:
      i. Induction treatment: 180 mg/kg/day divided every 8 or 12 hours for 14–21 days.
      ii. Maintenance therapy: 90–120 mg/kg/day as a single infusion once daily.
   b. Precautions:
      i. Use with caution in patients with kidney impairment, altered electrolyte levels, and neurologic or cardiac abnormalities.
      ii. Adjust dose for patients with abnormal kidney function.
      iii. Discontinue treatment if serum creatinine ≥250 μmol/L.
         - Restart therapy if serum creatinine ≤180 μmol/L.
      iv. Foscarnet is a venous irritant; infuse only into veins with adequate blood flow.
      v. Adequate hydration may reduce the risk of nephrotoxicity.
   c. Drug interactions:
      i. Pentamidine: Additive hypocalcemia.
      ii. Cyclosporine, aminoglycosides, amphotericin B, nonsteroidal anti-inflammatory agents: Additive nephrotoxicity.
      iii. Ciprofloxacin: Increased seizure potential.
5. IVIG:
   a. Addition of IVIG to antiviral treatment should be given in the following clinical situations:
      i. Tissue-invasive CMV disease.
      ii. Life-threatening disease, including CMV pneumonitis.
      iii. Hypogammaglobulinemia.
      iv. Drug-resistant virus.
   b. Use of CMV hyperimmune globulin is preferable.
   c. Dose regimen:
      i. Give daily for 1 week, then
      ii. Alternate day for 2 weeks or till clinical symptoms subside, then
      iii. Twice a week for 2 weeks, then
      iv. Weekly for 1 month, then
      v. Alternate week for 1 month, then
      vi. Monthly for 2–3 months.
      vii. Total treatment duration is 4–6 months depending on clinical severity and treatment response.

d. Preparations:

IVIG Preparation	Purification	Sugar	Osmolarity* (mOsm/kg)	CMV Titer (Paul-Ehrlich U/ml)	Equivalent Dose to ≥35 Paul-Ehrlich U/ml
Gammagard (5%*)	Solvent-detergent	Glucose 20 g/L	636 mOsm/kg	35–45	500 mg/kg/dose
Intragam (6%)	Solvent-detergent	Maltose 10 g/dL	Isotonic (actual osmolarity unknown)	No data	650 mg/kg/dose
Flebogamma (5%)	Cold alcohol fractionation, PEG precipitation, ion exchange chromatography	D-sorbitol	240–370 mOsm/kg	32–34	650 mg/kg/dose
Intratect	Octanoic acid, solvent-detergent and nanofiltration	Glycine 270–330 mmol/L	280–350 (supplied <320) mOsm/kg	25	700 mg/kg/dose
Octagam (high CMV titer)	Solvent-detergent	Maltose 10g/dL	310–380 mOsm/kg	66	500 mg/kg/dose
Megalotect CP	Octanoic acid, solvent-detergent and nanofiltration	Glycine 270–330 mmol/L	280–350 (supplied <320) mOsm/kg	100	50 mg/kg/dose

*IVIG preparations with high osmolarity are contraindicated in transplantation.

6. Decrease immunosuppression:
   a. Cautious reduction in immunosuppression should be considered in transplant patients with:
      - CMV disease (especially if moderate to severe).
      - Severe lymphopenia.
      - Deficient nonspecific or CMV-specific T-cell function.
   b. May not be feasible in patients with recent rejection or at heightened risk of rejection episodes.
   c. Strategies of cautious reduction in immunosuppression:
      i. Decrease or discontinue anti-metabolites, including azathioprine or mycophenolate mofetil.
      ii. Consider changing mycophenolate to everolimus if there is a high risk of rejection.
      iii. Continue prednisolone and calcineurin inhibitors unless there is evidence of life-threatening infection.

III. Secondary prophylaxis:

1. After completing the full-dose antiviral treatment course, secondary prophylaxis with oral valganciclovir intended to prevent CMV relapse is not recommended as a routine practice for all patients.
2. May be considered for at least 3 months in subsets of high-risk patients:
   a. Patients with lymphopenia.
   b. Use of ATG.
   c. Donor CMV-positive, recipient CMV-negative (D+R-) state.
3. High-risk T-cell deficient patients should have secondary antiviral prophylaxis and further reduction in immunosuppression to allow for T-cell immune reconstitution.

E. Monitoring

1. Monitoring of CMV PCR should be done weekly during therapy till 2 consecutive negative tests, then fortnightly for one month, then monthly for 6 months.

2. Monitoring during antiviral therapy should include full blood count, liver panel, and kidney function and should be performed weekly during intravenous ganciclovir therapy.
3. Diffusing capacity of the lungs for carbon monoxide (DLCO) in CMV pneumonitis (improvement after 3 weeks).
4. Post-treatment monitoring for relapsing CMV disease include:
   a. Monthly clinical and virology assessment and absolute lymphocyte count for 6 months.
   b. CMV-specific and/or nonspecific T-cell immune monitoring.

F. Prevention of CMV Infection

1. Prophylactic strategy:
   a. Administration of an antiviral drug to all "at-risk" patients for a defined period after transplantation.
      i. Antiviral drugs with proven efficacy for CMV prophylaxis: Valganciclovir (preferred), IV ganciclovir, high-dose valacyclovir.
      ii. Addition of immunoglobulin preparations as an adjunct to antiviral prophylaxis may reduce severe CMV disease and mortality.
   b. Antiviral prophylaxis should generally be started within the first 10 days (preferably 48–72 hours) after transplantation.
   c. Duration of prophylaxis:
      i. 6 months in donor CMV-positive, recipient CMV-negative (D+R-) transplants.
      ii. 3 months in recipient CMV-positive (R+) or following the use of anti-lymphocyte depleting agents.
   d. Prophylaxis is associated with lower rates of allograft loss and may also prevent reactivation of Epstein–Barr virus.
   e. Post-prophylaxis delayed-onset CMV infection occurs commonly with prophylactic strategy in D+R- patients after prophylaxis is discontinued.
      i. Heightened risk of CMV disease within 3–6 months after stopping antiviral prophylaxis.
      ii. Monitoring after stopping antiviral prophylaxis:
         - CMV PCR at least once weekly for 3 months.
         - Immunological tests at baseline:

- Absolute lymphocyte count and CD4+/CD8+ T-cell subsets.
- Nonspecific (mitogen-stimulated) T-cell immune responses.
- CMV-specific CD8+ and/or CD4+ T cell immunity, e.g., interferon-gamma release assay, enzyme-linked immunosorbent spot (ELISPOT) assay.

Note: Immunologic monitoring at the end of antiviral prophylaxis suggests that lymphopenia (absolute lymphocyte count, CD4+ T-cell count) and the lack of CMV-specific (and nonspecific) T-cell response are associated with increased risks of post-prophylaxis delayed-onset CMV disease.

2. Preemptive strategy:
   a. Involves administration of antiviral drug only to asymptomatic patients with evidence of early CMV replication in order to prevent CMV disease.
      i. Do weekly CMV PCR for 12 weeks after transplantation (consider a longer duration for highly immunocompromised hosts).
      ii. If a positive CMV threshold is reached, start oral valganciclovir (preferred) or IV ganciclovir at treatment dose.
      iii. Treat until "negative" threshold is achieved (2 consecutive negative weekly CMV PCR).
      iv. Resume weekly monitoring until Week 12 or for the duration of being highly immunocompromised.
   b. Not recommended for D+R- kidney transplant patients if the results of the CMV PCR cannot be made available on the same day of testing.
      - Failure to detect CMV replication early and institute appropriate intervention may occur due to the rapid CMV viral kinetics.
   c. May be considered an alternative approach to CMV prevention in patients with acute rejection treated with anti-lymphocyte antibody or high-dose steroids.
   d. Viral load threshold for starting preemptive antiviral therapy is assay-specific, center-specific, and risk-specific.

e. Advantages of preemptive therapy:
   i. Reduces exposure to drug-adverse effects.
   ii. May allow subclinical CMV replication before antiviral treatment, resulting in the generation of CMV-specific T-cells, and potentially a lower incidence of delayed onset CMV disease.

3. Hybrid approach:
   - Short-term antiviral prophylaxis is followed by CMV surveillance and preemptive therapy during the period of CMV disease risk.

Recommended Reading

1. Aw MM, Murugasu B, Tan AW, Seah CC, Balakrishnan V, Yap HK. (2000) Quantitation of peripheral blood cytomegalovirus DNA for monitoring recurrent cytomegalovirus retinitis in pediatric solid organ transplant recipients. *Pediatr Transplant* **4**:100–106.
2. Razonable RR, Humar A. (2019) Cytomegalovirus in solid organ transplant recipients — Guidelines of the American Society of Transplantation Infectious Diseases Community of Practice. *Clin Transplant* **33**:e13512.
3. Santos CAQ, Vella J, Brennan DC. (2020, updated) Clinical manifestation, diagnosis and management of cytomegalovirus disease in kidney transplant recipients. Edited by: Murphy B, Marr KA, Lam AQ, Bond S. *UpToDate ONLINE.* http://www.uptodateonline.com.
4. Zachary KC. (2020, updated) Ganciclovir and valganciclovir: An overview. Edited by: Hirsch MS, Mitty J. *UpToDate ONLINE.* http://www.uptodateonline.com.

12 Management of Epstein–Barr Virus-Associated Infection and Post-Transplant Lymphoproliferative Disease in Pediatric Kidney Transplantation

Koh LJ, Teo S, Lau PYW, Ng KH, Yeo WS and Yap HK

A. Epstein–Barr Virus (EBV)-Associated Disease

1. EBV infection in pediatric kidney transplantation is highly associated with B-cell post-transplant lymphoproliferative disorder (PTLD).
2. PTLD encompasses a wide spectrum of lymphoproliferative disorders, ranging from infectious mononucleosis and lymphoid hyperplasia to highly invasive malignant lymphoma.
3. PTLD has been reported in 1.2–10.1% of pediatric kidney transplant recipients, with 47% of cases occurring within 6 months, 62% within 1 year, and 90% within 5 years of the transplant.

B. WHO Classification of PTLD

Categories of PTLD	Subtypes
Non-destructive PTLDs	• Plasmacytic hyperplasia. • Infectious mononucleosis. • Florid follicular hyperplasia.
Polymorphic PTLD	• Polyclonal. • Monoclonal.

(*Continued*)

(*Continued*)

Categories of PTLD	Subtypes
Monomorphic PTLD	• B-cell lymphomas, diffuse large B cell lymphoma, Burkitt/Burkitt-like lymphoma, plasma cell myeloma, plasmacytoma-like, others. • T cell/NK cell lymphomas, peripheral T cell lymphoma, hepatosplenic T cell lymphoma, others.
Classic Hodgkin lymphoma-like PTLD	

C. Risk Factors for PTLD

1. EBV seronegative recipient status:
   a. Single most important risk factor in the development of PTLD.
      - Incidence of PTLD is 25–50 times higher in EBV-naive recipients.
      - Relative risk of PTLD is approximately 20-fold higher in EBV-seronegative recipients than in EBV-seropositive recipients, in the first year post-transplant.

   b. Transplant recipients who acquire primary EBV infection are at a greater risk of developing PTLD, with the source of virus from the donor organ.
   c. Seronegative recipients are also at risk of developing late PTLD from community-acquired EBV infection.
   d. Seropositive recipients under 12 months of age should be considered seronegative due to the presence of maternally derived EBV antibodies.
2. Potent immunosuppression regimen:
   a. Reports suggest a higher incidence of PTLD with the use of more potent immunosuppression, including a high cumulative dose of anti-thymocyte globulin (ATG), OKT3, belatacept, and alemtuzumab.
   b. More recent reports have not shown an increased risk with use of tacrolimus, mycophenolate mofetil (MMF), or the combined use of tacrolimus and MMF.
3. Simultaneous cytomegalovirus (CMV) disease:
   a. CMV disease may contribute to the net state of immunosuppression, possibly resulting in an increased risk of PTLD.

4. Human Leukocyte Antigen (HLA) mismatch:
   a. Number of HLA-B mismatches was independently associated with the development of diffuse B-cell PTLD.
5. Age:
   a. Pediatric patients who are EBV seropositive have a higher risk of PTLD compared to adults.
   b. This may be due to recent infection with incompletely developed immune responses.

D. Diagnostic Work-Up of PTLD

1. The diagnostic work-up of PTLD primarily involves:
   a. Confirmation of diagnosis
   b. Determining the extent of involvement of the disease.
2. Blood investigations and serology:
   a. Full blood count.
   b. Blood urea, creatinine, sodium, potassium, chloride, bicarbonate, calcium, phosphate, and uric acid.
   c. Liver function test with gamma-glutamyltransferase (GGT).
   d. Lactate dehydrogenase.
   e. EBV serology:
      i. Anti-EBV viral capsid antigen (VCA) IgM (positive = acute infection, ≥four-fold rise = re-activation)
      ii. Anti-EBV VCA IgG.
      iii. Anti-EB nuclear antigen (EBNA):
         - Increased anti-EBV VCA IgG and falling or lack of anti-EBNA IgG signify chronic infection: High risk of acquiring PTLD.

EBV infection	EBV DNA >1000 copies/ug DNA
Primary EBV infection	Anti-EBV VCA IgM positive
EBV reactivation	Four fold or greater increase in anti-EBV VCA IgM in seropositive patients
Chronic EBV infection	Increased anti-EBV VCA IgG and a lack of anti-EBNA IgG

   f. EBV/CMV PCR (to be sent to Paeds Lab) (significant variability between assays for EBV DNA. Trends using the same assay in the same patient are more useful than a single value).
   g. EBV genome sequencing.
3. Imaging:
   a. Ultrasound of relevant regions.
   b. Contrast-enhanced computed tomography (CT) or magnetic resonance imaging (MRI) of the chest, abdomen and pelvis.
   c. PET-CT (whole body) to measure disease activity.
   d. Bone marrow aspiration and biopsy suggested for patients with cytopenias.
   e. MRI if suspicious of central nervous system involvement.
4. Histology/Cytology:
   a. Excision of lymph nodes/tonsils.
   b. Liver biopsy (if hepatomegaly).
   c. Bilateral bone marrow aspirate and trephine (consider flow cytometry and cytogenetics) if patient has cytopenias.
   d. Lumbar puncture (if extra-nodal involvement suspected).
   e. Epstein–Barr virus-encoded small RNAs (EBER) staining in all biopsy specimens (to determine the presence of EBV in cells) and staining of lambda and kappa light chains (to determine the clonality of cells) as per Pathologist's protocol.
   f. CD20 expression on biopsy specimens.

E. Screening for PTLD in High-Risk Recipients

1. Monthly EBV PCR until 1 year post-transplant, then 3 monthly in the second year, then 6-monthly untill seroconversion in seronegative patients.
2. Monthly liver panel, GGT for the first year post-transplant.
3. Annual hepatobiliary ultrasound scan.

F. Prevention of PTLD in High-Risk Recipients

1. Recommended prophylaxis according to the table below:
   - For dosing, refer to chapter "Sequential Immunosuppression Protocol for Kidney Transplantation".

Risk Factors		Recommended Prophylaxis		
EBV Status	**ATG**	**CMV Hyperimmune Globulin**	**IV Ganciclovir**	**Oral Valganciclovir**
Negative donor to Negative recipient + blood transfusion (leukocyte filtered)	Y	Y (single dose)		
Positive donor to Positive recipient	Y	Y (single dose)		3 months
Negative donor to Positive recipient	Y	Y (single dose)		3 months
Positive donor to Negative recipient	Y/N	Y	10 days	6 months (Prolong to 1 year if lymphopenic)

2. Treatment of asymptomatic recipients with EBV-positive PCR:
   a. Indication for treatment:
      - EBV PCR ≥1000 copies/μg DNA on 2 occasions.
   b. Consider reduction of basal immunosuppression.
   c. Start CMV hyperimmune globulin (Megalotect CP®):
      - Dose: 50 mg/kg/dose (1 ml/kg/dose) 2-weekly for a total of 6 doses.
   d. IV ganciclovir treatment dose for 3 weeks followed by oral valganciclovir treatment dose for a total of 3 months, and then oral valganciclovir prophylactic dose for a further 3 months.
   e. Consider IV Rituximab 375 mg/m^2 in high-risk patients.

G. Treatment of PTLD

1. Reduction of basal immunosuppression:
   a. Maintain only glucocorticoids OR
   b. Decrease calcineurin inhibitors (CNI) by at least 50% AND stop anti-proliferative agents
   c. Consider mammalian target of rapamycin inhibitor (mTORi) protocol with CNI.

2. Antiviral treatment for EBV-positive B-cell lymphoma:
   a. Antiviral treatment with IV ganciclovir for 3 weeks, followed by
   b. Treatment dose of valganciclovir for at least 3 months or longer according to the blood level of EBV replication (EBV PCR).
   c. CMV hyperimmune globulin 50 mg/kg/dose should also be initiated 2-weekly for 6 doses.
   d. Prophylaxis with valganciclovir should be continued for up to a further 6 months after EBV PCR is negative.
3. Eradication of *Helicobacter pylori (H. pylori)* in the case of lymphomas from mucosal-associated lymphoid tissue with positive *H. pylori*:
   - Full eradication of *H. pylori* should be carried out with subsequent *H. pylori* prophylaxis instituted to avoid relapse.
4. Rituximab in CD20-positive lymphomas:
   - IV Rituximab 375 mg/m^2 weekly for 4 weeks or 750 mg/m^2 weekly for 2 weeks (see chapter "Anti-CD20 Monoclonal Antibody Therapy for Nephrotic Syndrome" for the infusion protocol).
5. Chemotherapy for diffuse lymphomas or unsatisfactory response to previous treatment:
   - CHOP chemotherapy (cyclophosphamide, doxorubicin, vincristine, and prednisolone) is used alone or in combination with Rituximab.
6. Cessation of immunosuppression should be considered in patients refractory to chemotherapy, with or without graft nephrectomy.

H. Post-treatment Monitoring

1. Monthly EBV PCR for 1 year (for EBV positive patients) then 3–6 monthly if EBV PCR becomes negative.
2. PET-CT scan (whole body) at diagnosis of PTLD and 1-month post-completion of Rituximab course or chemotherapy and yearly if EBV PCR remains positive.

Recommended Reading

1. Dharnidharka VR. (2018) Comprehensive review of post-organ transplant hematologic cancers. *Am J Transplant* **18**:537–549.
2. Allen UD, Preiksaitis JK; AST Infectious Diseases Community of Practice. (2019) Post-transplant lymphoproliferative disorders, Epstein-Barr virus infection, and disease in solid organ transplantation: Guidelines from the American Society of Transplantation Infectious Diseases Community of Practice. *Clin Transplant* **33**:e13652.
3. Negrin RS, Brennan DC. (2020, updated) Treatment and prevention of post-transplant lymphoproliferative disorders. Edited by: Chao NJ, Freedman AS. *UpToDate ONLINE.* http://www.uptodateonline.com.

13 Management of BK Virus Disease in Kidney Transplantation

Lau PYW, Teo S, Ekhambaram S and Yap HK

A. Definitions

1. BK polyomavirus (BKPyV) viruria: Presence of BKPyV in the urine.
2. BKPyV viremia: Presence of virus in the blood or plasma.
   - Upper limit of normal plasma BKPyV load is 250 copies/ml.
3. The clinical diagnosis of BK polyomavirus-associated nephropathy (PyVAN) can be **possible, probable, presumptive**, or **proven** depending on the detection of BKPyV in the urine, plasma and/or kidney allograft biopsy.
   a. Possible: High-level BKPyV viruria in the absence of BKPyV-DNAemia and histological evidence of PyVAN.
   b. Probable: Plasma BKPyV-DNAemia sustained >1000 copies/ml (>3 $\log_{10}$ copies/ml) in the absence of histological evidence of PyVAN.
   c. Presumptive: Plasma BKPyV-DNAemia increased >10000 copies/ml (>4 $\log_{10}$ copies/ml) in the absence of histological evidence of PyVAN.

Specimen	Marker (*comments on test*)	Clinical Diagnosis of PyVAN			
		Possible	Probable	Presumptive	Proven
Urine	"High-level viruria": • Decoy cells (*check if inflammation and/or clots*). • BKPyV urine DNA load >7 $\log_{10}$ copies/ml. • BKPyV VP1 mRNA load ≥6.5 $\log_{10}$ copies/ngRNA. • PyV particles (*check if in clusters or "Haufen"*).	+	+	+	+
Plasma	"BKPyV-DNAemia": • Plasma load >3 $\log_{10}$ copies/ml (sustained in 2 measurements in <3 weeks). • Plasma load >4 $\log_{10}$ copies/ml (increased in 1 of 2 measurements in <3 weeks).	–	+ +	+ +	+
Biopsy	"Polyomavirus-associated nephropathy": • Viral cytopathic changes • Inflammatory infiltrates/tubulitis. • More than mild interstitial fibrosis/tubular atrophy.	–	–	–	+
Treatment *(recommendations need to account for the risk-benefit balance in each patient)*		No	(Yes)	Yes	Yes

B. Risk Factors of PyVAN

1. Primary infection with BKPyV occurs in the first decade of life via a respiratory or oral route, as evidenced by increase in BKPyV sero-prevalence to ≥90% with age, followed by long-lived latency in the uroepithelium and renal tubular cells.
2. BKPyV infection in kidney transplant recipients:
   - Viruria/decoy cells tend to occur first within 2–6 months post-transplant.
   - 25–40% of patients with viruria/decoy cells will progress to the viremia stage after a few weeks.
   - In the absence of any intervention, BKPyV viremia progresses to histologically proven PyVAN, affecting graft function and increasing the risk of graft loss from <10% to >90%.
3. The preferential occurrence of PyVAN in kidney transplant recipients compared to other non-kidney solid organ transplants suggests that factors specific to transplanting kidneys of BKPyV latency are of importance.
4. Risk factors:

Donor-related	Recipient-related	Transplant-related
• HLA mismatches. • Deceased donation. • BKPyV viruria. • High BKPyV antibody titers (marker of recent viral exposure and possibly a higher viral graft load). • Female.	• Older age. • Younger age. • Male. • Highly sensitized status. • ABO incompatibility. • History of hemodialysis as opposed to peritoneal dialysis. • ANCA antibodies. • 1,25-dihydroxy-vitamin D_3 deficiency. • Interferon-γ gene polymorphisms. • Low or absent BKPyV antibody titers. • Low or absent BKPyV-specific T-cell responses.	• Acute tubular necrosis. • Acute rejection and anti-rejection treatment. • Steroid exposure. • Lymphocyte-depleting antibodies. • Higher immuno-suppressive drug levels. • Immunosuppressive regime: Tacrolimus (Tac)-mycophenolate (MPA) higher risk compared to cyclosporin (CsA)-MPA or mTOR inhibitor combinations. • Ureteric stents. • Re-transplantation after graft loss due to PyVAN.

- Intensity of immunosuppression rather than the type of immunosuppression is the most important modifiable risk factor.

C. Surveillance for PyVAN

I. Principles:

1. Because effective and safe antiviral therapies are lacking, screening for BKV replication has become the key recommendation to initiate and guide a stepwise reduction of immunosuppression.
   - Allows for expanding BKPyV-specific cellular immune responses to stop BKPyV replication in the graft and clear BKPyV viremia.
2. PyVAN is usually diagnosed in the first 6 months post-transplant but can be delayed beyond the first year post-transplant.
3. Clinically silent viruria always precedes PyVAN, thus allowing identification of patients at risk for PyVAN and creating a window of opportunity for pre-emptive measures.

II. Pre-transplant screening:

1. Donor testing prior to kidney transplant for BKPyV viruria:
   - Virus genotyping or BKPyV VLP/Vp1-IgG antibody levels are not recommended at present.
2. Recipient testing prior to kidney transplant for BKPyV viruria, virus genotyping, BKPyV VLP/Vp1-IgG antibody levels, BKPyV (subtype)-neutralizing IgG levels, or BKPyV-specific T-cell quantity or function is not recommended at present.

III. Screening for BKV replication:

1. Screening tools:

Screening Test	Threshold	Comments*
Urine cytology for decoy cells (per cytospin)	≥10 (1 log_{10}) cells	• Cheap and rapid. • PPV 27–90%, NPV 99–100%. • Recommended 2-weekly for the first 3 months post-transplant, then monthly until 9 months post-transplant, then every 3 months until 2 years post-transplant. • If detected, testing for BKPyV-DNAemia should be done for decision-making.
Urine BKPyV DNA PCR (copies/ml)	$\geq 10^7$ (7 log_{10}) cells	• More sensitive. • PPV 67%, NPV 100%. • If detected, testing for BKPyV-DNAemia should be done for decision-making. • Viruria usually seen about 6–12 weeks prior to detection of viremia. • Viruria fluctuates and is often self-limiting, requiring no intervention. • Delayed decline of the urinary BKV load in response to reduced immunosuppression.
Urine BKPyV VP1 mRNA RT-PCR (copies/ng RNA)	$\geq 6.54 \times 10^5$ (5.82 log_{10}) cells	• PPV 75%, NPV 97%. • Research tool (inadequate clinical data).
Urine direct negative staining EM	PyV in clusters "Haufen"	• PPV and NPV >90%. • Not widely available.
Plasma BKPyV DNA PCR (copies/mL)	$\geq 10^4$ (4 log_{10}) cells	• More sensitive. • PPV 50–85%, NPV 100%. • Viremia seen about 2–6 weeks prior to detection of PyVAN. • 50% are transient.

*PPV = positive predictive value, NPV = negative predictive value.

2. Plasma BKPyV DNA PCR is the preferred screening test to identify kidney transplant recipients for preemptive treatment for PyVAN.
3. Frequency of post-transplant screening using plasma BKPyV DNA PCR:
   - Monthly for the first 9 months post-transplant.
   - Subsequently 3 monthly during the first 2 years post-transplant.
   - Annually after the first 2 years post-transplant.
   - Screening for BKPyV replication should also be done when there is allograft dysfunction or when patients undergo kidney allograft biopsy for surveillance or cause/indication.
4. If plasma BKPyV DNA PCR is positive, repeat plasma BKPyV DNA PCR within 3 weeks:
   a. If there is sustained plasma BKPyV DNA PCR 1000–10000 copies/ml within 3 weeks, probable PyVAN is suspected.
   b. If plasma BKPyV DNA PCR increases to >10000 copies/ml within 3 weeks, presumptive PyVAN is suspected.
5. This allows for:
   a. Identification of patients spontaneously clearing BKPyV-DNAemia.
   b. Exclusion of laboratory errors.
   c. Capturing BKPyV replication dynamics.
   d. Balancing the competing risk of precipitating acute rejection after reducing immunosuppression.

IV. Kidney allograft biopsy:

1. In kidney transplant patients with BKPyV viremia, kidney allograft biopsy is not required prior to reducing immunosuppression, if the kidney allograft function is at baseline and there is no increased risk of acute rejection.
2. Kidney allograft biopsy is recommended in the following situations where BKPyV viremia is accompanied by:
   a. Elevation in serum creatinine.
   b. Highly sensitized status with panel-reactive antibodies.
   c. Donor-specific antibodies.
   d. Past allograft rejection.
   e. Re-transplantation.
   f. Other causes of allograft dysfunction such as recurrence of original kidney disease, or if drug toxicity is suspected.

   g. High-level viremia >10000 (4 $\log_{10}$) copies/ml persists despite reduction of immunosuppression.
3. Diagnosis of proven PyVAN on kidney biopsy is based on:
   a. Demonstrating PyV cytopathic changes in allograft tissue.
   b. Confirmation by immunohistochemistry with antibodies against the large T-antigen of the Simian virus 40 (clone PAb 416, Calbiochem) or in-situ hybridization ("proven PyVAN").
4. Biopsy sampling:
   a. Minimum of 2 biopsy cores, preferentially containing medullary tissue.
      - BKPyV replication in the kidney may be focal.
      - Allograft biopsy for proven PyVAN may be false negative in 10–30% of the BKPyV-DNAemia positive cases, especially when the biopsies are taken early after DNAemia onset and lack medullary tissue.
   b. Negative biopsy results cannot rule out early focal PyVAN with certainty.
5. Acute allograft rejection can be concurrent with PyVAN and should be considered in the presence of the following:
   a. Endarteritis.
   b. Fibrinoid vascular necrosis.
   c. Glomerulitis.
   d. C4d deposits along peritubular capillaries.
6. The histological findings of proven PyVAN should be semi-quantitatively assessed using the American Society of Transplantation-Infectious Disease Community of Practice (AST-IDCOP) 2013 as well as the Banff 2017 Study Group classification.
   a. AST-IDCOP 2013 classification: Histopathology patterns by Drachenberg criteria.

Histological Pattern	Features	Graft Function	Risk of Graft Loss
PyVAN-A	Viral cytopathic changes: ≤25%. Interstitial inflammation: ≤10%. Tubular atrophy: ≤10%. Interstitial fibrosis: ≤10%.	Mostly baseline	<10%

(*Continued*)

Histological Pattern	Features	Graft Function	Risk of Graft Loss
PyVAN-B	Viral cytopathic changes: 11 to >50%. Tubular atrophy: <50%. Interstitial fibrosis: <50%.	Mostly impaired	50%
B1	+ Interstitial inflammation: 11–25%	Slightly above baseline	25%
B2	+ Interstitial inflammation: 25–50%	Significantly impaired	50%
B3	+ Interstitial inflammation: >50%	Significantly impaired	75%
PyVAN-C	Viral cytopathic changes variable. Interstitial inflammation variable. Tubular atrophy: >50%. Interstitial fibrosis: >50%.	Significantly impaired; Progressive failure	>80%

b. Banff 2017 histologic classification system of proven PyVAN*:
   i. Histologic classes of proven PyVAN are defined by the intra-renal PyV load (PyVL) and Banff *ci* scores.
   ii. The PyVL scores are assigned according to the extent of viral induced tubular changes.
   iii. A tubule with intranuclear viral inclusion bodies (Type 1 or 2) and/or a positive immunohistochemistry reaction for SV40 T antigen in ≥1 cells per tubular cross-section is considered a "positive tubule".
   iv. The overall percentage of positive tubular cross-sections is estimated in the entire biopsy sample (all available cores, cortex and medulla):
      - PyVL 1: ≤1% of all tubules/ducts with viral replication.
      - PyVL 2: >1% to ≤10% of all tubules/ducts with viral replication.
      - PyVL 3: >10% of all tubules/ducts with viral replication.

PyVAN Class-1		PyVAN Class-2		PyVAN Class-3	
PyVL	Banff *ci* Score	PyVL	Banff *ci* Score	PyVL	Banff *ci* Score
1	0–1	1	2–3	–	–
–	–	2	0–3	–	–
–	–	3	0–1	3[a]	2–3

*Note:

- As defined in the Banff Study Group Proposal, biopsies with moderate-severe fibrosis can be designated as class-3 only if the viral tissue involvement is PyVL-3.
- In practice, many biopsies with severe fibrosis have low PyVL scores and do not fall in this class despite the expected poor prognosis.

7. Prognostic value (Drakenberg):
   a. Children with ≥50% decline of GFR showed PyVAN histopathology pattern B3, and plasma BKPyV load were more likely $>2.5 \times 10^6$ (6.4 $\log_{10}$) copies/ml.
   b. Children with <50% GFR decline showed better histology (pattern A and B1), and plasma BKPyV load $<2.5 \times 10^5$ (6.4 $\log_{10}$) copies/ml.
8. JC polyomavirus-mediated PyVAN should be considered in kidney transplant patients with histological signs of PyVAN, declining kidney function, and absence of BKPyV in blood, urine or graft tissue.

D. Treatment Principles

I. Principles:

1. The mainstay of therapy for significant BKPyV replication and PyVAN in kidney transplant recipients without concurrent acute rejection is **reducing the immunosuppression** when:
   a. Sustained BKPyV DNAemia $>10^3$ ($>3 \log_{10}$) copies/ml in 2 measurements within 3 weeks.
   b. Presumptive PyVAN.
   c. Positive PyV cytopathic changes on allograft biopsy (proven PyVAN).
2. Clearance of BKPyV-DNAemia following reduced immunosuppression is more readily achieved if BKPyV-DNAemia is sustained

between 10^3–10^4 (3–4 log) copies/ml (probable PyVan, as compared to presumptive PyVAN or proven PyVan).

3. Reduction of immunosuppression has been reported to be safe and effective for preventing PyVAN and clearing BKV viremia with subsequent acute rejections ranging from 8–12%, which should respond to steroid treatment.
4. More advanced disease may require other interventions and a longer time for recovery, and may result in a permanent loss of kidney function.

II. Strategies to reduce immunosuppression:

1. Dose reduction of calcineurin inhibitor (CNI) and antiproliferative drug (MPA or azathioprine):

	Strategy 1	Strategy 2
Step 1	Reduce CNI dose by 25–50% in 1–2 steps.	Reduce antiproliferative drug by 50%.
Step 2	Reduce antiproliferative drug by 50%.	Reduce CNI dose by 25–50%.
Step 3	Stop antiproliferative drug.	Stop antiproliferative drug.
Targets	a. Oral prednisolone should be tapered to ≤10 mg/day. b. Target of Tac trough levels: <6 ng/ml (3 ng/ml may be more appropriate from recent evidence). c. Target of CsA trough levels: <150 ng/mL (100 ng/mL may be more appropriate from recent evidence). d. Target of sirolimus trough levels: <6 ng/mL.	

2. Additional strategies:
   a. Switch Tac to low-dose CsA.
   b. Switch CNI to low-dose sirolimus.
      - Meta-analyses have shown decreased incidence rates of BKPyV-DNAemia and/or PyVAN for mTOR inhibitor combinations, which could potentially be harnessed in primary treatment or for refractory or advanced stages of PyVAN.
   c. Switch MPA to leflunomide or low-dose sirolimus.

3. After reducing immunosuppression, monitor until:
   a. Serum creatinine 2-weekly stable, then monthly.
   b. Plasma BKPyV DNA PCR 2-weekly followed by further reduction of immunosuppression until clearance of BKPyV DNAemia, then monthly for 6 months, then 3-monthly for at least 2 years.
4. Consider returning to routine maintenance immunosuppression after successful clearance of BKPyV-DNAemia.

III. Adjunctive therapy:

1. Principles:
   a. Adjunctive therapy may be considered in patients with sustained high-level plasma BKPyV load despite adequately reduced immunosuppression.
   b. There are no randomized controlled trials providing evidence that adjunctive therapy is superior to timely reduction of immunosuppression.
2. Intravenous immunoglobulin (IVIg):
   a. Valuable treatment option in patients with PyVAN and concurrent allograft rejection.
   b. Dose:
      i. PyVAN with acute rejection: 500 mg/kg daily for 7 consecutive days, followed by 2 g/kg monthly untill clearance of viremia.
      ii. PyVAN without rejection: 2 g/kg monthly untill clearance of viremia.
3. Cidofovir:
   a. Nucleoside analog, which inhibits viral replication in-vitro.
   b. Dose:
      i. Low dose of 0.25–1 mg/kg given at 2-week intervals for at least 4 doses (**maximum 8 doses**).
      ii. Give as an IV infusion in 500 ml 0.9% saline over 1 hour with pre- and post-hydration.
      iii. Do not give probenecid.
   c. Closely monitor serum creatinine, leukocyte counts, eye symptoms, and vision.
      - Anterior uveitis observed in 12–35% cases.
   d. Contraindicated in patients with baseline creatinine >300 μmol/L, pre-existing leucopenia or neutropenia, metabolic acidosis, proteinuria, and history of uveitis.

   e. Discontinue therapy if there is unexplained worsening of kidney function, proteinuria or metabolic acidosis, or changes in visual acuity.
   f. Conflicting results on its benefit in stabilization of kidney function.
4. Leflunomide:
   a. Given in place of MPA as it is an immunosuppressant with modest antiviral properties.
   b. Dose in children:
      i. Recommended loading dose: 100 mg/1.73m^2/day for 3 days.
      ii. Maintenance therapy:
         - Weight 10–20 kg: 10 mg daily.
         - Weight 20–40 kg: 15 mg daily (may be given as 20 mg and 10 mg doses on alternating days).
         - Weight >40 kg: 20 mg daily.
   c. Dose in adults:
      i. Loading dose: 100 mg daily for 5 days.
      ii. Maintenance dose: 40 mg daily.
   d. Total duration of therapy is 3–6 months.
   e. Target leflunomide blood levels (if available): 40–100 μg/ml.
   f. Monitor the following tests 2 weeks after starting leflunomide, then monthly:
      i. Full blood count:
         - Thrombotic microangiopathy.
         - Bone marrow suppression.
      ii. Liver function test.
      iii. Consider lung function test to detect pulmonary fibrosis:
         - Every 6 months while on leflunomide.
         - If the patient has a persistent cough that is non-infective.
   g. Dose may be decreased by 50% in the absence of leflunomide level monitoring in the presence of:
      i. Anemia: Hemoglobin <10 g/dL.
      ii. Thrombocytopenia: Platelet $<100 \times 10^9$/L.
      iii. Elevation in liver enzymes >2.5 times of normal values.
5. Fluoroquinolones such as ciprofloxacin:
   a. Inhibits viral replication.
      - Antiviral effect is modest and may not be effective in well established PyVAN.
   b. Dose of ciprofloxacin: 10–15 mg/kg/dose BD (maximum 500 mg BD).

c. Role in prophylaxis: Start ciprofloxacin when plasma BKPyV load >625 copies/ml, combined with a small reduction in immunosuppression (reduce CNI or MPA by 30%).
d. If plasma BKPyV load does not decrease within 2 months of ciprofloxacin treatment, switch ciprofloxacin to leflunomide and discontinue MPA.

6. The antiviral treatment (leflunomide and fluoroquinolone) can be stopped once BKPyV loads are not detected for 3 consecutive months.

IV. Management of acute rejection:

1. Acute rejection concurrent with PyVAN or after reduced immunosuppression for presumptive or proven PyVAN should be treated.
2. Anti-rejection treatment (pulse steroid therapy) and IVIg followed by reduction of immunosuppression 2 weeks later.
3. Administration of lymphocyte-depleting agents should be done after careful evaluation of the competing risks of failure to control rejection and recurrence of PyVAN.
4. Rituximab and plasmapheresis may be considered if acute antibody-mediated allograft rejection is present.

V. Re-transplantation:

1. Re-transplantation can be considered for patients after the loss of a first kidney allograft due to PyVAN.
2. Recurrent BKPyV infection can occur in as many as 20% of cases.
3. In case of re-transplantation of patients with persistent BKPyV-DNAemia, a significant decline of at least 100 (2 $\log_{10}$) copies/ml indicative of emerging BKPyV-specific immune control should be achieved, and nephrectomy of primary graft is recommended.
4. Management of re-transplant:
   a. Induction therapy is not contraindicated after the clearance of BKPyV replication.
   b. Avoid extended periods of intense maintenance immunosuppression.
   c. Frequent screening for BKPyV replication is recommended.

E. Algorithm for Screening and Management of BKPyV replication and PyVAN in Kidney Allograft Recipients

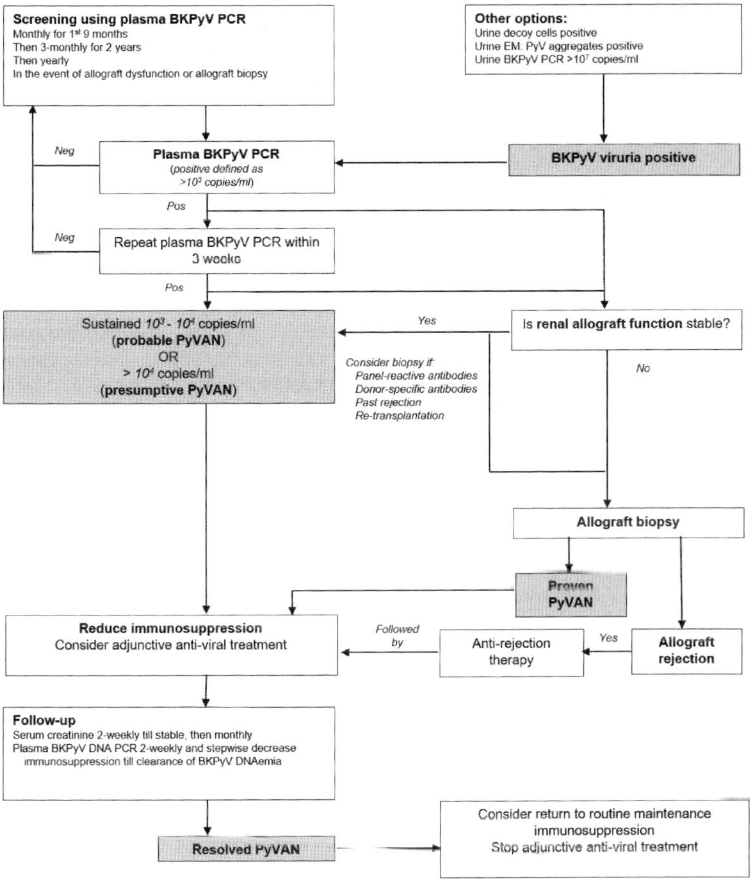

Recommended Reading

1. Blanckaert K, Vriese ASD. (2006) Current recommendations for diagnosis and management of polyoma BK virus nephropathy in renal transplant recipients. *Nephrol Dial Transplant* **21**:3364–3367.
2. Puliyanda DP, Toyoda M, Traum AZ, Flores FX, Jordan S, Moudgil A, Somers MJ. (2008) Outcome of management strategies for BK virus replication in pediatric renal transplant recipients. *Pediatr Transplant* **12**:180–186.
3. Kidney Disease: Improving Global Outcomes (KDIGO) Transplant Work Group. (2009) KDIGO clinical practice guideline for the care of kidney transplant recipients. *Am J Transplant* **9**(Suppl 3):S1–S157.
4. Araya CE, Garin EH, Neiberger RE, Dharnidharka VR. (2010) Leflunomide therapy for BK virus allograft nephropathy in pediatric and young adult kidney transplant recipients. *Pediatr Transplant* **14**:145–150.
5. Hirsch HH, Randhawa P; AST Infectious Diseases Community of Practice. (2013) BK polyomavirus in solid organ transplantation. *Am J Transplant* **1**(Suppl 4):179–188.
6. Zaman RA, Ettenger RB, Cheam H, Malekzadeh MH, Tsai EW. (2014) A novel treatment regimen for BK viremia. *Transplantation* **97**:1166–1171.
7. Hirsch HH, Randhawa PS; AST Infectious Diseases Community of Practice. (2019) BK polyomavirus in solid organ transplantation — Guidelines from the American Society of Transplantation Infectious Diseases Community of Practice. *Clin Transplant* **33**:e13528. doi:10.1111/ctr.13528

1 Kidney Biopsy Protocol

Ong J, Teo S and Yap HK

A. Evaluation of Kidney Biopsy

1. Light microscopy.
2. Immunofluorescence (or immunoperoxidase):
   - Should include evaluation of IgG, IgM, IgA, C3, C1q, albumin, fibrin, kappa, and lambda immunoglobulin light chains.
   - Special studies: Collagen chains (alpha 3, 4 and 5), phospholipase A2 receptor (PLA2R), amyloid A deposits, IgG subclasses.
3. Electron microscopy.

B. Contraindications

1. Absolute contraindications:
   a. Uncontrolled severe hypertension.
   b. Uncontrollable bleeding diathesis.
   c. Uncooperative patient.
   d. Active renal or peri-renal infection.
2. Relative contraindications:
   a. Small hyperechoic kidneys indicative of chronic irreversible disease.
   b. Solitary native kidney.
   c. Multiple, bilateral cysts.
   d. Malpositioned or horseshoe kidney.
   e. Renal tumor.

f. Hydronephrosis.
g. Skin infection over the biopsy site.

Note:

- Consider a biopsy by the interventional radiologist with an injection of gelatin sponge Gelfoam (R) to aid in hemostasis

OR

- Consider an open kidney biopsy rather than percutaneous, if it is important to obtain a histological diagnosis.

C. Patient Preparation

1. Review medications:
   a. Patient **must not** be on recent anti-platelet or anti-thrombotic agents including aspirin, dipyridamole, omega-3 fatty acids, or non-steroidal anti-inflammatory drugs (NSAIDs) for at least 1–2 weeks before the biopsy, and should not be restarted for another 1–2 weeks after the biopsy.
   b. Patients on heparin should stop the drug for AT LEAST 6 hours prior to the procedure, and the biopsy should only be performed only when the coagulation profile is normal.
   c. Patients on warfarin should stop the drug for at least 1 week until the international normalized ratio (INR) is <1.5, and this should not be restarted for at least a week after the procedure.
2. Blood pressure (BP) must be well controlled.
3. Obtain consent from parent/guardian.
4. Set intravenous (IV) cannula (preferably on upper limbs).
5. Pre-biopsy laboratory investigations to be done and the biopsy protocol form should be filled in with the following investigations:
   a. Full blood count.
   b. Urine microscopy.
   c. Urea, creatinine, sodium, potassium, chloride, bicarbonate, calcium, phosphate, and uric acid.
   d. Prothrombin time (PT) and activated partial thromboplastin time (aPTT).
   e. Bleeding time (in patients with azotemia) (optional).
   f. Group and cross match.
   g. Liver function test.

h. 24-hour urinary total protein or urine protein:creatinine ratio.
i. Creatinine clearance.
j. Lupus screen: Serum complements C3 and C4, anti-double-stranded DNA antibody (if indicated).
k. Hepatitis B surface antigen and antibody (if indicated).
l. Serum IgG, IgM and IgA (if indicated).

6. Keep patient fasted for 4 to 6 hours prior to biopsy.
7. Refer to the sedation team if the child has a history of difficult sedation, difficult airway, neuromuscular or respiratory disease, or is less than 1 year old.
8. Consider doing the biopsy in the pediatric intensive care unit (PICU) or high dependency unit if the child is less than 1 year old.

D. Biopsy Preparation

1. Inform the renal nurse/coordinator about the kidney biopsy.
2. Inform the laboratory technician about the kidney biopsy so that biopsy sample solutions and a dissecting microscope can be arranged for.
3. Arrange for an ultrasound machine with biopsy adaptors.
4. Inform the pediatric radiologist of the date and time of the kidney biopsy.
5. Consider the use of desmopressin (DDAVP) in patients with acute or chronic kidney failure where bleeding time is usually prolonged.
   - DDAVP 0.3 μg/kg (maximum dose 20 μg) given subcutaneously, or via IV infusion diluted in 1 ml/kg of normal saline and given over 30–60 minutes.

E. Biopsy Procedure

1. Biopsy is performed on the left kidney in general.
2. Position the patient in prone position with a sandbag under the costal margin.
3. Ultrasound of the kidneys:
   a. Ensure that both kidneys are present.
   b. Localization of the lower pole of the left kidney.
   c. Measure the depth of the lower pole of the kidney.

4. Infiltrate local anesthetic (1% lignocaine) deep to the renal capsule, before making a small incision over the biopsy entry point.
   - A 21-gauge spinal needle may be required for adequate infiltration of local anesthetic in large individuals.
5. Use a **16-gauge** biopsy needle.
6. Phase of respiration in which biopsy is performed:
   a. If the patient is not sedated: Perform the biopsy with the patient holding his breath in deep inspiration.
   b. If the patient is sedated: Perform the biopsy in expiration.
7. Limit entry into the kidney tissue to a maximum of 3 passes in a single setting.
8. Close the biopsy incision wound with a Steri-strip™ and cover with Tegaderm™ before placing the pressure dressing.

F. Post-Biopsy Care and Monitoring

1. Vital signs monitoring, including pulse rate, respiratory rate, oxygen saturation (SpO_2), and BP:
   a. Every 15 minutes for the 1st hour.
   b. Every 30 minutes for the next 4 hours.
   c. Hourly thereafter for the next 4 hours.
   d. Continue monitoring at least 4 hourly if urine is heavily bloodstained.
2. Complete bed (lie flat) for at least 4–6 hours.
3. Urine rack for inspection.
4. Inform pediatric nephrologist **immediately** if:
   a. Gross hematuria.
   b. Tachycardia.
   c. Hypotension.
      - Diastolic BP <60 mmHg
      - Systolic BP <80 mmHg or according to the formula below:

      Lowest systolic BP = 70 + [2 × (Age in years)] mmHg
5. Fluids: Oral or IV (if still sedated) at maintenance requirements.
6. Change biopsy site dressing to light dressing (do not remove Tegaderm™ on wound) the following day. Keep Tegaderm™ for at least one week.
7. Excuse from physical exercises for one month.

G. Complications of Kidney Biopsy

1. Bleeding:
   a. Sites:

Sites	Clinical Features
Collecting system	• Microscopic hematuria • Gross hematuria ± clots with ureteric obstruction
Subcapsular space	• Pressure tamponade • Pain
Perinephric space	• Hematoma • Marked decrease in hematocrit
Renal vasculature: • Renal artery, aorta, • Venous collaterals in patients with renal vein thrombosis • Arteriovenous fistula if the patient has had a previous biopsy	• Severe bleeding • Marked decrease in hematocrit

   b. Timing of bleed: Usually within 12 to 24 hours of the biopsy, but can occur up to a week later.
   c. Outcomes associated with post-biopsy bleeding:
      i. Transient macroscopic hematuria (3.5%).
      ii. Requirement for blood transfusion (0.9%).
      iii. Requirement for angiographic intervention to control bleeding (0.6%).
      iv. Requirement for nephrectomy to control bleeding (0.01%).
      v. Death (0.06%).
2. Pain lasting more than 12 hours (4%) due to:
   a. Ureteric obstruction by a blood clot in patients with gross hematuria.
   b. Stretching of the renal capsule by a subcapsular hematoma.
3. Arteriovenous fistulas (14%):
   a. Due to damage to the walls of an adjacent artery and vein.
   b. Usually clinically silent and resolve spontaneously over 1–2 years.

c. Symptomatic fistulae (rare) causing hematuria, hypotension or high-output heart failure require either transcatheter arterial embolization or surgical ligation.

4. Chronic hypertension due to the "Page kidney":
   - Due to pressure-induced ischemia from a large subcapsular hematoma leading to persistent activation of the renin-angiotensin system.
5. Infection of the peri-renal soft tissue (0.2%):
   - Usually occurs in patients with active renal parenchymal infection.

H. Sedation and Analgesia

I. Pre-sedation checklist:

1. Check the weight of the child. If child is obese, use the estimated lean body mass for the calculation of drug dosages.
2. Ensure child is well with no recent lower respiratory tract infection or wheeze.
3. Check for drug, latex and food allergies (e.g., soy, egg or nut).
4. Patent IV cannula *in-situ*.
5. IV drip set with 0.9% saline on standby.
6. Vital signs monitoring before sedation.
7. Dietary precautions:
   - Child <3 years: No solid or milk feeds × 4 hours
   - Child >3 years: No solid or milk feeds × 6 hours
8. Equipment on stand-by:
   - Cardiac monitor and SpO_2 monitor
   - Automated BP monitoring
   - Face-mask oxygen and suction equipment
   - Bag-valve-mask with oxygen tubing
   - Resuscitation trolley on standby
9. Positioning of the patient:

   a. Native kidney biopsy is performed with the patient in prone position.

   b. Careful management of the airway during the procedure is key.

      i. The head should be turned to one side and the neck slightly extended to open the airway.

ii. Ready access to suction, face-mask oxygen, and a bag-valve-mask should be prepared prior to the start of the procedure.

II. Medications for sedation/analgesia:

1. Topical EMLA™ cream to biopsy site 30–45 minutes before the procedure.
2. Local anesthetics:
   a. **Lignocaine** (1% Xylocaine): maximum 4 mg/kg or 0.4 ml/kg.
   b. **Lignocaine with adrenaline**: maximum 7 mg/kg or 0.7 ml/kg.
      - Dilute 0.05 ml of 1:1000 adrenaline to each 10 ml of 1% lignocaine to make 1:200000 concentration of adrenaline.
   c. **Bupivacaine** (0.5% Marcaine): maximum 2–3 mg/kg or 0.4–0.6 ml/kg.
   d. **Bupivacaine with adrenaline**: maximum 3–4 mg/kg or 0.6–0.8 ml/kg.
      - Dilute 0.05 ml of 1:1000 adrenaline to each 10 ml of 0.5% bupivacaine to make 1:200000 concentration of adrenaline.
3. IV medications:
   a. **Midazolam:** (5 mg/ml) 0.1–0.5 mg/kg/dose.
      i. Dilute 1 vial in 5 ml of 0.9% saline to make 1 mg/ml.
      ii. Use step-wise increments in dose (1–2.5 mg/dose) after at least 5 minutes, if the child shows no signs of being sedated.

      Antidote:
      i. IV flumazenil (Anexate) (500 μg/5 ml) 5 μg/kg/dose to be repeated every 60 seconds to a maximum of 40 μg/kg.
      ii. Respiratory depression may recur in a few minutes as flumazenil is short-acting.
   b. **Fentanyl:** (100 μg/2 ml) 1–2 μg/kg/dose (maximum 100 μg).
      i. Dilute 1 vial in 10 ml of 0.9% saline to make 10 μg/ml.
      ii. Rapid administration of fentanyl may cause chest wall rigidity.
         - Give the bolus over 5–10 minutes.

      Antidote for respiratory depression:
      i. IV naloxone (Narcan) 1–5 μg/kg/dose.
      ii. Repeat the dose at 2-minute intervals if there is no response.

***For total reversal for narcotic toxicity/cardiorespiratory arrest*:**

i. IV naloxone 0.1 mg/kg, maximum 2 mg at 2 minutes PRN.
ii. Respiratory depression may recur in a few minutes as naloxone is short-acting.
iii. Beware of rebound hypertension if fluid flush has been given for hypotension.
   - Give half the calculated dose and observe.

c. **Ketamine:** (50 mg/ml) 1–3 mg/kg.
   i. Dilute 1–2 ml in 5–10 ml 0.9% saline to give 10 mg/ml.
   ii. Start with 1 mg/kg/dose, repeat the dose after 5–10 minutes if inadequately sedated.
      - Doses at 2 mg/kg may cause apnea.
   iii. Give IV midazolam 0.1–0.2 mg/kg/dose for synergistic effect and prevention of emergence phenomena associated with ketamine in children.
   iv. Give IV atropine 0.02 mg/kg to reduce excessive salivation.
   v. Contraindicated in children with poorly controlled hypertension and raised intraocular pressure.

d. **Propofol:** (10 mg/ml, to be used neat).
   i. Indicated for children with poorly controlled hypertension or a history of difficult sedation.
   ii. Only to be used by experienced medical staff (refer to pediatric sedation team).
   iii. Preparation:
      - Draw up propofol into a 30-ml syringe.
      - Attach non-PVC tubing and prime the line with propofol.
   iv. Deliver 1–2 mg/kg of propofol as a bolus to induce sedation and then maintain at 1–10 mg/kg/hour using a syringe driver.
   v. Hypotension is a common side effect of propofol:
      - Stop the propofol infusion.
      - Flush 10 ml/kg of 0.9% saline.
      - If the BP improves, the sedation may continue at a lower rate of propofol infusion.
   vi. As propofol has no analgesic effects, local anesthetic at the biopsy site or IV fentanyl should be given.
      - If propofol is given in combination with fentanyl, there is a high risk of respiratory depression.

III. Management of complications associated with sedation:

1. Respiratory depression:
   a. Signs:
      i. Desaturation on pulse-oximeter.
      ii. Hypoventilation/apnea.
      iii. Stridor.
      iv. Cyanosis.
   b. Management algorithm:

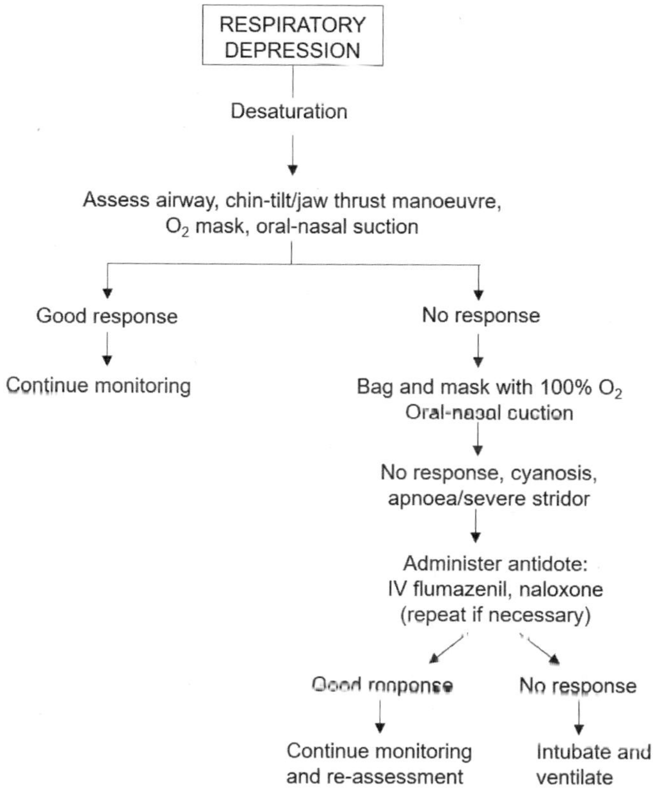

2. Hypotension:
   a. Prepare IV dopamine infusion in patients at high risk of hypotension, especially in transplant patients.
   b. Management algorithm:

HYPOTENSION

↓

Assess airway and breathing, O_2 mask

↓

IV 0.9% saline 10 ml/kg bolus

- → Good response → Continue monitoring
- → No response →
  - Repeat IV 0.9% saline bolus
  - IV phenylephrine 2-10 μg/kg/dose (maximum 500 μg)
  - IV dopamine infusion 5 μg/kg/min (titrate)
    - → Good response → Continue monitoring and re-assessment
    - → No response → Administer antidote: IV flumazenil, naloxone → No response → Abort procedure; Transfer to PICU for inotropic support

3. Hypertension:
   a. In patients at risk for hypertension, consider avoiding ketamine and use fentanyl and propofol instead.
   b. Ensure BP is normal before the start of sedation.
   c. Prepare IV glyceryl trinitrate (GTN) continuous IV infusion 1–10 μg/kg/min (maximum dose 400 μg/min) in patients at high risk for hypertension.

d. Consider using IV labetalol 0.2 mg/kg over 2 minutes.
   - If there is no response in 5–10 minutes, increase to 0.4–1.0 mg/kg (maximum bolus dose 20 mg).

Recommended Reading

1. Whittier WL, Korbet SM. (2020, edited) The Kidney biopsy. Edited by: Glassock RJ, Lam AQ. UpToDate ONLINE. http://www.uptodateonline.com

1 Reference Ranges for Urinary Solute Excretion

Lu L, Ng KH and Yap HK

A. Spot Urine Samples

1. Random urine samples correlate best with 24-hour urine values when taken as early morning specimens.
2. The 5th (P5) and 95th (P95) centiles of urinary solute:creatinine (Cr) ratios are:

Solute:Cr (mmol:mmol)	Age							
	1–6 months		6–12 months		1–2 years		2–3 years	
	P5	P95	P5	P95	P5	P95	P5	P95
Potassium:Cr	11	74	11	74	9	68	8	63
Calcium:Cr	0.09	2.2	0.00	2.2	0.07	1.5	0.06	1.4
Magnesium:Cr	0.4	2.2	0.4	2.2	0.4	1.7	0.3	1.6
Phosphate:Cr	1.2	19	1.2	19	1.2	14	1.2	12
Oxalate:Cr	0.07	0.22	0.06	0.17	0.05	0.13	0.04	0.1
Urate:Cr	0.8	1.6	0.7	1.5	0.5	1.4	0.47	1.3

Solute:Cr (mmol:mmol)	Age (Years)									
	3–5		5–7		7–10		10–14		14–17	
	P5	P95	P5	P95	P5	P95	P5	P95	P5	P95
Potassium:Cr	6.8	48	5.4	33	4.5	22	3.4	15	–	13
Calcium:Cr	0.05	1.1	0.04	0.8	0.04	0.7	0.04	0.7	0.04	0.7
Magnesium:Cr	0.3	1.3	0.3	1	0.3	0.9	0.2	0.7	0.2	0.6
Phosphate:Cr	1.2	8	1.2	5	1.2	3.6	0.8	3.2	0.8	2.7
Oxalate:Cr	0.03	0.08	0.03	0.07	0.02	0.06	0.02	0.06	0.02	0.06
Urate:Cr	0.4	1.1	0.3	0.8	0.28	0.56	0.2	0.44	0.2	0.4

B. 24-hour Urine Samples

1. Reliability of 24-hour urine collection:
   a. This can be confirmed in children >3 years of age by:
      - Urine creatinine excretion ≥0.18 mmol/kg/day (slightly higher in pubertal boys).
      - Urine volume >20 ml/kg/day.
   b. Decreased urinary creatinine excretion suggests:
      - 24-hour urine collection is not complete OR
      - Decreased muscle mass.
2. Reference ranges for 24-hour urine samples:

Solute	Normal Reference (per kg)	Normal Reference (per m^2 BSA)
Potassium		Adults: 25–125 mmol/day
Calcium	<0.1 mmol/kg/day (<4 mg/kg/day)	
Magnesium	≥0.05 mmol/kg/day (≥1.2 mg/kg/day)	≥3.6 mmol/1.73m²/day (≥88 mg/1.73m²/day)
Oxalate*		<0.5 mmol/1.73m²/day (<45 mg/1.73m²/day)
Urate		>1 year: <4848 µmol/1.73m²/day (<815 mg/1.73m²/day)
Citrate		>0.8–1.66 mmol/1.73m²/day (>140–320 mg/1.73m²/day)
Cystine**		<10 years: <55 µmol/1.73m²/day (<13 mg/1.73m²/day) >10 years: <200 µmol/1.73m²/day (<48 mg/1.73m²/day) Adults <250 µmol/1.73m²/day (<60 mg/1.73m²/day)

*Primary hyperoxaluria usually >0.7–1 mmol/1.73m²/day.
**Cystinuria usually >1.7 mmol/day (>400 mg/day).
Non-specific proximal renal tubule aminoaciduria ~1 mmol/day (250 mg/day).

C. Calcium

1. To convert spot urine calcium:creatinine ratio from mg/mg to mmol/mmol, multiply by 2.8.

2. In patients with decreased muscle mass, a spurious elevation of urine calcium:creatinine ratio can occur.
   - Consider using urine osmolality as the denominator to diagnose hypercalciuria:

$$\frac{\text{Urine calcium (mmol/L)}}{\text{Urine osmolality (mOsm/kg)}}$$

   - Normal urine calcium:osmolality ratio <0.00625.

D. Uric Acid

1. Simkin index:

$$\frac{\text{Urate excreted}}{\text{GFR}} = \frac{\text{PCr}}{\text{UCr}} \times \text{UUA}$$

GFR = Glomerular filtration rate
UUA = Urine uric acid (mmol/L)
UCr = Urine creatinine (mmol/L)
PCr = Plasma creatinine (mmol/L)

2. Normal values for urate excretion/GFR in children:

Age	Urate Excretion/GFR
<2 years	<0.18 mmol/L
>2 years	<0.035 mmol/L

E. Citrate

1. Age- and gender-specific references for urine citrate excretion:

	Boys		Girls	
	P5	P50*	P5	P50*
2 to <7 years:				
24-hour citrate (mg/kg)	4.2	13.5	5.2	15.1
24-hour citrate (mg/1.73 m²)	177	591	218	651
Citrate:Cr (mg/mmol)	27	86	33	98
Citrate:Cr (mg/g)	242	763	290	863

(*Continued*)

(*Continued*)

	Boys		Girls	
	P5	P50*	P5	P50*
7 to <13 years:				
24-hour citrate (mg/kg)	3.1	11.3	5.0	12.8
24-hour citrate (mg/1.73 m^2)	162	600	253	657
Citrate:Cr (mg/mmol)	16	62	30	78
Citrate:Cr (mg/g)	139	550	261	687
13 to <18 years:				
24-hour citrate (mg/kg)	2.2	7.7	4.2	12.3
24-hour citrate (mg/1.73 m^2)	130	476	248	729
Citrate:Cr (mg/mmol)	10	38	24	69
Citrate:Cr (mg/g)	89	340	216	611

*Patients at risk of nephrolithiasis should ideally have urine citrate excretion ≥P50.

2. Urine calcium:citrate ratio:
   - An elevated urine calcium:citrate ratio may better identify individuals at risk of hypercalciuria or calcium oxalate stone formation.

	Boys		Girls	
	P50	P95	P50	P95
2 to <7 years:				
Calcium:citrate (mg/mg)	0.15	0.48	0.13	0.42
Calcium:citrate (mmol/mg)	0.0037	0.012	0.0032	0.010
7 to <13 years:				
Calcium:citrate (mg/mg)	0.17	0.60	0.12	0.47
Calcium:citrate (mmol/mg)	0.0042	0.015	0.0030	0.012
13 to <18 years:				
Calcium:citrate (mg/mg)	0.22	0.80	0.16	0.60
Calcium:citrate (mmol/mg)	0.0055	0.020	0.0040	0.015

F. Phosphate

1. Urine phosphate excretion depends on serum phosphate levels.
   a. In cases of renal phosphate wasting, urine phosphate may be undetectably low in the presence of severe hypophosphatemia.
   b. Thus, in situations where pathology is likely, indices of urine phosphate excretion that take into account serum phosphate concentrations should be used.
   c. As serum phosphate levels are altered by dietary intake, samples should be collected in the fasting state.
2. Tubular maximum reabsorption rate of phosphate normalized to glomerular filtration rate (TMP/GFR):
   a. The maximal capacity of the kidney tubules to reabsorb phosphate can only be interpreted in the context of the rate of phosphate delivery to the kidney, which is determined by GFR and is thus quantified by the TMP/GFR.
   b. TMP/GFR (mmol/L) is equivalent to the renal threshold for phosphate, beyond which urine phosphate excretion is linearly proportionate to plasma phosphate concentration.
   c. Calculation of TMP/GFR:
      - Tubular phosphate reabsorption is assumed to be saturated when the tubular reabsorption of phosphate (TRP), which is given by 1-fractional excretion of phosphate, is ≤86%.
      - When TRP ≤86%, TMP/GFR = TRP × $P_{phosphate}$
      - When TRP >86%, TMP/GFR =

$$0.3 \times \frac{TRP}{1-(0.8 \times TRP)} \times P_{phosphate}$$

   d. Reference ranges for TMP/GFR:

Age	TMP/GFR (P5–P95, mmol/L)
Newborn	1.56–2.96
1 month to 2 years	1.08–2.22
2–15 years	1.15–2.44
25–35 years	1.00–1.35 (male) 0.96–1.44 (female)

G. Cystine

Age	Urine cystine:creatinine (mmol/mmol)
<1 month	<0.085
1–6 months	<0.053
>6 months	<0.018

H. Potassium

1. Trans-tubular potassium gradient (TTKG):
   a. TTKG is a measure of aldosterone-driven potassium secretion in the distal nephron.

$$TTKG = \frac{U_k \times P_{osm}}{P_k \times U_{osm}}$$

   where U_K = Urine potassium concentration
   P_K = Plasma potassium concentration
   U_{Osm} = Urine osmolality
   P_{Osm} = Plasma osmolality

   b. TTKG is only valid when urine sodium >25 mmol/L and $U_{Osm} > P_{Osm}$.
   In normotensive patients with hypokalaemia, TTKG >2 suggests renal potassium loss.

Recommended Reading

1. Matos V, Melle G Van, Boutat O, Markert M, Bachmann C, Guignard JP. (1997) Urinary phosphate/creatinine, calcium/creatinine, and magnesium/creatinine ratios in a healthy pediatric population. *J Pediatr* **131**:252–257.
2. Payne RB. (1998) Renal tubular reabsorption of phosphate (TmP/GFR): Indications and interpretation. *Ann Clin Biochem* **35**:201–206.
3. Matos V, Melle G Van, Werner D, Bardy D, Guignard JP. (1999) Urinary oxalate and urate to creatinine ratios in a healthy pediatric population. *Am J Kidney Dis* **34**:1–6.
4. Barth JH, Jones RG, Payne RB. (2000) Calculation of renal tubular reabsorption of phosphate: The algorithm performs better than the nomogram. *Ann Clin Biochem* **37**:79–81.

5. Richmond W, Colgan G, Simon S, Stuart-Hilgenfeld M, Wilson N, Alon US. (2005) Random urine calcium/osmolality in the assessment of calciuria in children with decreased muscle mass. *Clinical Nephrology* **64**:264-270.
6. Friedman A. (2009) Laboratory assessment and investigation of renal function. In: *Pediatric Nephrology*. Eds. Avner E, Harmon W, Niaudet P, Yoshikawa N.
7. Kirejczyk JK, Porowski T, Konstantynowicz J, Kozerska A, Nazarkiewicz A, Hoppe B, Wasilewska A. (2014) Urinary citrate excretion in healthy children depends on age and gender. *Pediatr Nephrol* **29**:1575–1582.
8. Noone D, Langlois V. (2016) Laboratory evaluation of renal disease in childhood. In: Pediatric Kidney Disease. Eds. Geary DF, Schaefer F. Springer. pp 76–105.
9. Smith J, Bruder Stapleton F. (2019, updated) Prevention of recurrent nephrolithiasis in children. Edited by: Baskin LS, Kim MS. *UpToDate ONLINE*. http://www.uptodate.com.

2 Reference Ranges for Urinary Catecholamine Metabolites Excretion

Sng A, Teo S, Ng KH and Yap HK

A. Urinary Catecholamine Metabolites Excretion

1. Urinary catecholamine metabolites/creatinine ratios:
   a. Age-specific 97.5th percentile reference standards for urinary catecholamine metabolites:creatinine ratios.
      - Values are in nmol/mmol (µg/g).

Age	Metanephrine	Normetanephrine	Epinephrine	Norepinephrine
0–3 months	496 (864)	2728 (4421)	43 (69)	182 (272)
3–6 months	389 (678)	1678 (2720)	46 (75)	132 (197)
6–12 months	267 (466)	1162 (1884)	37 (60)	130 (195)
1–2 years	216 (377)	592 (959)	24 (39)	93 (139)
2–5 years	213 (371)	455 (738)	23 (37)	61 (91)
5–10 years	178 (310)	287 (465)	18 (29)	48 (72)
10–15 years	131 (228)	209 (339)	11 (18)	35 (53)
15–20 years	72 (126)	170 (275)	7 (12)	35 (53)
20–25 years	83 (145)	190 (308)	9 (14)	35 (53)
Conversion factor*	0.574	0.617	0.617	0.669

*To convert µg/g to nmol/mmol (µmol/mol) creatinine, multiply by the conversion factor.

Age	Dopamine	Homovanillic acid (HVA)	Vanillymandelic acid (VMA)
0–3 months	1974 (2675)	21700 (35000)	10.8 (18.9)
3–6 months	1810 (2453)	19900 (32100)	12.4 (21.8)
6–12 months	1427 (1933)	19500 (31400)	9.6 (16.9)
1–2 years	1221 (1654)	17000 (27300)	8.9 (15.5)
2–5 years	853 (1156)	14600 (23500)	5.9 (10.3)
5–10 years	625 (847)	10200 (16500)	4.3 (7.6)
10–15 years	407 (552)	6000 (9700)	3.2 (5.6)
15–20 years	305 (413)	3600 (5800)	2.5 (4.3)
20–25 years	289 (391)	3200 (5200)	2.6 (4.6)
Conversion factor*	0.738	0.621	0.571

*To convert µg/g to nmol/mmol (µmol/mol) creatinine, multiply by the conversion factor.

b. Urinary dopamine:creatinine ratio:
- 0–2 years: 0–2.22 mmol/mol
- >2–5 years: 0–1.13 mmol/mol
- >5–10 years: 0–0.77 mmol/mol
- >10 years: 0–0.40 mmol/mol

c. Urinary VMA:creatinine ratio:
- 0–1 years: <10.7 mmol/mol
- 2–4 years: <6.3 mmol/mol
- 5–9 years: <4.7 mmol/mol
- 10–19 years: <4.7 mmol/mol
- >19 years: <3.4 mmol/mol

d. Urinary HVA:creatinine ratio:
- <1 year: <25.0 mg/g creatinine
- 1 year: <22.5 mg/g creatinine
- 2–4 years: <18.0 mg/g creatinine
- 5–9 years: <12.0 mg/g creatinine
- 10–14 years: <8.0 mg/g creatinine
- ≥15 years (adults): <8.0 mg/24 hours

2. 24-hour urinary catecholamine metabolites excretion:
   a. Urinary norepinephrine and epinephrine:

Age (years)	Norepinephrine (μg/day)	Age (years)	Epinephrine (μg/day)
0 to <1	<11	0 to <1	<2.6
1 to <2	1–17	1 to <2	<3.6
2 to <4	4–29	2 to <4	<6.1
4 to <7	8–45	4–9	0.2–10
7 to <10	13–65	10–15	0.5–20
≥10	15–80	≥16	<21

   b. Urinary metanephrine and normetanephrine:

Age (years)	Normetanephrines (μg/day)		Age (years)	Metanephrines (μg/day)	
	Male	Female		Male	Female
3–8	34–169	29–145	3–8	29–92	18–144
9–12	84–422	55–277	9–12	59–188	43–122
13–17	91–456	57–286	13–17	69–221	33–185
18–29	103–390	103–390	≥18	44–261	30–180

   c. Urinary dopamine:
      - 0 to <1 year: <86 μg/day
      - 1 to <2 years: 10–140 μg/day
      - 2 to <4 years: 40–260 μg/day
      - ≥4 years: 65–400 μg/day
   d. Urinary VMA:
      - Normal <8.0 mg/day
   e. Urinary HVA:
      - Normal <8.0 mg/day

f. Conversion table:

	Conventional Unit	Conversion Factor	SI Unit
Epinephrine	µg/day	5.91	nmol/day
Norepinephrine	µg/day	5.46	nmol/day
Dopamine	µg/day	6.53	nmol/day
Metanephrines	µg/day	5.07	nmol/day
Normetanephrines	µg/day	5.26	nmol/day

B. Procedure for Urine Collection for Catecholamine Metabolites:

1. Withhold interfering drugs for at least 2 weeks.
   a. Drugs that increase catecholamine secretion:
      - Cocaine, amphetamines, caffeine.
      - Sympathomimetics: Salbutamol, terbutaline, phenylephrine, dobutamine, isoprenaline, pseudoephedrine.
      - Alpha-2-blockers: Phenoxybenzamine, phentolamine (possibly due to effect of blocking negative feedback on presynaptic sympathetic endings).
      - L-dopa (precursor of catecholamines).
   b. Drugs that inhibit catecholamine reuptake or metabolism:
      - Tricyclic antidepressants.
      - Norepinephrine reuptake inhibitors: Bupropion, reboxetine, viloxazine.
      - Antipsychotics (increase normetanephrines, norepinephrine).
      - Monoamine oxidase inhibitors.
      - Prochlorperazine.
      - Reserpine.
   c. Drugs that influence the spectrometry measurements:
      - Labetalol, sotalol, isoproterenol.
      - Acetaminophen: structurally related (plasma metanephrines).

d. Other potential interference (minor influence, test can still be performed with these drugs onboard):
   - Calcium channel blockers (small effect on noradrenaline due to reflex sympathetic activation with short-acting drugs).
   - Beta-blockers (plasma metanephrines).
   - Co-trimoxazole (interferes with detection of HVA).

2. Dietary restrictions for 24 hours prior to urine collection:
   - No coffee, tea, bananas, cocoa products, vanilla products, curry, walnut, chili, pineapple, capsicum, and spices and food containing capsaicin.
3. Avoid stress and strenuous exercise during the urine collection.
4. Urine should be collected in a bottle containing added acid (to ensure stability of urinary catecholamines).
5. If the initial test is negative but suspicion is high, consider repeating the collection during symptomatic periods or send a serum sample for fractionated metanephrines or normetanephrines for confirmation.

Recommended Reading

1. O'Meara A, Tormey W, FitzGerald RJ, Fitzgibbon M, Kenny D. (1994) Interpretation of random urinary catecholamines and their metabolites in neuroblastoma. *Acta Pediatr* **83**:88–92.
2. Pussard E, Neveux M, Guigueno. (2009) Reference intervals for urinary catecholamines and metabolites from birth to adulthood. *Clin Biochem* **42**:536–539.
3. Mayo Clinic Laboratories. (2021) Rochester 2021 test catalog. Laboratory reference edition.

3 Total Body Water Nomograms Based on Morgenstern Equations

Teo S, Ng KH and Yap HK

Male Total Body Water (L) Nomograms:

Weight (kg) \ Height (cm)	50	54	58	62	66	70	74	78	82	86	90	94	98	102	106	110	114
2	1.6	1.7	1.8	1.9													
3	1.9	2.1	2.2	2.4													
4	2.2	2.4	2.6	2.8	3.0												
5	2.4	2.7	2.9	3.1	3.3												
6	2.6	2.9	3.1	3.4	3.6	3.9	4.1										
7	2.8	3.1	3.4	3.6	3.9	4.2	4.4	4.7	4.9								
8	2.9	3.2	3.5	3.9	4.1	4.4	4.7	5.0	5.3	5.5	5.8						
9				4.0	4.4	4.7	5.0	5.3	5.6	5.9	6.2	6.5	6.7				
10				4.2	4.6	4.9	5.2	5.6	5.9	6.2	6.5	6.8	7.1	7.4	7.7		
11				4.4	4.8	5.1	5.5	5.8	6.2	6.5	6.8	7.1	7.5	7.8	8.1	8.4	8.7
12				4.5	4.9	5.3	5.7	6.0	6.4	6.8	7.1	7.5	7.8	8.1	8.5	8.8	9.1
13								6.3	6.6	7.0	7.4	7.8	8.1	8.5	8.8	9.2	9.5
14								6.5	6.9	7.3	7.7	8.0	8.4	8.8	9.2	9.5	9.9
15								6.7	7.1	7.5	7.9	8.3	8.7	9.1	9.5	9.9	10.2
16								6.8	7.3	7.7	8.1	8.6	9.0	9.4	9.8	10.2	10.6
17											8.4	8.8	9.2	9.7	10.1	10.5	10.9
18											8.6	9.0	9.5	9.9	10.4	10.8	11.2
19											8.8	9.3	9.7	10.2	10.6	11.1	11.5
20											9.0	9.4	9.9	10.4	10.9	11.3	11.8

Male Total Body Water (L) Nomograms:

Weight (kg)	Height (cm) 106	110	114	118	122	126	130	134	138	142	146	150	154	158	162	166	170	174	178	182	186	190
20	10.9	11.3	11.8	12.3	12.7	13.2	13.6	14.0	14.5	14.9	15.3	15.7										
22	11.4	11.9	12.4	12.8	13.3	13.8	14.3	14.7	15.2	15.7	16.1	16.6										
24	11.8	12.3	12.9	13.4	13.9	14.4	14.9	15.4	15.9	16.4	16.8	17.3	17.8	18.3	18.7							
26	12.2	12.8	13.3	13.9	14.4	15.0	15.5	16.0	16.5	17.0	17.5	18.0	18.5	19.0	19.5							
28	12.6	13.2	13.8	14.4	14.9	15.5	16.0	16.6	17.1	17.7	18.2	18.7	19.3	19.8	20.3	20.8	21.3					
30	13.0	13.6	14.2	14.8	15.4	16.0	16.6	17.1	17.7	18.3	18.8	19.4	19.9	20.5	21.0	21.6	22.1					
32	13.3	14.0	14.6	15.2	15.8	16.5	17.1	17.7	18.3	18.8	19.4	20.0	20.6	21.2	21.7	22.3	22.9	23.4	24.0			
34	13.6	14.3	15.0	15.6	16.3	16.9	17.5	18.2	18.8	19.4	20.0	20.6	21.2	21.8	22.4	23.0	23.6	24.2	24.7			
36	13.9	14.6	15.3	16.0	16.7	17.3	18.0	18.7	19.3	19.9	20.6	21.2	21.8	22.4	23.1	23.7	24.3	24.9	25.5	26.1	26.6	
38	14.2	14.9	15.7	16.4	17.1	17.8	18.4	19.1	19.8	20.4	21.1	21.8	22.4	23.0	23.7	24.3	24.9	25.6	26.2	26.8	27.4	
40			16.0	16.7	17.4	18.1	18.8	19.5	20.2	20.9	21.6	22.3	23.0	23.6	24.3	24.9	25.6	26.2	26.9	27.5	28.1	28.8
42			16.3	17.0	17.8	18.5	19.2	20.0	20.7	21.4	22.1	22.8	23.5	24.2	24.9	25.5	26.2	26.9	27.5	28.2	28.8	29.5
44			16.6	17.3	18.1	18.9	19.6	20.4	21.1	21.8	22.6	23.3	24.0	24.7	25.4	26.1	26.8	27.5	28.2	28.8	29.5	30.2
46			16.8	17.6	18.4	19.2	20.0	20.8	21.5	22.3	23.0	23.8	24.5	25.2	26.0	26.7	27.4	28.1	28.8	29.5	30.2	30.9
48			17.1	17.9	18.7	19.5	20.3	21.1	21.9	22.7	23.5	24.2	25.0	25.7	26.5	27.2	27.9	28.7	29.4	30.1	30.8	31.5
50			17.3	18.2	19.0	19.8	20.7	21.5	22.3	23.1	23.9	24.7	25.4	26.2	27.0	27.7	28.5	29.2	30.0	30.7	31.5	32.2
52						20.1	21.0	21.8	22.6	23.5	24.3	25.1	25.9	26.7	27.5	28.2	29.0	29.8	30.6	31.3	32.1	32.8

Male Total Body Water (L) Nomograms:

Weight (kg)	Height (cm) 126	130	134	138	142	146	150	154	158	162	166	170	174	178	182	186	190
54	20.4	21.3	22.1	23.0	23.8	24.7	25.5	26.3	27.1	27.9	28.7	29.5	30.3	31.1	31.9	32.7	33.4
56	20.7	21.3	22.5	23.3	24.2	25.0	25.9	26.7	27.6	28.4	29.2	30.0	30.8	31.7	32.4	33.2	34.0
58	20.9	21.3	22.8	23.7	24.5	25.4	26.3	27.1	28.0	28.8	29.7	30.5	31.4	32.2	33.0	33.8	34.6
60	21.2	22.1	23.1	24.0	24.9	25.8	26.7	27.5	28.4	29.3	30.1	31.0	31.8	32.7	33.5	34.4	35.2
62	21.4	22.4	23.3	24.3	25.2	26.1	27.0	27.9	28.8	29.7	30.6	31.5	32.3	33.2	34.0	34.9	35.7
64	21.7	22.6	23.6	24.6	25.5	26.4	27.4	28.3	29.2	30.1	31.0	31.9	32.8	33.7	34.5	35.4	36.3
66				24.8	25.8	26.8	27.7	28.6	29.6	30.5	31.4	32.3	33.2	34.1	35.0	35.9	36.8
68				25.1	26.1	27.1	28.0	29.0	30.0	30.9	31.8	32.8	33.7	34.6	35.5	36.4	37.3
70				25.4	26.4	27.4	28.4	29.3	30.3	31.3	32.2	33.2	34.1	35.1	36.0	36.9	37.8
72				25.6	26.6	27.7	28.7	29.7	30.7	31.6	32.6	33.6	34.5	35.5	36.4	37.4	38.3
74				25.9	26.9	27.9	29.0	30.0	31.0	32.0	33.0	34.0	34.9	35.9	36.9	37.7	38.8
76				26.1	27.2	28.2	29.3	30.3	31.3	32.3	33.3	34.4	35.3	36.3	37.3	38.3	39.3
78				26.3	27.4	28.5	29.5	30.6	31.6	32.7	33.7	34.7	35.7	36.7	37.7	38.7	39.7
80				26.5	27.6	28.7	29.8	30.9	31.9	33.0	34.1	35.1	36.1	37.1	38.2	39.2	40.2

Female Total Body Water (L) Nomograms:

Weight (kg)	Height (cm)																
	50	54	58	62	66	70	74	78	82	86	90	94	98	102	106	110	114
2	2.0	2.1	2.2	2.4													
3	2.4	2.6	2.8	2.9													
4	2.8	3.0	3.2	3.4	3.6												
5	3.1	3.3	3.5	3.8	4.0												
6	3.3	3.6	3.8	4.1	4.3	4.6	4.8										
7	3.5	3.8	4.1	4.4	4.8	4.9	5.2	5.5	5.7								
8	3.7	4.0	4.3	4.6	4.9	5.2	5.5	5.8	6.1	6.4	6.6						
9				4.9	5.2	5.5	5.8	6.1	6.4	6.7	7.0	7.3	7.6				
10				5.1	5.4	5.8	6.1	6.4	6.8	7.1	7.4	7.7	8.0	8.3	8.6		
11				5.3	5.6	6.0	6.4	6.7	7.1	7.4	7.7	8.1	8.4	8.7	9.0	9.3	9.6
12				5.4	5.8	6.2	6.6	7.0	7.3	7.7	8.0	8.4	8.7	9.1	9.4	9.7	10.0
13								7.2	7.6	8.0	8.3	8.7	9.1	9.4	9.8	10.1	10.4
14								7.4	7.8	8.2	8.6	9.0	9.4	9.7	10.1	10.5	10.8
15								7.6	8.0	8.5	8.9	9.3	9.7	10.0	10.4	10.8	11.2

Female Total Body Water (L) Nomograms:

Weight (kg)	Height (cm)																				
	106	110	114	118	122	126	130	134	138	142	146	150	154	158	162	166	170	174	178	182	186	190
20	11.8	12.3	12.7	13.2	13.6	14.0	14.5	14.9	15.3	15.7	16.1	16.5										
22	12.3	12.8	13.3	13.7	14.2	14.7	15.1	15.6	16.0	16.4	16.9	17.3										
24	12.8	13.3	13.8	14.3	14.8	15.2	15.7	16.2	16.7	17.1	17.6	18.0	18.5	18.9	19.4							
26	13.2	13.7	14.2	14.8	15.3	15.8	16.3	16.8	17.3	17.8	18.3	18.7	19.2	19.7	20.1							
28	13.6	14.1	14.7	15.2	15.8	16.3	16.8	17.3	17.9	18.4	18.9	19.4	19.9	20.4	20.9	21.3	21.8					
30	13.9	14.5	15.1	15.7	16.2	16.8	17.3	17.9	18.4	18.9	19.5	20.0	20.5	21.0	21.5	22.0	22.5					
32	14.3	14.9	15.5	16.1	16.6	17.2	17.8	18.4	18.9	19.5	20.0	20.6	21.1	21.7	22.2	22.7	23.2	23.7	24.3			
34	14.6	15.2	15.8	16.4	17.0	17.7	18.2	18.8	19.4	20.0	20.6	21.1	21.7	22.3	22.8	23.4	23.9	24.4	25.0			
36	14.8	15.5	16.2	16.8	17.4	18.1	18.7	19.3	19.9	20.5	21.1	21.7	22.3	22.8	23.4	24.0	24.5	25.1	25.6	26.2	26.7	
38	15.1	15.8	16.5	17.1	17.8	18.4	19.1	19.7	20.3	21.0	21.6	22.2	22.8	23.4	24.0	24.6	25.1	25.7	26.3	26.9	27.4	
40			16.8	17.4	18.1	18.8	19.5	20.1	20.7	21.4	22.0	22.7	23.3	23.9	24.5	25.1	25.7	26.3	26.9	27.5	28.1	28.6
42			17.0	17.7	18.4	19.1	19.8	20.5	21.1	21.8	22.5	23.1	23.8	24.4	25.0	25.7	26.3	26.9	27.5	28.1	28.7	29.3
44			17.3	18.0	18.7	19.5	20.2	20.9	21.5	22.2	22.9	23.6	24.2	24.9	25.5	26.2	26.8	27.4	28.1	28.7	29.3	29.9
46			17.5	18.3	19.0	19.8	20.5	21.2	21.9	22.6	23.3	24.0	24.7	25.3	26.0	26.7	27.3	28.0	28.6	29.3	29.9	30.5
48			17.8	18.5	19.3	20.0	20.8	21.5	22.3	23.0	23.7	24.4	25.1	25.8	26.5	27.2	27.8	28.5	29.2	29.8	30.5	31.1
50			18.0	18.8	19.6	20.3	21.1	21.8	22.6	23.3	24.1	24.8	25.5	26.2	26.9	27.6	28.3	29.0	29.7	30.4	31.0	31.7
52						20.6	21.4	22.1	22.9	23.7	24.4	25.2	25.9	26.6	27.4	28.1	28.8	29.5	30.2	30.9	31.6	32.2

Female Total Body Water (L) Nomograms:

Weight (kg)	Height (cm)																
	126	130	134	138	142	146	150	154	158	162	166	170	174	178	182	186	190
54	20.8	21.6	22.4	23.2	24.0	24.8	25.5	26.3	27.0	27.8	28.5	29.2	29.9	30.7	31.4	32.1	32.8
56	21.1	21.9	22.7	23.5	24.3	25.1	25.9	26.6	27.4	28.2	28.9	29.7	30.4	31.1	31.9	32.6	33.3
58	21.3	22.1	23.0	23.8	24.6	25.4	26.2	27.0	27.8	28.5	29.3	30.1	30.8	31.6	32.3	33.1	33.8
60	21.5	22.4	23.2	24.1	24.9	25.7	26.5	27.3	28.1	28.9	29.7	30.5	31.3	32.0	32.8	33.5	34.3
62	21.7	22.6	23.4	24.3	25.2	26.0	26.8	27.7	28.5	29.3	30.1	30.9	31.7	32.4	33.2	34.0	34.8
64	21.9	22.8	23.7	24.6	25.4	26.3	27.1	28.0	28.8	29.6	30.4	31.3	32.1	32.9	33.6	34.4	35.2
66				24.8	25.7	26.5	27.4	28.3	29.1	30.0	30.8	31.6	32.4	33.2	34.1	34.9	35.7
68				25.0	25.9	26.8	27.7	28.6	29.4	30.3	31.1	32.0	32.8	33.6	34.5	35.3	36.1
70				25.2	26.1	27.0	27.9	28.8	29.7	30.6	31.5	32.3	33.2	34.0	34.9	35.7	36.5
72				25.4	26.4	27.3	28.2	29.1	30.0	30.9	31.8	32.7	33.5	34.4	35.2	36.1	36.9
74				25.6	26.6	27.5	28.4	29.4	30.3	31.2	32.1	33.0	33.9	34.7	35.6	36.5	37.3
76				25.8	26.8	27.7	28.7	29.6	30.6	31.5	32.4	33.3	34.2	35.1	36.0	36.8	37.7
78				26.0	27.0	27.9	28.9	29.9	30.8	31.7	32.7	33.6	34.5	35.4	36.3	37.2	38.1
80				26.2	27.2	28.1	29.1	30.1	31.1	32.0	33.0	33.9	34.8	35.7	36.7	37.6	38.5

Morgenstern BZ, Wuhl E, Nair KS, Warady BA, Schaefer F. (2006) Anthropometric prediction of total body water in children who are on pediatric peritoneal dialysis. *J Am Soc Nephrol* **17**:285–293.

	50% dose Q12h	50% dose Q24h	IHD: 10-20 mg/kg/dose Q24h AD PD: 10-20 mg/kg/dose Q24h	20-40 mg/kg/dose Q12h
lo change		4 mg/kg/dose Q6h	IHD: 4 mg/kg/dose Q6h PD: 4 mg/kg/dose Q6h	No change
	Not recommended because therapeutic concentrations are not attainable.			
	75% dose Q6h	20%-50% dose Q6h	IHD: 20%-50% dose Q6h AD PD: 20%-50% dose Q6h	75% dose Q6h
	No change			No recommendation
	70% dose Q8h		IHD: 50-75 mg/kg piperacillin Q12h AD PD: 50-75 mg/kg piperacillin dose Q12h	35-50 mg/kg piperacillin Q8h
	100% dose Q12h	Please Refer to ID		5 mg/kg TMP Q8h
	10mg/kg Q18-24h	10 mg/kg one time	10 mg/kg/dose, dosing frequency as per serum concentration	10 mg/kg/dose, dosing frequency as per serum concentration
	10mg/kg Q48h	10 mg/kg one time	10 mg/kg/dose, dosing frequency as per serum concentration	10 mg/kg/dose, dosing frequency as per serum concentration
	Adjust dose and frequency based on pre-trough levels. Target 10-20 mcg/ml.			
	100% dose Q24h	50% dose Q24h	IHD: 5 mg/kg/dose Q24h AD PD: 5 mg/kg/dose Q24h	10 mg/kg/dose Q12h
	100% dose 3x/day	50% dose Q12h	IHD: 50% dose Q12h AD PD: 50% dose Q12h	No recommendation
	100% dose Q24h	50% dose Q24h	IHD: 10 mg/kg/dose Q24h AD PD: 10 mg/kg/dose Q24h	No recommendation
	eGFR 28-35: 50 mg/kg Q24h eGFR <28: No recommendation	No recommendation	No recommendation	60-80 mg/kg Q24h
4h 4h 8h 8h	eGFR 28-35: 50-65 mg/kg Q48h eGFR <28: No recommendation			60-80 mg/kg Q48h
	eGFR 10-24: 1.25 mg/kg Q24h	1.25 mg/kg 3x/week	IHD: 1.25 mg/kg 3x/wk AD PD: 1.25 mg/kg 3x/wk	2.5 mg/kg Q24h
h	eGFR 10-24: 0.625 mg/kg Q24h	0.625 mg/kg 3x/week	IHD: 0.625 mg/kg 3x/wk AD PD: 0.625 mg/kg 3x/wk	1.25 mg/kg/dose Q24h
	eGFR 10-24: 50% dose Q48h	No recommendation OR use IV ganciclovir	IHD: 50% dose 3x/wk AD PD: No recommendation	50% dose Q24h
	eGFR 10-24: 50% dose 2x/week	No recommendation OR use IV ganciclovir	IHD: 50% dose 3x/wk AD PD: No recommendation	50% dose Q48h
	No change			
	total dose can be decreased by 50% or dose can be given every other day if renal dysfunction is due to the drug.			
	No change for loading dose.			
ly dose Q24h		50% of daily dose Q48h	IHD: 1.5-6 mg/kg/dose Q48h AD PD: 1.5-6 mg/kg/dose Q48h	6 mg/kg/dose Q24h
	No change			

Receiving Continuous Renal Replacement Therapy, Trotman 2005 (4) Drug Package Inserts

enzae strains. Maximum clavulanate dose 10 mg/kg/day; note the amoxicillin:clavulanate ratio varies for oral preparations.

ctively. **IHD**: intermittent hemodialysis. **PD**: peritoneal dialysis.

Antimicrobial Dosing in Ped

This card is intended for pa

Estimating Kidney Function

Estimated glomerular filtration rate (eGFR) is calculated in ml/min/1.73 m^2 for pediatric patients when using this guideline

Full-term infants (0-12 months) (eGFR) = (30.1 x L)/Cr — where eGFR is calculated in ml/min/1.73m^2

1 years - 18 years (eGFR) = (36.5 x L)/Cr — L = length/height measured in cm — Cr = c

Drug		Dosage for normal kidney function (MAX per dose)	eGFR 30 - ml/min/1.7
Amikacin	IV Usual	Traditional: IV 5-7.5 mg/kg Q8h (750mg) Extended: IV 15 mg/kg Q24h (1500mg)	If eGFR <50 ml
	IV CF	Traditional: IV 10 mg/kg Q8h (750mg) Extended: IV 30 mg/kg Q24h (1500mg)	If eGFR <50 ml/
Amoxicillin		PO 15-30 mg/kg Q8h (1g)	No chan
Amoxicillin/ Clavulanate	IV	IV 25 mg/kg amoxicillin Q8h	No char
	PO Usual	PO 15 mg/kg amoxicillin Q12h	
	PO High dose*	PO 20 mg/kg amoxicillin Q8h	100% dose
Ampicillin	IV Usual	IV 15 mg/kg Q6h (500mg)	No char
	IV Sepsis	IV 25 mg/kg Q6h (1g)	
	IV Meningitis	IV 50 mg/kg Q6h (2g)	
Ampicillin/ Sulbactam	IV	IV 25-50 mg/kg ampicillin Q6h (3g)	100% dos
	PO	<30 kg: PO 12.5-25 mg/kg sultamicillin Q12h (750mg)	
		≥30 kg: PO 375-750 mg sultamicillin Q12h (750mg)	
Azithromycin	IV/PO	10 mg/kg Q24h (500mg) D1 then 5 mg/kg Q24h (250mg) on D2-5	
Cefaclor		PO 10-15 mg/kg Q8h (500mg)	
Cefazolin	IV Usual	IV 25 mg/kg Q8h (1g)	No cha
	IV Severe	IV 30-50 mg/kg Q8h (2g)	
Cefepime	IV Usual	IV 50 mg/kg Q12h (2g)	100% dos
	IV Severe	IV 50 mg/kg Q8h (2g)	100% dos
Cefotaxime	IV Sepsis	IV 25-50 mg/kg Q6h (2g)	100% dos
	IV Meningitis	IV 75 mg/kg Q6h (2g)	
Ceftazidime	IV Usual	IV 30 mg/kg Q8h (2g)	100% dos
	IV Severe	IV 50 mg/kg Q8h (2g)	
Ceftriaxone	IV Sepsis	IV 50 mg/kg Q24h (2g)	
	IV Meningitis	IV 50 mg/kg Q12h (2g)	
	IV Typhoid	IV 80 mg/kg Q24h (2g)	
Cefuroxime axetil	PO Suspension	PO 10-15 mg/kg Q12h (500mg)	No cha
	PO Tablet	PO 250-500 mg Q12h (500mg)	
Cephalexin	PO Usual	PO 10-15 mg/kg Q6h (1g)	100% do
	PO Severe	PO 15-25 mg/kg Q6h (1g)	
Ciprofloxacin	IV	IV 10-15 mg/kg Q12h (400mg)	No ch
	P.aeruginosa	IV 10 mg/kg Q8h (400mg)	
	PO	PO 10-20 mg/kg Q12h (750mg)	
Clarithromycin		PO 7.5 mg/kg Q12h (500mg)	No ch
Clindamycin	IV/PO Mild-Moderate	IV/PO 5 mg/kg Q6h-Q8h (600mg)	
	IV/PO Severe	IV/PO 10 mg/kg Q6h-Q8h (600mg)	
Cloxacillin	IV/PO Usual	IV/PO 15 mg/kg Q6h (2g)	
	IV High dose	IV 25-50 mg/kg Q4h-Q6h (2g)	
Ertapenem	IV/IM	<13 years: IV/IM 15 mg/kg Q12h (500mg)	
		≥13 years: IV/IM 1000 mg Q24h (1000mg)	No C
Gentamicin	IV	Traditional: IV 2-2.5 mg/kg Q8h Extended: IV 6 mg/kg Q24h (360mg)	If estimated eGF
	IV Synergistic	Traditional: IV 1 mg/kg Q8h Extended: IV 3 mg/kg Q24h (360mg)	
Levofloxacin	IV/PO	<5 years: 5-10 mg/kg Q12h (750mg/day)	No c
		≥5 years: 5-10 mg/kg Q24h (750mg)	
Linezolid	IV/PO	<12 years: IV/PO 10 mg/kg Q8h (600mg)	
		≥12 years: IV/PO 10 mg/kg Q12h (600mg)	

atients with Kidney Dysfunction

month and <18 years ONLY

neasured in µmol/L

	eGFR 10 – 29 ml/min/1.73m²	eGFR <10 ml/min/1.73m²	Dialysis AD = after dialysis on HD days	CRRT
², then use traditional dose: 5-7.5 mg/kg/dose x1. Adjust dose & frequency based on levels. Re-dose when trough <10 mcg/ml. Traditional Peak 15-30 mcg/ml; Extended Peak 60-100 mcg/ml; trough <10 mcg/ml				
², then use traditional dose: 7.5-10 mg/kg/dose x1. Adjust dose & frequency based on levels. Re-dose when trough <10 mcg/ml. Traditional CF Peak 25-40 mcg/ml; Extended CF Peak 80-120 mcg/ml; trough <10 mcg/ml				
	100% dose Q12h	100% dose Q24h	IHD: 8-20 mg/kg/dose Q24h AD PD: 8-20 mg/kg/dose Q24h	No recommendation
	100% dose Q12h	100% dose Q24h	IHD: 8-20 mg/kg/dose Q24h AD PD: 8-20 mg/kg/dose Q24h	No recommendation
	100% dose Q8-12h	100% dose Q12h	IHD: 35-50 mg/kg/dose Q12h AD PD: 35-50 mg/kg/dose Q12h	35-50 mg/kg/dose Q6h
	100% dose Q12h	100% dose Q24h	IHD: 100% dose Q24h AD PD: 100% dose Q24h	CVVH: 100% dose Q12h CVVHD/HDF: 100% dose Q8h
No change				
change		50% dose Q8h	IHD: 50% dose Q8h AD PD: 50% dose Q8h	No recommendation
	100% dose Q12h 50% dose Q12h	100% dose Q24h 50% dose Q24h	IHD: 25 mg/kg/dose Q24h AD PD: 25 mg/kg/dose Q24h	25 mg/kg/dose Q8h
	100% dose Q24h	100% dose Q48h	IHD: 50 mg/kg/dose Q24h AD PD: 50 mg/kg/dose Q24h	50 mg/kg/dose Q12h
	100% dose Q12h	100% dose Q24h	IHD: 35-70 mg/kg/dose Q24h AD PD: 35-70 mg/kg/dose Q24h	35-70 mg/kg/dose Q12h
	100% dose Q24h	100% dose Q48h	IHD: 50 mg/kg/dose Q48h AD PD: 50 mg/kg/dose Q48h	50 mg/kg/dose Q12h
No change with dose <2 g/day. If concurrent kidney and hepatic dysfunction, use MAX 2 g/day.				50 mg/kg Q24h
	No change	100% dose Q24h	IHD: 15 mg/kg/dose Q24h AD PD: 15 mg/kg/dose Q24h	No recommendation
	100% dose Q12h	100% dose Q24h	IHD: 5-10 mg/kg/dose Q24h AD PD: 5-10 mg/kg/dose Q24h	No recommendation
	100% dose Q18h	100% dose Q24h	IHD: 10-15 mg/kg/dose Q24h AD PD: 10-15 mg/kg/dose Q24h	10-15 mg/kg/dose Q12h
	50% dose Q12h	50% dose Q24h	IHD: 4 mg/kg/dose Q24h AD PD: 4 mg/kg/dose Q24h	No recommendation
No change				
No change unless concurrent hepatic impairment.				
No recommendation				
	50% dose Q24h		IHD: 50% dose Q24h AD (N.B. A supplemental dose of 150 mg after hemodialysis is recommended if daily dose is given less than 6 hours before start of hemodialysis.) PD: 50% dose Q24h	No change
73m², then use traditional dose: 2-2.5 mg/kg/dose x1. Adjust dose & frequency based on levels. Re-dose when trough <2 mcg/ml. Traditional Peak 4-8 mcg/ml; Extended Peak 15-25 mcg/ml; trough <2 mcg/ml				
FR < 50 ml/min/1.73m², then use traditional dose: 1 mg/kg/dose. Adjust dose and frequency based on levels. Peak for synergy dosing 3-4 mcg/ml; Re-dose when trough <2 mcg/ml.				
	100% dose Q24h	100% dose Q48h	IHD: 5-10 mg/kg/dose Q48h PD: 5-10 mg/kg/dose Q48h	10 mg/kg/dose Q24h
No change			IHD: 10 mg/kg/dose Q12h PD: 10 mg/kg/dose Q12h	No change

Meropenem	IV Usual		IV 10 mg/kg Q8h (2g)	100% dose
	IV Severe		IV 20 mg/kg Q8h (2g)	
	IV Meningitis		IV 40 mg/kg Q8h (2g)	
Metronidazole			IV/PO 10 mg/kg Q8h (500mg)	
Nitrofurantoin			PO 1.25-1.75 mg/kg Q6h (100mg)	
Penicillin G	IV Usual		IV 30 mg/kg Q6h (2g)	No char
	IV Severe		IV 50 mg/kg Q6h (2g)	
Pencillin V	PO		PO 7.5-15 mg/kg Q6h (500mg)	
Piperacillin/ Tazobactam	IV Usual		IV 50-75 mg/kg piperacillin Q6h (4g piperacillin)	70% dos
	IV CF		IV 100 mg/kg piperacillin Q6h (4g piperacillin)	
Trimethoprim-Sulfamethoxazole (TMP/SMZ)	IV/PO Usual		PO 4 mg/kg TMP Q12h; IV 6 mg/kg TMP Q12h	No cha
	Stenotrophomonas		IV 5 mg/kg TMP Q8h	
	PCP		IV 5 mg/kg TMP Q6h-8h	
Vancomycin		<16 years	IV 15 mg/kg Q6h (1g)	10 mg/kg
		≥16 years	IV 15 mg/kg Q8h-Q12h (1g)	10mg/kg
Acyclovir	IV	Term - 3 mo	IV 20 mg/kg Q8h	100% dos
		3 mo - 12 years	IV 500 mg/m^2 Q8h	
		>12 years	IV 10 mg/kg Q8h	
	IV Chickenpox	All ages	IV 10 mg/kg Q8h	
	PO Chickenpox		≥2 years PO 20 mg/kg/dose 4x/day (800mg)	No cha
Valacyclovir			PO 20 mg/kg/dose Q8h (1000mg)	100% dos
Foscarnet	IV Induction (CMV)		IV 60 mg/kg Q8h	eGFR 71-98: 4 eGFR 57-70: 5(eGFR 43-56: 4(eGFR 36-42: 6(
	IV Maintenance (CMV)		IV 90-120 mg/kg Q24h	eGFR 71-98: 70- eGFR 57-70: 50- eGFR 43-56: 80-1 eGFR 36-42: 60-
Ganciclovir	IV Induction		IV 5 mg/kg Q12h	eGFR 50-69: 2. eGFR 25-49: 2.
	IV Maintenance		IV 5 mg/kg Q24h	eGFR 50-69: 2 eGFR 25-49: 1.
Valganciclovir	PO Induction		PO 15-18 mg/kg Q12h (900mg)	eGFR 40-59: 5 eGFR 25-39: 5
	PO Maintenance		PO 15-18 mg/kg Q24h (900mg)	eGFR 40-59: 5 eGFR 25-39: 5
Amphotericin	Liposomal (Ambisome)		IV 3-5 mg/kg Q24h	
	Amphotericin B		IV 0.25-1 mg/kg Q24h	
Caspofungin		<3 months	IV 25 mg/m^2 Q24h (No load)	No c
		≥3 months	IV Load: 70 mg/m^2 Q24h x 1 dose (70mg) IV Maint: 50 mg/m^2 Q24h (70mg)	
Fluconazole			IV/PO Load: 6-12 mg/kg x 1 dose (800mg)	
			IV/PO Maint: 3-12 mg/kg Q24h (800mg)	
Itraconazole			PO 2.5-5 mg/kg PO Q12h	

References

(1) Drug Prescribing in Renal Failure, Aronoff 2007 (2) Lexicomp Online (3) Antibiotic Dosing in Critically Il

Compiled by: Dr Tsingyi Koh, Dr Mas Suhaila Isa, Dr Ian Kai Zhi Tan *Vetted by: Dr Sok Hoon Lim, Dr L*

*High dose amoxicillin/clavulanate is indicated for otitis media or pneumonia with beta-lactamase positive or non-typeable *H*

IM: intramuscular. **IV**: intravenous. **PO**: per oral.

Q: every.

CRRT: continuous renal replacement therapy. **CVVH/HD/HDF**: continuous venovenous - hemofiltration/hemodialysis/hemoc

CF: cystic fibrosis. **CMV**: cytomegalovirus. **P. aeruginosa**: *Pseudomonas aeruginosa*. **PCP**: *Pneumocystis jirovecii* pneumo